the developing child

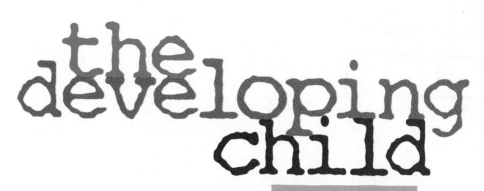

the developing child

eighth edition

Helen Bee

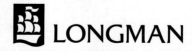 **LONGMAN**

An imprint of Addison Wesley Longman, Inc.

New York • Reading, Massachusetts • Menlo Park, California • Harlow, England
Don Mills, Ontario • Sydney • Mexico City • Madrid • Amsterdam

Acquisitions Editor: Rebecca Dudley
Developmental Editor: Rebecca Kohn
Project Editor: Donna DeBenedictis
Text and Cover Designer: Amy Trombat
Cover Photo: Nancy Sheehan/PhotoEdit
Art Studio: A Good Thing
Photo Researcher: Rosemary Hunter
Electronic Production Manager: Alexandra Odulak
Desktop Administrator: LaToya Wigfall
Manufacturing Manager: Hilda Koparanian
Electronic Page Makeup: Interactive Composition Corp.
Printer and Binder: Courier/Kendallville, Inc.
Cover Printer: The Lehigh Press, Inc.

For permission to use copyrighted material, grateful acknowledgment is made to the copyright holders on p. 541, which is hereby made part of this copyright page.

Library of Congress Cataloging-in-Publication Data

Bee, Helen L., 1939–
    The developing child / Helen Bee. — 8th ed.
      p. cm.
    Includes bibliographical references and index.
    ISBN 0-673-99990-4
    1. Child psychology. 2. Child development. I. Title.
  BF721.B336 1995
  155.4—dc20   96-4802
                                    CIP

ISBN 0-673-99990-4

12345678910—CRK—99989796

TO:

Sarah Brooks and Diane Edie

Thanks for all the music,
figurative as well as literal,
you have brought
into my life

Brief Contents

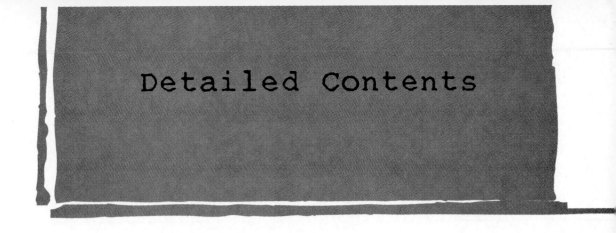

Detailed Contents

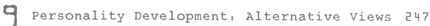

Part Five: The Social Child

Part Six: The Whole Child

13 The Ecology of Development: The Child Within the Family System   364

14 Beyond the Family: The Impact of the Broader Culture   395

Boxed Features

The Real World

To the student:

Hello and welcome. Let me invite you into the study of a fascinating subject—children and their development. This is a bit like inviting you into my own home, since I have lived in the world of the study of children for a great many years. Unfortunately, I cannot know each of you individually, but by writing this book as if it were a conversation between you and me, I hope I can make the reading and the studying of this subject as personal a process as possible.

Because such personal involvement is one of my goals, you will find that I often write in the first person and that I have included a number of anecdotes about my own life. It is for the same reason that I usually give you the full name of many of the researchers and theorists I quote—so that you will have some sense that these are real people doing the research and proposing the theories.

Welcome, too, to the adventure of science. From the very first edition of this book, one of my goals has been to try to convey a sense of excitement about scientific inquiry. I want each of you to take away some feeling for the way psychologists think, the kinds of questions we ask, and the ways we go about trying to answer those questions. I also want you to take away with you some sense of the theoretical and intellectual ferment that is part of any science. Think of psychology as a kind of detective story. We discover clues after hard, often painstaking work; we make new guesses or hypotheses; and then we search for new clues to check on those hypotheses.

Of course, I also want you to come away from reading this book with a firm grounding of knowledge in the field. There is much that we do not yet know or understand. But developmental psychologists have learned a lot, much of it fascinating, some of it surprising. These facts and observations will be of help to you professionally if you are planning (or are already in) a career with children—such as teaching, nursing, social work, medicine, or psychology; the information will also be useful to you as parents, now or in the future. There is much to be learned. In the midst of all that learning, though, I hope you enjoy the reading as much as I have enjoyed the writing.

Helen Bee

To the instructor:

Working on a revision of a book that has been through as many editions as has *The Developing Child* is a task with many pleasant benefits. The basic structure is familiar and well established; some sections become more and more polished over time and require little new work; editors have long since given up trying to make my writing style sound like anything other than what it is—personal and informal.

At the same time, the process of revising a text is not as simple as it may appear. One of the most difficult tasks is to decide how to deal with the massive, continuous inflow of new data, new theories, new concepts. I subscribe to 20 journals and read at least another dozen on a regular basis; my office overflows with new edited volumes. One cannot handle this new information simply by adding more sections to the text, edition after edition. One must cut and trim and reshape entire chapters to try to reflect the current state of our thinking and knowledge. In the process, one must work very hard not to get stuck in old ruts, to use old structures or patterns of talking about a particular subject simply because they are familiar, rather than adopting a newer structure that works better with current data. In this edition, for example, I have substantially revised Chapter 9, on personality development, by including a discussion of the "Big Five" personality factors and their links to temperament—a change that necessarily reverberated through the entire chapter.

In this edition I have also undertaken a deliberate "pruning" of citations—in a manner that I hope is analogous to the neural pruning that occurs in infants in the early years of life. My goal in each case has been to list those citations that would be most helpful to both students and instructors. Very often this means listing the most recent source on a given topic, because the reader can readily backtrack from a recent source to the earlier work on the same subject. Where there are several good, recent sources, I have sometimes listed several, but equally often I have chosen to list only the one that gives the broadest coverage of some subject. Finally, where there is a classic study on some topic, I have retained that citation, most often also providing a current citation on the same subject. Even with this pruning, the list of references is still long. But I hope you and your students will find that this edition is a little leaner, a bit less encrusted with parentheses.

Basic Goals

Throughout the process I keep my basic goals in mind:

1. To find that difficult but essential balance between theory, research, and practical application.
2. To make the study of child development relevant not just for psychologists but also for students in the many other fields in which this information is needed: nursing, medicine, social work, education, home economics.
3. To keep all discussions as current as humanly possible, so that students can encounter the very latest thinking, the most recent research.
4. To write to the student in as direct a way as possible, so that the book is more like a conversation than a traditional text; such a personal style need not clash with either theoretical clarity or research rigor, both of which I continue to work hard to achieve.

Additional Goals of the Eighth Edition

In this edition, several additional goals guided my work.

Increased Biological Emphasis. I wanted to add discussions of the biological aspects of development wherever I could, since this is a burgeoning and highly fruitful current area of research and theorizing. You will see this new emphasis in a number of places:

- A considerably expanded discussion of behavior genetics in Chapter 1

- An expanded discussion of synaptogenesis, dendrite formation, and pruning in Chapter 2

- An expanded discussion of the development of the nervous system in Chapter 4

- Discussion of the latest behavior genetic research on temperament and personality in Chapter 9

Increased Coverage of Emotion. I have also expanded the discussion of emotional development, which is covered in several chapters:

- Discrimination of the emotions of others in infancy and early childhood in Chapter 5

- An expanded discussion of "reading" others' emotions in Chapter 7, exploring the link between such an ability and the emerging theory of mind

- A new discussion of emotion regulation in Chapter 7

- An expanded discussion of the child's own expression of emotion in Chapter 10

- A discussion of both the universality and cultural variations in emotional expression in Chapter 12

Further Strengthening the Emphasis on Culture. In the seventh edition, one of my primary goals was to infuse the entire book with a multicultural or cross-cultural flavor—to search for those basic developmental processes that are the same across cultures and to try to understand the ways in which culture and subculture shapes an individual child's development. In this edition, I have tried to add to this process, such as by emphasizing the contrast between cultural *individualism* and *collectivism.* I have introduced this distinction in Chapter 1, in an expanded discussion of the concept of culture, and have then carried the concepts through the book.

I have also struggled, as do all social scientists, with the problem of terminology and labels for various cultural and ethnic groups. Should one use *black* or *African-American?* Should one say *Hispanic* or *Latino?* And how should one label the dominant white cultural group: *White, Caucasian, Anglo,* or *Euro-American?* Some authors have resolved the dilemma by choosing one label from each set and then using those labels consistently. I have rejected that solution because there just seems to me to be still too much flux, too much variability of usage by members of these groups as well as by social scientists and other writers. I have opted instead for a less elegant solution that I think better reflects the way things are at the moment: I have used all the alternative terms at various times, as the occasion seemed to demand. For example, when I report results from the Census Bureau's wide-ranging research, I typically use the terms *white* and *black,* because these are the labels the Census Bureau uses; when I talk about studies of Hispanic children, I have generally used the word *Anglo* to refer to the contrasting white culture, because this is the term most often used by Hispanics themselves. And when I need to emphasize the European origin of the dominant white culture in the United States, I have used the term *Euro-American,* especially in contrast to other hyphenated American groups, such as African-Americans or Asian-Americans. Sometimes, I confess, I have used the briefer terms simply because the repeated use of hyphenated labels becomes cumbersome.

Updating Figures and Tables. A fourth specific goal in this edition has been to find really current research examples of key points, especially research results that could be displayed in clear figures. This search has led not only to the updating of virtually every table, but also to the addition of 20 completely new figures and four new tables, many of them replacing older data. You will still see some figures in this edition based on research done in the 1970s and 1980s; often there is simply nothing newer available that makes the same point as clearly as does an older piece of research. But in many areas there are fascinating new studies that illustrate important points.

Other Changes in the Eighth Edition

New or Expanded Coverage. In addition to the comprehensive updating that is part of any revision, I have added or revised several key sections:

- The discussion of health in Chapter 4 has been substantially increased, with a particular emphasis on adolescent risk-taking behavior.

- The description of vocabulary and grammar development in Chapter 8 has been greatly enriched with data from the first really large-scale cross-sectional data from Fenson et al. (1994). I also added a discussion of vocabulary development in elementary school to this chapter.

- Chapter 9 now opens with an extended discussion of the usefulness of the "Big Five" personality dimensions for describing child personality, as well as the links between temperament and the "Big Five." This change improves the structure of the whole chapter.

- An extended new discussion of self-concept in the school setting is now included in Chapter 10.

- Chapter 11 contains several completely new pieces: (1) an extended discussion of Bradford Brown's fascinating new work on adolescent crowds and cliques; (2) a discussion of "relational aggression," a form that is more common in girls than boys; and (3) data from a particularly fine new experimental study by van den Boom of the link between parental responsiveness and infants' security of attachment.

- A major new section has been added to Chapter 13 on the impact of single parenthood on long-term outcomes, drawing primarily from the work of McLanahan and Sandefur (1994).

- The discussion of the impact of schooling in Chapter 14 has been substantially expanded.

- Chapter 15 now includes a section specifically focused on delinquency, including a new box on delinquency in girls.

Tried-and-True Features

In addition to all these additions and changes, I have naturally tried to keep all the qualities and features that you have appreciated in earlier editions: the engaging and clear writing style; the critical thinking questions in the margins (which were a great hit in the seventh edition); the annotated lists of suggested readings; and boldfaced key terms, listed at the end of each chapter and defined in the glossary.

As in the last edition, there are also three types of boxes, each designed to explore a somewhat different kind of issue:

- *Research Reports* boxes give a more in-depth exploration of a particular research topic. Most often they describe a single study, or a program of studies, by a single researcher or research group, in some detail; in other cases they examine a body of research by a number of different investigators. They are intended to give students a feeling for how research is actually conducted and to introduce them to some of the significant researchers in the field.

- *Cultures and Contexts* boxes are aimed directly at the question of cultural influences on development. In many cases, these boxes describe cross-cultural research on basic developmental processes—research designed to tell us whether particular developmental patterns, observed in Western or Euro-American groups, are really universal. Other boxes look at differences between cultures, subcultures, or U.S. ethnic groups—differences in patterns of child rearing, differences in children's behavior, differences in ecological niches.

- *Real World* boxes examine highly applied questions. Many are aimed at students-as-parents or as prospective parents, providing them with quite specific advice based on research. Others examine questions of cultural or societal interest. All are designed to show students that such practical questions can indeed be addressed with research.

Supplements

Naturally, a variety of supplements are also available to the instructor and the student.

Instructor's Manual (ISBN 0-673-97350-6). The instructor's manual (IM) for this edition is an expansion and updating of the extensive manual prepared for the seventh edition. This IM, as did the earlier versions, lays out a whole course using *The Developing Child,* including preplanning, a sample syllabus, suggested organization of the lectures, and lecture material for each chapter. I have added new material for each chapter for this edition, including good new sources.

The IM also includes, as before, a set of transparency masters. Many of these are repeats of the ones provided with the seventh edition, but there are also 14 new transparencies, most of them of brand-new data. This ought to keep you from getting into a rut!

Finally, the integrated film/video guide has been updated for this edition.

Test Bank (ISBN 0-673-97354-9). Written by Carolyn Meyer of Lake Sumter Community College, the test bank contains approximately 2000 questions, 65 percent of which are new for this edition. Each of these multiple-choice, true/false, short answer, and essay questions is referenced to page number, topic, and skill.

Study Guide (ISBN 0-673-99992-0). Written by Betty Sunerton of Dawson

College, each chapter of the comprehensive study guide contains a brief chapter outline, learning objectives, a definition of key terms, lists of key concepts and individuals, and three practice tests containing multiple-choice, matching, and fill-in-the-blank questions with their answers.

SuperShell II Student Tutorial. Pam Griesler of Columbia University has written this interactive computerized tutorial for IBM-compatible (ISBN 0-673-97351-4) and Macintosh (ISBN 0-673-97854-0) computers. In addition to chapter outlines and glossary terms, SuperShell provides immediate correct answers to multiple-choice, true-false, and short-answer questions. All the material is referenced to the text page. It contains material not found in the study guide and provides a running score for students.

Software. Two forms of software are available with the test bank. TestMaster Computerized Testing System is a flexible, easy-to-master computerized test bank that includes all the test items in the printed test bank. The TestMaster software allows instructors to edit existing questions and add their own items. It is available in IBM (ISBN 0-673-97353-0) or Macintosh (ISBN 0-673-97352-2) formats.

QuizMaster is software, available to instructors, that allows students to take TestMaster-generated tests on computer. QuizMaster gives the students their scores right away as well as a diagnostic report at the end of the test. This report lets the students know what topics or objectives they may need to study to improve their scores. Test scores can be saved on disk, allowing instructors to keep track of scores for individual students, class sections, or whole courses.

Bouquets

My work on this edition, as with every edition, has been greatly aided by the criticism and commentary provided by colleagues, who took the time to look at earlier editions or early drafts. I am enormously appreciative of the thoughtful comments and suggestions made by

Janette B. Benson, University of Denver

Marvin W. Berkowitz, Marquette University

Rebecca Bigler, The University of Texas at Austin

Ken Bordens, Indiana University/Purdue University at Fort Wayne

Mary Lou Brotherson, St. Thomas University

Daniel J. Christie, The Ohio State University

Joan Cook, County College of Morris

Joan Coughlin, Palo Alto College

Kathleen Fox, Salisbury State University

Marlynn M. Griffin, Georgia Southern University

John Hensley, Tulsa Junior College

E. Romayne Hertweck, Mira Costa College

Harry W. Hoeman, Bowling Green State University

Sharon Hott, Allegany Community College

Robert J. Keller, Kishwaukee College

Rosemary Mills, University of Manitoba

Eleanor A. Ryan, Elmhurst College

Nicholas R. Santilli, John Carroll University

George Vesprani, University of Cincinnati

My work is also made enormously easier by the terrific team of people at Longman (formerly HarperCollins College)–the same team I have now worked with on several books. By now we know each other's strengths and weaknesses and the process has become remarkably smooth. Jill Lectka, who was my acquisitions editor, was efficient, charming, and ever helpful. (She even took me out to dinner at the best restaurant in Madison when she was in town.) Becky Kohn must be the best developmental editor on the face of the earth. She reads every chapter and makes helpful comments; she answers all my technical questions; sometimes she calls just to hear how things are going, which gives me a rare opportunity to agonize over whatever current dilemma is facing me. Not many people have the patience to listen to a writer's dilemmas! Becky also keeps the paperwork flowing and acts as a capable liaison with all the many departments at Longman. I couldn't get along without her. The third member of this team *extraordinaire* is Rosemary Hunter, the photo researcher who provides me with heaps of wonderful photos to choose from and searches out special pictures when we need them. Rosemary and I have now worked together four times and have so fully arrived at the same wavelength that we hardly need to talk to one another anymore. To all three, my deepest thanks.

Last but never least, there is my personal "convoy," who trucks along with me through each book. My husband, Carl de Boor, solves my computer puzzles and sometimes keeps me from tearing out my hair in clumps when deadlines become too tight or chapter structures defy solution. My local friends, especially Sarah Brooks and Diane Edie, drop in regularly just to say hi, to give me a hug, or to sing—a welcome break from the solitary exercise of writing. Sarah has also taken on the thankless task of organizing my files so that I can actually find my copy of that 1988 paper from the *New England Journal of Medicine* I need at some specific moment. Quite literally, I could not live without these very special people. Thank you.

Helen Bee

the developing child

Basic Questions

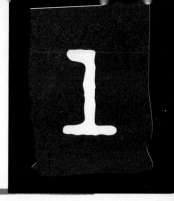

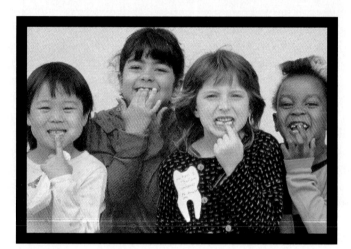

Each summer, I spend several months at an unusual camp in the state of Washington, where adults of all ages as well as families with young children come each year to live for a short time in a kind of temporary community. Because many of the same people come back year after year, bringing their children (and often later their grandchildren), I see these growing children in once-a-year snapshots. When a family arrives, I am quite naturally struck by how much the children have changed, and I find myself saying to the kids, "Good grief, you've grown a foot," or, "Last time I saw you, you were only this big." (I say these things, even remembering full well how much I hated it when people said these things to me at the same age. Of course I had grown. And because I was always taller than anyone my age, I didn't like to be reminded of this peculiarity.)

At the same time, I am also struck by the consistency in these kids from year to year. Sweet-tempered young Malcolm and ebullient Crystal always give me many hugs; Malcolm's older brother Elliot, far shyer, still gazes at me silently from some measured distance. He warms up as the days go by, but his behavior is quite different from his brother's, and remains noticeably constant from year to year. Even 14-year-old Stacey, now clearly in the midst of adolescence, is in many ways the same dreamy and slow-moving child he was at age 4 or 7 or 10. Each of these children has a particular style, a particular set of skills, a particular personality, and these qualities appear to be at least somewhat consistent from year to year, perhaps even into adult life.

These simple examples illustrate one of the key points about human development: It involves both change and continuity. To understand development, we will need to look at both. Equally important, we need to understand which developmental changes, and which types of consistency or continuity, are shared by individuals in all cultures and which are unique to a given culture, to a group within a culture, or to a particular individual. For example, you probably know that in the first weeks after they are born, babies do not sleep through the night; they wake every two hours or so to be fed. But by about 6 weeks of age most babies are able to string several two-hour stretches together, and begin to show something approximating a day/night sleeping pattern (Bamford et al., 1990). That certainly sounds like a basic biological change, one that would occur pretty much regardless of the child's environment. But according to one study (Super & Harkness, 1982), babies in rural Kenya who are carried about by their mothers in a sling all day and fed on demand at night do not show any shift toward a nighttime sleep pattern over the first eight months of life. Instead they continue to wake intermittently throughout the 24-hour period. So what seems like a universal, biological process turns out not to be universal at all. It is affected by culture—by attitudes and values expressed through variations in care and handling. This issue of what is universal and what is not will be a persistent theme.

This example also illustrates the point that to understand how development works, we will need to explore both *nature* and *nurture,* both biology and environment, and how they interact to explain both consistency and change. Throughout these chapters, I will be trying to sort out the relative impact of nature and nurture in each domain of development and at each age. That task will be a great deal easier if you have at least a grounding in some of the basic concepts and theories that form the framework for such an analysis. So let me take you on a quick tour of current ideas about nature and nurture, and an equally brief look at the major theoretical approaches to explaining both consistency and individuality in development.

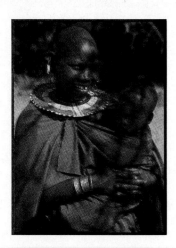

In many parts of Kenya, babies are carried in slings all day and allowed to nurse on demand at night. This cultural pattern, quite different from what we see in most Western societies, seems to have an effect on the baby's sleep/wake cycle.

Nature and Nurture: An Ancient Debate

The argument about nature versus nurture, also referred to as *heredity versus environment* or *nativism versus empiricism,* is one of the oldest and most central theoretical issues within philosophy as well as psychology. When asked by developmental psychologists, the question is basically whether a child's development is governed by a pattern built in at birth or whether it is shaped by experiences after birth. Historically, the nativist/nature side of the controversy was represented principally by Plato and (in the more modern era) René Descartes, both of whom believed that at least some ideas were innate. On the other side of the philosophical argument was a group of British philosophers called "empiricists," such as John Locke, who insisted that at birth the mind is a blank slate—in Latin, a *tabula rasa*. All knowledge, they argued, is created by experience.

No developmental psychologist today would cast this issue in such black-and-white terms. We agree that a child's development is a product of some interaction of nature and nurture. In every culture, puberty occurs sometime between roughly age 9 and age 16, but the timing is affected by such environmental factors as diet. Some temperamental patterns may be inherited, but they can be and are modified by the parents' style of caregiving. And so on. *No* aspect of development is entirely one or the other. Nonetheless, there is still a good deal of disagreement about the relative importance of these two factors. Because of this disagreement, and because it is easier to introduce the various concepts separately, I'll begin by talking about each of the two halves of this dichotomy, saving for later the question of how nature and nurture interact.

Think about your own patterns of behavior for a moment. Which ones do you think are the *most* governed by basic human biology (nature)? Which ones seem to be most a product of your environment, including your upbringing?

The Nature Side of the Equation

Until fairly recently, the theoretical pendulum was well over toward the environmental end of the continuum. Most of our research, and most of our theorizing, focused on environmental effects of one type or another. But in the last decade or so, there has been a notable swing in the other direction. Within developmental psychology there is now a growing emphasis on the biological roots of behavior and of development itself. In part, this shift has grown out of new technology that allows physiologists and psychologists to study the functioning of the brain in much greater detail, as well as the development of new statistical techniques that make it possible to study genetic influences in new ways. But the shift may also have occurred because it became clear that we needed more balance in our explanations of development. Whatever the reasons, it is clear that a resurgence of interest in the biological roots of behavior has occurred.

Inborn Biases and Constraints

One example of this resurgence is in the concept of "inborn biases" or "constraints" on development. The argument, which is in some ways a modern descendant of Descartes' notion of inborn ideas, is that the baby is "programmed" in some fashion to pay more attention to certain kinds of information or to respond in particular ways to objects. For example, Dan Slobin (Slobin, 1985b), who studies early language learning, proposes that children are born with certain "operating principles" that govern the way they listen to and try to make sense out of the flow of sounds coming at them. One such principle, according to Slobin, is the tendency to pay special attention to the beginnings and ends of strings of sounds. Similarly, in the study of infants' cognitive development, researchers such as Elizabeth Spelke (1991) have concluded that babies come into the world with certain "preexisting conceptions" or constraints in their understanding of objects and the way they behave. Very young babies already seem to understand that objects will move downward if they are not supported and that a moving object will continue to move in the same direction unless it encounters an obstacle. Unlike Descartes, current theorists do not propose that these built-in response patterns are the end of the story; rather, they see them as the starting point. What then develops is a result of experience filtered through these initial biases. But those biases *constrain* the number of developmental pathways that are possible (Campbell & Bickhard, 1992).

Maturation

Nature can shape processes after birth in other ways as well, most clearly through genetic programming that may determine whole sequences of later development. This is not a new idea; Arnold Gesell (Gesell, 1925; Thelen & Adolph, 1992) proposed such an idea 70 years ago. He used the term **maturation** to describe such genetically programmed sequential patterns of change, and this term is still uniformly used today. Changes in body size and shape, changes in hormones at puberty, changes in muscles and bones, and changes in the nervous system all may be programmed in this way. You can probably remember your own physical changes during adolescence. The timing of these pubertal changes differs from one teenager to the next, but the basic sequence is essentially the same for all children. Such sequences, which begin at conception and continue until death, are shared by all members of our species. The instructions for these sequences are part of the specific hereditary information that is passed on at the moment of conception.

Any maturational pattern is marked by three qualities: It is universal, appearing in all children, across cultural boundaries; it is sequential, involving some pattern of unfolding skill or characteristics; and it is relatively impervious to environmental influence. In its purest form, a maturationally determined developmental sequence occurs regardless of practice or training. You don't have to practice growing pubic hair; you don't have to be taught how to walk. In fact, it would take almost herculean efforts to *prevent* such sequences from unfolding. But even confirmed maturational theorists agree that experience has some effect. These powerful, apparently automatic, maturational patterns require at least some minimal environmental support, such as adequate diet and opportunity for movement and experimentation.

Modern research also tells us that specific experience interacts with maturational patterns in intricate ways. For example, Greenough (1991) notes that one of the proteins required for the development of the visual system is controlled by a gene whose action is only triggered by visual experience. So *some* visual experience is needed for the genetic program to operate. In normal development, of course, every (nonblind) child will have some such experience. But examples like this one tell us that maturational sequences do not simply "unfold" automatically. The system appears to be "ready" to develop along particular pathways, but it requires experience to trigger the movement.

I should point out that the term *maturation* does not mean quite the same thing as *growth,* although the two terms are sometimes used as if they were synonyms. *Growth* refers to some kind of step-by-step change in quantity, as in size, and it can occur either with or without an underlying maturational process. A child's body could grow because her diet has significantly improved, or it could grow because she is getting older. The first of these has no maturational component, while the second does. To put it another way, the term *growth* is a *description* of change, while the concept of maturation is one *explanation* of change.

Behavior Genetics

The idea of inborn biases and the concept of maturation are both designed to account for patterns and sequences of development that are the *same* for all children. But nature can also contribute to variations from one individual to the next, since genetic inheritance is individual as well as collective. The study of genetic contributions to individual behavior, called **behavior genetics,** has become a particularly vibrant and influential research area in recent years and has contributed greatly to the renewed interest in the biological roots of behavior.

Using two primary research techniques, the study of identical and fraternal twins, and the study of adopted children (described more fully in the *Research Report* on page 6), behavior geneticists have shown that specific heredity affects a remarkably broad range of behaviors. Included in the list are not only obvious physical differences such as height, body shape, or a tendency to skinniness or obesity, but also cognitive abilities such as general intelligence (about which I will have a great deal more to say in Chapter 6), and more specific cognitive skills or problems such as spatial visualization ability or reading disability (Rose, 1995). Newer research is also showing that many aspects of pathological behavior are genetically influenced, including alcoholism, schizophrenia, excessive aggressiveness or antisocial behavior, even anorexia (Gottesman & Goldsmith, 1994; McGue, 1994). Finally, and importantly, behavior geneticists have found a significant genetic influence on children's temperament, including such dimensions as emotionality (the tendency to get distressed or upset easily), activity (the tendency toward vigorous, rapid behavior), and sociability (the tendency to prefer the presence of others to being alone) (Plomin et al., 1993).

Recent behavior genetic research even shows that the child's *environment* is affected by heredity (Plomin, 1995), via either of two routes. First, the child inherits her genes from her parents, and those same parents create the environment in which the child is growing up. For example, parents who themselves have higher IQs are not only likely to pass their "good IQ" genes on to their children, they are also likely to create a richer, more stimulating environment for their child.

Second, the child creates her own influences. Because children begin life with varying genetically patterned qualities, they *elicit* different behavior from parents and others. Cranky children thus encounter a different set of experiences than do sunny-dispositioned children; large and robust children elicit different kinds of caregiving than do frail children. Furthermore, children and adults also choose, and then interpret, their experiences. These choices and interpretations are affected by all the individual's inherited tendencies, including not only IQ but also temperament or pathologies. For example, in their study of twins and stepchildren, Robert Plomin and his colleagues (1994) have found that identical twin adolescents describe their parents, or their friends, in more similar terms than do fraternal twins. Furthermore, full siblings describe their parents more similarly than do genetically unrelated stepsiblings. It appears that identical twins are *experiencing* their parents, and their family environment, in more similar ways. This does *not* mean that there is somehow an "experiencing the environment" gene. Rather, the full genetic pattern of each child or adult affects the way he or she experiences and interprets. Because identical twins have the same genetic makeup, they experience and interpret more similarly.

Research of this kind has forced developmental psychologists to rethink some long-held assumptions about the effects of environment. At the same time, I want to emphasize that no behavior geneticist is saying that heredity is the *only* cause of behavior, or even the most central one in many cases. Indeed, as Robert Plomin points out, behavior genetic research has been as important in showing the significant effect of environment as in proving the centrality of heredity (Plomin, 1995). Certainly, genetic influences are totally dominant for some characteristics, such as inherited diseases. But for most aspects of development, such as variations in personality or intellectual abilities, the effect of a particular

Research Report

How Do Behavior Geneticists Identify Genetic Effects?

Investigators can search for a genetic influence on a trait in either of two primary ways: They can study identical and fraternal twins, or they can study adopted children. Identical twins share exactly the same genetic patterning, because they develop from the same fertilized ovum. Fraternal twins each develop from a separate ovum, separately fertilized. They are therefore no more alike than are any other pair of siblings, except that they have shared the same prenatal environment and grow up in the same sequential niche within the family. If identical twins turn out to be more like one another on any given trait than fraternal twins, that would be evidence for the influence of heredity on that trait.

A powerful variant of the twin strategy is to study twins who have been reared apart. If identical twins are still more like one another on some dimension, despite having grown up in different environments, we have even clearer evidence of a genetic contribution for that trait.

In the case of adopted children, the strategy is to compare the degree of similarity between the adopted child and his birth parents (with whom he shares genes but not environment) with the degree of similarity between the adopted child and his adoptive parents (with whom he shares environment but not genes). If the child should turn out to be more similar to his birth parents than to his adoptive parents, or if his behavior or skill is better predicted by the characteristics of his birth parents than by characteristics of his adoptive parents, that would again demonstrate the influence of heredity.

In very recent years, behavior geneticists have devised a method that combines some of the elements of the twin and adoption strategies by studying twins along with children growing up in stepfamilies. Stepfamilies can include full siblings, half siblings, and stepsiblings. Thus, it is possible to see whether the degree of similarity on some trait matches the degree of genetic similarity in any pair of children.

Let me give you two examples, both from studies of IQ. Bouchard and McGue (1981, p. 1056, Fig. 1) have combined the results of dozens of twin studies on the heritability of IQ scores, with the following results:

Identical twins reared together	.85
Identical twins reared apart	.67
Fraternal twins reared together	.58
Siblings (including fraternal twins) reared apart	.24

The numbers here are correlations—a statistic I'll explain more fully later in this chapter. For now you need to know only that a correlation can range from 0 to +1.00 or −1.00. The closer it is to 1.00, the stronger the relationship it describes. In this case, the number reflects how similar the IQs are of the two members of a twin pair. You can see that identical twins reared together have IQs that are highly similar, much more similar than what occurs for fraternal twins reared together. You can also see, though, that environment plays a role, since identical twins reared apart are less similar than are those reared together.

The same conclusion comes from two well-known studies of adopted children, the Texas Adoption Project (Loehlin, Horn, & Willerman, 1994) and the Minnesota Transracial Adoption Study (Scarr, Weinberg, & Waldman, 1993). In both studies, the adopted children were recently given IQ tests at roughly age 18. Their scores on this test were then correlated with the earlier-measured IQ scores of their natural mothers and of their adoptive mothers and fathers:

	Texas	Minnesota
With the natural mother's IQ	.44	.29
With the adoptive mother's IQ	.03	.14
With the adoptive father's IQ	.06	.08

In both cases, the children's IQs were at least somewhat predicted by their natural mothers' IQs, but *not* by the IQs of their adoptive parents, with whom they had spent their entire childhood. Thus, the adoption studies, like the twin studies of IQ, tell us that there is indeed a substantial genetic component in what we measure with an IQ test.

genetic pattern is more a matter of probability than certainty. We know there is *some* genetic effect because identical twins are a lot more alike in personality, IQ, or many specific behavior patterns than are fraternal twins. But even identical twins are not identical in these characteristics. For example, studies of adult criminals done in the U.S., Germany, Japan, Norway, and Denmark show that if one of a pair of identical twins has been jailed for some criminal act, the probability that the other twin has also been jailed is about 50 percent. Among fraternal twins, this "concordance rate" is only 23 percent. This shows a clear genetic effect, but the role of environment is also obvious. In virtually every case, specific outcomes for a given child depend on the interaction of that child's genetic patterning with the particular environment the child encounters and creates. Given that basic agreement, what we now need is a great deal more knowledge about the types of environmental factors that foster or inhibit the emergence of some genetic pattern.

The Nurture Side of the Equation

Models of Environmental Influence

Concepts on the nurture side of this ancient dispute have also become considerably more subtle and complex. In a particularly helpful analysis, Richard Aslin (1981a) suggests five models of influence, shown schematically in Figure 1.1. In each drawing the dashed line represents the path of development of some skill or behavior that would occur without a particular experience; the solid line represents the path of development if the experience were added.

For comparison purposes, the first of the five models actually shows a maturational pattern with *no* environmental effect. The second model, which Aslin calls *maintenance,* describes a pattern in which some environmental input is necessary to sustain a skill or behavior that has already developed maturationally. For example, kittens are born with full binocular vision, but if you cover one of their eyes for a period of time, binocular skill declines. Similarly, muscles will atrophy if not used.

The third model shows a *facilitation* effect of the environment in which a skill or behavior develops earlier than it normally would because of some experience. For example, children whose parents talk to them more often and with more complex sentences in the first 18 to 24 months of life appear to develop two-word sentences and other early grammatical forms somewhat earlier than do children whose parents talk to them less. But less-talked-to children catch up shortly thereafter, so there is no permanent advantage in grammatical complexity.

When a particular experience does lead to a permanent advantage, Aslin would call it *attunement.* For example, kids growing up in families in which their parents talk to them a great deal have slightly higher IQs later than do kids who receive less early verbal stimulation. That is, being talked to a lot in early childhood has at least two rather different effects: It speeds up early grammar (a facilitation effect), and it promotes a persistently higher IQ (an attunement effect).

Aslin's final model, *induction,* describes a pure environmental effect: Without some experience a particular behavior would not develop at all. Giving a child tennis lessons or exposing him to a second language would fall into this category.

These five models illustrate the greater complexity of current thinking about the nurture side of the nature/nurture issue. But they still do not take us far enough. At least

Another example: New behavior genetic evidence (McGue & Lykken, 1992) shows that the concordance rate for divorce is about .45 among adult identical twins but only .30 among adult fraternal twins. This difference occurred whether the twins' parents had been divorced or not. What are the implications of this finding for our understanding of the effect of divorce on children?

Several decades ago, educators devised the preschool program called Head Start to improve the school preparation of children growing up in poor families. Which of Aslin's models do you think best describes what the designers of Head Start thought (or hoped) would be the result of the program? Does it make any difference for public policy if Head Start has a "facilitation" effect rather than an "attunement" effect?

FIGURE 1.1 Aslin's five models of possible relationships between maturation and environment. The top model shows a purely maturational effect; the bottom model (induction) shows a purely environmental effect. The other three show interactive combinations: *maintenance,* in which experience prevents the deterioration of a maturationally developed skill; *facilitation,* in which experience speeds up the development of some maturational process; and *attunement,* in which experience increases the ultimate level of some skill or behavior above the "normal" maturational level. (*Source:* Aslin, 1981a, p. 50.)

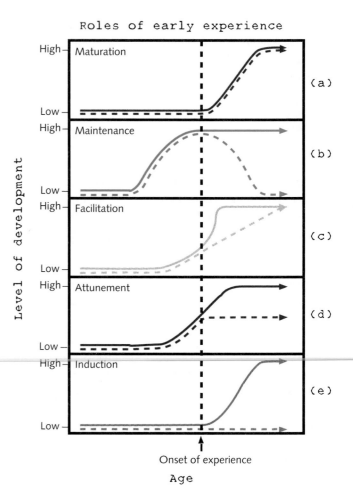

three other aspects of the environmental side of the equation are also significant in current thinking about development: the timing of experience, the child's own interpretation of experience, and the total ecological/cultural system in which experiences occur.

The Timing of Experience

Just as the importance of nature may vary from one time in development to another, so the timing of specific experiences may matter as well. At 6 months of age the impact of day care on an infant may be quite different than that at 16 months; moving from one school to another during puberty may have a different effect than moving during another stage; and so forth.

Our thinking about the importance of timing was stimulated, in part, by research on other species that showed that specific experiences had different or stronger effects at some points in development than at others. The most famous example is that baby ducks will become *imprinted* (become attached to and follow) on any duck or any other quacking, moving object that happens to be around them 15 hours after they hatch. If nothing is moving or quacking at that critical point, they don't become imprinted at all (Hess, 1972). So the period just around 15 hours after hatching is a **critical period** for the duck's development of a proper following response.

We can see similar critical periods in the action of various **teratogens** in prenatal development. A teratogen is some outside agent, such as a disease organism or chemical, that, if present during prenatal development, adversely affects the process of that development. While some teratogens can have negative consequences at any time in gestation, most have effects only during some critical period. For example, if a mother contracts the disease *rubella* (commonly called German measles) during a narrow range of days in the first three months of pregnancy, some damage or deformity occurs in the fetus. Infection with the same virus after the third month of pregnancy has no such effect.

In the months after birth too there seem to be critical periods in brain development—specific weeks or months during which the child needs to encounter certain types of stimulation or experience for the nervous system to develop normally and fully (Hirsch & Tieman, 1987).

The broader and somewhat looser concept of a **sensitive period** has also been widely used. A sensitive period is a span of months or years during which a child may be particularly responsive to specific forms of experience, or particularly influenced by their absence. For example, the period from 6 to 12 months of age may be a sensitive period for the formation of a core attachment to the parents. Other periods may be particularly significant for intellectual development or language (Tamis-LeMonda & Bornstein, 1987).

Internal Models of Experience

Another concept appearing more and more prominently in our theoretical repertoire is that of an internal model of experience. The key idea is that the effect of some experience lies in an individual's *interpretation* of it, the *meaning* the individual attaches to it, rather than in any objective properties of the experience. You can easily come up with everyday examples from your own life. For instance, suppose a friend says to you, "Your new haircut looks great. I think it is a lot more becoming when it's short like that." Your friend intends it as a compliment, but what determines your reaction is how you *hear* the comment, not what is intended. You might hear the compliment, but you might also hear an implied criticism. ("Your hair used to look awful. . . .") If you regularly hear criticism in other people's comments, we would say that you have an internal model of yourself and others that includes a basic expectation that might be something like this: "I usually do things wrong, so other people criticize me."

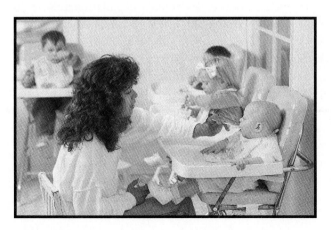

If the first year of life is a sensitive period for the establishment of a secure attachment (as some contend), then is it risky for a child of this age to be in day care, separated from her parents every day? There is a hot debate among psychologists on this point.

Theorists who emphasize the importance of such meaning systems argue that each child creates a set of internal models—a set of assumptions or conclusions about the world, about himself, and about relationships with others—through which all subsequent experience is filtered (Epstein, 1991). John Bowlby expressed this idea when he talked about the child's "internal working model" of attachment (1969; 1980). A child with a secure model of attachment may assume that someone will come when he cries and that affection and attention are reliably available. A child with a less secure model may assume that if a grown-up frowns it probably means she will be yelled at. Of course these expectations are based on actual experiences, but once formed into an internal model, they generalize beyond the original experience and affect the way the child interprets future experiences. A child who expects adults to be reliable and affectionate will be more likely to interpret the behavior of new adults in this way and will re-create friendly and affectionate relationships with others outside the family; a child who expects hostility will read hostility into otherwise fairly neutral encounters.

Such a view of the pathway or mechanism of environmental effects is not dominant in developmental psychology, but it has gained importance in recent years.

The Ecological Perspective

A third facet of current thinking about environmental effects is a growing emphasis on casting a wider environmental net. Until quite recently, most research on environmental influences focused on a child's family (frequently only the child's mother), perhaps on playmates or on some proximate inanimate stimulation such as toys. If we looked at a larger family context at all, it was usually in terms of the general wealth or poverty of the family.

In the past 10 or 15 years, however, there has been a strong push to widen our scope, to consider the *ecology* or *context* in which each child develops. Urie Bronfenbrenner, one of the key figures in this area (1979; 1989), emphasizes that each child grows up in a complex social environment (a social ecology) with a distinct cast of characters: brothers, sisters, one or both parents, grandparents, baby-sitters, pets, schoolteachers, friends. And this cast is itself embedded within a larger social system: The parents have jobs that they may like or dislike; they may have close and supportive friends, or they may be quite isolated; they may be living in a safe neighborhood or one full of dangers; the local school may be excellent or poor; and the parents may have good or poor relationships with the school. Bronfenbrenner's argument is that we must not only include descriptions of these more extended aspects of the environment in our research, but also understand the ways in which all the components of this complex system interact with one another to affect the development of an individual child.

A particularly impressive example of research that examines such a larger system of influences is Gerald Patterson's work on the origins of antisocial (highly aggressive) behavior in children (Patterson, DeBarsyshe, & Ramsey, 1989). His studies show that parents who use poor disciplinary techniques and poor monitoring of the child are more likely to have noncompliant or antisocial children. Once established, however, the child's antisocial behavior pattern has repercussions in other areas of his life, leading both to rejection by peers and to academic difficulty. These problems, in turn, are likely to push the young person toward a deviant peer group and still further delinquency (Dishion et al., 1991; Vuchinich, Bank, & Patterson, 1992). So a pattern that began in the family is maintained and exacerbated by interactions with peers and with the school system.

How would you describe the "ecology" of your own childhood? What sort of family? What sort of neighborhood and school? What other significant people were in your life? What significant events affected your parents' lives?

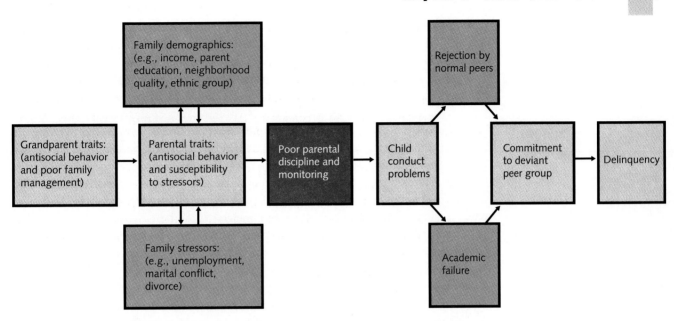

FIGURE 1.2 Patterson's model describes the many factors that influence the development of antisocial behavior. The core of the process, in this model, is the interaction between the child and the parent (the green box). One might argue that the origin of antisocial behavior lies in that relationship. But Patterson argues that larger ecological or contextual forces are also "causes" of the child's delinquency. (*Source:* Patterson, DeBaryshe, & Ramsey, 1989, Figures 1 and 2, pp. 331, 333.)

But Patterson does not stop there. He argues that the family's good or poor disciplinary techniques are not random events but are themselves shaped by the larger context in which the family exists. He finds that those parents who were raised using poor disciplinary practices are more likely to use those same poor strategies with their children. But he also finds that even parents who possess good basic child-management skills may fall into poor patterns when the stresses in their own lives are increased. A recent divorce or period of unemployment increases the likelihood that parents will use poor disciplinary practices and thus increases the likelihood that the child will develop a pattern of antisocial behavior. Figure 1.2 shows Patterson's conception of how these various components fit together. Clearly, by taking into account the larger social ecological system in which the family is embedded, our understanding of the process is greatly enhanced.

Cultural Influences

What is missing from both Bronfenbrenner's and Patterson's formulations is an emphasis on the still broader concept of **culture.** This term has no commonly agreed-upon definition, but in essence it describes some *system of meanings and customs,* including values, attitudes, goals, laws, beliefs, morals, and physical artifacts of various kinds, such as tools, forms of dwellings, and the like. Furthermore, to be called a culture, this system of meanings and customs must be *shared by some identifiable group,* whether that group is a subsection of some population or a larger unit, and *transmitted from one generation of that group to the next* (Betancourt & Lopez, 1993; Cole, 1992). Families and children are clearly embedded in culture, just as they are located within an ecological niche in the culture.

My awareness of the power of even quite small cultural variations was greatly enhanced by a year spent in Germany. My goal had been to learn German, which is my husband's native tongue, but I learned as much about culture as about language. The two cultures—German and American—are outwardly quite similar. But even quite small variations often left me feeling dislocated and uncertain. One fairly trivial example: In the parts of the U.S. where I have lived, it is very common for people to admire and talk to a stranger's baby, such as in a grocery store checkout line, or while out walking. In Germany, this is considered an invasion of privacy and is greeted with body language that conveys some combination of surprise, annoyance, and even fear. Indeed, strangers in Germany almost never speak to one another in casual situations. I experienced these behaviors as coldness and rejection of my friendliness and felt increasingly isolated, even when my logical mind told me these were merely cultural differences and not anything personal. Experiences like this convinced me that Sapir was right when he said, "The worlds in which different societies live are distinct worlds, not merely the same world with different words attached" (1929, p. 209).

Individualism and Collectivism. One major dimension on which cultural worlds differ from one another is that of **individualism** versus **collectivism.** Cultures with an individualistic emphasis assume that the world is made up of independent individuals. In such a culture, the family is clearly not seen as unimportant for the child's rearing. A nurturing family is essential. But the underlying assumption is that achievement and ultimately responsibility are individual rather than collective (Greenfield, 1994; Kim & Choi, 1994). Most European cultures are based on such individualistic assumptions, as is the Euro-American culture. But Patricia Greenfield points out that roughly 70 percent of the world's population operates with a collectivist belief system. Here the emphasis is on collective rather than individual identity, on group solidarity, sharing, duties and obligations, and group decision making. A child growing up in such a system is integrated into a strong, cohesive group that protects and nourishes that individual throughout his life. Both achievement and responsibility are shared. Collectivism is the dominant theme in most Asian countries, as well as in many African and South American cultures. Among minority groups in the U.S., collectivism is central to the cultural beliefs of most Native Americans, African-Americans, Mexican-Americans, and Asian-Americans.

Greenfield (1995) gives a wonderful example of how this difference can affect actual child-rearing practices as well as our judgments of others' child rearing. She notes that mothers from the Zinacanteco Maya culture maintain almost constant bodily contact with their young babies and do not feel comfortable when they are separated from the infants. They believe that their babies *require* this contact to be happy. When these mothers saw a visiting anthropologist put her own baby down, they were shocked and blamed the foreign baby's regular crying on the fact that he was separated from his mother so often. Greenfield argues that the constant body contact of the Mayan mothers is a logical outgrowth of their collectivist approach because their basic goal is *inter*dependence rather than independence. The American anthropologist, in contrast, operates with a basic goal of independence for her child and so emphasizes more separation. And each group judges the other's form of child rearing to be less optimal or even inadequate.

This example makes it clear that the distinction between individualism and collectivism provides a useful conceptual hook on which we may be able to hang some of our analyses of cultural differences and cultural effects. But Greenfield's analysis, and her example, also makes it clear that developmental psychology, as a scientific endeavor, has been almost entirely embedded in an individualistic cultural system. We have assumed that children develop as individuals, according to some lawful process. Even when we acknowledge that development may be influenced by context and culture, our unit of study and analysis is almost always the individual, not the family or the village or some other collective. Now we must begin to try to look at development through collectivist eyes as well.

Two Basic Reasons for Studying Cultural Variations. As I see it, there are two fundamental reasons why we need to study cultural variations, one that is primarily "individualistic" and the other "collectivist." First, I continue to assume that there *are* some developmental patterns or processes that are inherent in the individual and thus are truly universal. But to uncover them it is not enough to study white American middle-class children and assume that what we see in their development is true for all children. When we think we have uncovered some basic sequence or process, we need to observe or test other children, from other subcultural or cultural groups, from as wide an array of cultures as possible, so that the presumed universality of the developmental pattern is tested directly.

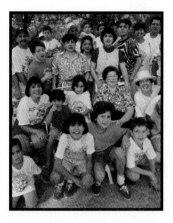

In the Hispanic-American subculture, families like the Limons, shown here at their annual reunion, are tightly knit, with frequent contact and support. Their interactions are based on a *collectivist* belief system. Such a cultural pattern may have wide repercussions.

We can also search for universals in the relationship between environment and child outcome. For example, in a recent study in Egypt, Ted Wachs and a group of Egyptian colleagues (Wachs et al., 1993) found that children in families in which the parents talked a lot to their babies were later rated as more competent. This result closely parallels the relationship between these two variables found in studies in the United States, which points us toward some possibly universal link between levels of language stimulation and the child's cognitive development.

But in other cases, the same relationships may *not* hold across cultures or subcultures. For example, the relationship between the availability of prenatal care and the rate of infant mortality is not the same in the Mexican-American subculture as in the African-American subculture (Albrecht, Miller, & Clarke, 1994; Lambert, 1993). Among Mexican-Americans, poverty is *not* associated with high infant mortality, while among African-Americans it is. Such a difference obviously has implications not only for our understanding of culture, but also at a practical level for any attempt to design an appropriate intervention to reduce infant mortality.

The "collectivist" argument for studying culture is simply to understand culture itself and its impact on the child's development. How is children's development changed by cultural variations, as in the example of "sleeping through the night" I already mentioned? How do variations in individualism and collectivism affect the way children experience their childhood and adolescence? For instance, some have argued that one consequence of individualism in U.S. culture, with its emphasis on individual freedom, is a much higher level of tolerance of aggression and violence than in collectivist cultures (Lore & Schultz, 1993).

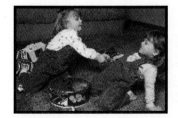

American researchers have concluded that this kind of physical aggression is normal among 2-year-olds like Laura and Megan. But it may be more likely in "individualistic" cultures than in "collectivist" cultures. How could you find out?

To achieve understanding of cultural variations it will not be enough simply to catalog a whole series of cultural patterns and describe the children in each setting. Ultimately, we will need to develop theories about the *ways* cultural variations affect children.

Fortunately, our store of cross-cultural research is growing steadily. In a few areas, such as the study of language, moral development, and attachment, we already have a fair amount of information about developmental patterns in myriad cultures. In many other areas our research is still highly Eurocentric, but I will bring in cross-cultural or subcultural research wherever I can find it.

Interactions of Nature and Nurture

The ecological/cultural approach underlines the importance of understanding the interactions among many different environmental influences. Equally, we need to understand the interactions among various internal and external influences, between nature and nurture.

We could look at this interaction in at least two ways. On the one hand, we could look for the common or normative patterns of interaction between nature and nurture. Every baby is born with certain common skills and every baby matures following some shared maturational pathway. At the same time, virtually every environment has common characteristics as well. Babies are fed, held, talked to. How do these common patterns of nature and nurture interact to produce the pattern of behavior we then see? This is basically the approach taken by most of those who have studied perceptual development and language development and by some who have studied cognitive development. I'll be describing the current conclusions drawn from this work in later chapters.

Alternatively, we might look for ways in which nature/nurture interactions *vary* from one child to another. The basic idea is that the same environment may have quite different effects on children who are born with different characteristics. One influential approach of this type is the study of *vulnerable* and *resilient* children.

Vulnerability and Resilience

A baby born weighing only 2 pounds, a child born into a highly impoverished family, a baby who has an unusually cranky or difficult temperament, all seem to start life with several strikes against them, while a child with a particularly sunny disposition begins the developmental journey with certain advantages. In recent years, theorists and researchers such as Norman Garmezy and Michael Rutter (Garmezy, 1993; Garmezy & Rutter, 1983; Rutter, 1987) have argued that such variations in children's qualities or assets are vitally important, making some children vulnerable to the stresses of childhood while buffering others from the worst consequences.

In their writings, Garmezy and Rutter have largely emphasized social origins of vulnerability, such as inadequately loving relationships with parents. Frances Horowitz uses the same term but focuses primarily on inborn kinds of vulnerability, such as premature birth, or a "difficult" temperament. In Horowitz's model, shown in Figure 1.3, the child's inborn vulnerability or resilience interacts in a particular way with the "facilitativeness" of the environment (Horowitz, 1987; 1990). A highly facilitative environment is one in which the child has loving and responsive parents and is provided with a rich array of stimulation. If the relationship between vulnerability and facilitativeness were merely additive, we would find that the best outcomes occurred for resilient infants reared in optimum environments, the worst outcomes would be found for vulnerable infants in poor environments, and the other combinations would lie somewhere in between. But that is not what Horowitz proposes. Instead she is suggesting that a resilient child in a poor environment may do quite well, since such a child can take advantage of all the stimulation and opportunities available; similarly, she suggests that a vulnerable child may do quite well in a highly facilitative environment. According to this model it is only the double whammy—the vulnerable child in a poor environment—that leads to really poor outcomes for the child.

In fact, as you will see throughout the book, a growing body of research shows precisely this pattern. For example, very low IQ scores are most common among children who were

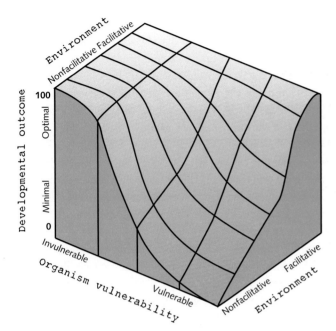

FIGURE 1.3 Horowitz's model describes one possible type of interaction between the vulnerability of the child and the quality of the environment. The height of the surface is the goodness of the developmental outcome (such as IQ or skill in social relationships). In this model, only the combination of a vulnerable infant and a nonfacilitative environment will result in really poor outcomes. (*Source:* Horowitz, 1987, Figure 1.1, p. 23.)

low-birth-weight *and* reared in poverty-level families, while low-birth-weight children reared in middle-class families have essentially normal IQs, as do normal-weight infants reared in poverty-level families (Werner, 1986). And among low-birth-weight children who are reared in poverty-level families, those whose families show "protective" factors (such as greater residential stability, less crowded living conditions, and more acceptance, more stimulation, and more learning materials) turn out better than do equivalently low-birth-weight children reared in the least optimum poverty conditions (Bradley et al., 1994). The key point here is that the same environment can have quite different effects, depending on the qualities or capacities the child brings to the equation.

Another possible variation of this same idea: Do you think it is possible that girls and boys, beginning in infancy, respond differently to the *same* environments? If this is true, what would be the ramifications of such a pattern?

The Nature of Developmental Change

The nature/nurture controversy is not the only "big question" in developmental psychology. An equally central dispute concerns the nature of developmental change itself: Is a child's expanding ability just "more of the same," or does it reflect a new kind of activity? For example, a 2-year-old is likely to have no individual friends among her playmates, while an 8-year-old is likely to have several. We could think of this as a *quantitative* change (a change in amount) from zero friends to some friends. Or we could think of it as a *qualitative* change (a change in kind or type) from disinterest in peers to interest, or from one *sort* of peer relationship to another. Where a given researcher or theorist stands on this question has a profound effect on the way he or she perceives children and their behavior. Does a child simply get better and better at things, such as walking or running, or reading? That is, are the *processes* the same and only the efficiency or the speed different, or are there different processes at different ages? Do older children use different strategies, develop different understandings, organize their behavior differently? These issues are particularly central in discussions of cognitive development, which I'll be talking about in Chapters 7 and 12.

Stages and Sequences

An important related question, also especially relevant to discussions of cognitive development, concerns the existence of *stages* in the course of development. If development consists only of additions (quantitative change), then the concept of stages is not needed. But if development involves reorganization or the emergence of wholly new strategies or skills (qualitative change), then the concept of stages may become attractive. Certainly we hear a lot of "stagelike" language in everyday conversation about children: "He's just in the terrible twos," or, "It's only a stage she's going through."

Although there is not always agreement on just what would constitute evidence for the existence of discrete stages, the usual description is that a stage shift involves not only a change in skills but also some discontinuous change in underlying *structure* (McHale & Lerner, 1990). The child in a new stage approaches tasks differently, sees the world differently, is preoccupied with different issues.

As we move through the following chapters, you will see that stage theories are common in studies of development, although the concept has come under considerable recent attack. John Flavell, a major thinker in the area of cognitive development, points out that research on children's thinking in the past several decades has yielded only limited evidence of stages. What one does see are *sequences* of development in each of a large number of content areas—sequences in the development of concepts of gender, sequences in the development of memory strategies, sequences in the acquisition of language skills. Each of these sequences appears to be common across children and to reflect qualitative as well as quantitative changes, but the many sequences do not seem to be organized into cohesive wholes that we might think of as broad stages (Flavell, 1985; 1992). A child might be very advanced in one sequence and only average in several others, for example, rather than being equally fast or slow in all areas. Thus, the idea of stages of development, which seems at first blush to be a tidy way of organizing information, a simple way of describing changes with age, has turned out to be slippery and difficult to sustain. You should keep that in mind as you encounter the various stage theories that are still part of our theoretical language. You should also note, however, that it is not necessary to assume stages in

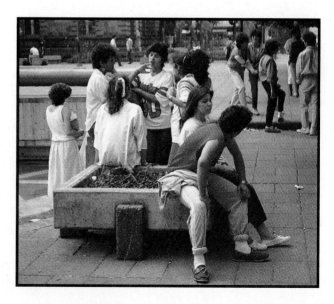

Are these Costa Rican teenagers hanging out together in a group because this is a normal "stage" in adolescence? What other explanations of this behavior could you think of?

order to argue that the nature of developmental change is qualitative as well as (or instead of) quantitative. Qualitative change may be gradual as well as abrupt, sequential rather than stagelike.

Theories of Development

In principle, any of the many logical combinations of answers to the various questions I have been asking about nature versus nurture, or about the nature of development, might form the basis of a theory of development. But certain patterns of answers have been much more prominent than others. Of these, four families of theories have been most influential—not just in studies of development but also in psychology as a whole: biological, learning, psychoanalytic, and cognitive-developmental theories. Since I will be examining all four in much greater detail in later chapters, let me describe them only briefly here, pointing out the ways in which they differ in their answers to the key questions.

Biological Theories

The most basic proposition of biological theories of development is that both our common patterns of development and our unique individual behavioral tendencies have their roots in the genes, or in hormone patterns, or in maturationally governed changes in the brain. Biologically oriented theorists do not argue that environment is unimportant—no one takes such an extreme position. But behavior genetic research has made it clear that genetic programming is a powerful framework, affecting both shared and individual patterns of development—a point I will return to repeatedly.

Learning Theories

Learning theorists have started from the other end of the nature/nurture argument, emphasizing the dominant role of experience. Albert Bandura, a leading theorist of this school, puts it this way:

> Human nature is characterized by a vast potentiality that can be fashioned by direct and vicarious experience into a variety of forms within biological limits. (Bandura, 1989, p. 51)

Clearly, Bandura is not rejecting biology, any more than biological theorists reject environment. But he sees human behavior as enormously plastic, shaped by predictable processes of learning. Two of those processes are classical conditioning and operant conditioning. If you have encountered these concepts in earlier courses, you can skim the next section. But for those of you who lack such a background, a brief description is needed.

Classical Conditioning.   This type of learning, made famous by Pavlov's experiments with his salivating dog, involves the acquisition of new signals for existing responses. If you touch a baby on the cheek, he will turn toward the touch and begin to suck. In the technical terminology of **classical conditioning,** the touch on the cheek is the **unconditioned stimulus;** the turning and sucking are **unconditioned responses.** The baby is already programmed to do all that; these are automatic reflexes. Learning occurs when some *new* stimulus is hooked into the system. The general model is that other stimuli that are present just before or at the same time as the unconditioned stimulus will eventually trigger the same responses. In the typical home situation, for example, a number of stimuli occur at about the same time as the touch on the baby's cheek before feeding. There is the sound of the mother's footsteps approaching, the kinesthetic cues of being picked up, and the tactile cues of being held in the mother's arms. All these stimuli may eventually become **conditioned stimuli** and may trigger the infant's response of turning and sucking, even without any touch on the cheek.

Classical conditioning is of special interest in our study of child development because of the role it plays in the development of emotional responses. For example, things or people present when you feel good will become conditioned stimuli for that same sense of goodwill, while those previously associated with some uncomfortable feeling may become conditioned stimuli for a sense of unease or anxiety. This is especially important in infancy, since a child's mother or father is present so often when nice things happen—when the child feels warm, comfortable, and cuddled. In this way mother and father usually come to be conditioned stimuli for pleasant feelings, a fact that makes it possible for the parents' mere presence to reinforce other behaviors as well. But a tormenting older sibling might come to be a conditioned stimulus for angry feelings, even after the sibling has long since stopped the tormenting. These classically conditioned emotional responses are remarkably powerful. They begin to be formed very early in life, continue to be created throughout childhood and adulthood, and profoundly affect each individual's emotional experiences.

Operant Conditioning. The second major type of learning is most often called **operant conditioning,** although you will also see it referred to as *instrumental conditioning.* Unlike classical conditioning, which involves attaching an old response to a new stimulus, operant conditioning involves attaching a new response to an old stimulus, achieved by the application of appropriate principles of reinforcement. Any behavior that is reinforced will be more likely to occur again in the same or in a similar situation. There are two types of reinforcements. A **positive reinforcement** is any event that, following some behavior, increases the chances that the behavior will occur again in that situation. Certain classes of pleasant consequences, such as praise, a smile, food, a hug, or attention, serve as reinforcers for most people most of the time. But strictly speaking, a reinforcement is defined by its effect; we don't know something is reinforcing unless we see that its presence increases the probability of some behavior.

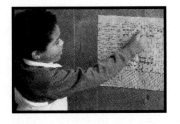

A daily achievement chart, like this one for 5-year-old Aaron, can be highly reinforcing for many children.

The second major type is a **negative reinforcement,** which occurs when something an individual finds *unpleasant* is *stopped.* Suppose your little boy is whining and begging you to pick him up. At first you ignore him, but finally you do pick him up. What happens? He stops whining. So your picking-up behavior has been *negatively reinforced* by the cessation of his whining, and you will be *more* likely to pick him up the next time he whines. At the same time, his whining has probably been *positively reinforced* by your attention, so he will be more likely to whine on similar occasions.

Both positive and negative reinforcements strengthen behavior. **Punishment,** in contrast, is intended to weaken some undesired behavior. Sometimes punishments involve eliminating nice things (like "grounding" a child, taking away TV privileges, or sending her to her room). Often they involve administering unpleasant things such as a scolding or a spanking. What is confusing about the idea of punishment is that it doesn't always do what it is intended to do: It does not always suppress the undesired behavior. If your child has thrown his milk glass at you to get your attention, spanking him may be a positive reinforcement instead of the punishment you intended.

In laboratory situations, experimenters can be sure to reinforce some behavior every time it occurs, or to stop reinforcements completely so as to produce extinction of the response. But in the real world, consistency of reinforcement is the exception rather than the rule. Much more common is a pattern of **partial reinforcement,** in which some behavior is reinforced on some occasions but not others. Studies of partial reinforcement show that children and adults take longer to learn some behavior under partial reinforcement conditions, but once established, such behaviors are much more resistant to extinction. If you smile at your daughter only every fifth or sixth time she brings a picture to show you (and if she finds your smile reinforcing), she'll keep on bringing pictures for a very long stretch, even if you quit smiling altogether.

Additional Processes in Bandura's Theory. Bandura, whose variation of learning theory is by far the most influential among developmental psychologists today, suggests several other key forms of learning (1977; 1982; 1989). First, he argues that learning does not always require direct reinforcement. Learning may also occur merely as a result of watching someone else perform some action. Learning of this type, called **observational learning** or **modeling,** is involved in a wide range of behaviors. Children learn ways of hitting from watching other people in real life and on TV. They learn how to be generous by watching others donate money or goods.

Bandura also calls attention to another class of reinforcements called **intrinsic reinforcements** or *intrinsic rewards,* such as pride or discovery. These are reinforcements internal to the individual, such as the pleasure a child feels when she finally figures out how to draw a star, or the sense of satisfaction you may experience after strenuous exercise.

Finally, and perhaps most important, Bandura has gone far toward bridging the gap between learning theory and cognitive-developmental theory by emphasizing important *cognitive* (mental) elements in observational learning. Indeed, he now even refers to his theory as "social cognitive theory" (1986; 1989). For example, Bandura now stresses the fact that modeling can be the vehicle for learning abstract as well as concrete skills or information. The observer extracts a rule that may be the basis of the model's behavior, and learns the rule as well as the specific behavior. In this way a child or adult can acquire attitudes, values, ways of solving problems, even standards of self-evaluation through modeling.

Collectively, these additions to traditional learning theory make the system far more flexible and powerful, although it is still not a strongly *developmental* theory. That is,

Think again about your own upbringing. What values or attitudes do you think you learned through modeling? How were those values and attitudes displayed (modeled) by your parents or others?

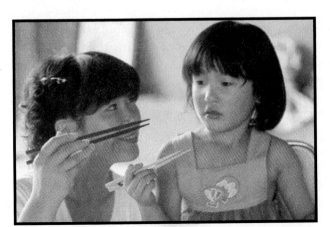

Learning to use chopsticks through modeling is only one of the myriad skills, attitudes, beliefs, and values that are learned in this way.

Bandura has little to say about changes with age in what or how a child may learn from modeling. In contrast, psychoanalytic theories are strongly developmental, emphasizing sequential, often stagelike qualitative change.

Psychoanalytic Theories

In Greek, the word *psyche* refers to the soul, spirit, or mind. So psychoanalysis is the analysis of the mind or spirit. All the theorists in this general tradition have been interested in explaining human behavior by understanding the underlying processes of the mind and the personality. And nearly all psychoanalytic theorists have begun by studying and analyzing adults or children who are disturbed in some way. Many believed they could come to understand the normal processes by analyzing how they had gone wrong.

As with learning theories, a whole family of theories is called "psychoanalytic," beginning with Freud's and continuing with theories by Carl Jung (1916; 1939), Alfred Adler (1948), Erik Erikson (1963; 1980), and many others.

Sigmund Freud (1905; 1920) is usually credited with originating the psychoanalytic approach, and his terminology and many of his concepts have become part of our intellectual culture, even while his explicit influence on developmental psychologists has waned. Among current theorists in this tradition, Erik Erikson is probably the most influential, although the work of other important thinkers, such as John Bowlby and Jane Loevinger, has been strongly influenced by psychoanalytic theory.

The most distinctive and central assumption of the psychoanalytic approach is that behavior is governed by *unconscious* as well as conscious processes. Some of these unconscious processes are present at birth; others develop over time. For example, Freud proposed the existence of a basic unconscious, instinctual sexual drive he called the **libido.** He argued that this energy is the motivating force behind virtually all our behavior. Freud also proposed that unconscious material is created over time through the functioning of the various defense mechanisms—those automatic, normal, unconscious strategies for reducing anxiety that we all use daily, such as repression, denial, or projection.

A second basic assumption is that personality has a structure, and that this structure develops over time. Freud proposed three parts, the **id,** which is the center of the libido; the **ego,** a much more conscious element, the executive of the personality; and the **superego,** which is the center of conscience and morality, since it incorporates the norms and moral strictures of the family and society. In Freud's theory, these three parts are not all present at birth. The infant and toddler is all id, all instinct, all desire, without the restraining influence of the ego or the superego. The ego begins to develop in the years from 2 to about 4 or 5 as the child learns to adapt his instant-gratification strategies. Finally, the superego begins to develop just before school age, as the child incorporates the parents' values and cultural mores.

Psychoanalytic theorists also see development as fundamentally stagelike, with each stage centered on a particular form of tension or a particular task. The child moves through these stages, resolving each task, reducing each tension as best as he can. There is direction to this development, an ideal sequence.

The stages themselves are conceived somewhat differently in the various theories in this tradition. Freud thought they were strongly influenced by maturation. In each of Freud's five *psychosexual stages,* the libido is invested in that part of the body that is most sensitive at that age. In a newborn, the mouth is the most sensitive part of the body, so libidinal energy is focused there. The stage is therefore called the *oral* stage. As neurological

The Real World

We All Use Defense Mechanisms Every Day

I suspect that when many of you hear the phrase "defense mechanisms," you think of some kind of abnormal or deviant behavior. It is important for you to understand, though, that Freud conceived of them not only as unconscious but also as entirely normal. Their primary purpose is to help us protect ourselves against anxiety. Since we all feel anxious some of the time, we all use some form of defense.

Suppose I send a paper to a professional journal and it comes back with a rejection letter. To deal with the anxiety I naturally feel after such a rejection, I resort (unconsciously) to some kind of defense mechanism.

All defense mechanisms distort reality to some extent, but they vary in the amount of distortion involved. At one extreme end is *denial*. I might deny that I had ever submitted the paper or that it had ever been rejected. A notch less distorting are mechanisms like *projection*, in which I push my feelings onto someone else. ("Those people who rejected this paper are really stupid! They don't know what they're doing.") In this way, I ascribe to others the qualities I fear may be true for me—in this instance, stupidity. I might also *repress* my feelings, insisting that I really don't mind at all that my paper is rejected; later, I might simply forget that I had ever submitted that paper. Or I could use *intellectualization*, in which I consider, in emotionally very bland terms, all the reasons why the paper was rejected. Intellectualization sounds quite rational and open, as if there were no defense involved. But what has been pushed away is the emotion.

Among the least distorting defenses is *suppression*, in which I allow myself to be aware of my distress but still shove it away for a while by saying, *à la* Scarlett O'Hara, "I'll think about it tomorrow." So I push it away, but not so firmly into the unconscious as is true for repression.

Not long ago I was reminded very forcibly of just how powerful these defensive processes can be. I received a phone call at noon one day from a friend, who told me of the death from AIDS of a man who was very dear to me. I said all the right things at the time, finished my lunch, and went back to work, pressing to meet a deadline. At dinner that evening, I had this vague feeling that there was some important news I meant to tell my husband, but I *couldn't remember what it was.* I went to a choir rehearsal that evening and was unbearably grumpy and irritable but couldn't figure out why. As I got into my car to drive home, the memory of my friend's death suddenly returned, and I burst into tears in the parking lot. This is a perfect example of repression. I couldn't deal with the news when it first arrived, so I pushed it out of my conscious memory long enough to get me through the day.

Can you think of equivalent examples in your own life? When was the last time something uncomfortable happened to you? How did you handle it? Bear in mind that these defenses are entirely normal.

---

development progresses the infant has more sensation in the anus (hence the *anal* stage), and later the genitalia (the *phallic* and eventually the *genital* stages).

The stages Erikson proposes, called **psychosocial stages,** are influenced much less by maturation and much more by common cultural demands for children of a particular age, such as the demand that the child become toilet trained at about 2 or that the child learn school skills at age 6 or 7. In Erikson's view, each child moves through a fixed sequence of tasks or dilemmas, each centered on the development of a particular facet of identity. For example, the first task, central to the first 12 to 18 months of life, is to develop a sense of basic trust. If the child's caregivers are not responsive and loving, however, the child may develop a sense of mistrust, which will affect her responses at all the later stages.

In both theories, however, the critical point is that the degree of success a child experiences in meeting the demands of these various stages will depend very heavily on the interactions he has with the people and objects in his world. This *interactive* element in Freud's and all subsequent psychoanalytic theories is absolutely central. Basic trust cannot be developed unless the parents or other caregivers respond to the infant in a loving, consistent way. The oral stage cannot be fully completed unless the infant is given sufficient gratification of the desire for oral stimulation. And when one stage is not fully resolved, the old patterns or the unmet need are carried forward, affecting the individual's ability to handle later tasks or stages. So, for example, a young adult who developed a sense of mistrust in the first years of life may have a more difficult time establishing secure intimate relationships with a partner or friends—a pattern that has now been found in a growing number of studies (e.g., Hazan & Shaver, 1990; Senchak & Leonard, 1992; Simpson, 1990).

Does this make sense to you—this idea that one carries unresolved issues forward into adulthood? Can you think of any examples in your own experience?

Cognitive-Developmental Theories

In psychoanalytic theories, the quality and character of a child's relationships with a few key people are seen as central to the child's whole development. The child's encounters with the inanimate world—with toys and objects, with sights and sounds—are rarely discussed. Cognitive-developmental theorists, whose interest has been primarily in cognitive development rather than personality, reverse this order of importance, emphasizing the centrality of the child's explorations of objects. But cognitive-developmental theorists share with their psychoanalytically inclined colleagues the assumption that the cause or source of change is internal to the child as well as external. The child is an active participant in the process of development.

The central figure in cognitive-developmental theory has been Jean Piaget (1952; 1970; 1977; Piaget & Inhelder, 1969), a Swiss psychologist whose theories shaped the thinking of several generations of developmental psychologists. Piaget, along with other early cognitive theorists such as Lev Vygotsky (1962) and Heinz Werner (1948), was struck by the great regularities in the development of children's thinking. He noticed that all children seemed to go through the same kinds of sequential discoveries about their world, making the same sorts of mistakes and arriving at the same solutions. For example, 3- and 4-year-olds all seem to think that if you pour water from a short, fat glass into a tall, thin one, there is more water in the thin glass, since the water level is higher there than it was in the fat glass. But most 7-year-olds realize that the amount of water is the same in either case. If a 2-year-old loses her shoe, she may look for it briefly and haphazardly, but she does not undertake a systematic search. A 10-year-old, in contrast, is likely to use such good strategies as retracing her steps or looking in one room after another.

Piaget's detailed observations of children's thinking led him to several assumptions, the most central of which is that it is the nature of the human organism to *adapt* to its environment. This is an active process. In contrast to many learning theorists, Piaget does not think that the environment *shapes* the child. Rather, the child (like the adult) actively seeks to understand his environment. In the process, he explores, manipulates, and examines the objects and people in his world.

The process of adaptation, in Piaget's view, is made up of several important subprocesses—*assimilation, accommodation,* and *equilibration*—all of which I will define fully in Chapter 7. What you need to understand at this preliminary point is that Piaget thought that the child develops a series of fairly distinct "understandings" or "theories" about the way the world works, based on her active exploration of the environment. Each of these "theories" comprises a specific stage. Since Piaget thought that virtually all infants begin with the same skills and built-in strategies, and since the environments children encounter are highly similar in important respects, he believed that the stages through which their thinking moves are also similar. Piaget proposed a fixed sequence of four ma-

Table 1.1
Comparison of Developmental Theories on Some of the Key Questions About Development

Issue	Biological Theory	Learning Theory	Psychoanalytic Theory	Cognitive-Developmental Theory
What is the major influence on development?	Primarily nature	Primarily nurture	Both	The child's own internal processing of experience
Is developmental change qualitative or quantitative?	Both	Both in Bandura's version	Qualitative	Qualitative
Are there stages or sequences?	Sequences	No stages; some sequences	Stages	Piaget said stages
Examples of research questions emerging from that theoretical tradition	Temperamental differences and their effects; role of heredity and environment in intelligence	Impact of TV on behavior; origins of social behaviors such as aggression	Attachment; fantasies	Development of logic; gender concepts; moral development

jor stages, each growing out of the one that preceded it, and each consisting of a more or less complete system or organization of concepts, strategies, and assumptions.

Contrasting the Theories

No doubt by now your head is swimming with theories. But we can make some order out of the array by returning to some of the central issues I discussed earlier in the chapter and by looking at how the various theories differ along these dimensions—an analysis you can see in Table 1.1. In this table, as in my descriptions of the theories, I have intentionally made the contrasts as great as possible to help you keep the alternatives clearly separate. But as we go along you will find that many current theories involve very interesting mixtures of these approaches. You've already seen this in the cognitive elements now contained in Bandura's theories and in the ecological concepts added to a basic learning theory approach in Patterson's work. But other examples are easy to find, such as newer theories of the child's attachment to her parents that combine basic psychoanalytic concepts with clearly cognitive themes such as the notion of an internal working model. And in virtually every area of study we see a return to an emphasis on biological roots. Having distinctly separate theories may be tidy, but I find the new blends, the new syntheses, far more intriguing.

Finding the Answers: Research on Development

I've asked an enormous number of questions already in this chapter. But before you can understand the answers—before I can get to the really interesting stuff you are probably most curious about—you need one more tool, namely, at least a modicum of familiarity with the methods researchers use when they explore questions about development. You'll need such a familiarity to make sense out of the research I'll be talking about throughout this book, and you'll need it in the future if you are going to be an intelligent consumer of research information provided through newspapers and magazines.

Let me walk you through the various alternative methods by using a concrete example with clear practical ramifications. Imagine that you are a social scientist. One day you get a call from your local state representative. She has become seriously concerned about the apparently rising levels of crime and lawlessness among teenagers and wants to propose new legislation to respond to this problem. First, though, she wants to have some answers to a series of basic questions:

1. Does the same problem exist everywhere in the world, or only in the United States? If the latter, then what is it about our culture that promotes or supports such behavior?

2. At what age does the problem begin to be visible?

3. Which kids are most at risk for such delinquent behavior, and why?

How would you, could you, go about designing one or more studies that might answer such questions? You would face a number of decisions:

- To answer the question about the age at which delinquent acts begin, should you compare groups of children and teenagers of different ages, or should you select a group of younger children and follow them over time, as they move into adolescence? And should you study young people in many settings or cultures, or in only one setting, such as inner-city youth in the U.S.? These are questions of *research design*.

- How will you measure delinquent behavior? Can you observe it? Can you ask about it? Can you rely on official records? What other things about each young person might you want to know to begin to answer the "why" question? Family history and relationships? Relationships with peers? Self-esteem? These are questions of *research methodology*.

- How will you analyze the data you collect and how will you interpret your findings? Suppose you find that young people whose families live in poverty are considerably more likely to be delinquent. Would you be satisfied to stop there, or would you want to analyze the results separately for each of several ethnic groups, for children growing up with single mothers, or in other ways that might clarify the meaning of your results? These are questions of *research analysis*.

Research Design

Choosing a research design is crucial for any research, but especially so when the subject matter you are trying to study is change (or continuity) with age. You have basically three choices: (1) You can study different groups of people of different ages, called a **cross-sectional design.** (2) You can study the *same* people over a period of time, called a **longitudinal design.** (3) Or you can combine the two in some fashion, using what is called a **sequential design** (Schaie, 1983). And if you want to know whether the same patterns hold across different cultures or contexts, you will need to do some kind of

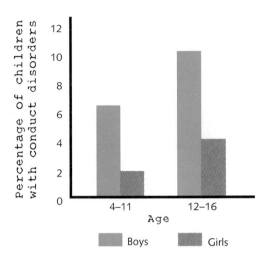

FIGURE 1.4 In this cross-sectional comparison from the Ontrio study of conduct disorders, boys and teenagers showed higher rates of problem behavior. (*Source:* Offord, Boyle, & Racine, 1991, from Table 2.4, p. 40.)

cross-cultural research, in which equivalent or parallel methods are used in more than one context.

Cross-sectional Designs

The key feature of a cross-sectional design is that the researcher assesses separate age groups, with each subject tested only once. To study delinquency cross-sectionally you might select groups of subjects at each of a series of ages, such as 8, 10, 12, 14, and 16. You would then measure each child or teen's delinquent behavior, along with whatever other characteristics you had decided were important. To get some feeling for what the results from such a study might look like, take a look at Figure 1.4, which shows the rate of "conduct disorders" in a large random sample of all children between the ages of 4 and 16 in the province of Ontario, Canada (Offord, Boyle, & Racine, 1991). (A conduct disorder is akin to what is often called delinquency in everyday language.) It is clear that conduct disorders in this sample were far more common in adolescents and in boys. Such a pattern of results is typical of studies in a number of Western countries, in which this work has been done.

Cross-sectional research is often enormously useful. It is relatively quick to do, and when age differences are indeed found, it may suggest new hypotheses about developmental processes. When the investigators collect a rich array of additional information about each subject, it can also yield highly interesting results. In the Ontario study, for example, Offord and his colleagues found that the probability of a conduct disorder was four times as high in low-income families, nearly three times as high in "dysfunctional" families, three times as high in families with domestic violence, and so forth. Thus, a research design of this type can begin to tell us *which* children are at risk and give us some hints about whys.

At the same time, cross-sectional designs have three major problems or limitations. The first of these is the "cohort problem."

The Cohort Problem. Social scientists use the word **cohort** to describe groups of individuals born within some fairly narrow band of years who share the same cultural/historical experiences at the same times in their lives. Within any given culture, successive cohorts may have quite different life experiences. For example, the 4-year-olds in the Offord study were born in 1979; the 16-year-olds were born in 1967. In that span of 12 years in the U.S., the percentage of children whose mothers were working rose about 14

Make a list of all the differences you can think of between the likely childhood experiences of the cohort born (in your country) in 1960 and the cohort born in 1990. How might those differences affect the behavior of the children in each group?

points; the proportion of children living in single-parent families increased from about 11 percent to about 19 percent (Hernandez, 1994). Assuming that similar trends (albeit probably less extreme) have also been true of Canada, then the two age groups in Figure 1.4 differ not just in age, but also in family experiences. Is the higher level of delinquency in the older group linked to age per se or to changes in culture? When we compare different age groups in a single study, as we do in any cross-sectional design, we are also inevitably comparing cohorts to some degree. Thus, *cohort* and *age* are totally confounded, and we cannot tell whether some apparent age difference is really attributable to age or only to cohort differences. When the age groups we are comparing are close in age, as is true in most studies of children, this is not usually a major problem, since we can assume roughly similar life circumstances. But over age ranges of as much as 10 years, the cohort differences may be significant.

The Time of Measurement Problem. A related difficulty is that any study is done at some specific time, and the results may simply not generalize to other time periods. The Ontario study was done in 1982 and 1983. Would we find the same results if we were to repeat the study today? Might all the problem rates be higher? Would the same family characteristics predict conduct disorders now as predicted them then? This problem of generalizing across time periods is especially acute in any society or culture undergoing rapid change, as is the case in many Western cultures today.

Origins, Sequences, and Consistency. Finally and perhaps most important, cross-sectional research cannot tell us much about *sequences* of development or about the cumulative development of some pattern over time. The Ontario study doesn't tell us what happens—in children or in families—to lead to increased rates of conduct disorders in adolescence. It also doesn't tell us if there is some typical sequence through which a child passes, such as from minor misbehavior to more serious lawlessness. To give you another example, a cross-sectional study of children's gender concepts might show that 2-year-olds have a different idea of gender than 4-year-olds. But this won't tell us whether there are steps in between or whether every child acquires this concept in the same sequence.

Similarly, cross-sectional studies will not tell us anything about the consistency of individual behavior over time. For example, it won't tell us if the children who show conduct disorders at 6 or 7 or 8 are likely to show the same kind of problem in adolescence.

Longitudinal Designs

Two of these three problems can be addressed with longitudinal designs, in which the *same* individuals are studied over a period of time. They allow us to look at sequences of change and individual consistency or inconsistency over time. And because they compare performances by the same people at different ages, they get around the cohort problem. Because of these advantages, they have become extremely common in developmental research.

As one example, Patterson's model of the development of aggressive and delinquent behavior, laid out in Figure 1.2, is buttressed by a number of longitudinal studies in which boys at high risk for later delinquency were followed from fourth grade through junior high school (Patterson, Capaldi, & Bank, 1991; Vuchinich et al., 1992).

But longitudinal designs are not a panacea. Because they are time-consuming and expensive, researchers often study quite small samples, so that it is hard to generalize the findings to broader groups. This design also does not solve the time of measurement problem, because each study involves only one group, growing up in a particular historical context.

One solution to this problem is to repeat a longitudinal study several times, each time with a new cohort. This particular strategy, called a *cohort-sequential design,* is one of a family of research designs, called sequential designs, that involve either combinations of cross-sectional or combinations of longitudinal designs, or both. I know of no large cohort-sequential studies in which cohorts as widely apart as 10 or more years have been followed through childhood, but shorter-term versions of this design are becoming much more common.

Cross-cultural or Cross-context Designs

Finally, when we want to address the questions of universality or cultural specificity, we need to compare across cultures—a task that researchers have approached in several ways.

One way is with what anthropologists call an **ethnography**—a detailed description of a single culture or context, based on extensive observation. Often the observer lives within the culture for a period of time, perhaps as long as several years. Information from several different ethnographies may then be compared, to see if similar developmental patterns exist in varying cultures (Whiting & Edwards, 1988). For example, are girls and boys given different tasks in every culture and are those gender assignments similar from one context, one culture, to the next?

Alternatively, researchers can use standardized assessment instruments or methods to study some aspect of children's development or behavior in other cultural settings and then can compare their results to existing U.S. or Western data. This is precisely what Wachs and his colleagues did in the Egyptian study I mentioned earlier. As such a body of research in any one area accumulates, it is possible to compare results across many cultures.

Finally, there are studies in which the same investigator compares two or more samples of children or families, each from a different culture or context, using the same or comparable instruments or measures or direct translations of those measures. Such comparative research has become quite common within the United States, involving comparisons of children or families in several different ethnic groups or neighborhoods. Cross-national comparisons are also beginning to appear with greater regularity, although they are still comparatively rare (e.g., Kagan et al., 1994). I've described one example in the *Cultures and Contexts* box on page 28.

This is immensely difficult research to do well. Among the many difficulties, perhaps the most troublesome is the problem of equivalence of measurement. Is it enough just to translate some test into another language? Will the same measure or assessment technique be equally valid in all cultures? Do behaviors have the same *meaning* in other contexts, other cultures? For example, Anne-Marie Ambert (1994) makes the point that when Western researchers study parent behavior, they begin with the assumption that the mother is the most central figure in a child's upbringing. But in many cultures in the world, multiple mothering is the rule, and the biological mother may do relatively little nurturing. If we then try to measure the "quality" of the mother's caregiving behavior by counting the number of nurturing acts or the frequency of smiles or verbal interactions, we may come to quite erroneous conclusions.

What other problems can you think of that would make it hard to do good cross-cultural research?

Experimental Designs

Most of the research designs I have described so far are alternative ways to look at changes with age. But if we are interested in examining a basic process—such as learning or memory—or in *explaining* any observed phenomena, we may do **experiments.**

Cultures and Contexts

An Example of a Cross-cultural Comparison Study

Mark Bornstein and his colleagues (Bornstein, Tal, & Tamis-LeMonda, 1991; Bornstein et al., 1992) videotaped 24 mothers in each of three countries—Japan, France, and the United States—interacting in their homes with their 5-month-old infants. They noted that the *babies* behaved very similarly, which suggests that any differences in the mothers' behaviors can't be attributed to varying signals or responses from the babies. And in some ways, the mothers responded similarly. In particular, they all showed similar rates of nurturance toward their infants and similar levels of imitation. Nonetheless, there were some intriguing differences.

First of all, American mothers simply provided much more stimulation to their babies than did either Japanese or French mothers. They pointed, named, described, touched, and positioned their babies more. Furthermore, mothers in these three cultures gave different weight to various types of stimulation. American mothers and French mothers were more likely to focus efforts on getting their babies to interact with objects and less likely to concentrate on getting their babies to interact with Mom. For Japanese mothers, the two were nearly in balance. A third difference was that American mothers were a lot more likely to use a special, high-pitched sort of speech toward their infants—a form of speech sometimes called "motherese." Both the French and Japanese mothers used motherese occasionally, but much less often than the American mothers. French and Japanese mothers were more likely to talk to their babies using ordinary adult conversational tones. Such a finding does not—or does not necessarily—mean that the *process* of development is different in these different cultures. Babies in every culture may respond similarly to motherese, for example. Rather, these results suggest some of the subtle but significant ways that babies may be shaped into the cultural pattern in which they are growing.

An experiment is normally designed to test a specific hypothesis, a particular causal explanation. For example, Patterson hypothesized that the beginning of the chain of causal events implicated in aggressive and delinquent behavior lies in the family discipline patterns. To test this, he could devise an intervention experiment in which some families of aggressive children are given training in better discipline techniques and other families, with similar children, are given no training. He could then check at the end of the training, and perhaps some months or years later, to see if the children whose families had had the training were less likely to show aggression or delinquency.

A key feature of an experiment, then, is that subjects are assigned *randomly* to participate in one of several groups. Subjects in the **experimental group** receive the treatment the experimenter thinks will produce an identified effect, while those in the **control group** receive either no special treatment or a neutral treatment. The presumed causal element in the experiment is called the **independent variable.** In the mythical Patterson experiment, the training is the independent variable. Any behavior that independent variable is expected to influence is called a **dependent variable.** In the example I'm using, later levels of aggression or delinquency are dependent variables.

Problems with Experiments in Studying Development.   Experiments like this are essential for our understanding of many aspects of development. But two special problems in studying child or adult development limit the use of experimental designs.

First, many of the questions we want to answer have to do with the effects of particular unpleasant or stressful experiences on individuals—abuse, prenatal influences such as the mother's drinking, family poverty, or parental unemployment. For obvious ethical reasons, we cannot manipulate these variables. We cannot ask one set of pregnant women to have two alcohol drinks a day and others to have none; we cannot randomly assign adults to become unemployed. So to study the effects of such experiences we must rely on nonexperimental designs, including longitudinal and sequential studies.

Second, the independent variable in which we are often most interested is age itself, and *we cannot assign subjects randomly to age groups.* We can compare 4-year-olds and 6-year-olds in their approach to a particular task, such as searching for a lost object, but the children differ in a host of ways in addition to their ages. Older children have had more and different experiences. Thus, unlike psychologists studying other aspects of behavior, developmental psychologists *cannot* systematically manipulate many of the variables we are most interested in.

To get around this problem, we can use any one of a series of strategies that are sometimes called *quasi experiments,* in which we compare groups but do not assign the subjects randomly. Cross-sectional comparisons are a form of quasi experiment. So are studies in which we select naturally occurring groups that differ in some dimension of interest, such as children whose parents choose to place them in day-care programs compared to children whose parents rear them at home, or children in single-parent families versus those in two-parent families.

Such comparisons have built-in problems, because groups that differ in one way are likely to be different in other ways as well. Families who place their children in day care, compared to those who rear them at home, are also likely to be poorer, may more often be single-parent families, and may have different values or religious backgrounds. If we find that the two groups of children differ in some fashion, is it because they have spent their daytime hours in different places or because of these other differences in their families? We can make such comparisons a bit cleaner if we select our comparison groups initially so that they are matched on those variables we think might matter, such as income or marital status or religion. But quasi experiments, by their very nature, will always yield more ambiguous results than will a fully controlled experiment.

Research Methods

Choosing a research design is only the first crucial decision an investigator must make. Equally important is to decide what subjects to study and how to study them.

Choosing the Subjects.   Because we would like to uncover basic developmental patterns that are true for all children, all adolescents, or all adults, the ideal strategy would be to choose and study a random sample of all people in the world. This is clearly impractical, so some kind of compromise is necessary. One compromise, becoming more and more common in today's research, is to select large samples that are representative of some subgroup or population—such as the Ontario study I've already described. This is a widely used strategy in sociology and epidemiology, and it can be very fruitful in psychology as well. But because it is difficult to collect highly detailed information from or about large numbers of subjects, we frequently trade off depth for breadth.

The other alternative, very common in psychological research on children, is to focus on studying a smaller group of subjects in greater depth and detail, in an attempt to uncover very basic processes. For instance, Alan Sroufe and his colleagues (Sroufe, 1989; Sroufe, Egeland, & Kreutzer, 1990) have studied a group of 267 children and families, beginning before the birth of the child. Families were deliberately chosen from among those thought to be at high risk for later caregiving problems, such as low-education single mothers with unplanned pregnancies. The children have now been repeatedly studied, each time in considerable detail. The sample is not representative of the population as a whole, but the results are enormously informative nonetheless and may tell us more about the process of emotional and social development than we could possibly glean from larger samples studied more broadly. Neither strategy is better than the other; both are useful. In either case, we need to remember that the conclusions we can draw will be limited by the sample we studied and by the type of information we could obtain.

The two time-honored ways of gathering information about individuals are observation and asking questions. Because infants and young children are not particularly good at answering questions, observation has been an especially prominent research strategy among developmental psychologists.

Observation. Any researcher planning to use observation to collect information about children or their environments will have to make at least three further decisions: What shall I observe? Where shall I observe? How shall I record the observations?

The decision about what to observe can be divided still further: Should you try to observe everything a child does or focus only on selected behaviors? Should you observe only the child or also the immediate environment—such as the responses of the people around the child—or the quality of the home? Which I choose will depend largely on the basic question I am trying to address. If I am interested in the child's first words I would not need to pay much attention to how close the child was sitting to an adult or to whether the child exchanged mutual gazes with the adults in his vicinity. But I might want to make note of what the child was playing with, whether other people were present, and what they said to the child. On the other hand, if I were interested in the development of attachment, I would want to make note of mutual gazes as well as how close or far away from the parent the child might be standing or sitting.

It is also no simple matter to decide *where* we will observe. We can observe in a natural setting, such as a child's home or school, in which case we are introducing an enormous amount of variability into the system and increasing the complexity of the observation immensely. Or we can choose a controlled setting, keeping it the same for each child observed. For example, the most commonly used measure of the security of a child's attachment to an adult is obtained in what is called the Strange Situation: The child is observed in a series of episodes in a laboratory setting, including periods with the mother, with the mother and a stranger, alone with a stranger, and reunited with the mother. By standardizing the situation, we gain the enormous advantage of having comparable information for each child, but we may lose some ecological validity. We cannot be sure that what we observe in this strange laboratory is representative of the child's behavior in more accustomed settings.

Questionnaires and Interviews. Among researchers studying older children, questionnaires and interviews provide an excellent alternative to observation. They have been widely used in studies of children's moral development, for example (which you'll read about in Chapter 12), as well as in studies of peer relationships among elementary-school- and high-school-age children. Assessments of parent-child relationships are also often done with questionnaires.

Each of these alternatives has costs and benefits. Structured laboratory tests give the experimenter excellent control over the situation so that each subject is confronted with the same task, the same stimuli. But because they are artificial, such tests may not give us an accurate portrayal of how individuals behave in the more complex natural environment. Interviews, especially very open-ended ones in which the subject is only guided toward general topics, may give a rich picture of an individual's thoughts and feelings, but

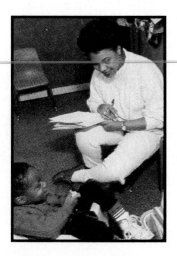

Careful observation of children in both natural and experimentally created settings has formed the backbone of our knowledge about early development.

Research Report

Ethical Issues in Research on Development

Anytime we try to understand human behavior by observing, testing, and asking questions, we are probing into personal lives. If we go into a home to observe the way the parents interact with their children, we are invading their privacy. We may even inadvertently give the impression that there must be something wrong with the way they are raising their family. If we give adults or children laboratory tests, some subjects will do very well, others will not. How will the less-successful subject interpret this experience? What is the risk that some subject will become depressed over what he perceives as a poor performance?

Any research on human behavior involves some risks and raises some ethical questions. Because of this, psychologists and other social and biological scientists have established clear procedures and guidelines that must be followed before any observation can be undertaken or any test given. In every university or college—the setting in which most such research is done—a committee of peers must approve any research plan involving human subjects. The most basic guideline is that subjects must always be protected from any potential mental or physical harm. More specific principles include:

Informed Consent. Each adult subject must give written consent to participate. When research involves children, informed consent must be obtained from the parent or guardian. In every case, the procedure and its possible consequences must be explained in detail. If there are potential risks, these must be described. For example, if you were studying patterns of communication between teenagers and their parents, you might want to observe each family while they talked about some unresolved issue between them. As part of your informed consent request, you would have to explain to each family that while such discussions often lead to greater clarity, they also occasionally increase tension. And you would need to provide support and debriefing at the end of the procedure, to assist any family who found the task stressful or destabilizing.

Right of Privacy. Subjects must be assured that highly personal information they may provide will be kept entirely private—including information about income, attitudes, or illegal behavior like drug taking. Researchers can use the information *collectively*, but they cannot report it individually in any way that will associate a subject's name with some piece of data—unless the subject has specifically given permission for such use.

In virtually all cases, it is also considered unethical to observe through a one-way mirror without the subject's knowledge or to secretly record behavior.

Testing Children. These principles are important for any research, but particularly so for research on children. Any child who balks at being tested or observed must *not* be tested or observed; any child who becomes distressed must be comforted; any risk to the child's self-esteem must be avoided.

how do you reduce the answers to a set of scores that will allow you to compare groups or individuals with one another? Questionnaires solve some of this problem, but the trade-off may be the richness and individuality of replies. Often the best strategy—although one not always possible because of cost in time or money—is to collect many different kinds of information from or about each subject.

Research Analysis

Finally, you need to analyze the results of your research. In studies of development, we see two broad forms of analysis.

First, we can compare different age groups by simply calculating the average score of each group on some measure, just as the Ontario researchers did in comparing rates of conduct disorders for each age or gender group in the results shown in Figure 1.4. You will see *many* examples of exactly this kind of analysis as you go through the book.

A second strategy allows us to look at relationships between two separate variables, most often using a statistic called a **correlation.** A correlation is simply a number ranging from –1.00 to +1.00 that describes the strength of a relationship between two variables. A zero correlation shows no linear relationship between those variables. For instance, you might expect to find a zero or near-zero correlation between the length of big toes and IQ. People with toes of all sizes have high IQs, and those with toes of all sizes have low IQs. The closer a correlation comes to –1.00 or +1.00, the stronger the relationship being described. If the correlation is positive, it indicates that high scores on the two dimensions tend to go together and that low scores tend to go together, such as length of big toes and shoe size. Height and weight are also strongly positively correlated, as are age and memory span.

If the correlation is negative, it describes a relationship in which high scores on one variable are associated with low scores on the other. For example, there is a negative correlation between the amount of disorder and chaos in a family and the child's later IQ: High chaos is associated with lower IQ, and low chaos with higher IQ.

Perfect correlations (–1.00 or +1.00) do not happen in the real world, but correlations of .80 or .70 do occur, and correlations of .50 are common in psychological research, indicating a relationship of moderate strength.

Correlations are an enormously useful descriptive tool. If you test or measure the same people several times over a period of time, a correlation can tell you how consistent or inconsistent their behavior is on some dimension, such as aggression. Or a correlation can describe links between two environmental variables or between the child's behavior and some experience he may have had. Useful as they are, though, correlations have a major limitation: They do not tell us about *causal* relationships. For example, several researchers have found a moderate positive correlation between the "difficultness" of a child's temperament and the amount of punishment the child receives from his parents: The more difficult the temperament, the more punishment the child experiences. But which way does the causality run? Do difficult children *elicit* more punishment? Or does a greater rate of punishment lead to a more difficult temperament? Or is there some third factor that may cause both, such as perhaps some genetic contribution both to the child's difficultness and to the parent's personality? The correlation alone does not allow us to choose among these alternatives. Stating the point more generally: No correlation, standing alone, can prove causality. A correlation may point in a particular direction or suggest possible causal links, but to discover the causes, we must explore such possibilities with other techniques, including experiments.

A Final Word

It may seem to you that these details about research design are of interest and value only to professional researchers. But that is not true. You will find that knowledge of this kind has many practical, daily applications, even if you never take another course in psychology. An example:

An issue of *Time* magazine several years ago included an article about a system for providing stimulation for the unborn baby. The pregnant woman is supposed to wear a belt full of audio equipment, on which tapes of various complex patterns of heartbeat sounds are played. The article reported that the maker of this gadget had done some "research" to demonstrate that this procedure produces smarter, faster-developing babies. To quote *Time:* "Last year 50 of the youngsters [whose mothers had worn the belt], ranging in age from six months to 34 months, were given standardized language, social and motor-skills tests. Their overall score was 25% above the national norm" (September 30, 1991, p. 76).

I hope you would not go out and buy this apparatus on the basis of that finding! After reading what I've said about research design, you should to be able to see immediately that self-selection is a major problem here. What kind of mothers will buy such a gadget? How are they likely to differ from mothers who would not buy it? In fact, this reported "research" tells us nothing. It isn't even a quasi experiment because there is no comparison group. Equivalent reports of research on children, on adolescents, on adults appear in the newspapers and popular magazines every day. Obviously, I want you to be critical analysts of the research I'll talk about in this book. But if nothing else, I want you to become very critical consumers of popularly presented research information. Some of it is very good. A lot of it is bunk, or at the very least inconclusive. I hope you are now in a better position to tell the difference.

Summary

1 To understand children's development, we must understand both change and consistency, both universality and individuality.

2 Both nature and nurture, biology and culture, are involved in all aspects of development, although there has been long-standing disagreement on the relative importance of these factors.

3 Current thinking about the nature side of the equation not only emphasizes the role of maturation but also points to potential inborn strategies of perceiving or responding to the environment.

4 Genetic differences also clearly play a significant role in a great many patterns of behavior.

5 Current thinking about the nurture side of the equation emphasizes not only the potential importance of the timing of some experience and the significance of a child's interpretation of some experience, but also the importance of examining the entire ecological system in which development occurs, including culture.

6 One important dimension along which cultures vary widely is individualism versus collectivism. Most Western cultures emphasize individualism, while Asian, Latin, and African cultures are more likely to emphasize collectivism.

7 Nature and nurture may not interact in precisely the same way for each child. Children with different inborn qualities (vulnerability or resilience) may be affected differently by the same environment.

8 Another key question concerns the nature of developmental change itself, whether it is qualitative or quantitative, continuous or stagelike.

9 Four families of theories represent different combinations of positions on these issues: biological, learning, psychoanalytic, and cognitive-developmental.

10 Biological theorists, such as Gesell or behavior geneticists, generally assume that the most significant influences on development are internal (nature) and that developmental change is primarily quantitative.

11 Learning theorists generally place strongest emphasis on environmental influences, thought to produce largely quantitative change. Bandura's influential version of learning theory includes more cognitive elements and the crucial concept of modeling.

12 Psychoanalytic theorists such as Freud and Erikson have primarily studied the development of personality, emphasizing the interaction of internal instincts and environmental influences in producing

shared stages of development as well as individual differences in personality.

13 Cognitive-developmental theorists such as Piaget and his many followers emphasize the child's own active exploration of the environment as a critical ingredient leading to shared stages of development. They strongly emphasize qualitative change.

14 A first major question in planning research is the basic research design. Cross-sectional studies compare different children of different ages; longitudinal studies observe the same children as they develop over time; sequential studies combine some of these features; and cross-cultural studies compare children, their rearing, or nature/nurture relationships in differing cultures or subcultures.

15 Each of these designs has particular strengths and drawbacks.

16 To study causal connections, researchers normally use experimental designs. In an experiment, the researcher controls (manipulates) one or more relevant variables and assigns subjects randomly to different treatment and control groups.

17 In a quasi experiment, subjects are not randomly assigned to separate groups; rather, existing groups are compared. Quasi experiments are needed in developmental research because subjects cannot be randomly assigned either to age groups or to experience such negative treatments as poverty or abuse or poor attachment.

18 Decisions about research methods include the choice of subjects to be studied and the methods to be used to observe or assess them.

19 When research results are analyzed, the two most common methods are comparing average scores between groups and describing relationships among variables with the statistic called a correlation. It can range from +1.00 to −1.00 and describes the strength of the relationship.

Key Terms

behavior genetics (p. 4)

classical conditioning (p. 17)

cohort (p. 25)

collectivism (p. 12)

conditioned stimulus (p. 18)

control group (p. 28)

correlation (p. 32)

critical period (p. 8)

cross-cultural research (p. 25)

cross-sectional design (p. 24)

culture (p. 11)

dependent variable (p. 28)

ego (p. 20)

ethnography (p. 27)

experiment (p. 27)

experimental group (p. 28)

id (p. 20)

independent variable (p. 28)

individualism (p. 12)

intrinsic reinforcements (p. 19)

libido (p. 20)

longitudinal design (p. 24)

maturation (p. 4)

modeling (p. 19)

negative reinforcement (p. 18)

observational learning (p. 19)

operant conditioning (p. 18)

partial reinforcement (p. 19)

positive reinforcement (p. 18)

psychosocial stages (p. 21)

punishment (p. 18)

sensitive period (p. 9)

sequential design (p. 24)

superego (p. 20)

teratogen (p. 9)

unconditioned response (p. 17)

unconditioned stimulus (p. 17)

Suggested Readings

Bornstein, M. H. (Ed.). (1987). *Sensitive periods in development. Interdisciplinary perspectives.* Hillsdale, NJ: Erlbaum.

Bornstein's own paper in this collection of reports is an excellent introduction to the concept of sensitive periods, but the book also contains a number of reports of research exploring potential sensitive periods both in humans and in other animals.

Cole, M. (1992). Culture in development. In M. H. Bornstein & M. E. Lamb (Eds.), *Developmental psychology: An advanced textbook* (3rd ed.) (pp. 731–738). Hillsdale, NJ: Erlbaum.

Not at all easy reading, but one of the best analyses I have yet seen on this very complicated subject.

Greenfield, P. M., & Cocking, R. R. (Eds.). (1994). *Cross-cultural roots of minority child development.* Hillsdale, NJ: Erlbaum.

One of the central themes in this excellent collection of papers is the impact of individualism and collectivism on the lives of children in different cultural contexts.

Plomin, R., & McClearn, G. E. (Eds.). (1993). *Nature, nurture & psychology.* Washington, DC: American Psychological Association.

If you think the "great debate" about nature and nurture is an old issue, this book will quickly persuade you otherwise. The controversy is alive and well, although the papers in this book reflect the efforts of many people to recast it in more useful terms.

Rowe, D. C. (1994). *The limits of family influence: Genes, experience, and behavior.* New York: Guilford Press.

A clear, well-reasoned book arguing that developmental psychologists have greatly exaggerated the effects of "nurture" on personality, intelligence, and other characteristics and greatly underestimated the effects of heredity. This is another good introduction to some current thinking on the nature/nurture controversy.

Seitz, V. (1988). Methodology. In M. H. Bornstein & M. E. Lamb (Eds.), *Developmental psychology: An advanced textbook* (2nd ed.). Hillsdale, NJ: Erlbaum.

A very good source for a further exploration of various methods of research. Well organized and clearly written.

Thomas, R. M. (Ed.). (1990). *The encyclopedia of human development and education. Theory, research, and studies.* Oxford: Pergamon Press.

This is a very useful volume. It includes brief descriptions of virtually all the theories I have described in this chapter as well as a helpful chapter on the concept of stages. Each chapter is quite brief but covers many of the critical issues.

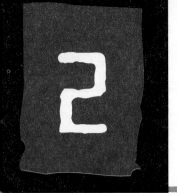

Prenatal Development

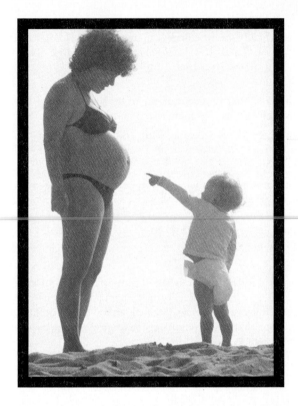

At a family gathering a decade or so ago, my then four-months-pregnant sister-in-law Nancy complained of a headache. Having heard warnings about the possible ill effects of various kinds of drugs during pregnancy, she was very reluctant to take any aspirin. We tried all the usual home remedies (shoulder rubs, warm baths, herb tea), but the headache persisted. Finally, she took a nonaspirin pain medicine, which did the trick.

This incident brought home to me very clearly just how sensitized most women are today to the various hazards (*teratogens*) during pregnancy, including drugs. I was impressed by Nancy's determination to avoid doing anything harmful. Even more, I was struck by how long the list of "don'ts" had become and how hard it is for a conscientious woman to be sure of what is okay and what is not.

So what do we now know? What does the list of dos and don'ts look like today? It's an important practical question for any of you who plan to be parents, and to answer it I need to explore what we know about the basic processes of development from conception to birth, as well as what we have learned about what can interfere with those basic processes. And of course beyond this practical issue, it is also essential for any complete understanding of child development that we begin our search at the beginning—at conception and pregnancy.

Conception

The first step in the development of a single human being is that moment of conception when a single sperm cell from the male pierces the wall of the ovum of the female—a moment captured in the photo in Figure 2.1. Ordinarily, a woman produces one **ovum** (egg cell) per month from one of her two ovaries. This occurs roughly midway between two menstrual periods. If it is not fertilized, the ovum travels from the ovary down the **fallopian tube** toward the **uterus,** where it gradually disintegrates and is expelled as part of the next menstruation.

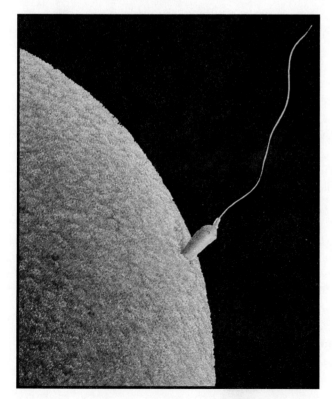

FIGURE 2.1 The moment of conception when a single sperm has pierced the shell of the ovum.

But if a couple has intercourse during the crucial few days when the ovum is in the fallopian tube, one of the millions of sperm ejaculated as part of each male orgasm may travel the full distance through the woman's vagina, cervix, uterus, and fallopian tube, and penetrate the wall of the ovum. A child is conceived. The now fertilized ovum then continues on its journey down the fallopian tube, where instead of disintegrating, it implants itself in the wall of the uterus. Interestingly (and perhaps surprisingly to you), only about half of such "conceptuses" are likely to survive to birth, and such survival is rarer for male conceptuses than for female. About a quarter are lost in the first few days after conception, often because of a flaw in the genetic material. Typically, these women do not even know that they are pregnant. Another quarter are spontaneously aborted ("miscarried") at a later point in the pregnancy (Wilcox et al., 1988).

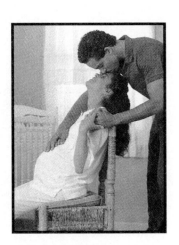

Most parents find the nine months of a pregnancy to be a time of delighted anticipation. It is also a time in which the genetic patterning for the child (the genotype) is established and in which complex maturational sequences unfold.

The Basic Genetics of Conception

It is hard to overstate the importance of the genetic events accompanying conception. The combination of genes from the father in the sperm and from the mother in the ovum creates a unique genetic blueprint—the **genotype**—that characterizes each individual. To understand how that occurs, I need to back up a few steps.

The nucleus of each cell of our bodies contains a set of 46 **chromosomes** arranged in 23 pairs. These chromosomes include all the necessary genetic information, including not only genetic information that controls highly individual characteristics like hair color, height, body shape, temperament, and aspects of intelligence, but also all those characteristics shared by all members of our species, such as patterns of physical development or "built-in biases" of various kinds.

The only cells that do *not* contain 46 chromosomes are the sperm and the ovum, collectively called **gametes** or germ cells. In the early stages of development, gametes divide as do all other cells (a process called *mitosis*), with each set of 23 chromosome pairs "unzipping" and duplicating itself. But in gametes there is a final step, called *meiosis,* in which each new cell receives only one chromosome from each original pair. Thus, each gamete has only 23 chromosomes, instead of 23 *pairs.* When a child is conceived, the 23 chromosomes in the ovum and the 23 in the sperm combine to form the 23 *pairs* that will be part of each cell in the newly developing body.

The chromosomes, in turn, are composed of long strings of molecules of a chemical called **deoxyribonucleic acid** (DNA). In an insight for which they won the Nobel Prize, James Watson and Francis Crick (1953) deduced that DNA is in the shape of a *double helix,* a kind of twisted ladder. The remarkable feature of this ladder is that the rungs are made up in such a way that the whole thing can "unzip" and then each half can guide the duplication of the missing part, thus allowing multiplication of cells, so that each new cell contains the full set of genetic information.

The string of DNA that makes up each chromosome can be further subdivided into segments, called **genes,** each of which controls or influences a particular feature or a portion of some developmental pattern. A gene controlling some specific characteristic, such as your blood type or your hair color, always appears in the same place (the *locus*) on the same chromosome in every individual of the same species. The locus of the gene that determines whether you have type A, B, or O blood is on chromosome 9; the locus of the gene that determines whether you have the Rh factor in your blood is on chromosome 1;

and so forth. Geneticists have made remarkable strides in recent years in mapping the loci for a great many features or characteristics—a scientific achievement that has allowed similarly giant strides in our ability to diagnose various genetic defects or inherited diseases before a child is born.

Dominant and Recessive Genes

Because each individual inherits *two* of each chromosome (one from each parent), the genetic instructions at any given locus may be either the same (*homozygous*) or contradictory (*heterozygous*). If you receive a gene for blue eyes from both parents, your inheritance is homozygous and you will have blue eyes. But what if you receive heterozygous information, such as a gene for blue eyes from one parent and a gene for brown eyes from the other?

Heterozygosity is resolved in several different ways, depending on the particular genes involved. Sometimes the two signals appear to blend, resulting in some intermediate characteristic. For example, the children of one tall parent and one short parent generally have height that falls in between. A rarer outcome is that the child expresses *both* characteristics. For example, type AB blood results from the inheritance of a type A gene from one parent and a type B gene from the other. The most common outcome of heterozygosity, however, is that one of the two genes is *dominant* over the other, and only the dominant gene is actually expressed. The "weaker" gene, called a *recessive* gene, continues to be part of the genotype and can be passed on to the individual's offspring through meiosis, but it has no effect on the individual's visible characteristics or behavior.

A large number of specific diseases appear to be transmitted through the operation of dominant and recessive genes, such as Tay-Sachs disease, sickle-cell anemia, and cystic fibrosis. Figure 2.2 shows how this might work in the case of sickle-cell anemia, which is caused by a *recessive* gene. For an individual to have this disease, she or he must inherit the disease gene from *both* parents. A "carrier" is someone who inherits the disease gene from only one parent. Such a person does not actually have the disease but can pass the disease gene on to his or her children. If two carriers have children together (example 3 in the figure) or if a carrier and someone with the disease have children (example 4 in the figure), their offspring may inherit disease genes from both parents and thus have the disease.

Unlike this simple example, most human characteristics are affected by many more than one gene. Temperament, intelligence, rate of growth, even apparently simple characteristics such as eye color, all involve the interaction of multiple genes. Very exciting new genetic research has also pointed toward totally unexpected additional complexities. For example, researchers studying muscular dystrophy, a recessive gene disease, have observed that this disease often becomes more severe from one generation to the next, apparently through some kind of multiplication of the DNA in the section of the chromosome that signals the disease (Fu et al., 1992). Other genetic researchers have discovered that, contrary to the long-accepted theory, the outcome may be different if a particular gene comes from the mother rather than from the father, even though the genes appear to signal precisely the same genotypic characteristic (McBride, 1991; Rogers, 1991). Research like this is beginning to unlock the secrets of genetic transmission, but our understanding is still far from complete.

In the inheritance of eye color, brown is dominant over blue. Can you figure out what your parents' genotype for eye color has to be, based on the color of your eyes, your siblings' eyes, and that of your grandparents? What is your *own* eye color genotype likely to be?

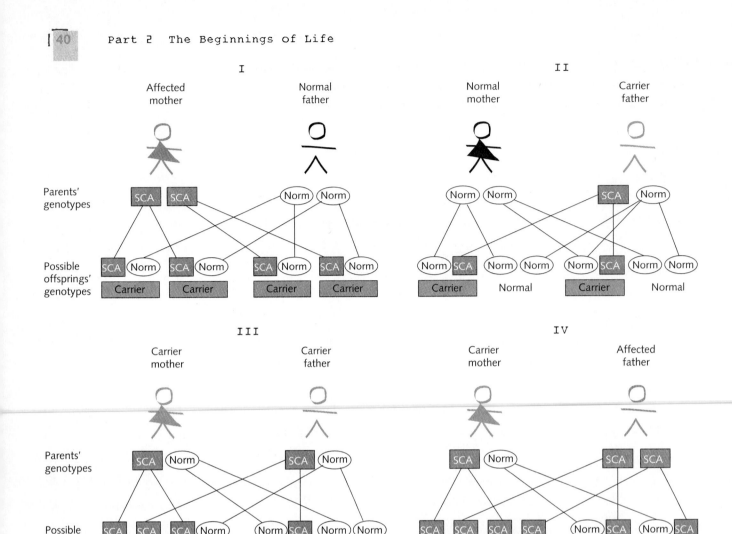

FIGURE 2.2 Some examples of how a recessive gene disease, like sickle-cell anemia, is transmitted. In section I, a mother who has the disease passes her sickle-cell disease gene to all her children, but since her partner is normal, the children are all carriers and do not actually express the disease. In section II, a normal mother and a carrier father have no children with the disease, but each of their children has a 50/50 chance of inheriting the SCA gene from the carrier mother. The child can inherit the actual disease either of three ways: with two carrier parents (section III), with one carrier parent and one affected parent (section IV), or with two affected parents (not shown in the figure).

Males and Females

Still another complexity comes from the fact that there are actually two types of chromosomes. In 22 of the pairs, called **autosomes,** the members of the pair look alike and contain exactly matching genetic loci. The twenty-third pair, however, operates differently. The chromosomes of this pair, which determine the child's gender and are therefore called the **sex chromosomes,** come in two types, referred to by convention as the X and the Y chromosomes. A normal human female has two X chromosomes on this twenty-third pair (an XX pattern), while the normal human male has one X and one Y (an XY pattern). The X chromosome is considerably larger than the Y and contains many genetic loci not matched on the Y.

Note that the sex of the child is determined by the X or Y chromosome from the sperm. Since the mother has *only* X chromosomes, every ovum carries an X. But the father has both X and Y chromosomes. When the father's gametes divide, some sperm will carry an X, some a Y. If the sperm that fertilizes the ovum carries an X, then the child inherits an XX pattern and will be a girl. If the fertilizing sperm carries a Y, then the combination is XY and the infant will be a boy.

Geneticists have pushed this understanding a step further, discovering that only one very small section of the Y chromosome actually determines maleness—a segment referred to as *TDF, or testis-determining factor* (Page et al., 1987). Fertilized ova that are genetically XY but that lack the TDF develop physically as female. This finding is one of many that led geneticists to conclude that the fetus is inherently female. To put it another way, the female form has been seen as the "default option" in prenatal development. According to this argument, femaleness is a kind of passive process, occurring in the absence of any specific signal, while maleness requires the additional genetic signal of TDF. But very recent work calls this widely accepted description into question. A number of scientists (Arn et al., 1994; Bardoni et al., 1994) have found indications that a "femaleness" gene may also exist, or perhaps a whole collection of genes required to stimulate the appropriate development of female genitalia and internal reproductive organs. As in so many areas of science, the more we discover, the more complex we see the process really is.

Incidentally, the mother does have some indirect effect on the likelihood of an XX or an XY conception because the relative acidity or alkalinity of the mucus in the vagina affects the survival rate of X-carrying or Y-carrying sperm. This chemical balance varies both from one woman to the next and during the course of each woman's monthly cycle. So a woman's typical chemical balance or the timing of intercourse can sharply alter the probability of conceiving a child of a particular gender, even though it is still true that the X or Y in the sperm is the final determining factor.

One important consequence of the difference between X and Y chromosomes is that a boy inherits many genes from his mother on his X chromosome that are not matched or counteracted by equivalent genetic material on the Y chromosome. Among other things, this means that recessive diseases or other recessive characteristics that have their loci on the nonmatched parts of the X chromosome may be inherited by a boy directly from his mother, a pattern called *sex-linked* transmission, illustrated in Figure 2.3 with the disease hemophilia.

You can see that for females, sex-linked recessive genes operate just as they do in other recessive diseases: The girl will have the characteristic only if she inherits the recessive gene from both parents. But a male will inherit the characteristic by receiving the recessive gene only from his mother. Since his Y chromosome from his father contains no parallel loci for these characteristics, the boy has no counteracting instructions and the mother's recessive gene causes the disorder or other characteristic. For sex-linked characteristics like muscular dystrophy or hemophilia, half the sons of women who carry the recessive disease gene will have the disease, and half the daughters will be carriers of the gene. These daughters, in turn, will pass the disease on to half their sons.

Twins and Siblings

In the great majority of cases, babies are conceived and born one at a time. But multiple births occur roughly once in 100 cases. The most common type of multiple birth is *fraternal twins,* when more than one ovum has been produced and both have been fertilized, each by a separate sperm. Such twins, also called *dizygotic* twins, are no more alike genet-

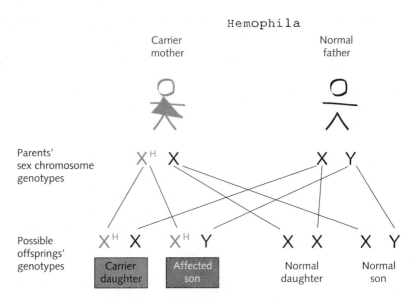

FIGURE 2.3 Compare the pattern of sex-linked transmission of a recessive disease with the patterns already shown in Figure 2.2. In the inheritance of a sex-linked disease such as hemophilia, a carrier mother will, on average, pass on the disease to half her sons because there is no offsetting gene on the Y chromosome. But a daughter of a carrier mother will not inherit the disease itself unless her father has it.

ically than any other pair of siblings and need not even be of the same sex. In rarer cases, a single fertilized ovum may divide and each half may develop into a separate individual. These are *identical* or *monozygotic* twins and have identical genetic heritages because they come from precisely the same original fertilized ovum. You'll remember from Chapter 1 that comparisons of the degree of similarity of these two types of twins is one of the two major research strategies in the important field of behavior genetics.

Genotypes and Phenotypes

Using such strategies, behavior geneticists have made great strides in identifying those skills, characteristics, or traits that are influenced by heredity. But no geneticist proposes that an inherited combination of genes fully *determines* any outcome for a given individual. Geneticists (and psychologists) make an important distinction between the genotype, which is the specific set of "instructions" contained in a given individual's genes, and the **phenotype,** which is the actual observed characteristics of the individual. The phenotype is a product of three things: the genotype, all the environmental influences from the time of conception onward, and the interaction between the environment and the genotype. A child might have a genotype associated with high IQ, but if his mother drinks too much alcohol during pregnancy the fetal nervous system may be damaged, resulting in mild retardation. Another child may have a genotype for a "difficult" temperament but have parents who are particularly sensitive and thoughtful, so that the child learns other ways to handle herself.

This distinction between the genotype and the phenotype is crucial. Genetic codes are not irrevocable signals for this or that pattern of development or this or that disease. The eventual developmental outcome is also affected by the specific experiences the individual may have from conception onward.

Can you think of other examples where the phenotype would be different from the genotype?

Development from Conception to Birth

If we assume that conception takes place two weeks after a menstrual period, when ovulation normally occurs, then the period of gestation of the human infant is 38 weeks (about 265 days). Most physicians calculate gestation as 40 weeks, counting from the last menstrual period. However, all the specifications of weeks of gestation I've given here are based on the 38-week calculation, counting from the presumed time of conception.

These 38 weeks have been subdivided in several different ways. Physicians typically talk in terms of three equal three-month periods, called *trimesters*. In contrast, biologists and embryologists typically divide the weeks of gestation into three unequal subperiods, linked to specific changes within the developing organism. These stages are the *germinal,* which lasts roughly 2 weeks; the *embryonic,* which continues until about 8 to 12 weeks after conception; and the *fetal,* which makes up the remaining 26 to 30 weeks.

The Germinal Stage: From Conception to Implantation

Some time during the first 24 to 36 hours after conception, cell division begins; within two to three days there are several dozen cells and the whole mass is about the size of a pinhead. This initial mass of cells is undifferentiated until about four days after conception. At that point the organism, now called a *blastocyst,* begins to subdivide. A cavity begins to appear within the ball of cells, and the mass divides into two parts. The outer cells will form the various structures that will support the developing organism, while the inner mass will form the **embryo** itself. When it touches the wall of the uterus, the outer shell of cells in the blastocyst breaks down at the point of contact. Small tendrils develop and attach the cell mass to the uterine wall, a process called *implantation.* When implantation occurs, normally 10 days to 2 weeks after conception, the blastocyst has perhaps 150 cells (Tanner, 1978). You can see this whole sequence schematically in Figure 2.4.

The Embryonic Stage

The embryonic stage begins when implantation is complete and continues until the various support structures are fully formed and all the major organ systems have been laid down in at least rudimentary form, a process that normally takes another 6 to 10 weeks.

Development of Support Structures. Two of the key support structures that develop out of the outer layer of cells are the **amnion,** which is the sac or bag, filled with liquid (amniotic fluid), in which the baby floats, and that marvelous organ, the **placenta,** a platelike mass of cells that lies against the wall of the uterus. The placenta is fully developed by about four weeks after conception and serves as liver, lungs, and kidneys for the embryo and fetus. The embryo's circulatory system is connected to the placenta through a third support structure, the *umbilical cord.* Thus, the placenta lies between the mother's

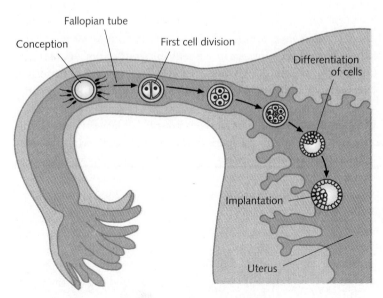

FIGURE 2.4 This schematic shows the normal progression of development for the first 10 days of gestation, from conception to implantation.

Fallopian tube

Conception

First cell division

Differentiation of cells

Implantation

Uterus

FIGURE 2.5 You can see here how the various structures are organized during the fetal period. Note especially the placenta and the umbilical cord, and the fact that the fetus floats in the amniotic fluid.

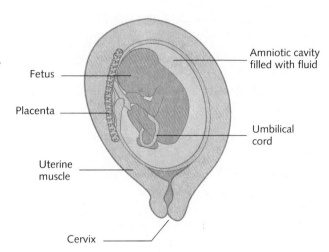

circulatory system and the embryo's, and can serve as a sort of filter. Nutrients such as oxygen, proteins, sugars, and vitamins from the maternal blood can pass through the placental filter, while digestive wastes and carbon dioxide from the infant's blood pass back through to the mother, whose own body can eliminate them (Rosenblith, 1992). At the same time, many (but not all) harmful substances, such as viruses the mother may carry, are filtered out because they are too large to pass through the various membranes in the placenta. The same is true of most of the mother's hormones. Most drugs and anesthetics, however, do pass through the placental barrier, as do some disease organisms. You can see all these separate structures in Figure 2.5.

Development of the Embryo. While these support structures are developing, the mass of cells that will form the embryo is itself differentiating further into several types of cells that form the rudiments of skin, sense receptors, nerve cells, muscles, circulatory system, and internal organs. Such differentiation is remarkably swift. By the eighth week of gestation, the embryo is roughly 1½ inches long and has a heart that beats, a primitive circulatory system, the beginnings of eyes and ears, a mouth that opens and closes, legs, arms, and a primitive spinal cord. When this *organogenesis* is complete, a new stage, that of the **fetus,** begins.

The Fetal Stage

The seven months of the fetal stage involve primarily a process of refining all the primitive organ systems already in place, much like what happens in constructing a house: The framework is created quickly, but the finishing work is lengthy. You can get some feeling for the rapidity of the changes by looking at Table 2.1, which lists some of the milestones of fetal development.

Development of the Nervous System. The nervous system is one of the least-well-developed elements at the end of the embryonic period. It is composed of two basic types of cells, **neurons** and **glial cells.** The glial cells are the glue that holds the whole system together, providing firmness and structure to the brain, helping to remove debris after neuronal death or injury, and segregating neurons from one another. The neurons do the job of receiving and sending messages from one part of the brain to another or from one part of the body to another.

Neurons have four main parts, which you can see in the drawing in Figure 2.6 (p. 46): (1) a cell body; (2) branchlike extensions of the cell body called **dendrites,** which are the major *receptors* of nerve impulses; (3) a tubular extension of the cell body called the **axon,**

Table 2.1
Major Milestones of Fetal Development

Gestational Age	Major New Developments
12 weeks	Sex of child can be determined; muscles are developed more extensively; eyelids and lips are present; feet have toes and hands have fingers.
16 weeks	First fetal movement is usually felt by the mother at about this time; bones begin to develop; fairly complete ear is formed.
20 weeks	Hair growth begins; fetus is very human looking at this age, and thumb-sucking may be seen.
24 weeks	Eyes are completely formed (but closed); fingernails, sweat glands, and taste buds are all formed; some fat deposit beneath skin. The fetus is capable of breathing if born prematurely at this stage, but survival rate is still low for those born this small.
28 weeks	Nervous system, blood, and breathing systems are all well enough developed to support life, although prematures born at this stage have poor sleep/wake cycles and irregular breathing.
29–40 weeks	Interconnections between individual nerve cells (neurons) develop rapidly; weight is added; general "finishing" of body systems takes place.

which can extend as far as 1 meter in humans (about 3 feet); and (4) terminal fibers at the end of the axon, which form the primary *transmitting* apparatus of the nervous system. Because of the branchlike appearance of dendrites, physiologists describe these structures in a language intriguingly reminiscent of botany, speaking of the "dendritic arbor" or of "pruning" of the arbor.

The point at which two neurons connect, either where dendrites from two neurons come into contact or where the axon's transmitting fibers come into close contact with another neuron's dendrites, is called a **synapse.** The communication at the synapse is accomplished with chemical *neurotransmitters.* The number of such synapses in a single human is vast. One cell in the part of the brain that controls vision, for instance, may have as many as 10,000 to 30,000 synaptic inputs to its dendrites (Greenough, Black, & Wallace, 1987).

Glial cells begin to develop at about 13 weeks after conception and continue to be added until perhaps two years after birth. The great majority of neurons are apparently formed between 5 and 18 weeks of gestation (Huttenlocher, 1994; Todd et al., 1995), and—with rare exceptions—these are all the neurons the individual will ever have. Neurons lost later are not replaced.

In these early weeks of the fetal period, neurons are very simple. They consist largely of the cell body with short axons and little dendritic development. It is in the last two months before birth and in the first few years after birth that the lengthening of the axons and the major growth of the "dendritic arbor" occurs. Indeed, as the dendrites first develop in the eighth and ninth months of gestation, they appear to be sent out in a kind of exploratory system; many of these early dendrites are later reabsorbed, with only the useful expansions remaining. In these final fetal months, however, synapse formation is

Can you think of any practical consequences of the fact that all the neurons one is ever going to have are present by about 20 weeks of gestation?

FIGURE 2.6 The structure of a single developed neuron. The cell bodies are the first to be developed, primarily between 10 and 20 weeks of gestation. Axons and dendrites begin to develop in the last two months of gestation and continue to increase in size and complexity for several years after birth.

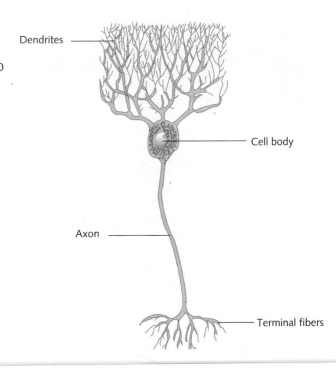

Dendrites

Cell body

Axon

Terminal fibers

much slower; most synapses are formed after birth. For example, in the part of the brain involved in vision, babies have about ten times the number of synapses at 6 months as they had at birth (Huttenlocher, 1994).

Development of Length and Weight. Similarly, the major growth in fetal size occurs late in the fetal period, with the gain in length occurring earlier than the major gain in weight. The fetus is about half her birth length by about 20 weeks gestation, but she does not reach half her birth weight until nearly three months later, at about 32 weeks.

An Overview of Prenatal Development

One of the most important points about prenatal development is how remarkably regular and predictable it is. If the embryo has survived the early, risky period, development usually proceeds smoothly, with the various changes occurring in what is apparently a fixed order, at fixed time intervals. Maturation seems clearly at work. The fetus doesn't learn to grow fingernails, nor does it have to be stimulated from the outside to grow them. The eyes, the ears, the internal organs, the nervous system are all apparently controlled in some fashion by the developmental codes contained in the genes.

However, this sequence of development is not immune to modification or outside influence, as you'll soon see in detail. Indeed, as psychologists and biologists have looked more carefully at various kinds of teratogens, it has become clear that the sequence is more vulnerable than had earlier appeared. But before I begin talking about the various things that can go wrong, I want to make sure to state clearly that the maturational system is really quite robust. Normal prenatal development requires an adequate environment, but "adequate" seems to be a fairly broad range. *Most* children are quite normal. The list of things that can go wrong is long and getting longer as our knowledge expands. Yet many of these possibilities are quite rare, many are partially or wholly preventable, and many need not have permanent consequences for the child. Keep this in mind as you read through the next few pages.

The potential problems can be grouped into two classes: genetic errors and those damaging environmental events called teratogens. Genetic errors occur at the moment of conception and cannot be altered. Teratogens may affect development at any time from conception onward.

Genetic Errors

In perhaps 3 to 8 percent of all fertilized ova, the genetic material itself contains errors because either the sperm or the ovum has failed to divide correctly, so that there are either too many or too few chromosomes. Current estimates are that perhaps 90 percent of these abnormal conceptuses are spontaneously aborted. Only about 1 percent of live newborns have such abnormalities.

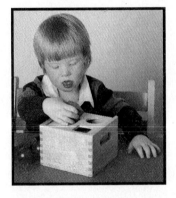

Note the distinctive facial characteristics of this Down syndrome child.

More than 50 different types of chromosomal anomaly have been identified, many of them very rare. The most common is **Down syndrome** (also called *mongolism* and *trisomy 21*), in which the child, because of a failure of proper meiosis in either sperm or ovum, has three copies of chromosome 21 rather than the normal two. Other forms of trisomy also occur, of course, but Down syndrome is by far the most frequent. Estimates of the incidence of this abnormality differ, but the frequency is somewhere between 1 in 600 and 1 in 1000 (Nightingale & Goodman, 1990). These children have distinctive facial features (as you can see in the photo) and are typically retarded.

The risk of bearing a child with this deviant pattern is greatest for mothers over 35. Among women ages 35 to 39, the incidence of Down syndrome is about 1 in 280 births; among 40-year-olds it is roughly 1 in 100; and for mothers age 45 it is 1 in 30 births (D'Alton & DeCherney, 1993). Research by epidemiologists also suggests a link between exposure to environmental toxins of various kinds and the risk of having an offspring with Down syndrome. For example, one large study in Canada shows that men who work as mechanics, farm laborers, or sawmill workers, all of whom are regularly exposed to solvents, oils, lead, and pesticides, are at higher risk for fathering Down syndrome children than are men who work in cleaner environments (Olshan, Baird, & Teschke, 1989). Findings like these suggest that chromosomal anomalies may not be purely random events but may themselves be a response to various teratogens.

Sex-Chromosome Anomalies

A second class of anomalies is associated with an incomplete or incorrect division of either sex chromosome, which occurs in roughly 1 out of every 400 births (Berch & Bender, 1987). As a general rule, children with sex-chromosome anomalies are not as severely affected as what we see in Down syndrome, but they do show unusual physical features and some cognitive deficits.

The most common sex-chromosome anomaly is an XXY pattern, called Klinefelter's syndrome, which occurs in roughly 1 or 2 out of every 1000 males. Affected boys most often look quite normal, although they have underdeveloped testes and, as adults, a scarcity of sperm. Most are not mentally retarded, but language and learning disabilities are common.

Not quite as common is the XYY pattern. These children also develop as boys, are typically unusually tall, and have mild retardation. A single-X pattern (XO), called Turner's syndrome, and a triple-X pattern (XXX) may also occur, and in both cases the child develops as a girl. Girls with Turner's syndrome are exceptions to the usual rule that embryos with too few chromosomes do not survive. These girls show stunted growth and are usually sterile. Without hormone therapy, they do not menstruate or develop breasts at puberty. These girls also show an interesting imbalance in their cognitive skills; they of-

The Real World
Prenatal Diagnosis of Genetic Errors

Not so many years ago children were born with whatever deformities, diseases, or anomalies happened to come along. The parents had no choices. Today, parents have access to many types of genetic information and tests to detect fetal abnormalities, which increase choice but may also create difficult decisions.

Prepregnancy Genetic Testing. Prepregnancy blood tests can tell you and your spouse whether you are carriers of genes for those diseases for which the loci are known, such as Tay-Sachs or sickle-cell anemia. This may be an important step if you and your spouse belong to a subgroup known to be likely to carry particular recessive genes.

Prenatal Diagnosis of the Fetus. Four prenatal diagnostic strategies are now available to test the embryo or fetus to see if the developing child has any abnormality. Two of these, the **alpha-fetoprotein test** (AFP) and ultrasound, are primarily used to detect problems in the formation of the *neural tube,* the structure that becomes the brain and spinal cord. If the tube fails to close at the bottom end, a disability called *spina bifida* occurs. Children with this defect are often partially paralyzed, and many (but not all) are retarded.

Alpha-fetoprotein is a substance produced by the fetus and detectable in the mother's blood. If the blood test, normally done between 16 and 18 weeks of gestation, shows an abnormally high AFP level, it suggests that there may be some problem with the spinal cord or brain. It does not mean a problem definitely exists; it means there is a higher *risk* of problems and further tests are indicated.

One such further test is **ultrasound,** which involves the use of sound waves to provide an actual "moving picture" of the fetus. With this method it is frequently possible to detect, or rule out, neural tube defects or other physical abnormalities. The procedure is not painful and gives parents an often delightful chance to see their unborn child moving, but it cannot provide information about the presence of chromosomal anomalies or inherited diseases.

If you want the latter information, you have two choices: **amniocentesis** or **chorionic villus sampling**

(CVS). In both cases, a needle is inserted and cells are taken from the developing embryo. In CVS, the sample is taken from cells in the membrane surrounding the embryo, called the chorion; in amniocentesis, the sample is from the amniotic fluid. Of the two, amniocentesis was developed earlier and is the more widely used. Its major drawback is that the amniotic sac must be large enough to allow a sample of fluid to be taken with very little danger to the fetus, so the test cannot be done until the sixteenth week of gestation and the results are not typically available for several more weeks. If the test reveals an abnormality and the parents decide to abort, it is quite late for an abortion to be performed. CVS, in contrast, is normally done between the ninth and eleventh weeks of gestation.

Neither of these procedures is without risk. Both procedures sometimes cause miscarriages (CVS at a slightly higher rate), and there has been a recent flurry of concern about *possible* links between CVS and slight increases in limb defects in the infant (Report of National Institute, 1993). Because of these risks, both procedures are recommended only for women known to be at high risk, such as those older than 35 or those who have borne a previous child with defects or chromosomal anomaly.

By the time you are facing this choice, there may be still newer and safer options using maternal blood samples; for example, researchers have reported that they can identify 89 percent of Down syndrome fetuses with a combination of three blood tests, including an alpha-fetoprotein test (Haddow et al., 1994). But no matter what technique you may select, the moral and ethical choices you may be called upon to make are far from easy.

For example, consider the case of diseases that can occur in mild or moderate as well as severe forms, such as sickle-cell anemia. Prenatal tests can tell you if the child will inherit the disease, but they cannot tell you how severely the child will be affected. Genetic counselors may play a very helpful role, but ultimately each couple has to make its own decisions.

ten perform particularly poorly on tests that measure spatial ability but perform at or above normal levels on tests of verbal skill (Golombok & Fivush, 1994). Girls with an XXX pattern are of normal size but are slower than normal in physical development. In contrast to Turner's syndrome girls, they have markedly *poor* verbal abilities (Rovet & Netley, 1983). We obviously have much to learn about why numbers and combinations of sex chromosomes would have such varying effects on cognitive abilities.

Fragile-X Syndrome

A quite different type of genetic anomaly, occurring in about one out of every 1250 males (Rose, 1995), involves not an improper number of chromosomes, but an abnormal section of DNA at a specific location on the X chromosome (Dykens, Hodapp, & Leckman, 1994) and is referred to as a "fragile X." This is an *inherited* disorder, following the sex-linked inheritance pattern illustrated earlier in Figure 2.3. Thus, both boys and girls may inherit a fragile X (ordinarily from a carrier mother), but boys, lacking the potentially overriding influence of a normal X, are much more susceptible to the negative intellectual or behavioral consequences. The affected child appears to have a considerably heightened risk of mental retardation; current estimates are that among males, 5 to 7 percent of all retardation is caused by this syndrome (Zigler & Hodapp, 1991).

Single-Gene Defects

As I have already indicated, problems can also occur at conception if the child inherits a gene for a specific disease. In a few cases, such diseases may be caused by a dominant gene. The best-known example is Huntington's disease, a severe neurological disorder resulting in rapid loss of both mental and physical functioning, with symptoms usually appearing only at midlife. Dominant-gene diseases are relatively rare because the affected parent would almost always know that he or she was suffering from the disorder and would be unable or unwilling to reproduce. (An exception to this general statement is Huntington's disease, because the affected individual does not show symptoms until midlife, typically well after the childbearing years.)

A diagnostic test for the presence of the gene for Huntington's disease is now available. If you came from a family in which this disease was present, would you want to be tested, so that you would know whether you would later develop the disease? Think about it carefully; the answer isn't as straightforward as it first seems.

Far more common are *recessive*-gene diseases, some of which I've listed in Table 2.2. The few examples listed in the table do not begin to convey the diversity of such disorders. Among known causes of mental retardation, for example, are 141 diseases or disorders with known genetic loci and 361 more whose loci have not yet been identified (Wahlström, 1990).

Geneticists estimate that the average adult carries genes for four different recessive diseases or abnormalities (Scarr & Kidd, 1983), but for any one disease the distribution of genes is not random. For example, sickle-cell genes are more common among blacks; Tay-Sachs is most common among Jews of Eastern European origin.

Teratogens: Diseases and Drugs

Deviant prenatal development can also result from variations in the environment in which the embryo and fetus are nurtured. I pointed out in Chapter 1 that the effect of any teratogen depends heavily on the *timing* of the intervention or interference, an example of *critical periods,* or *sensitive periods.* The general rule is that each organ system—the nervous system, heart, ears, reproductive system, and so on—is most vulnerable to disruption when it is developing most rapidly (Moore & Persaud, 1993). At that point it is maximally sensitive to outside interference, whether that be from a disease organism that passed through the placental barrier, inappropriate hormones, drugs, or whatever. Since the most rapid development of

Table 2.2
Some of the Major Inherited Diseases

Phenylketonuria	A metabolic disorder that prevents metabolism of a common amino acid (phenylalanine). Treatment consists of a special phenylalanine-free diet. The child is not allowed many types of food, including milk. If not placed on the special diet shortly after birth, the child usually becomes very retarded. Affects only 1 in 8000 children. Diagnostic tests for this disorder are now routinely given at birth; cannot be diagnosed prenatally.
Tay-Sachs disease	An invariably fatal degenerative disease of the nervous system; virtually all victims die within the first three to four years. This gene is most common among Jews of Eastern European origin, among whom it occurs in approximately 1 in 3500 births. Can be diagnosed prenatally with amniocentesis or chorionic villus sampling.
Sickle-cell anemia	A sometimes fatal blood disease, with joint pain, increased susceptibility to infection, and other symptoms. The gene for this disease is carried by about 2 million Americans, most often blacks. Can now be diagnosed prenatally through amniocentesis or chorionic villus sampling.
Cystic fibrosis	A fatal disease affecting the lungs and intestinal tract. Many children with CF now live into their twenties. The gene is carried by more than 10 million Americans, most often whites. Carriers cannot be identified before pregnancy, and affected children cannot be diagnosed prenatally. If a couple has had one CF child, however, they know that their chances of having another are 1 in 4.
Muscular dystrophy	A fatal muscle-wasting disease, carried on the X chromosome, and thus found almost exclusively among boys. The gene for the most common type of MD, Duchenne's, has just been located, so prenatal diagnosis may soon be available.

most organ systems occurs during the first 12 weeks of gestation, this is the period of greatest risk. Figure 2.7 shows the maximum times of vulnerability for different parts of the body.

Because most organ systems develop most rapidly during the first 12 weeks of gestation, this is the period of greatest risk from most teratogens. Of the many teratogens, the most critical are probably drugs the mother may take and diseases she may have or may contract during the pregnancy.

Diseases of the Mother

A disease in the mother can affect the embryo or fetus via any of three mechanisms. Some diseases, particularly viruses, can attack the placenta, reducing the nutrients available to the embryo. Others have molecules small enough to pass through the placental filters and attack the embryo or fetus directly. Examples of this type include rubella and rubeola (both forms of measles), cytomegalovirus (CMV), syphilis, diphtheria, influenza, typhoid, serum hepatitis, and chicken pox. The third transmission method occurs during birth: Disease organisms present in the mucous membranes of the birth canal may infect the infant. Genital herpes, for example, is transmitted this way. Current research suggests that AIDS is transmitted in both the second and third ways, as well as through breast milk after birth

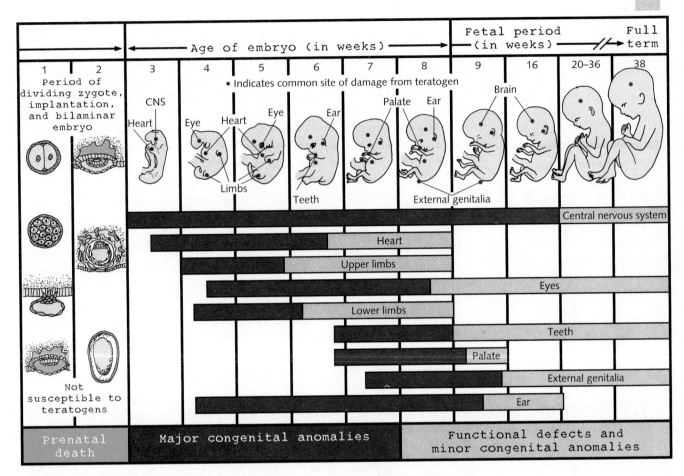

FIGURE 2.7 Critical periods in the prenatal development of various body parts. The blue portion of each line signifies the period during which any teratogen is likely to produce a major structural deformity in that particular body part. The yellow part of each line shows the period in which more minor problems may result. The embryonic period is generally the time of greatest vulnerability. (*Source:* Moore and Persaud, 1993, Figure 8–13, p. 156.)

(Van de Perre et al., 1991). Among the riskiest of these diseases for the infant are rubella, AIDS, CMV, and genital herpes.

Rubella Rubella (also called *German measles*) is most risky during the first few weeks of gestation. Most infants exposed in the first four to five weeks show some abnormality, compared to 20 percent of those exposed in the first trimester and only about 10 percent among those exposed in the final six months of the pregnancy (Moore & Persaud, 1993). Deafness, cataracts, and heart defects are the most common abnormalities.

Fortunately, rubella is preventable. Vaccination is available and should be given to all children as part of a regular immunization program. Adult women who were not vaccinated as children can be vaccinated later, but this must be done at least three months before pregnancy to provide complete immunity.

AIDS. Worldwide, an estimated 3 million women are infected with HIV, the virus that causes AIDS, and the number of infected women of childbearing age is rising everywhere. In the United States today, approximately 7000 infants are born each year to mothers infected with HIV. In areas with a high population of drug users, as many as 3 to

Women readers: Have you been vaccinated for rubella? If you don't know, find out; if you have not been, arrange for such a vaccination—but only if you are sure you are not pregnant!

5 percent of all pregnant women are now HIV infected (Heagarty, 1991), and roughly one-half of 1 percent of babies test positive for the AIDS virus at birth. Indeed, AIDS is now the seventh leading cause of death in children ages 1 to 4 in the U.S., up from ninth in 1988 (Centers for Disease Control, 1994a).

These are grim numbers, but there are two bits of good news amid all this depressing information. First, only a minority of infants born to HIV-infected mothers become infected themselves. Estimates from various studies range from 15 to about 40 percent, but most experts now suggest a transmission rate of about 20 to 25 percent (Annunziato & Frenkel, 1993). Transmission appears to be more likely when the mother's HIV disease is in an advanced stage, but beyond that, physicians have not been able to predict with any accuracy (Peckham, 1994).

The second piece of good news is that very recent research shows that mothers who are treated with the drug AZT during their pregnancies have a markedly lower risk of transmitting the disease to their children—as low as 8 percent (Centers for Disease Control, 1994a).

CMV. A much less well known but remarkably widespread and potentially serious disease is cytomegalovirus (CMV), a virus in the herpes group. As many as 60 percent of *all* women have antibodies to CMV, but most have no recognized symptoms. One to 2 percent of babies whose mothers have CMV antibodies become infected prenatally. When the mother's disease is in an active phase, the transmission rate is more like 40 to 50 percent (Blackman, 1990). As with AIDS, researchers have not yet uncovered all the details of the mechanisms of transmission. Nor have they understood why only about 5 to 10 percent of babies infected prenatally show clear symptoms of the disease at birth. But the 2500 babies

Given these new findings, should all pregnant women be required to be tested for HIV infection, so that they can be given the appropriate drug? Medical ethicists have offered strong arguments on both sides of this question. What do you think?

The Real World

Rh Factor: Another Type of Genetic Problem

Another possible problem, Rh factor incompatibility, is neither a genetic defect nor a teratogenic effect, but an interesting interaction of heredity and environment. One of the many factors in the blood is the presence or absence of a red cell antigen, called the Rh factor because rhesus monkeys have it. Humans who have this factor are called Rh+ (Rh positive), while those who lack it are Rh− (Rh negative). Only about 15 percent of whites and 5 percent of blacks in the United States are Rh−; this condition is quite rare among Asians and Native Americans.

Problems arise if the mother is Rh− and the baby is Rh+. Because Rh+ is dominant, a baby with an Rh+ father could inherit an Rh+ gene from him, even though the mother is Rh−. If the mother's and fetus's blood mix in the uterus, the mother's body considers the baby's Rh+ factor to be a foreign substance, and her immune system tries to fight it off by producing antibodies. These antibodies cross the placenta and attack the baby's blood, producing a chemical substance in the baby called bilirubin. Babies

with high levels of bilirubin look quite yellow; if the condition is untreated, brain damage can occur.

Without treatment, the risk of damage to the fetus increases with each succeeding pregnancy in which an Rh− mother carries an Rh+ baby. Normally, the placenta keeps the two blood systems separate, but during birth some mixing usually occurs. So after the first baby, the mother produces some antibodies. With a second incompatible baby, these antibodies attack the infant's blood, producing negative effects.

This problem used to be treated with rather heroic measures, such as complete exchange of the infant's blood shortly after birth to remove all the antibodies. Fortunately, scientists have now discovered a much simpler and safer treatment. Within 3 days of the birth of her first child, an Rh− mother with an Rh+ baby can be injected with a substance called rhogam, which prevents the buildup of antibodies and thus protects subsequent infants, even if they are also Rh+.

born each year in the United States who do display symptoms of the disease have a variety of serious problems, often including deafness and widespread damage to the central nervous system. Most are mentally retarded. In fact, CMV is now thought to be the single most important known infectious cause of both congenital mental retardation and deafness.

I am aware, by the way, that what I have just said about CMV is potentially alarming, given the high rate of silent infection. However, keep the statistics correctly in mind: If the mother's disease is not active, only 1 to 2 percent of babies become infected, and of this number, only at most 10 percent show symptoms of the disease—which means that at most 2 out of every 1000 infants whose mothers carry an inactive antibody will show any effect.

Herpes Simplex. Like CMV, this form of herpes, also known as *genital herpes,* may be transmitted to the fetus during delivery if the mother's disease is in the active phase at that time. Not only will the child then periodically experience the genital sores characteristic of the disease, but other complications are also possible, most notably a potentially serious inflammation of the brain and spinal cord called *meningoencephalitis.* Because of this increased risk, many physicians now recommend surgical delivery (cesarean section) of infants of mothers with herpes, although vaginal delivery is possible if the disease is inactive.

Drugs Taken by the Mother

Two decades ago, the average pregnant woman in the U.S. took six to seven prescribed drugs and another three or four over-the-counter drugs (such as aspirin) during the course of her pregnancy (Stewart, Cluff, & Philp, 1977). Today that number is lower, but it is not zero. Virtually all women take at least one or two over-the-counter drugs during the course of a pregnancy—cough medicine, aspirin for fever or headaches, drugs for constipation, and so on (de Jong-van den Berg et al., 1993). What are the effects of any of these drugs on the embryo or fetus?

A vast amount of research has been done on the effects of prenatal drugs, involving everything from aspirin to antibiotics to alcohol and cocaine. Sorting out their effects has proven to be an immensely challenging task, not only because it is clearly impossible to assign women randomly to various drug groups, but also because in the real world most women who use one drug are highly likely to use others as well. Women who drink alcohol are also more likely to smoke; those who use cocaine are also likely to take other illegal drugs or to smoke or drink to excess. The task is made still more difficult by the fact that the effects of drugs may be subtle, visible only many years after birth in the form of minor learning disabilities or increased risk of behavior problems. Still, we are creeping toward some fairly clear conclusions in several areas. Let me give you some examples.

Smoking. One of the most extensive bodies of research is on the effects of smoking. One consistent result stands out: Infants of mothers who smoke are on average about half a pound lighter at birth than are infants of nonsmoking mothers (Floyd et al., 1993). This does not mean that every mother who smokes has a very small or early baby. It does mean that the risk of such an outcome is higher for mothers who smoke.

The causal mechanism seems to work this way: Nicotine constricts the blood vessels, which reduces blood flow to the placenta, in turn reducing nutrition to the fetus. In the long term, such nutritional deprivation seems to increase slightly the risk of learning problems or poor attention span at school age. There are also some signs of higher rates of behavior problems among children whose mothers smoked heavily during pregnancy (Fergusson, Horwood, & Lynsky, 1993).

Before you read further, make a list of all the drugs you have taken in the past year, including over-the-counter drugs (aspirin? decongestants?), prescription drugs, and such "recreational" drugs as alcohol, nicotine, or cocaine. How many are there? How hard would it be to give them all up if you were pregnant?

Although research on the effects of smoking is not always easy to interpret, because women who smoke are likely to differ in other ways from those who do not, the moral seems clear: The safest plan is not to smoke during pregnancy. Smokers who quit smoking early in their pregnancy have the same rates of preterm or low-birth-weight infants as do those who did not smoke at all (Ahlsten, Cnattingius, & Lindmark, 1993). The research also shows a relationship between the "dose" (the amount of nicotine you are taking in) and the severity of consequences for the child. So if you cannot quit entirely, at least cut back.

Drinking. Recent work on the effects of maternal alcohol ingestion on prenatal and postnatal development also carries a clear message: To be safe, don't drink during pregnancy.

The effects of alcohol on the developing fetus range from mild to severe. At the extreme end of the continuum are children who exhibit a syndrome called **fetal alcohol syndrome (FAS).** Mothers of these children are heavy drinkers or alcoholics, and the infants themselves are generally smaller than normal, with smaller brains. They frequently have heart defects, and their faces are distinctively different (as you can see in Figure 2.8). As children, adolescents, and adults, they continue to be shorter than normal, have smaller heads, and IQ scores in the range of mild mental retardation. Indeed, FAS is the leading known cause of retardation in the United States, exceeding even Down syndrome (Streissguth et al., 1991).

But the effects of alcohol during pregnancy are not confined to cases in which the mother is clearly an alcoholic or a very heavy drinker. Recent evidence also points to milder effects of moderate or "social" drinking, such as two glasses of wine a day. Children of mothers who drank at this level during pregnancy have an increased risk of an IQ below 85 and show poorer attention spans. I've given some details about one of the best studies in the *Research Report* on page 56, so you can get some feeling for how investigators have gone about studying this problem.

We do not yet know if there is any safe level of alcohol consumption during pregnancy, although most of those who work in this field are convinced that there is a linear relationship between the amount of alcohol ingested and the risk for the infant. This means that even at low dosage there is *some* increased risk. Probably it also matters when in the pregnancy the drinking occurs, and it *clearly* matters how many drinks the mother takes on any one occasion. Binge drinking (usually defined as five or more drinks on any one occasion) is significantly riskier than regular smaller doses (Olson et al., 1992; Streissguth, Barr, & Sampson, 1990). In the face of our remaining ignorance, the *safest* course is not to drink at all.

Cocaine. Significant numbers of pregnant women in the United States (and presumably elsewhere in the world) also take various illegal drugs, most notably cocaine, al-

FIGURE 2.8 These two children, from different countries and different racial backgrounds, have been diagnosed as having fetal alcohol syndrome (FAS). Both are mentally retarded and have relatively small heads. Note also the short nose and low nasal bridge typical of FAS children. (Copyright George Steinmetz.)

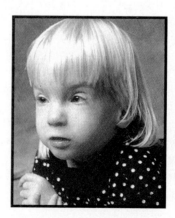
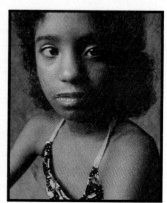

Research Report

Streissguth's Study of Prenatal Alcohol Exposure

The best single study of the consequences of prenatal alcohol exposure has been done by Ann Streissguth and her colleagues (Olson et al., 1992; Streissguth et al., 1980, 1981, 1984, 1989, 1990), who have followed a group of more than 500 women and children beginning in early pregnancy. Since the study was begun before there were widespread warnings about the possible impact of alcohol during pregnancy, the sample includes many well-educated, middle-class women with good diets who did not take many other recreational drugs but who did drink alcohol in moderate or even fairly heavy amounts while pregnant—a set of conditions that would be impossible to duplicate today, at least in the United States or other countries in which the risks are well advertised.

Streissguth tested the children repeatedly, beginning immediately after birth, again later in infancy, at age 4, at school age, and again at age 11. She found that the mothers' alcohol consumption in pregnancy was associated with sluggishness and weaker sucking in infancy, lower scores on a test of infant intelligence at 8 months, lower IQ at 4 and 7 years, and problems with attention and vigilance at 4, 7, and 11. Teachers also rated the 11-year-olds on overall school performance and on various behavior problems. On both measures those whose mothers had consumed the most alcohol during pregnancy were rated significantly worse.

Streissguth also was careful to obtain information about other drug use in pregnancy, including smoking, and asked mothers about their diet, their education, and their life habits. She found that the links between alcohol consumption and poor outcomes for the child hold up even when all these other variables are controlled statistically.

Setting aside those cases in which the child was diagnosed with the full fetal alcohol syndrome, the effects of moderate levels of alcohol use during pregnancy are not large in absolute terms, but they have significant practical consequences. For example, the difference in IQ scores at age 7 between children of abstainers and children of women who drank 1 ounce or more of alcohol per day during their pregnancies (roughly equivalent to 2 ounces of hard liquor or one 8-ounce glass of wine) was only about 6 points in Streissguth's sample (Streissguth et al., 1990). But this relatively small absolute difference means that three times as many alcohol-exposed children have IQs below 85 than is true among children of abstainers. Alcohol-exposed children are thus greatly overrepresented in special classes in schools and probably also appear in overlarge numbers among high school dropouts and the underemployed in adulthood—although those links remain for longer-term longitudinal studies to confirm.

though it is of course difficult to know exactly how prevalent the problem is, because many women are understandably reluctant to reveal such information to researchers or physicians. The best current estimates are that roughly 3 percent of all babies born in the U.S. have been prenatally exposed to cocaine. The risk is far higher among babies born to poor, inner-city mothers. In these groups, by some estimates, as many as 20 or 30 percent of mothers use cocaine (Hawley & Disney, 1992).

Cocaine appears to cross the placental barrier quite readily, but unlike alcohol, it creates no regular or recognizable syndrome of abnormalities. About a third of all cocaine-exposed babies are born prematurely, and among those born after a normal gestation period, many more are lower than normal in birth weight—a pattern that is very similar to what we see with smoking during pregnancy. In addition, they are three times as likely to have a very small head circumference. Some cocaine-exposed babies also show significant withdrawal symptoms after birth, such as irritability, restlessness, shrill crying, and tremors. Whether any long-term consequences can be ascribed clearly to prenatal cocaine exposure, however, is not yet clear. Some studies show long-term effects, while others do not (Griffith, Azuma, & Chasnoff, 1994; Richardson & Day, 1994). My sense is that we will eventually find that, as with alcohol exposure, the effects of cocaine are subtle and long-lasting, but that remains to be shown.

Other Teratogens

There are a great many other teratogens, including excess amounts of vitamin A, methylmercury, and lead, and many drugs or chemicals about which we have insufficient information are suspected of being teratogens. These include anticonvulsant medication taken by epileptics, polychlorinated biphenyls (PCBs, compounds widely used in electrical transformers and paint), radiation at high doses, aspirin, some antidepressants, some artificial hormones, and some pesticides (Vorhees & Mollnow, 1987). I don't have room to go into detail about what we know (or don't know) in each case, but let me say just a word about several of the more practically significant of the items on this list.

Diethylstilbestrol (DES). DES is a synthetic estrogen that at one time was commonly given to pregnant women to prevent miscarriages. The daughters of such women have been found to have higher rates of some kinds of cancers, and as many as 30 percent of the sons have been found to be infertile (Rosenblith, 1992).

Aspirin. One of the most widely used drugs, aspirin is teratogenic in animals when given in high doses. Humans rarely take high enough doses to produce such effects directly, but it turns out that aspirin in moderate amounts can have negative effects on the human fetus if it is ingested along with benzoic acid, a chemical widely used as a food preservative, such as in ketchup. This combination, especially in the first trimester, seems to increase the risk of physical malformations in the embryo/fetus.

Lead. In most industrialized countries, adults are exposed to fairly high dosages of lead, although the introduction of unleaded gasoline has had a significant impact on dosages, as has the elimination of lead-based paint. We have known for some time that high exposure to lead, such as from lead-based paints in old houses, has highly negative consequences for children, particularly for their intellectual development and functioning. But a newer set of studies shows that even quite low levels of lead in the blood of newborns or toddlers—levels previously classified as "safe" by U.S. federal guidelines and found in children who live in houses without lead-based paint—are associated with slightly lower IQ scores at later ages than we see in children with still lower lead levels (Tesman & Hills, 1994). Several longitudinal studies show that the effects are still detectable at ages 7 to 10 (Bellinger, Stiles, & Needleman, 1992). Because of this new evidence, the Centers for Disease Control changed its guidelines so that much lower blood lead levels are defined as dangerous.

As the study of teratogens expands, psychologists have realized that prenatal development is less insulated, less fully protected than we had first thought. In particular, many chemicals associated with modern industrial societies may have unforeseen effects on the fetus.

Other Influences on Prenatal Development

Diet. Another risk for the fetus is poor maternal nutrition, although it is crucial here to distinguish between chronic *sub*nutrition and acute *mal*nutrition. When a woman experiences severe malnutrition during pregnancy—such as we have seen during wartime in many countries—she has a greatly increased risk of stillbirths, low birth weight, and infant death during the first year of life (Stein et al., 1975). The effects seem to be worse when malnutrition occurs during the last half of the pregnancy, particularly in the final three months. Babies whose mothers suffer severe malnutrition during the final trimester are lighter at birth and have a greatly increased risk of dying during the first year.

The effects of subnutrition or less severe malnutrition, such as the chronic protein-energy malnutrition common in many populations around the world, have been far harder to establish. Most researchers have assumed that subnutrition should have a particularly large effect on the development of the nervous system. Animal studies confirm this. Rats whose caloric intake has been severely restricted during the fetal and early postnatal periods show a pattern described as *brain stunting,* with both the weight and volume of the brain reduced. They also show less dendritic development and less rich synaptic formation (Pollitt & Gorman, 1994). But whether these findings can be extended directly to humans has been very difficult to tease out.

When the prenatal malnutrition is severe enough to cause the death of the fetus or newborn, effects very similar to those in the rat studies have been observed. These infants have smaller brains, fewer and smaller brain cells (Georgieff, 1994). But when a baby experiences less-lethal subnutrition prenatally, the parallel is not so obvious. For one thing, such children are highly likely to encounter mal- or subnutrition after birth as well as prenatally, frequently accompanied by lower levels of stimulation in the home. How do we then sort out the effects of the *pre*natal nutrition? At the moment, most experts in this area have abandoned the previously widely held notion that typically observed levels of prenatal subnutrition have some direct, irremediable, negative effect on the developing brain (Ricciuti, 1993). Instead, what seems to happen is some variation of the interaction pattern I described in Chapter 1 (recall Figure 1.3): Malnutrition may make the infant more "vulnerable," perhaps because it makes him less energetic or responsive, or less able to learn from his experiences. In a nonstimulating environment such a vulnerable child is likely to do poorly. But a stimulating environment can overcome the vulnerability.

This pattern is illustrated nicely in the results of a small study by Philip Zeskind and Craig Ramey (1981). They have looked at the outcomes for a small group of 10 infants, all born to poverty-level mothers and all extremely thin at birth—usually a sign of prenatal malnutrition. Half of these babies happened to have been assigned randomly to a special enriched day-care program beginning when they were 3 months old. The other five malnourished babies received nutritional supplements but were reared at home in much less-stimulating circumstances. Other children in the day-care center had been of normal weight at birth, as were other home-reared children included in the study. Table 2.3 gives

Table 2.3
IQ Scores of 3-Year-Old Children

Experience After Birth	Prenatal Nutritional Status	
	Malnourished	Well Nourished
Enriched day care	96.4	98.1
Home-reared	70.6	87.7

Source: Zeskind & Ramey, 1981, p. 215.

the IQ scores of these four groups of children when they were 3 years old. As you can see, the results match Horowitz's model very well. Malnourished infants did well in the stimulating environment of the day-care center but extremely poorly in a less-supportive environment. Well-nourished infants also did better in the day-care environment than at home, but the difference was not nearly so large. Thus, malnutrition appeared to create a "vulnerability" that could only be overcome by an enriched environment.

The Mother's Age. One of the particularly intriguing trends in modern family life in the U.S. and many other industrialized countries is the increasing likelihood that women will postpone their first pregnancy into their late twenties or early thirties. In 1992, 23.5 percent of first births in the United States were to women over 30, more than double the rate in 1970 (U.S. Bureau of the Census, 1994). Of course women have many reasons for such decisions, chief among them being the increased need for second incomes in families and the desire of young women to complete job training and early career steps before bearing children. I'm not going to debate all the pros and cons. But I do want to explore the question that is relevant for the subject of this chapter, namely the impact of maternal age on the mother's experience of pregnancy and on the developing fetus. Here the recent data paint a somewhat different picture than does older evidence.

Current research suggests that mothers over 30 (particularly those over 35) are at increased risk for several kinds of problems, including miscarriage (McFalls, 1990); complications of pregnancy such as high blood pressure or bleeding (Berkowitz, et al., 1990); and death during pregnancy or delivery (Buehler et al., 1986).

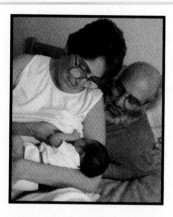

Older mothers, like this one, are becoming much more common in the U.S. and in other industrialized countries. Mothers over 30 (especially those over 35) and their infants have *slightly* increased risks of problems during pregnancy and delivery.

For example, in one large study of nearly 4000 women in New York, all of whom had received adequate prenatal care, Gertrud Berkowitz and her colleagues (1990) found that women 35 and older during their first pregnancies were almost twice as likely as women in their twenties to suffer some pregnancy complication. These effects of age are even greater if the mother has not had adequate prenatal care or has poor health habits. For example, the negative effects of maternal smoking on birth weight are considerably *greater* among women over 35 than among young women (Wen et al., 1990).

Whether the infants born to these older mothers also have higher risk of problems is not so clear. The evidence is conflicting. Older mothers appear to be only slightly more likely to have low-birth-weight infants (Berkowitz et al., 1990; Cnattingius, Berendes, & Forman, 1993) and may well have no heightened risk for bearing a child with birth defects—other than the well-established risk of chromosomal anomalies such as Down syndrome (Baird, Sadovnick, & Yee, 1991). However, researchers in Sweden, where mothers of all ages receive remarkably comprehensive and equal prenatal care, have recently reported higher rates of late-pregnancy miscarriage and heightened infant mortality for infants born to older mothers, especially for first births to mothers over 35 (Cnattingius et al., 1993). Given these varying results, the experts have been unable to reach a clear conclusion about risks for babies born to older mothers.

At the other end of the age continuum, the results of many studies seemed to be converging on the conclusion that if poverty and prenatal care are held constant, young mothers and their babies are at no greater risk for complications or abnormalities (McCarthy & Hardy, 1993; Osofsky, Hann, & Peebles, 1993). In absolute terms, of course, problem rates are higher among young mothers. But many researchers have argued that this higher rate occurs not because the mother is young, but because young mothers are more likely to live in poverty and to have inadequate prenatal care than are older mothers. But it now turns out that this may be an overly optimistic conclusion. An

The Real World

Weight Gain and Diet During Pregnancy

Life-styles have been changing; slimness and fitness in women are perhaps more highly valued now than before, especially among younger women of childbearing age. And all women want to give their unborn children the best possible start in the world. So questions about weight gain and diet during pregnancy are of vital concern to many women.

Weight Gain

As recently as 1950, the standard advice to pregnant women was to gain no more than 20 pounds over the 9 months. In the 1970s, however, new data accumulated showing that such low levels of gain were associated with higher risk of low birth weight and neurological impairment in the infant. This prompted a new recommendation from the American College of Obstetricians and Gynecologists and the American Academy of Pediatrics for a gain of between 22 and 27 pounds. More recently still, in 1990, the National Institute of Medicine issued new guidelines that base the recommended gain on a woman's prepregnancy weight-for-height (Taffel, Keppel, & Jones, 1993):

- A woman whose weight is normal for her height should gain between 25 and 35 pounds;
- A woman who is unusually lightweight for her height should gain 28 to 40 pounds;
- A woman who is heavy for her height should gain 15 to 25 pounds, and an obese woman should gain no less than 15 pounds.

Unfortunately, the very women who are otherwise at highest risk for various kinds of problems, including bearing a low-birth-weight infant, are also most likely to gain an insufficient amount: Those who are lightweight for their height before pregnancy, women older than 35, those with low education, and those whose birth attendant was neither a physician nor a midwife (Centers for Disease Control, 1992d) need to gain the most. Women who are very thin before their pregnancies are least likely to gain at a sufficient rate and are therefore at highest risk of bearing a low-birth-weight baby.

Interestingly, it begins to look as if variations in maternal weight gain during pregnancy may be one contributor

to the large difference between African-American and U.S. whites in neonatal mortality—a pattern I'll talk about in Chapter 3. The connective chain goes like this: Black women in the United States are, on average, heavier than white women of comparable social class and are more likely to be obese. Because of this, they are more likely to be (badly) advised, or they themselves choose, to restrict their weight gain during pregnancy, which in turn increases the likelihood of low birth weight in the infant (Kempe et al., 1992; Luke & Murtaugh, 1993). In fact, it looks as if for black women, even more than for white women, the optimum weight gain is one that is at the *upper* end of the range appropriate for their prepregnancy weight (Hickey et al., 1993).

A Good Diet

Pure poundage is not enough to ensure optimal development for the child. It also matters *what* the mother eats. Caloric requirements go up 10 to 20 percent (perhaps 300 calories a day beyond your maintenance level), but protein needs appear go up much more markedly. The usual current recommendation is that a pregnant woman of 19 or older needs to take in 1.3 grams of protein per kilogram (2.2 pounds) of her weight. As an example, this would mean that a woman weighing 125 pounds would require about 75 grams of protein per day. For teenagers, the protein requirement is still higher because they are still growing. (Since one egg has about 7 grams of protein, while one cup of cottage cheese has 33 grams, even this heightened requirement is not difficult to meet.) Requirements for most vitamins and minerals also increase during pregnancy. Calcium needs rise 50 percent (from 800 mg to 1200 mg daily), and iron requirements also rise, to perhaps 75 mg daily (Winick, 1980). Adequate folic acid is also critical. This nutrient, found in such foods as orange juice, spinach, and broccoli, helps to prevent neural tube defects such as spina bifida. Because the neural tube is forming in the first weeks of prenatal life, folic acid intake is especially important during the period immediately before pregnancy and in the first 6 weeks of pregnancy. Four to 8 milligrams per day is adequate, a level found in most multivitamins (Centers for Disease Control, 1992c).

unusually well designed new study points to increased risks for teenage mothers, even when they have good prenatal care and low economic or social risk.

Alison Fraser and her colleagues have studied 135,088 white girls and women, ages 13 to 24, who gave birth in Utah between 1970 and 1990 (Fraser, Brockert, & Ward, 1995). This is an unusual sample for studies on this subject: Almost two-thirds of the teenage mothers in this group were married, and most had adequate care; 95 percent remained in school. These special conditions have enabled Fraser to disentangle the effects of ethnicity, poverty, marital status, and mother's age—all of which are normally confounded in studies of teenage childbearing. Overall, Fraser found higher rates of adverse pregnancy outcomes among the teenage mothers (age 17 and younger) than among the mothers in their twenties. The rate of preterm births was twice as high; the incidence of low birth weight was almost twice as high. And these differences were found even when Fraser looked only at teenage mothers who were married, in school, and given adequate prenatal care. Outcomes were riskier still among teenage mothers who lacked adequate prenatal care, but this excellent study indicates that good care alone does not eliminate the heightened risk of problems linked to teenage birth. Just why such a heightened risk should exist is not entirely clear. The most likely possibility is that there is some biological consequence of pregnancy in a girl whose own growth is not complete. But whatever the underlying reason, these new results raise a variety of red flags.

The Mother's Emotional State. Finally, the mother's state of mind during the pregnancy may be significant, although the research findings are decidedly mixed (Istvan, 1986). Results from infrahuman studies are clear: Exposure of the pregnant female to stressors such as heat, light, noise, shock, or crowding significantly increases the risk of low birth weight as well as later problems in the offspring (Schneider, 1992). Studies of humans, however, have not pointed to such a clear conclusion, in part because researchers have not agreed on how one ought to measure such potentially relevant maternal states as anxiety or stress. Many investigators have found no link at all between their measures of the mother's overall life stress and either complications of her pregnancy or problems in the infant. Other investigators have found such links for some groups and not others. For example, Emmy Werner (1986) found that among middle-class women in her longitudinal study in Kauai, Hawaii, those who had negative feelings about their pregnancy or who were generally anxious or experienced some psychological trauma during the pregnancy had more birth complications and more infants with low birth weight or in poor condition than was true among middle-class women with lower stress or anxiety. But these same patterns did not hold among poor women in this study, many of whom lived in states of chronic stress or disorganization. Thus, it may be that long-term, chronic stressors have less impact on a specific pregnancy, while significant *increases* in anxiety or stress during a pregnancy may have more deleterious effects.

Folklore in virtually all cultures certainly points to a causal link between the mother's emotional experiences during her pregnancy and the outcome for the child. But at the moment the best I can do is to say that the hypothesis is still plausible, but not proven. Better epidemiological studies are needed if we are to go further.

An Overview of Risks and Long-Term Consequences of Prenatal Problems

Every time I write this chapter I am aware that the list of things that can go wrong seems to get longer and longer and scarier and scarier. Physicians, biologists, and psychologists keep learning more about both the major and the subtle effects of prenatal environmental

---

Another possible influence on prenatal development is the level of the mother's exercise. What kind of study would you have to do to figure out whether it is okay for pregnant women to maintain high levels of exercise, such as running 30 miles a week?

Before you read the next section, think about everything you have read so far in this chapter. See if you can figure out what three pieces of advice you would give to a pregnant friend, based on the information you have read. Why those three?

variations, so the number of warnings to pregnant women seems to increase yearly, if not monthly. One of the ironies of this is that too much worry about such potential consequences can make a woman more anxious, and anxiety is on the list of warnings! So before you begin worrying too much, let me try to put this information into perspective.

First, let me say again that *most* pregnancies are normal and largely uneventful, and most babies are healthy and normal at birth.

Second, any woman can take specific preventive steps to reduce the risks for herself and her unborn child. She can be properly immunized; she can quit smoking and drinking; she can watch her diet and make sure her weight gain is sufficient; and she and the child's father can have genetic counseling. In addition, she can get early and regular prenatal care. Many studies show that mothers who receive adequate prenatal care reduce the risks to themselves and their infants. Just one example: Jann Murray and Merton Bernfield (1988), in a study of more than 30,000 births, found that the risk of giving birth to a low-birth-weight infant was more than three times as great among women who had received inadequate prenatal care as among those receiving adequate care, and this pattern held among both blacks and whites. Unfortunately, inadequate care remains common in the U.S. In 1992, 22 percent of all mothers did not begin their prenatal care until at least the second trimester, and 5.2 percent either had no care at all or saw a health care provider only in the final few months (Wegman, 1994). Inadequate care was twice as common among black mothers as among whites (4.2 percent and 9.9 percent, respectively), and in both groups inadequate care was more common among mothers living in poverty and among teenage mothers.

Given such statistics, it is perhaps unsurprising that the U.S. continues to have a relatively high rate of infant mortality. The good news is that this rate has been declining steadily over the past decades, dropping from 20.0 infant deaths per 1000 births in 1970 to 8.3 in 1993 (Wegman, 1994). The bad news is that infant mortality is more than twice as high for blacks as for whites (16.3 and 6.8, respectively, in 1992) and that even an overall rate of 8.3 places the U.S. twenty-second in the world. Virtually all European countries, where prenatal care is typically free or low cost and universally available, have lower infant mortality rates, as do Japan (with the lowest rate in the world), Hong Kong, and Singapore.

The black/white difference in infant mortality is so significant a facet of U.S. culture that I need to say a further word about it. This difference has existed at least since record keeping began (in 1915) and has *not* been declining. It is found even when researchers compare only infants born to college-educated mothers (Schoendorf et al., 1992). Physicians and physiologists do not yet understand all the reasons for this discrepancy, although it is clear that one significant factor is that infants born to African-American mothers are much more likely to be born before the full gestational period is completed, and thus have low birth weight (Luke et al., 1993). When only full-term, normal-weight babies are compared, infant mortality is about the same in the two groups. But saying that only pushes the explanation back one step. We still need to know why blacks in the U.S. have more preterm, low-birth-weight babies, and the answer to this question is still unclear.

A third point to be made about prenatal problems is that if something does go wrong, chances are good that the negative consequences to the child will be short term rather than permanent. And many physical defects can be treated successfully after birth.

Of course some negative outcomes *are* permanent and have long-term consequences for the child. Chromosomal anomalies, including Down syndrome or deviations in sex-chromosome patterns, are permanent and nearly always associated with lasting mental retardation or school difficulties. Some teratogens also have permanent effects, such as fetal alcohol syndrome or deafness resulting from rubella. And as you'll see in Chapter 3, *very*-low-birth-weight infants (those under about 1500 grams, about $3\frac{1}{2}$ pounds) have an increased risk of persistent, long-term learning problems or low IQ, regardless of the richness of the environment in which they are reared.

But many of the effects I have talked about in this chapter may be detectable only for the first few years of the child's life, and then only in certain families. The relationship between prenatal problems and long-term outcomes, in fact, generally follows the same pattern I talked about with regard to malnutrition: We are more likely to see persisting problems if the child is reared in an unstimulating or unsupportive environment than if he grows up in a more optimal family situation. Claire Kopp puts it this way:

> To use an analogy, some perinatal risks (e.g., infections, anoxia, low-birth-weight) appear to act like a jolt to the system in which the system is hurt but is not irreparably damaged. With care and nurturance the system can fully mend in time whereas in the absence of adequate care, the system only partially recovers. (Kopp, 1994, p. 19)

So it is not the prenatal problem by itself that is the cause of the later difficulties; it is the combination of a prenatal problem and a relatively poor early environment that seems to produce long-term negative effects. So don't despair when you read the long list of cautions and potential problems. The story isn't as gloomy as it first seems.

Sex Differences in Prenatal Development

Because nearly all prenatal development is controlled by maturational codes that are the same for all members of our species—male and female alike—sex differences in prenatal development are not numerous. But there are a few, and they set the stage for some of the physical differences we'll see at later ages.

- Sometime between four and eight weeks after conception, the male hormone *testosterone* begins to be secreted by the rudimentary testes in the male embryo. If this hormone is not secreted or is secreted in inadequate amounts, the embryo will be "demasculinized," even to the extent of developing female genitalia. Girls do not secrete any equivalent hormone prenatally. However, the accidental presence of the male hormone, androgen, at the critical time (such as from some drug the mother may take or from a genetic disease called *congenital adrenal hyperplasia*) acts to "defeminize" or masculinize the female fetus, sometimes resulting in malelike genitalia.

- Such prenatal hormones also appear to affect the pattern of brain development as well as the development of genitalia, resulting in subtle brain differences that affect patterns of growth-hormone secretions in adolescence, levels of physical aggression, or relative dominance of the right and left hemispheres of the brain (Todd et al., 1995). The research evidence on such points is still fairly sketchy; it is clear that whatever role prenatal hormones play in brain architecture and functioning is highly complex. But the possibilities are intriguing—and yet another example of the growing importance of biological explanations of children's development.

- Girls are a bit faster in some aspects of prenatal development, particularly skeletal development. They are about 1 to 2 weeks ahead in bone development at birth (Tanner, 1978).

- Despite the more rapid development of girls, boys are heavier and longer at birth (Tanner, 1978).

- Boys are considerably more vulnerable to all kinds of prenatal problems. Many more boys than girls are conceived—on the order of about 120 to 150 male embryos to every 100 female—but more of the males are spontaneously aborted. At birth, there are about 105 boys for every 100 girls. Boys are also more likely to experience injuries at birth (perhaps because they are larger), and they have more congenital malformations (Zaslow & Hayes, 1986). Among those infants who experience severe complications during delivery, boys are more likely to die (Werner, 1986).

The striking sex difference in vulnerability is particularly intriguing, especially since it seems to persist. Older boys are more prone to problems as well, as are adult men. Males have shorter life expectancy, higher rates of behavior problems, more learning disabilities, and usually more negative responses to major stresses, such as divorce. One possible explanation for at least some of this sex difference may lie in the basic genetic difference. The XX combination affords the girl more protection against the fragile-X syndrome and against any "bad" genes that may be carried on the X chromosome. For instance, geneticists have found that a gene affecting susceptibility to infectious disease is carried on the X chromosome (Brooks-Gunn & Matthews, 1979). Because boys have only one X chromosome, such a gene is much more likely to be expressed phenotypically in a boy.

Social Class Differences

I will be talking much more fully about social class differences in development in Chapter 14, but I cannot leave this chapter without saying a word about the impact of social class on the risks of pregnancy and birth.

The basic sequence of fetal development is clearly no different for children born to poor mothers than for children born to middle-class mothers. But many of the problems that can affect prenatal development negatively are more common among the poor. For example, in the United States, mothers who have not graduated from high school are about twice as likely as mothers with a college education to have a low-birth-weight infant or to have a stillborn infant. Poor women are also likely to have their first pregnancy earlier and to have more pregnancies overall, and they are less likely to be immunized against such diseases as rubella. They are also less likely to seek prenatal care, or they seek it much later in their pregnancies. A significant portion of this difference could be overcome in the U.S. if we were willing to devote the resources needed to provide good, universal prenatal care. We could significantly reduce not only the rate of infant death but also the rate of physical abnormalities and perhaps even mental retardation. But equal access to care is not the only answer. In the Nordic countries, for example, in which such care is universally available, social class differences in low-birth-weight deliveries and in infant mortality rates remain (Bakketeig, Cnattingius, & Knudsen, 1993). Nonetheless, I am still convinced that access to good-quality prenatal care is a minimum goal. Among other things, it would create cost savings over the long run, because it costs a great deal less to provide prenatal care than it does to care for a low-birth-weight infant or a child with significant learning disabilities. Ultimately, though, the argument is broader than that: Every child, in my view, has a *right* to begin with the best possible start in life.

Summary

1   At conception, the 23 chromosomes from the sperm join with 23 from the ovum to make up the set of 46 that will be reproduced in each cell of the new child's body.

2   Each chromosome consists of a long string of deoxyribonucleic acid (DNA), divisible into specific segments called genes.

3   The child's sex is determined by the twenty-third pair of chromosomes, a pattern of XX for a girl and XY for a boy.

4   Geneticists distinguish between the genotype, which is the pattern of inherited characteristics, and the phenotype, which is the result of the interaction of genotype and environment.

5   During the first days after conception, called the germinal stage of development, the initial cell divides (mitosis), travels down the fallopian tube, and is implanted in the wall of the uterus.

6   The second stage, the period of the embryo, includes the development of the various structures that support fetal development, such as the placenta and the amnion, as well as primitive forms of all organ systems.

7   The final 30 weeks of gestation, called the fetal period, are devoted primarily to enlargement and refinements in all the organ systems.

8   All the neurons an individual will ever have are developed between 10 and 20 weeks gestation, but the axon and dendrites on each neuron develop in the final two months of gestation and in the first few years after birth.

9   Normal prenatal development seems heavily determined by maturation—a "road map" contained in the genes. Disruptions in this sequence can occur; the timing of the disruption determines the nature and severity of the effect.

10 Deviations from the normal pattern can be caused at conception by any of a variety of chromosomal anomalies, such as Down syndrome, or by the transmission of genes for specific diseases.

11 Prior to conception, it is possible to test parents for the presence of genes for many inherited diseases. After conception, several diagnostic techniques exist that identify chromosomal anomalies or recessive-gene diseases in the fetus.

12 Some diseases contracted by the mother may affect the child, including rubella, AIDS, CMV, and genital herpes. These may (but do not invariably) result in disease or physical abnormalities in the child.

13 Alcohol, nicotine, and cocaine all appear to have significantly harmful effects on the developing fetus; the greater the dose, the greater the potential effect appears to be.

14 The mother's diet is also important. If she is severely malnourished, there are increased risks of stillbirth, low birth weight, and infant death during the first year of life. Long-term consequences of milder subnutrition, however, have been more difficult to establish.

15 Older mothers and very young mothers also run slightly increased risks, although these risks are greatly reduced if the mother is in good health and receives adequate prenatal care.

16 Among other teratogens, prenatal lead exposure has been shown to be associated with lower IQs in infancy and early childhood.

17 High levels of anxiety or stress in the mother may also increase the risk of complications of pregnancy or difficulties in the infant, although the research findings here are mixed.

18 Some difficulties in prenatal development can produce permanent disabilities or deformities, such as Down syndrome or deafness from rubella. Other lasting problems, such as learning disabilities, may also be caused by teratogens. But many disorders associated with prenatal problems can be overcome if the child is reared in a supportive and stimulating environment.

19 During the embryonic period, the XY embryo secretes the hormone testosterone, which stimulates the growth of male genitalia and shifts the brain into a "male" pattern. Without that hormone, the embryo develops as a girl, as do normal XX embryos.

20 Other sex differences in prenatal development are few. Boys are slower to develop, bigger at birth, and more vulnerable to most forms of prenatal stress.

21 Nearly all potential problems of prenatal development are more common among poor women, but these increased risks can be greatly reduced with good diet and adequate prenatal care.

Key Terms

alpha-fetoprotein test (**p. 48**)	dendrites (**p. 44**)	gametes (**p. 38**)	rubella (**p. 51**)
amniocentesis (**p. 48**)	deoxyribonucleic acid (**p. 38**)	gene (**p. 38**)	sex chromosomes (**p. 40**)
amnion (**p. 43**)	Down syndrome (**p. 47**)	genotype (**p. 38**)	synapse (**p. 45**)
autosomes (**p. 40**)	embryo (**p. 43**)	glial cells (**p. 44**)	ultrasound (**p. 48**)
axon (**p. 44**)	fallopian tube (**p. 37**)	neuron (**p. 44**)	uterus (**p. 37**)
chorionic villus sampling (**p. 48**)	fetal alcohol syndrome (FAS) (**p. 54**)	ovum (**p. 37**)	
chromosome (**p. 38**)	fetus (**p. 44**)	phenotype (**p. 42**)	
		placenta (**p. 43**)	

Suggested Readings

The Boston Women's Health Collective. (1992). *The new our bodies, ourselves: A book by and for women.* New York: Simon & Schuster.

This recent revision of a popular book is really focused on the adult female's body, rather than on prenatal development, but it has an excellent discussion of health during pregnancy. This is a strongly feminist book. Some of you may not be entirely in sympathy with all the political views included, but it is nonetheless a very good, compact source of information on all facets of pregnancy and childbirth.

Moore, K. L., & Persaud, T. V. N. (1993). *The developing human: Clinically oriented embryology* (5th ed.). Philadelphia: Saunders.

A highly technical book aimed at medical students that may give more detail than you want, but I guarantee it will tell you anything you might want to know about prenatal development—and then some!

Nightingale, E. O., & Goodman, M. (1990). *Before birth: Prenatal testing for genetic disease.* Cambridge, MA: Harvard University Press.

A clearly written small book, addressed to prospective parents who are looking for practical guidance. It includes detailed descriptions of common genetic anomalies and inherited diseases and of diagnostic procedures. It also discusses ethical questions.

Nilsson, L. A. (1990). *A child is born.* New York: Delacorte Press, Seymour Lawrence.

A remarkable book, full of marvelous photographs of the embryo and fetus. It also has a good basic text describing prenatal development and problems of pregnancy.

Rosenblith, J. F. (1992). *In the beginning: Development in the first two years of life* (2nd ed.). Newbury Park, CA: Sage.

A first-rate text covering prenatal development and infancy. Much less technical than the Moore and Persaud book listed earlier, it would be an excellent next step in your reading if you are interested in this area.

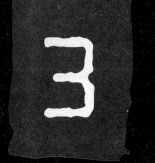
Birth and the Newborn Child

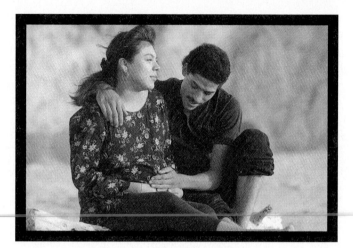

Try to imagine that you are a woman nine months pregnant with your first child. The long months of prenatal life are over and the baby is about to be born. If you are like many of today's mothers, you and your partner have explored your options for the location and conditions for your delivery; both of you may have taken prenatal classes; you have tried to prepare yourselves for what the baby will be like and how the advent of this new member of the family will change your life. You are a little apprehensive about the process of delivery and a bit uncertain about what to expect from the baby and about your own abilities to cope, but you are eager for the whole adventure to begin.

In this chapter I want to try to answer some of the questions that new parents reasonably ask about birth and about newborn babies. Does it make a difference whether the baby is born in a hospital or at home? Does it matter if the father is present or not? What happens if the birth is too early, or if something else goes wrong? I also want to describe the beginnings of the child's independent life so that you can have a clear picture of the qualities and skills with which the infant begins the long developmental journey. In the past few decades, researchers have discovered that the apparently helpless newborn really has a wide range of quite remarkable abilities. This knowledge has changed not only the information given out to new parents but also our theories of development.

Birth

The Stages of Labor

Labor progresses through three stages of unequal length.

The First Stage of Labor. Stage 1 covers the period during which two important processes occur: dilation and effacement. The cervix (the opening at the bottom of the uterus) must open up like the lens of a camera (**dilation**) and flatten out (**effacement**). At the time of actual delivery of the infant, the cervix must normally be dilated to about 10 centimeters (about 4 inches). This part of labor has been likened to putting on a sweater with a neck that is too tight. You have to pull and stretch the neck of the sweater with your head in order to get it on. Eventually, the neck is stretched wide enough so that the widest part of your head can pass through.

A good deal of the effacement may actually occur in the last weeks of the pregnancy, as may some dilation. It is not uncommon for women to begin labor 80 percent effaced and 1 to 3 centimeters dilated (Biswas & Craigo, 1994). The contractions of the first stage of labor, which are at first widely spaced and later more frequent and rhythmical, serve to complete both processes.

Customarily, stage 1 is itself divided into phases. In the *early* (or *latent*) phase, contractions are relatively far apart and are typically not too uncomfortable. In the *active* phase, which begins when the cervix is 3 to 4 centimeters dilated and continues until dilation has reached 8 centimeters, contractions are closer together and more intense. The last 2 centimeters of dilation are achieved during a period usually called the *transition* phase. It is this period, when contractions are closely spaced and strong, that women typically find the most painful. Fortunately, transition is relatively brief, especially in second or later pregnancies.

You can see the comparative length of these various phases for first births and for later births in Figure 3.1. The times are longer for women receiving anesthesia than for those delivering with natural childbirth, but in all groups there is quite a lot of variability. In one study, for example, Kilpatrick and Laros (1989) found a range of 3 to 19 hours in stage 1 for a group of women delivering a first infant without anesthesia.

Second Stage of Labor. At the end of the transition phase the mother will normally have the urge to help the infant out by "pushing." When the birth attendant (physician or midwife) is sure the cervix is fully dilated, she or he will encourage this pushing, and the second stage of labor—the actual delivery—begins. The baby's head moves past the stretched cervix, into the birth canal, and finally out of the mother's body. Most women find this part of labor markedly less distressing than the transition phase. It typically lasts less than an hour and rarely takes longer than two hours.

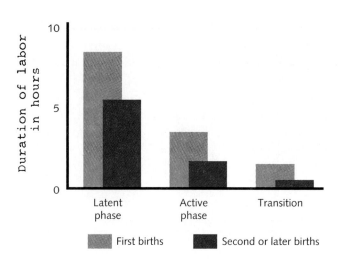

FIGURE 3.1 Typical pattern of timing of the phases of stage 1 of labor for first births and for subsequent births. The relatively long latent phase shown here counts from zero centimeters dilated, which increases the total hours somewhat. The total length of stage 1 ranges from 8 to 12 hours for a first birth and from 6 to about 8 hours for later births. (*Source:* Based on Biswas & Craigo, 1994, from Figures 10–16, p. 216, and 10–17, p. 217.)

Most infants are delivered head first, facing down toward the mother's spine. Three to 4 percent, however, are oriented differently, either feet first or bottom first (called *breech* presentations) (Brown, Karrison, & Cibils, 1994). Several decades ago most breech deliveries were accomplished with the aid of medical instruments such as forceps; today nearly four-fifths of breech presentations are delivered by cesarean section—a procedure I'll discuss more fully in a moment.

The Third Stage of Labor. Stage 3, typically quite brief, is the delivery of the placenta (also called the "afterbirth") and other material from the uterus. You can see all these steps schematically in Figure 3.2.

The First Greeting

The brief description I've just given does not begin to convey the emotional impact of the experience of childbirth for the mother or for the father, if he is present. Many women (and men) experience a time of intense joy as they greet the infant for the first time: laughter, exclamations of delight at the baby's features, first tentative and tender touching. Here's an excerpt from one mother's greeting (Macfarlane, 1977, pp. 64–65):

> *She's big, isn't she? What do you reckon? [Doctor makes a comment.] Oh look, she's got hair. It's a girl—you're supposed to be all little. Gosh. Oh, she's lovely. Oh, she's opened her eyes [laughs]. Oh lovely [kisses baby].*

Most parents are intensely interested in having the baby look at them right away. They are delighted if the baby opens her eyes, and they will try to stimulate her to do so if she doesn't. The parents' first tentative touches also seem to have a pattern to them: The parent first touches the infant rather gingerly with the tip of a finger and then proceeds gradually to stroking with the full hand (Klaus & Kennell, 1976; Macfarlane, 1977). Whether this same pattern holds in all cultures, I do not know. But the tenderness seen in most of these early encounters is striking.

Why do you think parents are so interested in having the baby look at them? Do you think this is a universal pattern?

Birth Choices

What I am going to say here about birth choices is necessarily specific to options and experiences in industrialized countries. In many other cultures there are no decisions to be

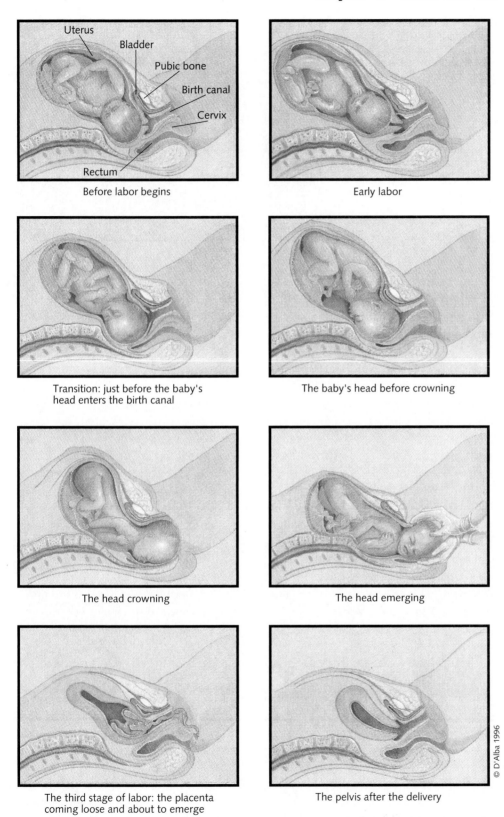

Before labor begins

Early labor

Transition: just before the baby's
head enters the birth canal

The baby's head before crowning

The head crowning

The head emerging

The third stage of labor: the placenta
coming loose and about to emerge

The pelvis after the delivery

© D'Alba 1996

FIGURE 3.2 The sequence of steps during delivery is shown clearly in these drawings.

At this point in the delivery, the baby's head is fully out. Notice that the father is present for this delivery, as is now the norm in the United States.

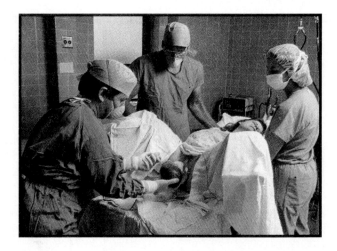

made about such questions as where the delivery will occur, whether the father should be present, or whether the mother should be given drugs to ease her pain. Custom dictates the answers. But in many Western industrialized countries, patterns and customs in this area continue to change rapidly, which leaves individual parents with decisions to make—decisions that may affect the child's health or the mother's satisfaction with the delivery. Because many of you will face these choices at some point in the future, I want to give you the best current information I have.

Drugs During Delivery.   One key decision concerns the use of drugs during delivery. Three types of drugs are commonly used: (1) *analgesics* (such as the common drug Demerol), which are given during the first stage of labor to reduce pain. All the analgesics in this group are members of the opium family of drugs; (2) *sedatives* or *tranquilizers* (such as Nembutol, Valium, or Thorazine), given during stage 1 labor to reduce anxiety; and (3) *anesthesia,* given during transition or the second stage of labor to block pain either totally (general anesthesia) or in portions of the body (local anesthesia). Of the three, anesthesia is least often used in the United States, although the use of one form of local anesthesia, the epidural block, has been increasing, with a current rate of up to 16 percent of all labors (Fields & Wall, 1993).

Studying the causal links between such drug use and the baby's later behavior or development has proven to be monumentally difficult. Controlled experiments are obviously not possible, since women cannot be randomly assigned to specific drug regimens. And drugs are given in myriad different combinations. But a few reasonably clear conclusions are possible.

First, we know that nearly all drugs given during labor pass through the placenta and enter the fetal bloodstream. Because the newborn lacks the enzymes necessary to break down such drugs quickly, the effect of any drug lasts longer in the baby than it does in the mother. Not surprisingly, then, drugged infants are slightly more sluggish, gain a little less weight, and spend more time sleeping in the first few weeks than do infants of nondrugged moms (Maurer & Maurer, 1988). These differences are quite small but have been observed repeatedly.

Beyond these first few days, however, psychologists have found no consistently observed effects from analgesics and tranquilizers, and only a few hints of long-term effects of anesthesia in a few studies (Rosenblith, 1992). Given such contradictory findings, only one specific piece of advice seems warranted: If you have received medication, you need to bear in mind that your baby is also drugged and that this will affect her behavior in the first few days. If you allow for this effect and realize that it will wear off, your long-term relationship with your child is likely to be unaffected.

The Location of Birth: Four Alternatives. A second choice parents must make is *where* the baby is to be born. Today in the U.S. there are typically four alternatives: (1) a traditional hospital maternity unit; (2) a hospital-based birth center or birthing room, which is located within a hospital but provides a more homelike setting, with labor and delivery both completed in the same room and family members often present throughout; (3) a freestanding birth center, like a hospital birth center except located apart from the hospital, with delivery typically attended by a midwife rather than (or in addition to) a physician; and (4) home delivery.

At the turn of the century, only about 5 percent of babies in the United States were born in hospitals; today the figure is 98.3 percent (U.S. Bureau of the Census, 1994). About 1 percent are born at home, and the remainder in birthing centers—a choice that is particularly common among Mexican-American mothers, especially in Texas. Because home deliveries are so uncommon in the U.S., much of what we know about them comes from research in Europe, where such deliveries are thought to be both more natural and less expensive for the medical care system. In countries where this pattern occurs, home deliveries are encouraged in uncomplicated pregnancies in which the woman has received good prenatal care. For example, in the Netherlands, a third of all deliveries are at home (Eskes, 1992). In this low-risk group, with a trained birth attendant present at delivery, the rate of delivery complications or infant problems is no higher in home or birth center deliveries than in hospital deliveries (Rooks et al., 1989; Tew, 1985). In contrast, infant mortality rates are significantly higher in *unplanned* home deliveries, in those without trained attendants, or in those where the mother had experienced some complication of pregnancy (Schramm, Barnes, & Bakewell, 1987).

Would you consider a home delivery for yourself? Why or why not? How much of your answer do you think is dictated by cultural patterns?

Incidentally, there is no evidence that babies born at home or in birthing centers are in any way off in the long run than are babies born in more traditional hospital settings. Assuming appropriate safety precautions, then, the choice should be based on what is most comfortable for the individual woman or couple.

The Presence of Fathers at Delivery. A third important decision is whether the father should be present at delivery. In the United States today this hardly seems like a "decision." As recently as 1972 only about a quarter of U.S. hospitals permitted the father to be present in the delivery room; by 1980, four-fifths of them did (Parke & Tinsley, 1984); and today the father's presence has become absolutely the norm—an illustration of how a cultural pattern surrounding an event as important as birth can undergo rapid change.

There have been several compelling arguments offered in favor of such a norm: The father's presence may lessen the mother's anxiety and give her psychological support; by coaching her in breathing and other techniques he may help her control her pain; and he may become more strongly attached to the infant by being present at the birth. At least some evidence supports the first two of these arguments, but—perhaps unexpectedly for some of you—the third has little support.

When fathers are present, mothers report lower levels of pain and receive less medication (Henneborn & Cogan, 1975). And when the mother has a coach (the father or someone else), the incidence of problems of labor and delivery goes down, as does the

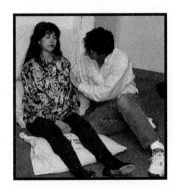

This couple, like so many today, is taking a prenatal class together. Having the father present at the delivery as coach seems to reduce the mother's pain and even shorten the length of labor.

duration of labor (Sosa et al., 1980). Furthermore, at least one study shows that women are more likely to report that the birth was a "peak" experience if the father was present (Entwisle & Doering, 1981).

What is far less clear is whether the father's relationship with his infant is affected positively by being present at delivery or by having an opportunity for early contact with the infant. In the 1970s and 1980s, most parents accepted the statements made by various psychologists and pediatricians that it was essential for the father's bonding with the baby for him to be present at the baby's birth. In fact, it was just such statements that led to the rapid increase in fathers' participation in births in the U.S. and elsewhere. But the evidence has failed to support the early arguments. On the plus side is some indication that those fathers whose birth experience has been particularly positive show signs of greater attachment to their infant throughout the first year (Peterson, Mehl, & Leiderman, 1979), but this seems to be true whether the father is actually present for the birth or not. Presence at delivery seems to have no magical effect. Thus, the father's presence may enhance the marital relationship but is neither necessary nor sufficient for the father's emerging attachment to his infant (Palkovitz, 1985).

This statement is not in any way intended as an argument against fathers' participation in the delivery process. The fact that the father's presence seems to help the mother control pain, reduce medication and labor duration, and may enhance the husband-wife relationship all seem to me to be compelling reasons for encouraging fathers to be present. In addition, of course, most fathers report powerful feelings of delight at being present at the birth of their children. Reason enough.

Have you read or heard before that a father wouldn't really "bond" with his baby unless he was present at delivery? Did you believe it? Why? Because it made sense to you, or because the evidence seemed especially good? Will you be more skeptical next time?

Problems at Birth

So far I have been discussing the process of normal, uncomplicated vaginal delivery. But as with prenatal development, some things can alter the normal pattern. The delivery itself may not proceed normally, leading to a surgical delivery through an abdominal incision, called a **cesarean section** (usually abbreviated C-section). Or the infant may not breathe immediately after birth or may be born too early, or even too late.

Cesarean Section Delivery. C-section deliveries occur for a variety of reasons, of which the most common are a breech position of the fetus, some sign of fetal distress, or a mother who has had a previous C-section. C-section deliveries are also more common among older mothers in the U.S.—a group that makes up an increasingly large proportion of all pregnancies (Adashek et al., 1993).

In virtually all industrialized countries, the frequency of C-sections rose in the 1970s and 1980s, a pattern illustrated in Figure 3.3. The particularly striking rise in the U.S. has actually been even greater than the figure suggests. In 1970, the cesarean rate in the U.S. was only 5.5. By 1985, this rate had quadrupled. The rate has now leveled off or even dropped a small amount, amid growing agreement that the current rate is substantially higher than medically necessary. In fact, the reduction of this rate to something closer to 12 to 15 percent is listed as a significant health objective for the year 2000 by the Centers for Disease Control (1993).

The rise has had many causes, both in the U.S. and in other countries. Fear of malpractice suits may be one element, particularly in the U.S. But much more of the increase appears to be due to changes in standard medical practice, such as requiring any woman

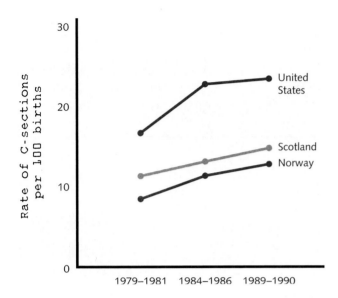

FIGURE 3.3 These findings illustrate the rise in the rate of cesarean section deliveries that occurred in virtually every industrialized country in the 1970s and early 1980s. (*Source*: Notzon et al., 1994, data from Table I, p. 496.)

who has had one C-section to have all subsequent deliveries the same way, as well as the widespread use of fetal monitors—equipment that allows the physician to hear the fetal heartbeat and thus to detect signs of fetal distress. Such signs of distress increasingly have been handled with C-sections, in order to reduce the apparent risk to the infant.

Both these practices have been questioned. For example, in Norway, Scotland, and Sweden, more than half of all women who have had one C-section delivery are able to have successful vaginal deliveries in subsequent pregnancies. In the U.S., only about 20 percent of such women have subsequent vaginal deliveries (Notzon et al., 1994), and this difference alone accounts for most of the much higher rate of C-sections in the U.S. compared with European countries. Similarly, some physicians (Levano et al., 1986) argue that fetal monitoring has led to many unnecessary C-sections, particularly in otherwise low-risk pregnancies.

I do not want to give you the impression that C-sections are never necessary. They clearly are. Breech position births, for example, appear to be safer if done by C-section than vaginally (Cheng & Hannah, 1993). But obstetricians worldwide agree that the rate has become too high and that it can be considerably reduced without added risk to mothers or infants. In Sweden, for example, after physicians made a collective decision to lower the rate, the rate dropped significantly in the late 1980s, and now stands at 10.7—without any increase in infant or maternal mortality (Notzon et al., 1994).

Anoxia (Lack of Oxygen). Another complication that can occur during delivery—and that may, in fact, be detected by a fetal monitor—is an insufficiency of oxygen for the infant. Such reduced oxygen supply is called **anoxia.** During the period immediately surrounding birth, anoxia may occur because the umbilical circulation system fails to continue the supply of blood oxygen until the baby breathes, or because the umbilical cord has been squeezed in some way during labor or delivery. Perhaps as many as 20 percent of newborns experience some degree of anoxia.

Long-term effects of anoxia have been hard to pin down. Prolonged anoxia is often (but not at all invariably) associated with such major consequences as cerebral palsy or

Low-birth-weight infants are kept in special isolettes, like this one, so that the temperature can be controlled. These babies are not only tiny, but also more wrinkled and skinny because the layer of fat under the skin has not fully developed.

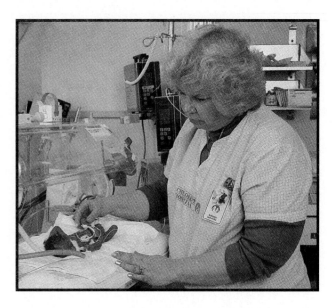

mental retardation. Briefer periods of oxygen deprivation appear to have little long-term effect, but that is still a tentative conclusion.

Low Birth Weight. Babies who weigh too little are at much higher risk for a whole range of other problems, including death during infancy and later learning problems. You already know from Chapter 2 that low birth weight is one of the common consequences of a variety of teratogens or other environmental factors, including the mother's smoking, some kinds of drugs, and low maternal weight gain. But I need to talk a bit more about the causes, varieties, and consequences of low birth weight.

Several different labels are used to describe infants with less than optimal weight. All babies below 2500 grams (about 5.5 pounds) are described with the most general term of **low birth weight (LBW).** Those below 1500 grams (about 3.3 pounds) are usually called *very low birth weight,* while those below 1000 grams are called *extremely low birth weight.* In 1991, 7.1 percent of all newborns in the U.S. were below 2500 grams—a total of about 290,000 infants each year (U.S. Bureau of the Census, 1994). About 15 percent of those babies weighed less than 1500 grams. Given what I said in Chapter 2, you will not be surprised to learn that low birth weight is considerably more common among blacks than among either Anglos or Hispanics in the U.S. In 1991, the respective rates were 13.6 percent, 5.8 percent, and 6.1 percent.

There are a variety of reasons for low birth weight, of which the most common is that the infant is born before the full 38 weeks of gestation. Any baby born before 36 weeks of gestation is labeled **preterm.** It is also possible for an infant to have completed the full 38-week gestational period but still weigh less than 2500 grams or to weigh less than would be expected for the number of weeks of gestation completed, however long that may have been. Such an infant is called **small for date.** Infants in this group appear to have suffered from prenatal malnutrition, such as might occur with constriction of blood flow caused by the mother's smoking or from other significant problems prenatally. As a group, these infants have poorer prognoses than do those of an equivalent weight who weigh an appropriate amount for their gestational age.

All low-birth-weight infants share some characteristics, including markedly lower levels of responsiveness at birth and in the early months of life. They are also more likely to experience respiratory distress in the early weeks and may be slower in motor development than their normal-weight peers.

About 80 percent of all low-birth-weight infants survive long enough to leave the hospital, but the lower the birth weight, the greater the risk of neonatal death. This pattern is especially clear in the results shown in Figure 3.4, which come from a study of a group of 1765 very-low-birth-weight infants born in seven different hospitals around the U.S. The limit of viability is about 500 to 600 grams, or about 23 weeks gestation. Babies born before 23 weeks rarely survive; those born at 23 or 24 weeks have at least a small chance of survival (Allen, Donohue, & Dusman, 1993).

Whether these really tiny babies survive or not depends a good deal on whether they receive state-of-the-art neonatal care. In hospitals with especially modern and aggressive neonatal intensive care units, as many as half of infants born weighing 500 to 1000 grams (1 to 2 pounds) may survive (Astbury et al., 1990).

You might think that all babies this small who do survive will have major developmental problems. But that is not the case. The long-term outcomes depend not only on the quality of care available to the infant, but also on just how small the baby was and what kind of family he or she grows up in (Bendersky & Lewis, 1994). Because medical advances in the care of LBW infants have been enormous in the past few decades, the more recently such a baby was born, the better the long-term prognosis seems to be (Perlman et al., 1995).

The great majority of those above 1500 grams who are not small for date catch up to their normal peers within the first few years of life. But those below 1500 grams, especially those below 1000, have significantly higher rates of long-term problems, including neurological impairment, lower IQs, smaller size, and greater problems in school (Breslau et al., 1994; Hack et al., 1994; Saigal et al., 1991). You can get a better sense of both the type and incidence of such problems from the data in Table 3.1, which lists the results for two studies, one from the U.S. and the other from Australia.

Three points are worth making about the findings from follow-up studies like those shown in the table. First, the smaller the infant at birth, the greater the likelihood of problems. Among the very small infants, significant difficulties are common. Second, some

If you were given the job of designing a program that would drastically reduce the incidence of low-birth-weight infants, what would you do, given what you now know? Where and how would you target your efforts?

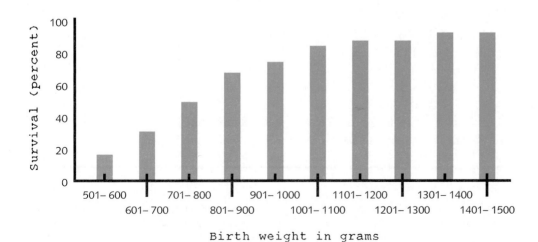

FIGURE 3.4 Among very-low-birth-weight infants, survival is clearly correlated with birth weight. (*Source*: Hack et al., 1991b, Figure 2, p. 590.)

Table 3.1
Two Examples of Long-Term Outcomes for Very-Low-Birth-Weight Infants

| | Australian Study[a] | U.S. Study[b] | |
	500–999 g	<750 g	750–1500 g
Number of babies followed	89	68	65
Age at testing	8 years	7 years	7 years
Percent with severe problems of some type (IQ below 70, deaf, blind, cerebral-palsied, etc.)	21.3	37.5	17.5
Additional percent with significant learning problem or IQ between 70 and 85	19.1	29	20

[a]Victorian Infant Collaborative Study Group, 1991. The study included all surviving children of 500–999 g born in a single state (Victoria) in Australia between 1979 and 1980. A total of 351 infants was born in this weight range, so only a quarter survived. With today's medical techniques, survival rates might be higher.

[b]Hack et al., 1994. The study includes the 68 survivors of a group of 243 children born in an area in Ohio from 1982 to 1986 with birth weights below 750 g, plus a comparison group born in the same period who were between 750 and 1500 g at birth.

problems do not appear until school age, when the child is challenged by a new level of cognitive task. Many surviving LBW children who appear to be developing normally at age 2 or 3 later show significant problems in school. Third (and much more optimistically), even in the extremely low-birth-weight group, some children seem to be fine. So it is not the case that *all* LBW children are *somewhat* affected; rather, *some* LBW children are significantly affected while others develop normally. Unfortunately, physicians and researchers have not yet found reliable ways to predict which babies are likely to have later difficulties, beyond the general correlation with birth weight itself. We do know that those babies who experience intraventricular hemorrhage (hemorrhage in the brain) in the weeks immediately after birth are more likely to have later problems (e.g., Bendersky & Lewis, 1994), but even in this group, significant deficits at school age are not universal. Our ignorance means that parents of LBW infants may be left in suspense for many years.

One piece of good news is that we do now know something about treatments that seem to improve the long-term chances of good functioning for LBW infants. Babies provided with special kinds of rhythmic stimulation while still in the hospital, such as water beds, rocking beds, heartbeat sounds, or body massage, are more alert, gain weight faster, and may even have higher IQs later than preterm babies receiving more typical hospital care (Barnard & Bee, 1983; Scafidi et al., 1990). And when special cognitive, emotional, and social supports are provided to such infants and to their families—such as helping the mothers to learn better skills for interaction with their babies or providing stimulating day care for the infants directly—the infants have a better chance of developing normally (Brooks-Gunn et al., 1993a; Spiker, Ferguson, & Brooks-Gunn, 1993).

Table 3.2
Evaluation Method for Apgar Score

Aspect of Infant Observed	Score Assigned		
	0	1	2
Heart rate	Absent	<100/min.	>100/min.
Respiratory rate	No breathing	Weak cry and shallow breathing	Good, strong cry and regular breathing
Muscle tone	Flaccid	Some flexion of extremities	Well flexed
Response to stimulation of feet	None	Some motion	Cry
Color	Blue; pale	Body pink, extremities blue	Completely pink

Source: Francis, Self, & Horowitz, 1987, pp. 731–732.

Assessing the Newborn

It has become customary in most hospitals to evaluate an infant's status immediately after birth and then again five minutes later, to detect any problems that may require special care. By far the most frequently used assessment system is something called an **Apgar score,** developed by a physician, Virginia Apgar (1953). The newborn is given a score of 0, 1, or 2 on each of five criteria, listed in Table 3.2. A maximum score of 10 is fairly unusual immediately after birth, because most infants are still somewhat blue in the fingers and toes at that stage. At the five-minute assessment, however, 85 to 90 percent of infants are scored as 9 or 10, meaning that they are getting off to a good start. Any score of 7 or better indicates that the baby is in no danger. A score of 4, 5, or 6 usually means that the baby needs help establishing normal breathing patterns; a score of 3 or below indicates a baby in critical condition, requiring active intervention. But the great majority of babies with such low Apgar scores have no long-term problems. Low scores are associated with long-term risk primarily when the infant grows up in nonoptimal circumstances. In stimulating and supportive environments, most children with low Apgar scores appear to develop normally (Breitmayer & Ramey, 1986).

Adapting to the Newborn

The baby is born and Mom, Dad, and infant return home and must now adapt to one another and to the massive changes in their lives occasioned by this new member of the family. For most adults, the role of parent brings profound satisfaction, a greater sense of purpose and self-worth, and a feeling of being grown up. And it may bring a sense of shared joy between husband and wife (Umberson & Gove, 1989). But it is also true that the birth of the first child signals a whole series of changes in parents' lives, and not all these changes are without strain.

In particular, marital satisfaction typically goes down in the first months and years after the first child is born (Glenn, 1990). Individuals and couples report a sense of strain made up partly of fatigue and partly of a feeling that there is too much to cope with, anxiety about not knowing how best to care for the child, and a strong sense of loss of time and intimacy in the marriage relationship itself (Feldman, 1987). In longitudinal studies in which couples have been observed or interviewed during pregnancy and then again in the months after the first child's birth, spouses typically report fewer expressions of love, fewer positive actions designed to maintain or support the relationship, and more expressions of ambivalence after the child's birth than before (Belsky, Lang, & Rovine, 1985). Such strains and reduced satisfaction are less noticeable when the child was planned rather than unplanned and among those couples whose marriage was strong and stable before the birth of the child. But virtually all couples experience some strain.

The Newborn: What Can He Do?

Who is this small stranger who brings both joy and strain? What qualities and skills does the newborn bring to this new interactive process? He cries, breathes, looks around a bit. But what else can he do in the early hours and days? On what skills does the infant build?

Reflexes

Infants are born with a large collection of **reflexes,** which are physical responses triggered automatically and involuntarily by a specific stimulus. Many of these reflexes are still present in adults, so you should be familiar with them, such as the knee jerk the doctor tests for or an automatic eye blink when a puff of air hits your eye.

The newborn's reflexes can be roughly grouped into two categories. First, many *adaptive reflexes* help the baby survive in the world into which he is born. Sucking and swallowing reflexes are prominent in this category. So is the rooting reflex—the automatic turn of the head toward any touch on the cheek, a reflex that helps the baby get the nipple into his mouth during nursing. These reflexes are no longer present in older children or adults but are clearly highly adaptive for the newborn.

Other adaptive reflexes persist over the whole life span, including a withdrawal reaction from a painful stimulus, the opening and closing of the pupil of the eye to variations in brightness, and many others. Finally, some reflexes were adaptive in evolutionary history and are still present in newborn humans, even though they are no longer helpful. The grasping reflex is one clear example. If you place your finger across a newborn baby's palm, he will reflexively close his fist tightly around your finger. If you do this with both palms, the baby's grasp is strong enough so that you can lift him up by his hands in this way. This reflex is also seen in monkeys and apes, for whom it is highly useful, since the infant must be able to cling to the mother's body while she moves about or to a tree branch or vine. Most observers assume that this reflex in humans is merely one residual from our evolutionary past.

A second category includes the *primitive reflexes,* so called because they are controlled by the more primitive parts of the brain, the medulla and the midbrain, both of which are close to being fully developed at birth. For example, if you make a loud noise or startle a baby in some other way, you'll see her throw her arms outward and arch her

The Real World

Postpartum Depression

An added difficulty for many women after the birth of a child is a period of depressed mood, often called the "maternity blues" or "postpartum blues." Estimates vary, but Western studies suggest that something between half and three-quarters of all women go through a brief period of crying often and feeling unexpectedly low in mood (Hopkins, Marcus, & Campbell, 1984). Most women pass through this depression in a few days and then return to a more positive and more stable mood state. But somewhere between 10 and 25 percent of women appear to experience a longer-lasting and more severe postpartum mood disturbance, commonly called a **postpartum depression**—a pattern found in studies in Australia, China, Sweden, and Scotland as well as in the U.S. (Campbell et al., 1992; Guo, 1993; Lundh & Gyllang, 1993; Webster et al., 1994).

Clinicians use the term *depression* or the phrase *clinical depression* to describe more than just the blues, although sadness or persisting low mood is one of the critical ingredients. To be diagnosed as suffering from a clinical depression, including postpartum depression, a person must also show at least half of the following additional symptoms: poor appetite, sleep disturbances (inability to sleep, or excessive sleep), loss of pleasure in everyday activities, feelings of worthlessness, complaints of diminished ability to think or concentrate, or recurrent thoughts of death or suicide.

You can see from this description that such a depressive episode is not a trivial experience. So the fact that as many as 2 women out of every 10 experience such feelings after the birth of a child is striking. Fortunately, postpartum depression is normally shorter than other forms of clinical depression. Six to eight weeks seems to be the typical duration, after which the woman gradually recovers her normal mood, although for perhaps 1 or 2 percent of women the depression persists for a year or longer.

The origins of these depressive episodes are not totally clear, although new research points to the likelihood that hormone patterns play a key role. Specifically, it looks as if women who have unusually high levels of steroid hormones in the late stage of their pregnancies are more likely to experience depression, apparently as a kind of withdrawal symptom from the rapid decline in hormones (Harris et al., 1994). Postnatal depression is also more common in women who did not plan their pregnancy, who were high in anxiety during the pregnancy, or whose partner is not supportive of them or is displeased with the arrival of the child (Campbell et al., 1992; O'Hara et al., 1992). When a woman has experienced high levels of life changes during the pregnancy and immediately after the birth—changes such as moving, death of someone close, loss of a job, or the like—her risk of depression also rises.

Understandably, mothers who are in the midst of a significant postpartum depression interact differently with their infants than do mothers whose mood is more normal. For example, Alison Fleming and her colleagues (1988) found that depressed mothers stroked and touched their infants with affection less frequently in the first three months after delivery than did nondepressed mothers. However, these differences did *not* persist after the mother's depression lifted; at 16 months, Fleming could find no differences in mother–child interaction between the mothers who had been depressed and those who had not.

I think it is quite common in our society to pass off a woman's postpartum depression as if it were a minor event, "just the blues." And of course for many women, it is. But for a minority, the arrival of a child ushers in a much more significant depressive episode, requiring at the very least a sympathetic and supportive environment, if not clinical intervention.

back, a pattern that is part of the *Moro* or *startle* reflex (shown in Figure 3.5). Stroke the bottom of her foot and she will splay out her toes and then curl them in, called the *Babinsky* reflex.

By about 6 months of age, when the portion of the brain governing such complex activities as perception, body movement, thinking, and language has developed more fully, these primitive reflexes begin to disappear, as if superseded by the more complex brain functions. When such reflexes persist past this age, it may signal the existence of

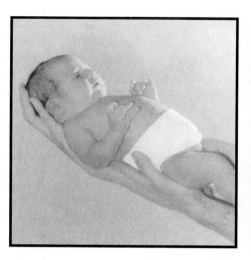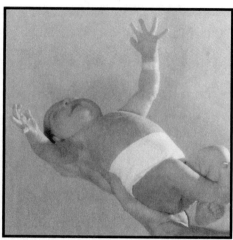

FIGURE 3.5 These two photos show the Moro reflex very well. In the photo on the left, the baby is fairly relaxed, but when the adult suddenly drops the baby (and catches him again), the baby throws his arms out and arches his back. This reflex is present for about the first six months.

some kind of neurological problem. The Babinsky, in particular, is used as a diagnostic tool by neurologists if they suspect the existence of some brain dysfunction in a child or adult.

These two categories of reflexes obviously overlap. Many adaptive reflexes—including the sucking and rooting reflexes—begin to fade late in the first year of life, indicating that they are controlled by the more primitive parts of the brain. But I think it is still helpful to distinguish between those reflexes that continue to have daily usefulness for the baby and those that are more purely reflections of the status of the nervous system, without other adaptive functions.

What would be different about development and about adult-baby interactions if babies were born *without* any reflexes but instead had to learn every behavior?

Perceptual Skills: What the Newborn Sees, Hears, and Feels

I'll be describing the infant's perceptual skills in detail in Chapter 5 and do not want to steal all that thunder. So let me merely summarize very briefly.

- The newborn can focus both eyes on the same spot, with 8 inches being roughly the best focal distance. Within a few weeks the baby can at least roughly follow a moving object with his eyes, and he can discriminate Mom's face from other faces almost immediately.

- He can easily hear sounds within the pitch and loudness ranges of the human voice; he can roughly locate objects by their sounds and can discriminate some individual voices, particularly the mother's voice.

- He can taste the four basic tastes (sweet, sour, bitter, and salty) and can identify familiar body odors. From birth, he can recognize his mother by her smell.

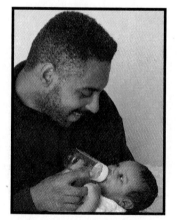

Newborns are pretty nearsighted, but they can focus very well at a distance of about 8 to 10 inches—just about the distance between 2-week-old Christian's eyes and his father's face when Dad holds him to give him a bottle.

Brief as this summary is, several points nonetheless stand out. First of all, newborns' perceptual skills are a great deal better than most parents believe—better than most psychologists or physicians believed until a few years ago. The better our research techniques have become, the more we have understood just how skillful the newborn baby really is.

Even more striking is how well adapted the baby's perceptual skills are for the interactions he will have with the people in his world. He hears best in the range of the human voice, and he can discriminate mother (or other regular caregiver) from others on the basis of smell, sight, or sound almost immediately. The distance at which he can focus his eyes best, about 8 inches, is roughly the distance between the infant's eyes and the mother's face during nursing.

You'll see in Chapter 5 that there is a long way to go in the development of sophisticated perceptual abilities. But the newborn begins life able to make key discriminations and to locate objects through various perceptual cues.

Motor Skills: Moving Around

In contrast, the motor skills of the newborn are not very impressive. She can't hold up her head; she can't coordinate her looking and her reaching yet; she can't roll over or sit up. These skills emerge only gradually in the early weeks. By 1 month, the baby can hold her chin up off the floor or mattress. By 2 months, she is beginning to swipe at objects near her with her hands.

One of the striking features of young babies' movements is how repetitively they perform their limited range of skills. They kick, rock, wave, bounce, bang, rub, scratch, or sway repeatedly and rhythmically. These repeated patterns become particularly prominent at about 6 or 7 months of age, although you can see some such behavior even in the first weeks, particularly in finger movements and leg kicking. These movements do not seem to be totally voluntary or coordinated, but they also do not appear to be random. For instance, Esther Thelen (1981) has observed that kicking movements peak just before the baby begins to crawl, as if the rhythmic kicking were a part of the preparation for crawling. Thelen's work has helped us see the patterns and order in the apparently random movements of the young infant. But even this understanding does not alter the fact that, by contrast with perceptual abilities, the baby's initial motor abilities are quite limited.

Learning and Habituation

It seems obvious that maturation must play a vital role in these early developmental processes. The body systems and parts of the nervous system required for many perceptual skills are largely complete at birth, while those needed for motor control are not.

But is maturation the only process involved? Can a newborn also learn from her experiences? This question has intrigued researchers for decades, for both theoretical and practical reasons. From a theoretical perspective the question is obviously crucial for understanding the relative influences of nature and nurture. From a practical point of view, the same question is also important, because the answer affects the sort of advice parents may be given about appropriate toys or stimulation for their child. For example, if a child's perceptual abilities develop largely through maturation rather than learning, then it doesn't make much sense to buy expensive mobiles to hang above the baby's crib. But if learning is possible from the earliest days of life, then various kinds of enrichment make much more sense.

What does the evidence tell us?

Classical Conditioning. The bulk of the research suggests that the newborn can be classically conditioned, although it is difficult. By 3 or 4 weeks of age, classical conditioning is quite easy to demonstrate in an infant. In particular, this means that the conditioned

Calves, foals, lambs, and newborns of virtually all mammals other than humans can stand and walk within a few hours of birth. Can you think of any useful evolutionary function for the greater motor helplessness of the human newborn?

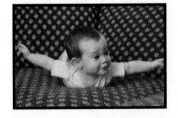

Young Lucy was 5 months old when this photo was taken, showing her "airplaning." By this age, you can see that she is able to hold not just her head but part of her chest off the ground—a big advance over the motor skills we see in newborns.

emotional responses I talked about in Chapter 1 may begin to develop as early as the first weeks of life. Thus, the mere presence of Mom or Dad or other favored person may trigger the sense of "feeling good," a pattern that may contribute to what we see as the child's attachment to the parent. Similarly, a child might develop various classically conditioned negative emotional responses that may be part of what we see as temperament.

Operant Conditioning. Newborns also clearly learn by operant conditioning. Both the sucking response and head turning have been successfully increased by the use of reinforcements, such as sweet-tasting liquids or the sound of the mother's voice or heartbeat (Moon & Fifer, 1990). At the least, the fact that conditioning of this kind can take place means that whatever neurological wiring is needed for learning to occur is present at birth. Results like this also tell us something about the sorts of reinforcements that are effective with very young children. It is surely highly significant for the whole process of mother-infant interaction that the mother's voice is an effective reinforcer for virtually all babies.

Schematic Learning. The fact that babies can recognize voices and heartbeats in the first days of life is also important because it suggests that another kind of learning is going on as well. This third type of learning, sometimes referred to as *schematic learning,* draws both its name and many of its conceptual roots from Piaget's theory. The basic idea is that from the beginning the baby organizes her experiences into expectancies, into "known" combinations. These expectancies, often called *schemas,* are built up over many exposures to particular experiences but thereafter help the baby to distinguish between the familiar and the unfamiliar. Carolyn Rovee-Collier (1986) has suggested that we might think of classical conditioning in infants as being a variety of schematic learning. When a baby begins to move her head as if to search for the nipple as soon as she hears her Mom's footsteps coming into the room, this is not just some kind of automatic classical conditioning, but the beginning of the development of expectancies. From the earliest weeks, the baby seems to begin to make connections between events in her world, such as the link between the sound of her mother's footsteps and the feeling of being picked up, or between the touch of the breast and the feeling of a full stomach. Thus, early classical conditioning may be the beginnings of the process of cognitive development.

Habituation. A related concept is that of **habituation.** Habituation is the automatic reduction in the strength or vigor of a response to a repeated stimulus. An example would probably help: Suppose you live on a fairly noisy street. The sound of cars going by is repeated over and over during each day. But after a while, you not only don't react to the sound, but quite literally *do not perceive it as being as loud.* The ability to do this—to dampen down the intensity of a physical response to some repeated stimulus—is obviously vital in our everyday lives. If we reacted constantly to every sight and sound and smell that came along, we'd spend all our time responding to these repeated events and not have energy or attention left over for things that are new and deserve attention.

The ability to *dishabituate* is equally important. When a habituated stimulus changes in some way, such as a sudden extra-loud screech of tires on the busy street by your house, you again respond fully. Thus, the reemergence of the original response strength is a sign that the perceiver—infant, child, or adult—notices some significant change.

It is very clear that a newborn is able both to habituate and to dishabituate. She will stop looking at something you keep putting in front of her face; she will stop showing a startle reaction (Moro reflex) to loud sounds after the first few presentations but will again show a startle response if the sound is changed. Such habituation itself is not a vol-

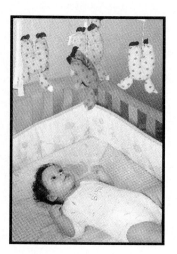

If you know that babies can see and respond to objects, you're much more likely to buy mobiles to hang over the crib, as 3-month-old Shina-Mira's parents have done.

untary process; it is entirely automatic. But for it to work, the newborn must be equipped with the capacity to "recognize" familiar experiences. That is, she must have, or must develop, schemas of some kind.

The existence of these processes in the newborn has an added benefit for researchers: It has enabled them to figure out what an infant responds to as "the same" or "different." If a baby is habituated to some stimulus, such as a sound or a specific picture, the experimenter can then present slight variations on the original stimulus to see the point at which dishabituation occurs. In this way, researchers have begun to get a picture of how the newborn baby or young infant experiences the world around him—a point I'll come back to in Chapter 5.

Social Skills

All the skills of the newborn I have described so far are important for the baby's comfort and survival. But human newborns, unlike those in many other species, are a very long way from being independent. If they are to survive, someone must provide consistent care over an extended period. So the infant's capacity to entice others into the caregiving role is critical. It is here that the "social" skills of infants come into play.

The newborn doesn't have a lot of obvious social abilities. He doesn't talk. He doesn't flirt. He smiles, but not often during the first weeks. Normal newborns nonetheless have a collection of behaviors that are remarkably effective for attracting and keeping the attention of adults. The reverse is also true, as I pointed out in talking about the baby's perceptual abilities: Adult faces and voices are remarkably effective for attracting and keeping the baby's attention too. It would seem from all this that the adult and the baby are programmed from the beginning to join in a crucial social "dance," one that forms the root of the developing relationship between parent and child and that is critical for the formation of the parent's bond to the child.

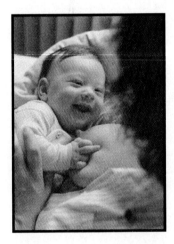

The baby's repertoire of social behaviors is quite limited, but these few behaviors appear to be very effective in eliciting nurturing. He cries when he needs something, which ordinarily brings someone to him to provide care. And then he responds to that care by being soothed, which is very reinforcing to the caregivers. He adjusts his body to yours when you pick him up; after the first few weeks, he gets quite good at meeting your eyes in a mutual gaze, or smiling—both of which are very powerful "hooks" for the adult's continued attention.

Who could resist this baby's smile and mutual gaze?

One other thing the baby does from the beginning, which seems to be critical for any social interaction, is to take turns. As adults, we take turns all the time, most clearly in conversations and eye contacts. In fact, it's very difficult to have any kind of social encounter with someone who does *not* take turns. Kenneth Kaye (1982) argues that the beginnings of this "turn taking" can be seen in very young infants in their eating patterns. As early as the first days of life, the baby sucks in a "burst-pause" pattern. He sucks for a while, pauses, sucks for a while, pauses, and so on. Mothers enter into this "conversation" too, often by jiggling the baby during the pauses. The eventual sequence looks something like this: Suck, pause, jiggle, pause, suck, pause, jiggle, pause. The rhythm of the interaction is really very much like a conversation. To be sure, we cannot be certain whether this conversational quality of very early interaction occurs because the adult figures out the baby's natural rhythm and adapts her own responses to the baby's timing or whether some mutual adaptation is going on. Nonetheless it is extremely intriguing that we can see this apparent turn taking in an infant 1 day old.

The Daily Life of Infants

Parents are obviously interested in the various skills and capacities of the newborn infant. They are delighted with his smiles and with each new ability as it emerges. But for most parents, the real questions are more practical: What is it like to live with a newborn? How is the infant's day organized? What sort of natural rhythms occur in the daily cycles? What can you expect from the baby as you struggle to adapt to and care for this new person in your life?

Researchers who have studied newborns have described five different states of sleep and wakefulness in infants, summarized in Table 3.3. Of these states, the least common in the newborn are the two awake states. At first, babies are awake and not fussing only about two to three hours each day.

The five main states tend to occur in cycles, just as your own states occur in a daily rhythm. Most infants move from deep sleep to lighter sleep to fussing and hunger and then to a brief period of alert wakefulness, after which they become drowsy and drop back into deep sleep. This cycle repeats itself roughly every two hours: Sleep, cry, eat, look; sleep, cry, eat, look. Because the first three parts of this repeating pattern—sleeping, crying, and eating—are so crucial for parents, let me say just a word more about each.

Sleeping

The child's sleep periods are important to parents because they provide breaks in what may otherwise seem like constant care. Newborns sleep as much as 90 percent of the time, as much in the daytime as at night (Whitney & Thoman, 1994). By 6 or 8 weeks of age, the total amount of sleep per day has dropped somewhat and we see signs of day/night sleep rhythms (called *circadian rhythms*)—at least among infants in Western countries, where regular sleep/wake cycles are more highly valued. Babies this age begin to string two or three two-hour cycles together without coming to full wakefulness, at which point we say that the baby

Table 3.3
The Basic States of Infant Sleep and Wakefulness

State	Characteristics
Deep sleep	Eyes closed, regular breathing, no movement except occasional startles
Active sleep	Eyes closed, irregular breathing, small twitches, no gross body movement
Quiet awake	Eyes open, no major body movement, regular breathing
Active awake	Eyes open, with movements of the head, limbs, and trunk; irregular breathing
Crying and fussing	Eyes may be partly or entirely closed, vigorous diffuse movement with crying or fussing sounds

Sources: Based on the work of Prechtl & Beintema, 1964; Hutt, Lenard, & Prechtl, 1969; Parmelee, Wenner, & Schulz, 1964.

can "sleep through the night." By 6 months, babies are still sleeping a bit more than 14 hours per day, but the regularity and predictability of the baby's sleep is even more noticeable—at least in Western samples. Not only do most 6-month-olds have clear nighttime sleep patterns, but they also begin to nap during the day at more predictable times.

I've given you the average figures, but of course babies vary a lot around these norms. Of the 6-week-old babies in one study, there was one who slept 22 hours per day and another who slept only 8.8 hours per day (Bamford et al., 1990). (Now there must be one tired set of parents!) And some babies, even in Western cultures, do not develop a long nighttime sleep period until late in the first year of life.

All these aspects of the baby's sleep pattern have implications for the emerging parent-infant interaction. Psychologists have also been interested in sleep patterns because marked irregularity of sleep patterns may be a symptom of some disorder or problem. Some babies born to mothers who used cocaine during pregnancy have difficulty establishing a regular pattern of sleeping and waking. Brain-damaged infants often have the same kind of difficulties, so any time an infant fails to develop clear sleep/waking regularity, it *may* be a sign of trouble.

Crying

Newborns actually cry less of the time than you might think. One researcher, studying normal newborns, found that the figure ranged from 2 to 11 percent of the time (Korner et al., 1981). Crying seems to increase over the first six weeks of life, and then it decreases. Initially, infants cry most in the evening; then they shift their crying more toward times just before feedings.

The basic function of the child's cry, obviously, is to signal need. Because babies can't move *to* someone to get taken care of, they have to *bring* someone to them, and crying is the main way they have to attract attention. In fact, infants have a whole repertoire of cry sounds, with different cries for pain or anger or hunger. The basic cry, which often signals hunger, is usually a rhythmical pattern: cry, silence, breath, cry, silence, breath, with a kind of whistling sound often accompanying the in-breath. An anger cry is typically louder and more intense, and the pain cry normally has a very abrupt onset—unlike the more basic kinds of cries, which usually begin with whimpering or moaning. However, not all infants cry in precisely the same way, so each parent must learn the specific sounds of his or her own baby. Alen Wiesenfeld and his colleagues (Wiesenfeld, Malatesta, & DeLoach, 1981) found that mothers (but not fathers) of 5-month-olds could discriminate between taped episodes of anger and pain cries in their own babies, while neither parent could reliably make the same discrimination with the taped cries of another baby.

In all of this, as with the nature of the cries themselves, there are wide individual differences. Fifteen to 20 percent of infants develop a pattern called *colic*, which involves daily, intense bouts of crying, totaling three or more hours a day. The crying is generally worst in late afternoon or early evening—a particularly inopportune time, of course, because parents are tired and needing time with one another then too. Colic typically appears at about 2 weeks of age and then disappears spontaneously at 3 or 4 months of age. Neither psychologists nor physicians know why colic begins or why it stops without any intervention. It is a difficult pattern to live with, but the good news is that it *does* go away.

One of the enduring practical questions for parents about a baby's crying is how they should respond to it. If they pick up the baby right away, every time he cries, will that simply reinforce the baby's crying, so that he will cry more? Or will such an immediate re-

How can you interpret the observation that mothers are better at discriminating among the various meanings of their baby's cries than are fathers? How could you design a study that would let you test your interpretation?

Research Report

Variations in Children's Cries

Parents have always known that some babies had cries that were particularly penetrating or grating; other babies seem to have much less noxious crying sounds. Researchers have confirmed this parental observation in a wide range of studies.

Many groups of babies with known medical abnormalities have different-sounding cries, including those with Down syndrome, encephalitis, meningitis, and many types of brain damage. In recent work, Barry Lester has extended this observation to babies who appear physically normal but are at risk for later problems because of some perinatal problem, such as preterm or small-for-date babies (Lester, 1987; Lester & Dreher, 1989). Such babies typically make crying sounds that are acoustically distinguishable from what you hear in a normal, low-risk baby. In particular, the cry of such higher-risk babies has a more grating, piercing quality. Interestingly, the cries of babies with colic also have some of these same qualities (Lester et al., 1992).

On the assumption that the baby's cry may reflect some basic aspect of neurological integrity, Lester also wondered whether one could use the quality of the cry as a *diagnostic* test. Among a group of high-risk babies, for example, could one predict later intellectual functioning from a measure of the gratingness or pitch of the baby's cry? The answer seems to be yes. Lester found that among preterms, those with higher-pitched cries in the first days of life had lower scores on an IQ test at age 5 years (Lester, 1987). The same kind of connection has also been found among both normal babies and those exposed to methadone prenatally. In all these groups, the higher the pitch and more grating the cry, the lower the child's later IQ or motor development (Huntington, Hans, & Zeskind, 1990).

Eventually, it may be possible for physicians to use the presence of such a grating or piercing cry as a signal that there may be some underlying physical problem with the infant or as a way of making better guesses about the long-term outcomes for individual babies at high risk of later problems, such as low-birth-weight babies.

sponse reassure the child, building the child's expectation that the world is a safe and reliable place?

Ten years ago I was confident that I knew the answer to this question, namely, always to respond immediately. Results from early studies gave no indication that such immediate responding increased the child's crying, and there was a lot of evidence that predictable responding was one ingredient in the development a secure attachment to the parent. More recent studies, though, make the answer less clear-cut. It now looks as if the parents' response may need to depend on the type of crying the child is doing. Intense crying, such as when the infant is hurt or significantly distressed—very hungry, very wet and uncomfortable, or the like—should be responded to immediately. But whimpering and milder crying, such as what a baby may do when she is put down for a nap, is another matter. When a parent responds immediately to all these milder cries, babies seem to learn to cry more often (Hubbard & van IJzendoorn, 1987). Thus, both reassurance and reinforcement seem to be involved, and it takes real sensitivity on the part of the parent to sort it out.

Eating

Eating is not a "state," but it is certainly something that newborn babies do frequently! Given the normal two-hour cycle of a newborn baby's day, the infant may eat as many as 10 times a day. By 1 month the average number is down to about five and a half feedings, with a very gradual decline from that number over the first year (Barnard & Eyres, 1979).

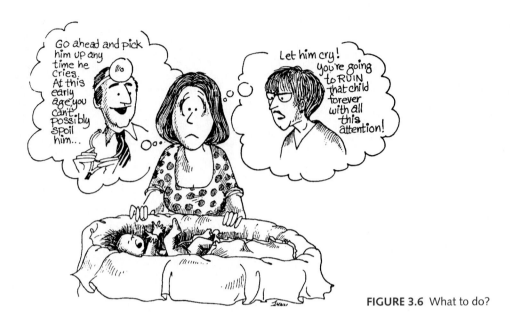

FIGURE 3.6 What to do?

Both breast-fed and bottle-fed babies eat about as frequently, but these two forms of feeding do differ in other important ways.

Breast- Versus Bottle-feeding. After several decades of extensive research in many countries, physicians and epidemiologists have reached clear agreement that breast-feeding is substantially superior nutritionally to bottle-feeding. Breast milk provides important antibodies for the infant against many kinds of diseases, especially gastrointestinal and upper respiratory infections (Cunningham, Jelliffe, & Jelliffe, 1991). Human breast milk also appears to promote the growth of nerves and intestinal tract, and may stimulate better immune system function over the long term.

Those women who find breast-feeding logistically difficult because of work or other demands may take some comfort from the fact that the research indicates that babies derive some protection from as little as one breast-feeding per day. There is also comfort in the observation that the *social* interactions between mother and child seem to suffer no ill effects from bottle-feeding. Bottle-fed babies are held and cuddled in the same ways as are breast-fed babies, and their mothers appear to be just as sensitive and responsive to their babies as are mothers of breast-fed infants (Field, 1977).

I do not want this set of statements to provoke intense guilt in those of you who find that you are physically or otherwise unable to breast-feed. Babies can and do thrive on formula. But it is clear that *if* you have a choice, babies will derive real benefits from breast-feeding.

What specific changes in policies or practices do you think would increase the rate of breast-feeding in the United States (or in your own country)?

Individual Differences Among Babies

Most of my emphasis in the past few pages has been on the many ways infants are alike. Barring some kind of physical damage, all babies have similar sensory equipment at birth and can experience the same kinds of happenings around them. They all sleep, eat, and cry. But babies also differ in important ways—in health, in temperament, even in their patterns of crying.

Cultures and Contexts

Cultural and Social Class Differences in Patterns of Breast-feeding

If you look at the incidence of breast-feeding in countries around the world over the past 40 or 50 years, you'll find some very curious patterns. In the 1950s and 1960s, breast-feeding declined dramatically in most Western countries, including the United States. By 1971, only 25 percent of U.S. women breast-fed even for a few weeks. At the same time, breast-feeding continued to be the normative method of infant feeding in non-Western countries, including virtually all Third World countries (World Health Organization, 1981).

In the succeeding two decades, these two trends reversed. Breast-feeding rose sharply in most industrialized countries as evidence of its importance has come to light; by 1984, 60 percent of U.S. women breast-fed for at least a few weeks (Ryan et al., 1991). In the same years an opposite trend occurred in most Third World and developing countries: Breast-feeding remained the most common mode of infant feeding, but rates and durations of breast-feeding began to drop in many countries, particularly among those living in urban settings.

One contributor to the decline of breast-feeding in less-industrialized countries appears to have been the marketing of infant formula. Manufacturers of formula often gave free samples or free feeding bottles to new mothers and assured women that formula is as good or better for babies, while frequently failing to provide adequate instruction on how formula should be used. Some women, knowing no better and faced with extreme economic hardship, diluted their infants' formula with water to make it stretch further. Sterilization procedures were also not well explained; for many women, proper sterilization was simply not feasible. Worldwide, the concern aroused by this change in normal feeding practices was sufficient to cause the World Health Organization to issue an "International Code of Marketing of Breast-milk Substitutes" in 1981. Marketing practices have since been modified. Yet the decline in breast-feeding has continued (Stewart et al., 1991).

Such a decline is cause for real concern, because bottle-fed babies in developing or Third World countries are at far higher risk of serious disease or death. In Bangladesh, for example, the risk of death from diarrhea is three times higher among bottle-fed than among breast-fed babies; in Brazil, the risk of death from various kinds of infections ranges from 2 1/2 to 14 times higher among the bottle-fed. In all these studies, the risk associated with bottle-feeding is far higher where the sanitary conditions are poorest (Cunningham et al., 1991). Breast-feeding is thus better for two reasons: It provides the baby with needed antibodies against infection, and it is likely to expose the baby to less infection in the first place.

Patterns in the U.S.

In view of such findings, it is disturbing to find that in the United States the trend line is again downward. Between 1984 and 1989 the percentage of women beginning breast-feeding dropped from 60 to 52 percent (Ryan et al., 1991). At both time points, it was the same subgroups that were more likely to breast-feed: older, well-educated, or higher-income mothers. Whites are also more likely than blacks or Hispanics to breast-feed. In 1989, the respective rates in the first weeks of the baby's life were 58, 23, and 48 percent (Ryan et al., 1991). In all three groups, however, better-educated mothers are more likely to breast-feed, while the less-educated and the poor are least likely to do so (MacGowan et al., 1991). This pattern is of special concern because rates of mortality and illness are already higher among infants born to poor mothers.

A mother's work status also makes some difference in her decision about breast- or bottle-feeding, but it is *not* the deciding factor in many cases. The majority of women who do *not* work also do not breast-feed, while many working women find creative ways to combine employment and breast-feeding (Ryan et al., 1991). If we had societal supports for such a combination, it could be made still easier.

Overall, it is clear that a large public health task still remains, not only in the United States but around the world, to educate women still further about the importance of breast-feeding and to create the cultural and practical supports needed to make breast-feeding easier.

Health and Death in the First Year

Virtually all babies get sick, most of them repeatedly. In the United States, the average baby has seven respiratory illnesses in the first year of life. (That's a lot of nose-wipes!) Interestingly, a whole series of studies shows that the incidence of such illnesses is higher among babies in day care than among those reared entirely at home, presumably because babies in group care settings are exposed to a wider range of germs and viruses (Hurwitz et al., 1991). In general, the more different people a baby is exposed to, the more often she is likely to be sick. But this is not the unmitigated negative that it may appear to be. Children reared entirely at home, with low exposure to others, have very high rates of illness when they first attend school. Attendance at day care simply means that the baby is exposed earlier to the various microorganisms that cause upper respiratory infections.

Infant Mortality. For a small minority of babies, though, the issue is not a few sniffles, but the possibility of death. I mentioned in the last chapter that in 1993, 8.3 babies out of every 1000 in the U.S. died before age 1. Almost two-thirds of these deaths occurred in the first month of life and were directly linked either to congenital anomalies or to low birth weight. In 1993, only about three deaths per 1000 births occurred in the remainder of the first year, and nearly half of those were cases of **sudden infant death syndrome (SIDS),** in which an apparently healthy infant dies suddenly and unexpectedly. In 1993, 4930 babies in the United States died of SIDS (Wegman, 1994).

SIDS is certainly not unique to the U.S. It occurs worldwide, although for unexplained reasons, the rate varies quite a lot from country to country. SIDS rates are particularly high, for example, in Australia and New Zealand, and particularly low in Japan and Sweden (Hoffman & Hillman, 1992).

Physicians have not yet uncovered the basic cause of these deaths. But we have learned a fair amount about the groups that are at higher risk: babies with low birth weight, males, blacks, those with young mothers, and those whose mothers smoked during pregnancy or after birth. SIDS is also more common in the wintertime and appears to be somewhat more common among babies who sleep on their stomachs (Hoffman & Hillman, 1992; Ponsonby et al., 1993), especially if the baby is sleeping on a soft or fluffy mattress, pillow, or comforter.

The growing evidence on the role of sleeping position persuaded pediatricians in many countries to change their standard advice to hospitals and families about the best sleeping position for babies. The American Academy of Pediatrics, for example, has been recommending since 1992 that when healthy infants are put down to sleep, they should be positioned on their sides or backs. This change in policy has been followed by a 12 percent drop in SIDS cases nationwide, with even more dramatic declines of as much as 50 percent in areas where the new recommendation has been widely publicized (Spiers & Guntheroth, 1994). Still, sleeping position cannot be the full explanation, because of course *most* babies who sleep on their stomachs do not die of SIDS.

The link between SIDS and maternal (or paternal) smoking is also becoming clearer and clearer: Babies whose mothers smoked during their pregnancy or who are exposed to smoke in the months after birth are about four times as likely to die of SIDS as are babies with no smoking exposure (Mitchell et al., 1993; Schoendorf & Kiely, 1992). One more powerful reason not to smoke. . . .

The higher risk of SIDS for African-American infants is part of a persistent pattern. You will remember from the last chapter that infant mortality is more than twice as high among black infants as among whites. An equivalent disadvantage exists for Native-American infants (Honigfeld & Kaplan, 1987). These persistent and disturbing differences appear to reflect not only variations in the availability of adequate prenatal care but also a lack of support for poor mothers and their infants after delivery. Poor infants, including both African-Americans and Native Americans, are less likely to receive appropriate immunizations, more likely to be ill, less likely to be seen by a doctor when they are ill, and four times as likely to die of such entirely preventable diseases as gastroenteritis (Starfield, 1991; Wegman, 1993).

Temperament

Another way babies differ, other than health, is in their *temperament.* Babies vary in the way they react to new things, in their typical moods, in their rate of activity, in their preference for social interactions or solitude, in the regularity of their daily rhythms, and in many other ways. I'll be talking about temperament at greater length in Chapter 9, but because the concept will come up often as we go along, it is important at this early stage to introduce some of the basic terms and ideas.

Psychologists who have been interested in these differences have proposed several different ways of describing the key dimensions of temperament. Buss and Plomin (1984; 1986) propose three dimensions: emotionality, activity, and sociability. Thomas and Chess (1977) describe nine dimensions, which they organize into three types: the easy child, the difficult child, and the slow-to-warm-up child.

As you'll see in Chapter 9, it is not yet clear whether one of these views, or some other, will eventually carry the theoretical day. But the Thomas and Chess formulation has been the most influential one thus far, so let me describe their three basic types for you.

The Easy Child. Easy children approach new events positively. They try new foods without much fuss, for example. They are also regular in biological functioning, with good sleeping and eating cycles, are usually happy, and adjust easily to change.

The Difficult Child. By contrast, the difficult child is less regular in body functioning and is slow to develop regular sleeping and eating cycles. These children react vigorously and negatively to new things, are more irritable, and cry more. Their cries are also more likely to have the higher-pitched, grating quality I talked about in the box on page 86 (Huffman et al., 1994). Thomas and Chess point out, however, that once the difficult baby has adapted to something new, he is often quite happy about it, even though the adaptation process itself is very difficult.

The Slow-to-Warm-Up Child. Children in this group are not as negative in responding to new things or new people as is the difficult child. They show instead a kind of passive resistance. Instead of spitting out new food violently and crying, the slow-to-warm-up child may let the food drool out and may resist mildly any attempt to feed her more of the same. These infants show few intense reactions, either positive or negative, although once they have adapted to something new, their reaction is usually fairly positive.

Interestingly, these temperamental features seem to occur in differing frequency in different cultures—a set of findings I've explored in the *Cultures and Contexts* box on the facing page. But in every culture some kind of temperamental variations can be seen in the very young infant and are at least somewhat persistent throughout childhood.

No psychologist studying temperament suggests that such individual differences are absolutely fixed at birth. Inborn temperamental differences are shaped, strengthened, bent, or counteracted by the child's relationships and experiences. What we do know is

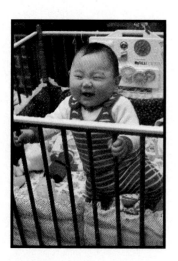

Young Genevieve is clearly delighted to have figured out how to pull herself up to a standing position. If her disposition is typically this sunny and accepting of new experiences, we would say she has an easy temperament.

Cultures and Contexts

Cultural Differences in Infant Temperament

Are infants all over the world alike in their temperaments? Are we just as likely to see a highly active infant in China, or among the Navaho, as among Caucasian infants? Several investigators have concluded that the answer is "no." There appear to be cultural differences in certain aspects of temperament, beginning as early as the first few months of life.

Daniel Freedman (1979) has observed newborn babies from four different cultures: Euro-American, Chinese, Navaho, and Japanese. Of the four, he found that the Euro-American babies were the most active and irritable and the hardest to console (the most "difficult" in Chess and Thomas's terms). Both the Chinese and the Navaho infants were relatively placid, while the Japanese infants responded vigorously but were easier to quiet than the Euro-American infants.

Jerome Kagan and his colleagues (1994) have replicated part of these results in their recent comparison of Chinese, Irish, and Euro-American 4-month-olds. They found that the Chinese infants were significantly less active, less irritable, and less vocal than were babies in the other two groups. The white American infants showed the strongest reactions to new sights, sounds, or smells.

Similarly, Chisholm has replicated Freedman's findings on Navaho babies, finding them to be significantly less irritable, less excitable, and more able to quiet themselves than Euro-American babies (1989).

Since such differences are visible in newborns they cannot be the result of systematic shaping by the parents. But the parents too bring their temperament and their cultural training to the interaction, which may tend to strengthen or perpetuate such temperamental differences. For instance, Freedman and other researchers have observed that both Japanese and Chinese mothers talk much less to their infants than do Caucasian mothers. These differences in mothers' behavior were present from their first encounters with their infants after delivery, so the pattern is not a response to the baby's quieter behavior. But such similarity of temperamental pattern between mother and child is likely to strengthen the pattern in the child, which would tend to make the cultural differences larger over time.

One of the key points from this research is that our notions of what is "normal" behavior for an infant may be strongly influenced by our own cultural patterns and assumptions.

that infants enter the world with somewhat different repertoires or patterns of behavior and that those differences not only affect the experiences the infant may choose, but also help to shape the emerging pattern of interaction that develops between infant and parents. For example, toddlers and preschoolers with difficult temperaments are more often criticized or physically punished by their parents than are easy children, presumably because the child's behavior *is* more troublesome (Bates, 1989). But once established, such a pattern of criticism and punishment itself is likely to have additional consequences for the child.

Nonetheless, not all parents of difficult children respond in this way. A skilled parent, especially one who correctly perceives that the child's "difficultness" is a temperamental quality and not a result of the child's willfulness or the parent's ineptness, can avoid some of the pitfalls and can handle the difficult child more adeptly.

Sex Differences

Finally, as I did in the last chapter, let me add at least a brief word about sex differences. Most of us, when we hear about a new baby's birth, immediately ask, "Is it a boy or a girl?" So this is clearly a highly salient issue for almost all of us. You might assume that such a preoccupation exists because boy and girl babies are really very different from one another. But in fact they are not. There are remarkably few sex differences among young infants. As was true at birth, girls continue to be a bit ahead in some aspects of physical maturity, and boys continue to be more vulnerable. For example, more boys die during the first year of life. Male infants also have more muscle tissue than do girls, and they may be slightly more physically active (Eaton & Enns, 1986), although the data here are quite inconsistent. But boys and girls do not seem to differ on the temperamental dimensions Thomas and Chess have described: Boys are not more often "difficult" in temperament, and girls are not more often "easy," even though that is what our stereotypes might lead us to expect. What dominates the system in these early months is not "boyness" or "girlness" but "babyness."

Summary

1 The normal birth process has three parts: dilation, delivery, and placental delivery.

2 The first "acquaintance" process after delivery may be an especially important one for parents. Most parents show an intense interest in the baby's features, especially the eyes.

3 Most drugs given to the mother during delivery pass through to the infant's bloodstream. They have short-term effects on infant responsiveness and on feeding patterns, but long-term effects are not yet well understood.

4 Home deliveries in uncomplicated pregnancies can be as safe as hospital deliveries.

5 The presence of the father during delivery appears to help reduce the mother's discomfort but appears not to be necessary for the establishment of the father's bond to the infant.

6 More than one-fifth of all deliveries in the U.S. today are by abdominal incision, called cesarean section, because of indications of fetal distress or other specific problems.

7 Several types of problems may occur at birth, including reduced oxygen supply (anoxia) to the infant or low birth weight.

8 Low-birth-weight infants have higher risk of death during the first year of life, but if they survive, most catch up to full-size peers by school age. Those with birth weights below 1500 grams or who are very small for date are more likely to show lasting problems.

9 Most parents experience delight and pleasure at their new role, but there are also strains. The majority of mothers have at least a brief period of "blues"; as many as one-tenth experience a more serious, longer depression. Marital satisfaction also typically declines.

10 The newborn has far more skills than most physicians and psychologists had thought, including excellent reflexes, good perceptual skills, and effective social skills.

11 The important infant reflexes include many crucial adaptive reflexes, such as rooting and sucking.

12 Perceptual skills include focusing both eyes, tracking slowly moving objects, discrimination of the mother by smell and sound, and general responsiveness to smells, tastes, and touch.

13 Motor skills, in contrast, are only rudimentary at birth.

14 Social skills, while rudimentary, are sufficient to bring people close for care and to keep them close for social interactions. The baby can meet a gaze and smile within the first month of life.

15 Newborns can learn from the first days of life and can habituate to repeated stimulation.

16 Cycles of sleeping, waking, crying, and eating are present from the beginning. Newborns sleep 16 to 18 hours per day, and eat roughly 10 times.

17 Breast-feeding has clear benefits to the baby, providing antibodies against diseases and reducing the risk of disease.

18 Other than death caused by low birth weight or congenital anomalies, sudden infant death syndrome is the most common cause of death in the first year. The risk of SIDS is higher in black infants, those with young mothers, or those whose mothers smoked. The cause is not yet understood.

19 Babies differ from one another on several dimensions, including vigor of response, general activity rate, restlessness, irritability, and cuddliness. These temperamental dimensions, which Thomas and Chess have grouped into "difficult," "easy," and "slow-to-warm-up" types, appear to be at least somewhat stable.

20 Male and female babies differ at birth on a few dimensions. Girls are more mature physically. Boys are more active, have more muscle tissue, and are more vulnerable to stress. No sex differences are found, however, on temperamental dimensions such as cuddliness or sootheability.

Key Terms

anoxia (**p. 73**)

Apgar score (**p. 77**)

cesarean section (**p. 72**)

dilation (**p. 67**)

effacement (**p. 67**)

habituation (**p. 82**)

low birth weight (LBW) (**p. 74**)

postpartum depression (**p. 79**)

preterm infant (**p. 74**)

reflexes (**p. 78**)

small-for-date infant (**p. 74**)

sudden infant death syndrome (SIDS) (**p. 89**)

Suggested Readings

Field, T. (1990). *Infancy.* Cambridge, MA: Harvard University Press.

Field reviews what we know about infancy in an engaging and clear style.

Maurer, D., & Maurer, C. (1988). *The world of the newborn.* New York: Basic Books.

An excellent description of the newborn written for the lay reader.

Osofsky, J. D. (Ed.). (1987). *Handbook of infant development* (2nd ed.). New York: Wiley-Interscience.

The material in this splendid collection of papers is considerably more technical than what you will find in Maurer and Maurer. But if you are interested in some specific aspect of infant development, this is an excellent source for a comprehensive review.

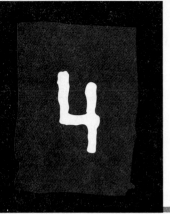

4

Physical Development

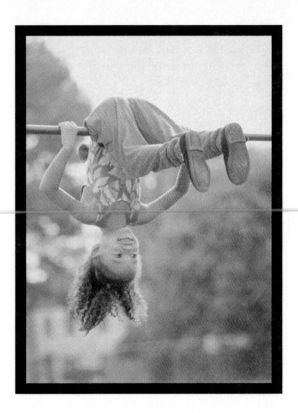

When my daughter (who is now 26) was about 8½, a lot of well-rehearsed family routines seemed to unravel. She was crankier than usual, both more assertive and more needful of affection, and alternately compliant and defiant. What on earth was happening? Had I done something dreadfully wrong? Was something going on at school? I mentioned my problems to several colleagues, many of whom told me their own tales about the special difficulties they had had with their daughters between ages 8 and 9. It finally occured to us all that there might be a physical explanation: Girls of 8 or 9 are actually beginning to experience the first hormone changes of puberty. Perhaps the inconsistent and uncomfortable behaviors I was seeing were one form of response to the changing hormones in the system.

It may amuse you to think of the clever psychologist missing such an obvious possibility. But in fact developmental psychologists have often placed too little emphasis on physical growth. We describe it briefly and then take it for granted. But I am convinced, both by the research literature on the effects of physiological change and by my observations as a parent, that an understanding of physical development is an absolutely critical first step in understanding children's progress, for at least four reasons.

Four Reasons for Studying Physical Development

The Child's Growth Makes New Behaviors Possible.   Specific physical changes are needed before the infant can crawl or walk. Similarly, the development of full reproductive capacity at adolescence is based on a complex sequence of physical changes. Thus, nonobvious physical changes are often the necessary underpinning of behavior change.

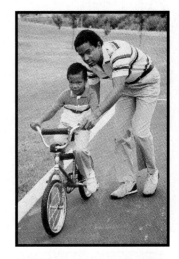

This 6-year-old is still unsteady on his bike. But once he masters this new physical skill, his life will change as he ranges more independently.

The flip side of this is that the *lack* of a particular physical development may set limits on the behaviors a child is capable of performing. An infant of 10 months cannot be toilet trained, no matter how hard parents may try, because the anal sphincter muscle is not yet fully mature. Toddlers cannot easily pick up raisins or Cheerios from their high chair trays until the muscles and nerves required for thumb-forefinger opposition have developed. Six-year-olds cannot reliably hit baseballs or throw basketballs through hoops, no matter how much their parents (or their coaches) may pressure them.

The Child's Growth Determines Experience.   A child's range of physical capacities or skills can also have a major indirect effect on cognitive and social development by influencing the variety of experiences she can have. An infant who is able to sit up can now reach more easily for objects around her; an infant who is able to crawl can explore still more widely, an experience that may have both positive and negative consequences. For example, Bennett Bertenthal and his colleagues (1994) have shown that several weeks after they learn to crawl, babies develop a fear of heights, but they also develop new skills in searching for lost objects. At an older age, a child who learns to ride a bike widens her horizons still further, as she explores her neighborhood on her own, perhaps for the first time.

The Child's Growth Affects Others' Responses.   The child's new physical skills also change the way others respond to her. For example, parents react quite differently to an infant who can crawl than to one who cannot. They begin to say "no" more often, put things out of reach, or put the baby in a playpen more often. Such changes in the pattern of interaction between parent and child may have both immediate and long-term consequences for the child's emotional or mental development.

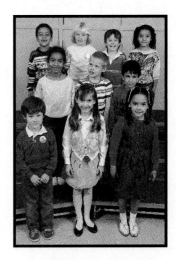

These Texas first graders are all the same age, but not all the same size. Because he is so much smaller, the little guy on the left in the front row is likely to be treated quite differently from his classmates.

Adults' expectations for children are also affected by the child's size and shape, attractiveness, or physical skills. Children who are pretty or tall or well coordinated are treated differently from those who are homely or petite or clumsy (Lerner, 1985). A Little League baseball coach may be more supportive of a child with advanced large-muscle coordination (good for home runs), while a classroom teacher may be especially appreciative of children whose small-muscle coordination is superior (good for writing and drawing).

Adults and children are also biased in favor of some specific body types. In the terminology introduced by Sheldon many years ago (1940), the most favored type is one that is well muscled and square in build, called *mesomorphic* by Sheldon. *Endomorphic* (rounded) and *ectomorphic* (skinny, tall, bony) body types are less preferred by both children and adults—a pattern of preferences that has been found not only in the U.S. but in samples of Japanese and Mexican children and adults as well (Lerner, 1985; 1987). Thus, individual differences in physical patterns, or speed of growth, can have profound effects on children's early experiences.

The Child's Growth Affects Self-concept. The final reason for us to pay close attention to physical development is that physical characteristics and physical skills (or lack of them) have a significant influence on a child's self-concept. I'll be talking about this topic much more fully in Chapters 9 and 10, but let me only point out here that this is another example of the importance of internal models, a concept I introduced in Chapter 1. A child's body image, which is part of her self-concept, is not simply a direct reflection of observable reality. Rather, it is an internal model shaped by a variety of things, including direct experience, what the child overhears from others, and the child's ideas about the then current cultural image of an ideal body. Like all internal models, the body image, once created, becomes relatively difficult to change. A child's choice of activities, her behavior in social situations, and her sense of self-worth are all likely to be affected throughout childhood and adolescence, perhaps even into adulthood, by the body image formed early in childhood. My own body image, for example, includes a strong element of "gawkiness," since I was always taller than everyone else and saw myself as uncoordinated. Whether that is *objectively* true is less important than the fact that I *believe* it to be true and base my behavior, my choices, my interpretations of my own behavior on that belief.

For all four of these reasons, I think it is important to begin our exploration of development with a fairly detailed look at physical growth and change.

Can you think of ways in which the same process has operated in your own life? Has your self-image been affected by your early growth or by your physical size or shape?

Basic Sequences and Common Patterns

Size and Shape

The most obvious thing about children's physical development is that kids get bigger as they get older. But even this simple statement may conceal some surprises. The biggest surprise for most people is the fact that at birth an infant is already one-third of his final height; by age 2 he is *half as tall* as he will be as an adult (hard to believe, isn't it?). Another possible surprise is the fact that growth from birth to maturity is neither continuous nor smooth. Figure 4.1 shows the four different phases in the development of height in boys and girls.

During the first phase, which lasts for about the first two years, the baby gains in height very rapidly, adding 10 to 12 inches in length in the first year and tripling his body weight in the same span. At about age 2, the child settles down to a slower but steady addition of 2 to 3 inches and about 6 pounds per year until adolescence.

The third phase is the dramatic "growth spurt," when the child may add 3 to 6 inches a year for several years, after which the rate of growth again slows until final adult size is reached. It is clear that this growth spurt is, on average, much larger for boys than for girls, but virtually all children show some increased rate of growth in this period.

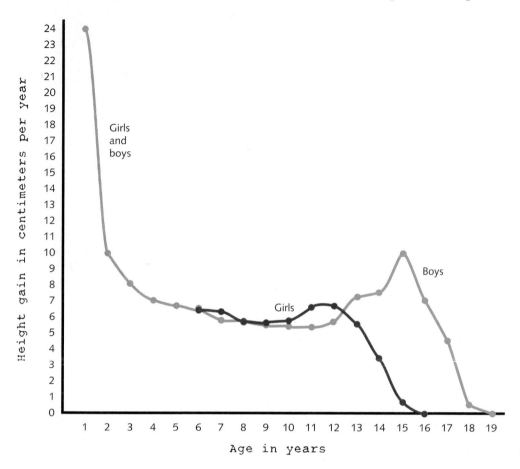

FIGURE 4.1 These curves show the gain in height for each year from birth through adolescence, based on recent data from many hundreds of thousands of American children. You can see the several clear phases: very rapid growth in infancy, slower growth in the preschool and elementary school years, a growth spurt at adolescence, and the cessation of growth at adulthood. (*Sources:* Tanner, 1978, p. 14; Malina, 1990; Lindsay et al., 1994; Baumgartner et al. 1986.)

At the same time, the shape and proportions of the child's body are changing. In an adult, the head is about one-eighth or one-tenth of the total height. But the toddler isn't built like that at all. In the 2-year-old, the head is about one-quarter of the total body length.

Individual body parts do not all grow at the same rate either. This is particularly striking at adolescence. During these years, a teenager's hands and feet grow to full adult size earliest, followed by the arms and legs, with the trunk usually the slowest part to grow. (In fact, a good signal for a parent that a child's puberty is beginning is a rapid increase in the child's shoe size.) Because of this asymmetry in the body parts, we often think of an adolescent as "awkward" or uncoordinated. Interestingly, research does not bear this out. Robert Malina, who has done extensive research on physical development, has found no point in the adolescent growth process at which teenagers become consistently less coordinated or less skillful in physical tasks (1990).

All these visible changes in size and shape are the result of changes on the inside in bones, muscles, and fat.

Bones

The hand, wrist, ankle, and foot all have fewer bones at birth than they will have at full maturity. For example, an adult has nine separate bones in his wrist. A 1-year-old has only three. The remaining six develop over the period of childhood, with complete growth by adolescence.

In one part of the body, though, the bones fuse rather than differentiating. The skull of a newborn is made up of several bones separated by spaces called **fontanels.** Fontanels allow the head to be compressed without injury during the birth process, and they give the brain room to grow. In most children, the fontanels are filled in by bone by 12 to 18 months, creating a single connected skull bone.

All the infant's bones are also softer, with a higher water content, than adults' bones. The process of bone hardening, called **ossification,** occurs steadily from birth through puberty, with bones in different parts of the body hardening in a sequence that follows two patterns that are characteristic of many physical developments in infancy and child-hood: from the head downward (**cephalocaudal**) and from the trunk outward (**proximodistal**). For example, spinal bones harden before those in the arms and legs, and bones of the hand and wrist harden before those in the feet.

You may well be thinking that bone hardening is pretty boring and unimportant stuff, but it has some fairly direct practical relevance. Soft bones are clearly needed if the fetus is going to have enough flexibility to fit into the cramped space of the uterus. But that very flexibility contributes to a newborn human's relative helplessness. Newborns are remarkably floppy; they cannot even hold their own heads up, let alone sit or walk. As the bones stiffen, the baby is able to manipulate his body more surely, which increases the range of exploration he can enjoy and makes him much more independent.

Muscles

In contrast to bones, muscle fibers are virtually all present at birth (Tanner, 1978). But like the infant's bones, muscle fibers are initially small and watery, becoming longer, thicker, and less watery at a fairly steady rate throughout childhood. At adolescence, mus-cles go through a growth spurt, just as height does, so that adolescents become quite a lot stronger in just a few years. Both boys and girls show this increase in muscle tissue and strength, but as you can see in Figure 4.2, the increase is much greater in boys. The re-searchers in this large Canadian cross-sectional study measured strength by having each child hang from a bar, with eyes level with the bar, for as long as possible. At age 9, boys could maintain this flexed arm hang for about 40 percent longer than could girls; by age 17, they could sustain it almost three times as long. This substantial difference in strength is one reflection of the sex difference in muscle tissue: Among adult men, about 40 per-cent of total body mass is muscle, compared to only about 24 percent in adult women.

The differences in muscle growth are, in turn, largely a product of variations in hor-mone patterns at adolescence. But we have at least a few hints that sex differences in exer-cise patterns or activity may also be involved. For example, boys have comparatively much greater arm strength, but the two sexes are more equal in leg strength (Tanner, Hughes, & Whitehouse, 1981). Such a pattern makes sense if we assume that all teenagers walk and use their legs a similar amount but that boys use their arm muscles in various sports activities more than girls do. Still, there does seem to be a basic hormonal

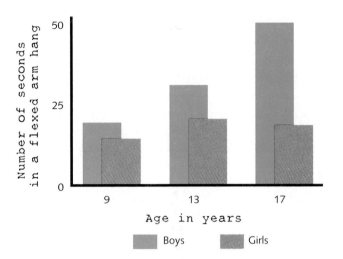

FIGURE 4.2 Both boys and girls get stronger between childhood and adolescence, but boys gain much more. (*Source:* Smoll & Schutz, 1990, from Table 1, p. 363.)

difference as well, because we know that very fit girls and women are still not as strong as very fit boys and men.

Fat

Another major component of the body is fat, most of which is stored immediately under the skin. This *subcutaneous fat* is first laid down beginning at about 34 weeks prenatally and has an early peak at about 9 months after birth (the so-called baby fat); the thickness of this layer of fat then declines until about age 6 or 7, after which it rises until adolescence.

Once again we see a sex difference in these patterns. From birth, girls have slightly more fat tissue than boys do, and this difference becomes gradually more marked during childhood. At adolescence, the difference grows still further. The size of the change is illustrated nicely in the results of the same Canadian study reflected in Figure 4.2 (Smoll & Schutz, 1990). Between ages 13 and 17, the percentage of body weight made up of fat rose from 21.8 to 24 percent among girls in this study but dropped from 16.1 to 14.0 percent among boys. So during and after puberty, proportions of fat rise among girls and decline among boys, while the proportion of weight that is muscle rises in boys and declines in girls.

Other Body Changes

Puberty also brings important changes in other body organs. In particular, the heart and lungs increase considerably in size and the heart rate drops. Both of these changes are more marked for boys than for girls—another of the factors that increase the capacity for sustained effort for boys relative to girls. Before puberty, boys and girls are fairly similar in physical strength, speed, and endurance, although even at these earlier ages, when a difference exists, it favors the boys. After puberty, boys have a clear advantage in all three (Smoll & Schutz, 1990).

Suppose you were a member of a local school board, faced with a decision about whether to have teenage boys and girls play on the same competitive teams, such as volleyball, soccer, or baseball. Given what you have read so far, how would you decide the issue, and why?

The Nervous System

Growth in height and weight involves changes you can see. Even the changes in muscles, bones, and fat can be detected fairly easily in the child's longer legs, greater strength, or softness or leanness of body. But two enormously important types of developmental changes in the body are not so easy to perceive—those in the nervous system and in hormones.

Composition of the Nervous System. Figure 4.3 shows the main structures of the brain. At birth, as I mentioned briefly in Chapter 3, the **midbrain** and the **medulla** are most fully developed. These two parts, both in the lower part of the skull and connecting to the spinal cord, regulate such basic tasks as attention and habituation, sleeping, waking, elimination, and movement of the head and neck (but not movement of the trunk or limbs)—all tasks a newborn can perform at least moderately well. The least-developed part of the brain at birth is the **cortex,** the convoluted gray matter that wraps around the midbrain and is involved in perception, body movement, and all complex thinking and language.

Recall from Chapter 2 that all these structures are composed of two basic types of cells, *neurons* and *glial cells.* Virtually all of both types of cells are already present at birth. The developmental process after birth is primarily the creation of synapses, which involves enormous growth of both the dendritic arbor and the axons and their terminal fibers. Most of that dendritic growth occurs in the cortex, primarily during the first year or two after birth, resulting in a tripling of the overall weight of the brain during those years (Nowakowski, 1987).

This remarkable brain development is not entirely smooth and continuous. Neurophysiologists have identified an initial burst of synapse formation in the first months after birth, followed by a "pruning" of synapses in each area of the brain, as redundant pathways and connections are eliminated and the "wiring diagram" is cleaned up (Huttenlocher, 1994).

For example, early in development each skeletal muscle cell seems to develop synaptic connections with several motor neurons in the spinal cord. But after the pruning process has occurred, each muscle fiber is connected to only one neuron. Some neurophysiologists, such as William Greenough (Greenough, Black, & Wallace, 1987), have suggested that the initial surge of development of the dendritic arbor and synaptic formation follows a built-in pattern; the organism is programmed to create certain kinds of neural connections and does so in abundance, creating redundant pathways. According to this argument, the pruning that then takes place, beginning at around 18 months or 2 years, is a response to specific experience, resulting in selective retention of the used or the most efficient pathways. Putting it briefly, "Experience does not create tracings on a blank tablet; rather experience erases some of them" (Bertenthal & Campos, 1987).

Greenough and his colleagues do not think that all synaptic development is governed by such built-in programming. He suggests that other synapses are formed entirely as a result of specific experience and that they go on being created throughout our lives as we learn new skills. But basic motor and sensory processes may initially follow built-in patterns, with pruning then based on experience.

Interestingly, pruning does not occur at the same time in all parts of the brain. For example, the maximum density of synapses in the portions of the brain that have to do with language comprehension and production occurs at about age 3 years, while the part of the cortex devoted to vision is maximally dense at 4 *months* of age, with rapid pruning thereafter (Huttenlocher, 1994).

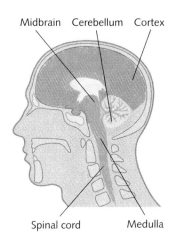

Midbrain   Cerebellum   Cortex

Spinal cord   Medulla

FIGURE 4.3 The medulla and the midbrain are largely developed at birth. In the first two years after birth it is primarily the cortex that develops, although increases in the dendritic arbor and in synapses also occur throughout the nervous system.

One of the most intriguing points about all this is that the combination of the early surge of synaptic growth and then pruning means that the 1-year-old actually has a *denser* set of dendrites and synapses than an adult does—a piece of information that has surprised many psychologists. Pruning also continues throughout childhood and adolescence. Even at age 4, when the early burst of pruning has occurred in all areas of the brain, synaptic density is about twice what we see in an adult's brain.

We can draw several important implications from all this new information about neurological development. First, we can see that a kind of "programmed plasticity" is built into the human organism. The brain has a remarkable ability to reorganize itself, to make the wiring diagram more efficient, or to find compensatory pathways following some injury. But this plasticity is greater in infancy than it is later. Perhaps paradoxically, the period of greatest plasticity is also the period in which the child may be most vulnerable to major deficits. Just as the time of most rapid growth of any body system prenatally is the time when the fetus is most vulnerable to teratogens, so the young infant needs sufficient stimulation and orderliness in his environment to maximize the early period of rapid growth and plasticity (de Haan et al., 1994). A really inadequate diet or a serious lack of stimulation in the early months may thus have subtle but long-range effects on the child's later cognitive progress.

At the same time, the new information about the continuation of the pruning process throughout childhood and adolescence has forced developmental psychologists to change our ideas about the links between brain development and behavior. If the brain was pretty much complete by age 2, as most of us were taught, it seemed logical to assume that whatever developments occurred after that age were largely the product of specific experience. But now we know that the brain changes significantly throughout childhood, which reopens all the questions about brain/behavior connections. Does language spurt between ages 2 and 3 because that is when the relevant portion of the brain is undergoing significant reorganization? Or is the reverse true? That is, do the synapses in the language centers of the brain get pruned later because that is when the child is learning language? Similarly, are the changes in thinking that we see at age 4, or at age 7, or at adolescence linked in some causal way to further changes in the brain? We do not yet have the data to answer such questions, but there is a very definite shift in the theoretical winds toward examining the neurological underpinnings of development in childhood and adolescence.

Myelinization. Another crucial process in neuronal development is the development of sheaths around individual axons, which electrically insulate them from one another and improve the conductivity of the nerve. This sheath is made up of a substance called **myelin;** the process of developing the sheath is called **myelinization.**

The sequence with which nerves are myelinized follows both cephalocaudal and proximodistal patterns. Thus, nerves serving muscle cells in the arms and hands are myelinized earlier than are those serving the lower trunk and the legs. Myelinization is most rapid during the first two years after birth, but it continues at a slower pace throughout childhood and adolescence. For example, the parts of the brain that govern motor movements are not fully myelinized until perhaps age 6 (Todd et al., 1995).

To understand the importance of myelin, it may help you to know that *multiple sclerosis* is a disease in which the myelin begins to break down. An individual with this disease gradually loses motor control, with the specific symptoms depending on the portion of the nervous system affected by the disease.

Hormones

A second crucial set of changes over the years of childhood and adolescence is in *hormones*—secretions of the various **endocrine glands** in the body. Hormones govern growth and physical changes in several ways, summarized in Table 4.1.

Of all the endocrine glands, the most critical is the pituitary, since it provides the trigger for release of hormones from other glands. For example, the thyroid gland only secretes thyroxine when it has received a signal to do so in the form of a specific thyroid-stimulating hormone secreted by the pituitary.

Hormones play a role at every stage of physical development, perhaps most strikingly at adolescence, but significantly at earlier stages as well.

Prenatal Hormones. Thyroid hormone (thyroxine) is present from about the fourth month of gestation and appears to be involved in stimulating normal brain development. Growth hormone is also produced by the pituitary, beginning as early as 10 weeks after conception. Presumably, it helps to stimulate the very rapid growth of cells and organs of the body. And as I mentioned in Chapter 2, testosterone is produced prenatally in the testes of the developing male and influences both the development of male genitals and some aspects of brain development.

Hormones Between Birth and Adolescence. Between birth and adolescence, physical growth is largely governed by thyroid hormone and pituitary growth hor-

Table 4.1
Major Hormones Involved in Physical Growth and Development

Gland	Hormone(s) Secreted	Aspects of Growth Influenced
Thyroid	Thyroxine	Normal brain development and overall rate of growth.
Adrenal	Adrenal androgen	Some changes at puberty, particularly the development of secondary sex characteristics in girls.
Testes (in boys)	Testosterone	Crucial in the formation of male genitals prenatally; also triggers the sequence of primary and secondary sex characteristic changes at puberty in the male.
Ovaries (in girls)	Estradiol	Development of the menstrual cycle and breasts in girls; has less to do with other secondary sex characteristics than testosterone does for boys.
Pituitary	Growth hormone, activating hormones	Rate of physical maturation; signals other glands to secrete.

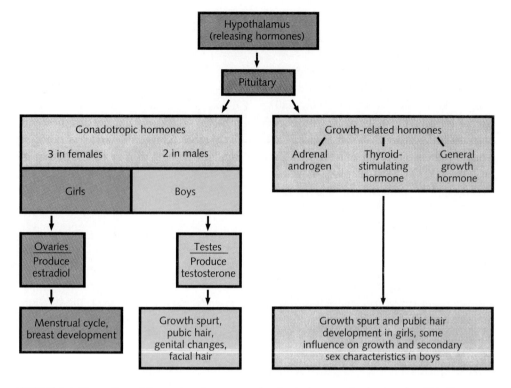

FIGURE 4.4 The action of the various hormones at puberty is exceedingly complex. This figure oversimplifies the process but gives you some sense of the sequence and the differences between the patterns for boys and girls.

mone. Thyroid hormone is secreted in greater quantities for the first two years of life and then falls to a lower level and remains steady until adolescence (Tanner, 1978), a secretion pattern that obviously matches the pattern of change in height you saw in Figure 4.1.

Secretions from the testes and ovaries, as well as adrenal androgen, remain at extremely low levels until about age 7 or 8, when adrenal androgen begins to be secreted—the first signal of the changes of adolescence (and possibly one of the sources of the changes I observed in my 8-year-old daughter) (Shonkoff, 1984).

Hormones in Adolescence. The early rise in adrenal androgen is only the first step in a complex sequence of hormone changes at adolescence, which you can see laid out schematically in Figure 4.4.

The timing of these changes varies a lot from one child to the next, but the sequence remains the same. At a signal from the hypothalamus, the pituitary gland begins secreting increased levels of **gonadotropic hormones** (two in males, three in females). These in turn stimulate the development of the glands in the testes and ovaries, which then begin to secrete more hormones, *testosterone* in boys and a form of **estrogen** called *estradiol* in girls. Over the course of puberty, the levels of testosterone increase 18-fold in boys, while levels of estradiol increase 8-fold in girls (Nottelmann et al., 1987).

At the same time, the pituitary also secretes three other hormones that affect growth and that interact with the specific sex hormones, although as you can see in Figure 4.4, the interaction is a little different for boys and girls. In particular, both the growth spurt and pubic hair development in girls are more influenced by adrenal androgen than is true for boys. Adrenal androgen is chemically very similar to testosterone, so it takes a "male" hormone to produce the growth spurt in girls.

Having said that, I need to add a caution: It is somewhat misleading to talk about "male" and "female" hormones. Both males and females have at least some of each. The difference is essentially in the relative proportion of the two. Within any one gender, these proportions differ as well, so some males have relatively more testosterone and less estrogen, while in others the two may be more balanced. Similarly, some girls may have a pattern of hormones that includes relatively more androgen, while others may have relatively little.

Development of Sexual Maturity

The physical result of the hormonal changes that take place during **puberty** is not only a spurt in height but also, more important, a set of physical changes that bring about full sexual maturity. Included are changes in the reproductive systems themselves (called *primary sex characteristics*), such as the testes and penis in the male, and the ovaries, uterus, and vagina in the female, as well as changes in *secondary sex characteristics:* the development of breasts in girls, changing voice pitch and beard growth in boys, and the growth of body hair in both sexes.

Each of these physical developments occurs in a defined sequence. Following the work of J. M. Tanner (1978), each sequence is customarily divided into five stages, with stage 1 always representing the preadolescent stage; stage 2, the first signs of pubertal change; stages 3 and 4, the intermediate steps; and stage 5, the final adult characteristic. Table 4.2 gives you two examples of these sequences, one for each sex. These stages have proven to be extremely helpful not only for describing the normal progress through puberty, but also for assessing the rate of development of individual youngsters.

Sexual Development in Girls

Studies of preteens and teens in both Europe and North America (Malina, 1990) reveal that for girls, the various sequential changes are interlocked in a particular pattern, shown schematically in Figure 4.5 (p. 106). The first steps are typically the early changes in breasts and pubic hair, followed by the peak of the growth spurt. Only then does first menstruation occur, an event called **menarche** (pronounced men-are-kee). Menarche typically occurs two years after the beginning of other visible changes and is succeeded only by the final stages of breast and pubic hair development. Among girls in industrialized countries today, menarche occurs, on average, between ages $12\frac{1}{2}$ and $13\frac{1}{2}$, with 95 percent of all girls experiencing this event between the ages of 11 and 15 (Malina, 1990).

Menarche does not signal full sexual maturity. It is possible to conceive shortly after menarche, but irregularity of ovulation is the norm for some time. In as many as three-quarters of the cycles in the first year and half the cycles in the second and third years after menarche, no ovum is produced (Vihko & Apter, 1980). Full adult fertility thus develops over a period of years.

The initial irregularity of both ovulation and the timing of menstrual cycles has some significant practical consequences for sexually active teenagers. For one thing, such irregularity no doubt contributes to the widespread (but false) assumption among early-teenage girls that they cannot get pregnant because they are "too young." At the same

Table 4.2
Examples of Tanner's Stages of Pubertal Development

Stage	Breast Development	Male Genital Development
1	No change except for some elevation of the nipple.	Testes, scrotum, and penis are all about the same size and shape as in early childhood.
2	Breast bud stage: elevation of breast and the nipple as a small mound. Areolar diameter is enlarged over stage 1.	Scrotum and testes are slightly enlarged. Skin of the scrotum is reddened and changed in texture but little or no enlargement of the penis.
3	Breast and areola both enlarged and elevated more than in stage 2 but no separation of their contours.	Penis slightly enlarged, at first mainly in length. Testes and scrotum are further enlarged.
4	Areola and nipple form a secondary mound projecting above the contour of the breast.	Penis further enlarged, with growth in breadth and development of glans. Testes and scrotum further enlarged and scrotum skin still darker.
5	Mature stage. Only the nipple projects, with the areola recessed to the general contour of the breast.	Genitalia are adult in size and shape.

Source: Petersen & Taylor, 1980, p. 127.

time the irregularity makes any form of rhythm contraception unreliable, even among teenagers who have enough basic reproductive knowledge to realize that the time of ovulation is normally the time of greatest fertility—knowledge that is not widespread.

Sexual Development in Boys

In boys, as in girls, the peak of the growth spurt typically comes fairly late in the sequence, as you can see in Figure 4.6. Malina's data suggest that on average a boy completes stages 2, 3, and 4 of genital development and stages 2 and 3 of pubic hair development before the growth peak is reached (Malina, 1990), with facial hair and the lowering of the voice coming only quite near the end of the sequence. Precisely when in this sequence the boy begins to produce viable sperm is very difficult to determine, although current evidence places this event some time between ages 12 and 14, usually *before* the boy has reached the peak of the growth spurt (Brooks-Gunn & Reiter, 1990).

Two things are particularly interesting about these sequences. First, if you compare Figures 4.5 and 4.6, you will see that boys begin the early stages of pubertal change only a short time later than do girls but that the growth spurt comes about two years earlier in girls. Most of you remember that period in late elementary school or junior high when all the girls were suddenly taller than the boys. (Do I remember that time! I *towered* over everyone.)

FIGURE 4.5 The figure shows the normal sequence and timing of pubertal changes for girls. The box on each black line represents the average age of attainment of that change, while the line indicates the range of normal times. Note the *wide* range of normality for all these changes. Also note how relatively late in the sequence the growth spurt and menarche occur. (*Sources:* Chumlea, 1982; Garn, 1980; Malina, 1990; Tanner, 1978.)

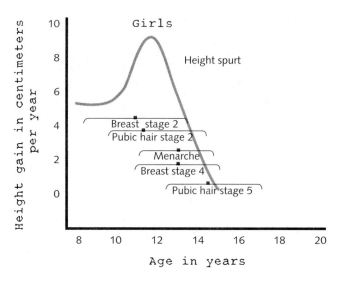

FIGURE 4.6 The sequence of pubertal changes begins about two years later for boys than for girls, but as for girls, the height spurt occurs relatively late in the sequence. (*Sources:* Chumlea, 1982; Malina, 1990; Tanner, 1978.)

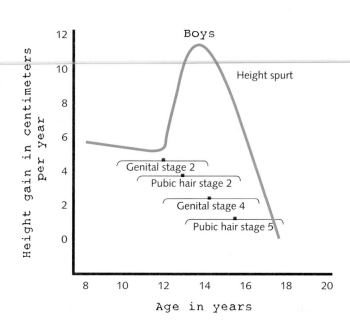

A second intriguing thing is that while the order of development seems to be highly consistent *within* each sequence (such as breast development or pubic hair development), quite a lot of variability occurs *across* sequences. I've given you the normative or average pattern, but individual teenagers often do not follow that normative pattern. For instance, a boy may be in stage 2 of genital development but already in stage 5 of pubic hair development; a girl might move through several stages of pubic hair development before the first clear breast changes, or experience menarche much earlier in the sequence than normal. So far physiologists have not figured out why this variation exists or what it might mean, but it is an important point to keep in mind if you are trying to make a prediction about an individual teenager.

Using the Body: The Effects of Physical Changes on Behavior

This brief picture of physical changes in the first 15 years of life should give you some sense of the alterations in muscles, fat, internal organs, and nervous system. But what this description does not convey is the impact of all those changes on the child's behavior. The effects are particularly striking at two time points: (1) in the first two or three years of life, when the baby develops the ability to sit up, crawl, walk, and then run, and to pick up and manipulate objects; and (2) at adolescence, when the rapid changes of puberty make mature sexual behavior possible.

Motor Development in the Early Years

Psychologists use the phrase **motor development** to describe the emergence of various abilities to move around and to use the body in skilled ways. Included are various *movement skills,* such as crawling, walking, running, and bike riding, as well as *manipulative skills,* such as grasping or picking up objects, throwing balls, holding a crayon or a pencil, or threading a needle. Nearly all the *basic* skills of both types are well developed by about 6 or 7 years of age. Beyond this age, motor development is mostly a question of refining the basic skills and integrating them into more and more complex movement sequences. So 6- and 7-year-olds can run, and they can probably dribble a basketball, but they can't yet do both at the same time. Table 4.3 lists some of the key milestones in these emerging abilities.

Table 4.3
Sequences of Development of Various Motor Skills

Age	Movement and Manipulative Skills
1 mo.	Lifts head. Holds object if placed in hand.
4–6 mos.	Sits with support. Holds head erect in sitting position. Reaches for and grasps objects.
7–9 mos.	Sits without support. Rolls over from stomach. Stands up using furniture. Transfers objects from one hand to the other.
10–12 mos.	Crawls. Walks grasping furniture. Walks without help (12–13 mos.).
13–18 mos.	Walks backward and sideways. Stacks two blocks. Puts objects into small containers and dumps them.
3–4 yrs.	Walks upstairs one foot per step. Pedals and steers tricycle. Catches large ball. Cuts paper with scissors. Holds pencil between thumb and first two fingers.
7–8 yrs.	Skips freely. Rides two-wheel bicycle. Plays ball games with some skill. Writes individual letters.

Sources: Connelly & Dalgliesh, 1989; Capute et al., 1984; The Diagram Group, 1977; Fagard & Jaquet, 1989; Mathew & Cook, 1990; Thomas, 1990a.

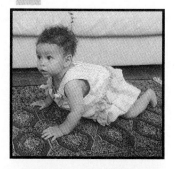

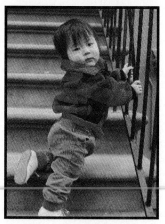

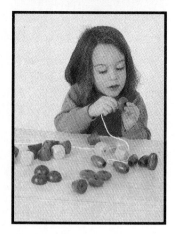

Some steps in motor development.

All these changes, particularly the early ones as the baby gradually shifts from sitting to crawling to walking, are normally a delight for parents to observe and encourage. But they have obvious practical ramifications as well. One example: Until a baby is able to crawl or walk, it is not necessary to put dangerous or fragile objects out of reach. When he begins to move around independently, childproofing the house becomes critical. Similarly, the types of toys you would buy or make for a child are obviously influenced by the child's motor skills. At about 1 year, stacking or nesting toys are likely to be big favorites (and ordinary objects, such as sets of measuring cups, probably work as well as expensive toys). In the second year of life, toys with wheels are very popular, but *push* toys are better than *pull* toys, because the child can see the object while it moves. By about age 2 or 3, the child may for the first time enjoy drawing with large crayons or pencils but cannot yet grasp smaller ones. For 5- and 6-year-olds, though, toys like jacks or marbles make good gifts, because a child this age has the small-muscle coordination needed to manipulate them.

The emergence of motor skills also has an impact on the timing of children's sports activities—an application I've explored in the *Real World* discussion on the facing page.

Adolescent Sexuality and Pregnancy

At adolescence, the underlying physical changes not only mean that the young person is stronger and faster and better coordinated than before, but also make mature sexual behavior possible. But unlike early motor development, which proceeds in pretty much the same way for all children, sexual behavior involves clear choices for the teenager. Should I or shouldn't I? What do we know about the choices teenagers make about their sexual activity?

As is usually the case, what I can tell you about this is almost entirely specific to the U.S. or to other industrialized countries. It is good to keep in mind that the whole question of adolescent sexuality is a central issue for those of us in such cultures in large part because we have created such a long delay between physical sexual maturity and social maturity: Young people are physically mature at 13 or 14, but they are not financially independent or fully trained until age 20 or later. In cultures in which 12- or 14-year-olds are considered ready to take on adult tasks and responsibilities, to marry and to bear children, adolescent sexuality is handled very differently. In the U.S., where adolescent pregnancy has become extremely common, it is perceived as a significant problem.

Adolescent sexual activity has increased fairly dramatically in the U.S. since the late 1950s (Miller, Christopherson, & King, 1993). By 1990, roughly half of teens reported they had had intercourse at least once (Centers for Disease Control, 1992b). You can see in Figure 4.7 that the percentage increases steadily with age and that at every age, more boys than girls report sexual activity.

The number of teens reporting multiple sexual partners has also risen in recent years. In the 1990 survey by the Centers for Disease Control, 20.6 percent of tenth-grade males and 38.5 percent of twelfth-grade males reported four or more partners. Among girls, the equivalent figures were 9.3 percent and 17.0 percent (Centers for Disease Control, 1992a).

At every age, we find consistent ethnic differences in all these figures: Hispanic-American and Caucasian youth are least likely to be sexually active and African-

The Real World

Sports for Children

In the U.S. and increasingly in other industrialized countries, children no longer play much in the street or in backyards; they play on organized teams and groups: soccer teams, Little League baseball, Pee Wee League football, swimming clubs, and the like. Many children begin such programs when they are 6 or 7, often with great enthusiasm. But participation peaks by age 10 or 11 and then declines rapidly. Why?

Kids drop out of such programs because the emphasis on competition and winning is so great (Harvard Education Letter, 1992). Amateur coaches often have poor understanding of the kinds of motor skills that are normal for a 6- or 7-year-old, so when they see a child who does not yet throw a ball skillfully or who kicks a ball awkwardly, they label this child as clumsy or uncoordinated. From then on, these perfectly normal kids get little playing time or encouragement. Only the stars—children with unusually good or early motor skill development—get maximum attention and exercise.

In fact, 6 or 7 is really too early for most children to be playing on full-sized playing fields or in competitive games (Kolata, 1992). It would be far better to wait until age 9 or 10—if then—for competitive games. In the earlier years, kids should spend their time learning and perfecting basic skills in activities that are fun regardless of their skill level and that involve as much movement as possible. One expert, Vern Seefeldt, the director of the Institute for the Study of Youth Sports at Michigan State University, says:

Children need to be in situations where their participation and ability to learn skills are maximized. In an adult game, you try to throw the ball so the batter can't hit it or kick the ball where it can't be retrieved. With kids, you need to do just the opposite. (Kolata, 1992, p. 40)

If children begin with organized sports activities as young as 6 or 7, the early experiences should be carefully selected. Soccer or swimming are particularly good, not only because everyone is likely to get at least some aerobic exercise, but also because the basic skills are within the abilities of children of this age. Baseball, in contrast, is *not* a good sport for the average 6- or 7-year-old, because it requires real eye–hand coordination to hit or catch the ball, and most 7-year-olds are not yet proficient at such coordination. By age 10 or so, many children will be ready to play sports such as basketball, but many organized sports, such as tennis, are still difficult for the average child of this age. (Jennifer Capriati, who began her professional tennis career at age 14 is, after all, an *exception*, and not the rule.) Only in adolescence do most young people have the strength and coordination for sports like football.

If you want to encourage your children to be involved in sports, choose carefully. Let the child try several sports to see which one or ones he or she may enjoy, and be sure to select programs in which *all* children are given skill training and encouragement and in which competition is initially deemphasized. And don't push too fast or too hard. If you do, your child is likely to drop out of any type of organized sport by age 10 or 11, saying—as many do—that he feels inadequate or that it isn't fun anymore.

American youth are most likely (Centers for Disease Control, 1992b). In the 1990 Centers for Disease Control survey, 72.3 percent of black high school students had had at least one experience of intercourse, compared to 53.4 percent of Hispanics and 51.6 percent of whites. The form and pattern of sexual activity also show ethnic differences in U.S. groups. Among both Anglos and Hispanics, sexual activity appears to move through a fairly typical sequence over time and within any one dating relationship, from hand-holding to kissing to stroking of breasts or genitals, to intercourse. So intercourse is considerably more likely in couples who are "going steady" and quite unlikely on a first date. Among blacks, at least in the U.S., this sequence does not appear to hold: They are more likely to move directly to intercourse (Miller et al., 1993).

FIGURE 4.7 These data, collected in the early 1990s, show that the likelihood of sexual activity increases steadily with age among this group of white teenagers. But the higher rate of intercourse among boys, typical of data from earlier decades, has nearly disappeared in this group. (*Source:* Luster & Small, 1994, from Table 1, p. 627.)

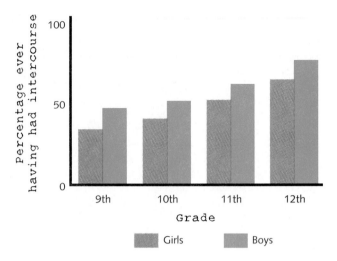

In boys the likelihood of sexual activity is somewhat correlated with the amount of testosterone in the blood (Halpern et al., 1993; Udry & Campbell, 1994). Among girls, hormones are somewhat linked to the girl's *interest* in sexuality but not to her likelihood of intercourse (Dyk, 1993). In both boys and girls, social factors are much better predictors of teen sexual activity than are hormones. Those who begin sexual activity early are more likely to live in poor neighborhoods in which young people have little monitoring by adults; they come from poorer families or from families in which sexual activity is condoned and dating rules are lax; they are more likely to use alcohol. Among girls, those who are sexually active are also more likely to have had early menarche, to have low interest in school, and to have a history of sexual abuse (Billy, Brewster, & Grady, 1994; Hovell et al., 1994; Small & Luster, 1994). In general, these same factors predict sexual activity among whites, blacks, and Hispanics. And in every group, the greater the number of these risk factors that are present in the life of an individual teenager, the greater the likelihood that he or she will be sexually active.

Despite their high levels of sexual activity, teenagers know remarkably little about physiology and reproduction. At best, only about half of white and a quarter of black teenagers can describe the time of greatest fertility in the menstrual cycle (Freeman & Rickels, 1993; Morrison, 1985). Many are convinced they cannot get pregnant because they are "too young." Perhaps in part because of such ignorance, contraceptive use is still relatively low—especially in comparison to most European countries, where teenage sexual behavior is as common but contraceptive information is far more widespread. Both Sweden and the Netherlands, for example, have very low teenage birth rates. In both, contraceptive information is widely available and contraceptive use is culturally acceptable (Jones et al., 1986). In the U.S., despite increases in contraceptive use in recent years, less than half of teenage girls use any type of contraceptives the first time they have intercourse, and fewer still regularly use effective methods, such as condoms or the pill (Jorgensen, 1993). Contraceptive use is even less likely among Hispanics than among Anglos (Fennelly, 1993), and in all groups is least likely among younger girls (Luster & Small, 1994).

Teenage Pregnancy. Given these facts, we shouldn't be surprised that the rate of teenage pregnancy is higher in the U.S. than in any other developed Western country

How many different reasons can you think of why teenagers would *not* use contraceptives? Which of those explanations might account for the lower use of contraception among Hispanic-Americans?

(Ambuel, 1995). In the Netherlands, for example, the pregnancy rate for girls between the ages of 15 and 19 is 14 per 1000 girls per year. In the United States it is 96 pregnancies per 1000 girls per year, of which four-fifths are unintended. The birth rate is about four times higher among African-American teen girls than among whites; Hispanic-Americans fall in between (Centers for Disease Control, 1993a). Sandra Hofferth estimates that fully 44 percent of all teenage girls in the U.S. will be pregnant at least once before the age of 20 (Hofferth, 1987a). About half of these pregnancies are carried to term.

Let me try to put these fairly astonishing numbers into some kind of context. Birth rates have actually dropped among the entire U.S. population in the past decades, *including among teenagers.* Indeed, the proportion of all births in the United States that were to teenagers has declined steadily since 1975. What has increased steadily since the 1960s is the rate of births to *nonmarried* teens. In 1988, 78 percent of all girls under 18 who gave birth in the U.S. were unmarried; among black girls, the rate was 95 percent (Furstenberg, 1991). Thus, it is not that more and more teenagers are bearing children, but that more and more pregnant teenage girls are choosing to rear their children without marrying.

Whether one sees this as a worrisome trend or not depends not only on one's religious or moral beliefs, but also on evidence about the long-term consequences of adolescent childbearing for the adult lives of the girls involved and for the lives of the children they bear. For the teenage mothers, the bulk of that evidence points to negative consequences, although it has been difficult to sort out which effects are due to early childbearing itself and which might be due to self-selection or the impact of poverty. Most studies indicate that teenage childbearing—whether married or unmarried—is associated with more children, more closely spaced, fewer years of total education throughout adult life, lower levels of occupational success, lower income in adulthood, and higher likelihood of divorce in adult life. These relationships are found among African-American, Hispanic, and Anglo teens, so these negative outcomes are not just ethnic differences in disguise (Astone, 1993; Hofferth, 1987b; Moore et al., 1993).

However, there are some mitigating facts. First of all, more than half of girls who become pregnant before age 18 nonetheless manage to complete high school by the time they are in their early twenties—a fact that runs counter to prevailing stereotypes (Upchurch, 1993). And many of those who struggle economically in their early adult years manage to recover in their thirties and forties, especially if they were able to complete at least high school (Upchurch, 1993; Werner & Smith, 1992). Despite these findings, though, teenage mothers as a group are still disadvantaged. For black inner-city girls in particular, the chances of moving out of poverty in adulthood seem to be far better for those who delay childbearing into their twenties (Freeman & Rickels, 1993).

For the children of these teenage mothers, the news is not good. These children are simply far more likely to grow up in poverty, with all the negative consequences that entail for the child's optimum development (Osofsky, Hann, & Peebles, 1993).

To avoid some of these negative consequences, we may need to take a page or two from pregnancy-prevention expertise developed in many other industrialized countries, especially about the appropriate timing and content of education about sex and/or contraception in the schools.

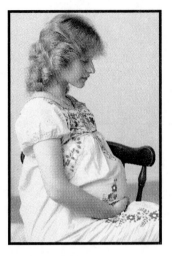

Teenage sexual activity is not more common in the U.S. than in most Western industrialized countries, but teen pregnancy is. Girls like this 14-year-old who give birth during their teens are more likely to have problems in adulthood, including lower income, less education, and higher risk of divorce.

Is it possible that these apparent consequences of teen childbearing are really caused by self-selection? That is, teenage mothers may simply be a different group to start with—less interested in school, from different kinds of homes. How could you figure out if that were the explanation?

The Real World
Which Teenage Girls Get Pregnant?

Whether a girl becomes pregnant during her teenage years depends on many of the same factors that predict sexual activity in general, including family background, educational aspirations, timing of sexual activity, and sub-cultural attitudes. Here are a few of the findings (Hayes, 1987):

- The younger a girl is when she becomes sexually active, the more likely she is to have at least one teen pregnancy.
- Girls who come from poor families, who are from single-parent families, or whose parents are relatively uneducated are more likely to become pregnant.
- Girls whose mothers became sexually active early and who bore their first child early are more likely to become pregnant as teens.
- Black and Hispanic teenagers are more likely than are Anglos to become pregnant, but for different reasons. Blacks are more likely to be sexually ac-

tive, while Hispanics, who have lower rates of sexual activity, are less likely to use contraception than are Anglos.

- The better a girl does in school and the stronger her educational aspirations, the more likely she is to use birth control consistently and the less likely she is to get pregnant.
- The more stable and committed the relationship between a teenage girl and her sexual partner, the *less* likely she is to become pregnant.
- Girls who have good communication about contraception with their mothers and whose mothers support the use of contraception are less likely to become pregnant.

The riskiest time for teen pregnancy is in the first year or so after a girl has become sexually active. It is during these early months that girls are least likely to seek out contraceptive information or to use contraception consistently.

Big or Fast Versus Slow or Small: Some Individual Differences in Physical Development

Although virtually all children and teenagers go through the various sequences of physical development in the same order, there are wide individual differences in the *rate* and *timing* of physical changes as well as in children's physical shape or skills. These differences are interesting in their own right, but they are also important because of the ways in which they can affect a child's self-image, her relationships with her peers, or her general contacts with the world around her.

Differences in Rate

Children vary *widely* in the speed with which they go through all the body and motor changes I have described. Some children walk at 7 or 8 months; others not until 18 months. Some are skillful soccer players at 7 or 8, others not until much later (if at all). These differences are most striking at puberty. Among 12- or 13-year-old girls, for example, some are already at stage 4 or 5 of breast development, and others are still clearly pre-pubescent. Some 14-year-old boys are already fully developed, with lowered voices and full beards, while others still have the narrow, slim bodies of children.

As a general rule, a child tends to be consistently early, average, or late in most aspects of physical development. The child who shows slower bone development is also likely to walk later and to have later puberty (Tanner, 1978). There are exceptions to this generalization, but what Tanner calls the *tempo of growth* is a powerful element in development.

Effects of Differing Rates on Mental Development. These differences in rate of development appear to have at least some small link to a child's mental development, so that children who are more rapid in physical development are also slightly ahead in mental development (Newcombe & Baenninger, 1989; Tanner, 1978). It is also true that taller children of any given age tend to score slightly higher on IQ tests than do shorter children of the same age (Dornbusch et al., 1987a; Humphreys, Davey, & Park, 1985), a pattern that has been found in studies in a number of countries, including Britain, Sweden, and the U.S.

The possible causes are myriad, including differences in prenatal environment, in pre- or postnatal diet, or in expectations and opportunities for short versus tall children. But whatever the cause, it is interesting that these differences persist into adulthood. That is, adults who were early developers as children still have a slight intellectual advantage over their slower-developing peers, even though the latter group has caught up in height, brain growth, and physical skill. The most likely explanation is that this carryover into adulthood is a consequence of the psychological effects of earliness or lateness rather than of the physiological effects.

Effects of Differences in Rate on Personality. Most of the research on the psychological effects of fast or slow growth has focused on only one age period: puberty. What happens to a girl who begins to menstruate at 10, or a boy who does not go through a growth spurt until age 16? Do they turn out differently?

The cumulative body of research on this question points to an interesting and complex hypothesis that once again underlines the importance of internal models. The general idea is that each young child or teenager has an internal model about the "normal" or "right" timing for puberty (Faust, 1983; Lerner, 1987; Petersen, 1987). Each girl has an internal model about the "right age" to develop breasts or begin menstruating; each boy has an internal model or image about when it is right to begin to grow a beard or for his voice to get lower. According to this hypothesis, it is the discrepancy between an adolescent's expectation and what actually happens that determines the psychological effect. Those whose development occurs outside the desired or expected range are likely to think less well of themselves and to be less happy with their bodies and with the process of puberty. They may also have fewer friends and experience other signs of distress.

In American culture today, most young people seem to share the expectation that pubertal changes will happen sometime between ages 12 and 14; anything earlier is seen as "too soon," anything later is thought of as late. If you compare these expectations to the actual average timing of pubertal changes, you'll see that such a norm includes girls who are average in development and boys who are *early*. So we should expect these two groups—normal-developing girls and early-developing boys—to have the best psychological functioning. Early-maturing boys are also more likely to be of the preferred *mesomorphic* body type, with wide shoulders and a large amount of muscle. Because boys with this body type tend to be good at sports, the early-developing boy should be particularly advantaged.

Figure 4.8 shows the specific predictions graphically. Because of the twin advantages of having puberty fall within the "normative" time and of having a more mesomorphic body type, early boys should be best off, followed by average boys and girls. The least well off should be late-developing boys and early-developing girls, both of whom are "off time."

FIGURE 4.8 According to this model of the effects of early and late puberty, the best position for girls is to be "on time," while for boys the best position is to be "early." For both sexes, however, it is the *perception* of earliness or lateness, and not the actual timing, that is thought to be critical. (*Source:* Adapted from Tobin-Richards et al., 1983, p. 137.)

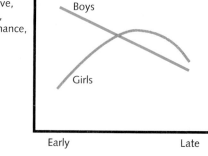

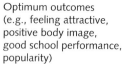

Teenager's perception of her or his pubertal timing

Research in the U.S. generally confirms these predictions. Girls who are early developers (before 11 or 12 for major body changes) show consistently more negative body images, such as thinking themselves too fat (Petersen, 1987; Simmons, Blyth, & McKinney, 1983). Such girls are also more likely to get into trouble in school and at home (Magnusson, Stattin, & Allen, 1986), are more likely to get involved with misbehaving peer groups (Silbereisen & Kracke, 1993), and are more likely to be depressed (Rierdan & Koff, 1993). Very late development in girls also appears to be somewhat negative, but the effect of lateness is not so striking for girls as it is for boys.

Among boys, as Figure 4.8 predicts, the relationship is essentially linear. The earlier the boy's development, the more positive his body image, the better he does in school, the less trouble he gets into, and the more friends he has (Duke et al., 1982).

In nearly all these studies, earliness or lateness has been defined in terms of the actual physical changes. The results are even clearer when researchers have instead asked teenagers about their internal model of earliness or lateness. For example, Rierdan, Koff, and Stubbs (1989) have found that the negativeness of a girl's menarcheal experience was predicted by her *subjective* sense of earliness; those who perceived themselves as early reported a more negative experience. But such a negative experience was *un*related to the actual age of her menarche.

This link between the internal model and the outcome is especially vivid in a study of ballet dancers by Jeanne Brooks-Gunn (1987; Brooks-Gunn & Warren, 1985). She studied 14- to 18-year-old girls, some of whom were serious ballet dancers studying at a national ballet company school. In this group, a very lean, almost prepubescent body is highly desirable. Brooks-Gunn therefore expected that among dancers, those who were very late in pubertal development would actually have a better image of themselves than those who were on time. And that is exactly what she found, as you can see in Figure 4.9. Among nondancers the same age, normal-time menarche was associated with a better body image than late menarche, but exactly the reverse was true for the dancers.

Thus, it seems to be the discrepancy or mismatch between the desired or expected pattern and a youngster's actual pattern that is critical, not the absolute age of pubertal development. Because the majority of young people in any given culture share similar expectations, we may see average effects of early or late development. But to predict the effect of early or late development in any individual teenager, we would need to know more about her or his internal model, or the culturally defined models that may be operating.

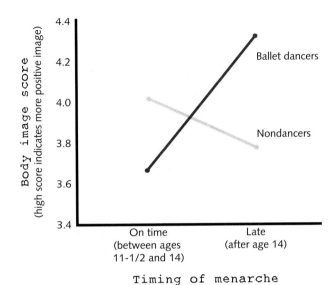

FIGURE 4.9 Serious ballet dancers clearly prefer to have a very late puberty. In this study, those dancers whose menarche was "on time" by ordinary standards actually had poorer body images than did those who were objectively quite late, while the reverse was true for nondancers. Thus, it is perception of timing and not actual timing that is critical. (*Source:* Brooks-Gunn & Warren, 1985, from Table 1, p. 291.)

Social Class and Racial Differences

As a group, poor children grow a bit slower and are a bit shorter than middle-class children, most probably because of dietary differences. Menarcheal age is also about six months later in girls growing up in less-affluent homes than in girls in middle-class homes (Garn, 1980).

Different racial groups too show somewhat different rates or patterns of development. Black infants and children appear to be slightly ahead of white children in some aspects of physical development. In fact, the gestational period for the black fetus seems actually to be slightly shorter than for the white fetus (Smith, 1978). Black babies also show somewhat faster development of motor skills, such as walking, and are slightly taller than their white counterparts, with longer legs, more muscle, and heavier bones (Tanner, 1978). In early and middle childhood, black children are slightly but consistently taller (Okamoto, Davidson, & Conner, 1993); at puberty, black girls have slightly earlier menarche as well (perhaps three months, on average). Thus, the tempo of growth appears to be somewhat faster in black children than in white.

Asian children also have a relatively rapid tempo of growth but are smaller, with long upper bodies and shorter final height.

Health and Illness

The study of both the common patterns and individual differences in normal physical growth forms the core of psychological research on physical development. But for parents, as well as for physicians and for society as a whole, another key aspect of a child's physical status is her health or illness.

Those of us who live in countries with relatively low infant and childhood mortality rates are used to thinking of childhood as a basically healthy time. But in a large fraction of the world's countries, as many as one out of every five children dies before age 5 (Wegman, 1992). In contrast, in the United States in 1992, fewer than 1 child out of 100 dies before age 5 (U.S. Bureau of the Census, 1994). Still, even in such advantaged circumstances, children do get sick; some die.

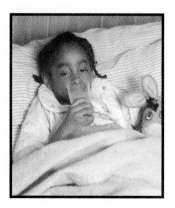

Most kids this age are sick in bed like this about six times a year.

Children who are sick a lot early in life have a higher risk of having health problems in adolescence and adulthood. How many different explanations can you propose to account for such a finding?

Health in Early and Middle Childhood

Brief sicknesses, such as colds or viruses (called *acute* illnesses by physicians) are common among young children. I mentioned in Chapter 3 that the average baby has seven or eight respiratory illnesses in the first year. Preschool children have perhaps six such illnesses per year, while in middle childhood the rate drops to perhaps four to six per year (Parmelee, 1986). In contrast, only about 10 percent of children have any kind of chronic illness (an illness lasting six months or longer) during childhood. The most common types are allergies, asthma, visual and hearing impairments, and diabetes (Starfield, 1991).

At every age, children who are experiencing high levels of stress or family upheaval are more likely to become ill. For example, a large nationwide study in the United States shows that children living in mother-only families have more asthma, more headaches, and a generally higher vulnerability to illnesses of many types than do those living with both biological parents (Dawson, 1991). Figure 4.10 shows one comparison from this study, using a "health vulnerability score." This score is the sum of nine questions answered by parents about their child's health. You can see in the figure that the average score is only about 1.0 out of a possible 9, which implies that most children are quite healthy. But it is clear that children living in more stressful family structures have higher health vulnerability—and this is true even when such other differences between the families as race, income, and mother's level of education are factored out.

Another danger for children is accidents. In any given year, about a quarter of all children under 5 in the U.S. have at least one accident that requires some kind of medical attention (U.S. Bureau of the Census, 1994). Accidents are also the major cause of death in preschool and school-age children (Starfield, 1991). At every age, accidents are more common among boys than among girls. They have more broken arms, more cuts and abrasions, presumably because of their more active and daring styles of play. Automobile accidents are a major contributor to the injury rate among children. Among very young children, the rate of serious injury and death from auto accidents has been dropping dramatically in recent years because of new laws mandating the use of restraint devices for infants and toddlers traveling in cars (Christophersen, 1989). Among teenagers, auto accidents continue to be the single most common cause of death, although here too the rate has been declining in the past two decades, as the use of seat belts has increased (Centers for Disease Control, 1993b).

Obesity. Accidents and disease are not the only health hazards for children. One significant additional risk in this age range is obesity. Estimates of the frequency of obe-

FIGURE 4.10 Dawson finds that children from single-parent and stepparent families are more likely to be sick, a fact that probably demonstrates the effect of stress on illness. (*Source:* Dawson, 1991, from Table 3, p. 577.)

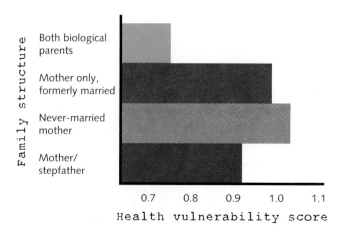

sity among children vary quite a lot, depending in part on how it is defined. One typical definition is a body weight 20 percent or more above the normal weight for height, and by this definition, 15 to 20 percent of U.S. youngsters are obese, with the incidence rising steadily in the past 30 years (Centers for Disease Control, 1994d; Gortmaker et al., 1987).

High rates of obesity are common in other Western countries as well. For example, researchers in Italy reported that among a large sample of 10-year-olds, 23.4 percent of the boys and 12.7 percent of the girls were classed as obese (Maffeis et al., 1993).

Obesity is *not* ordinarily more common among poor children, although the incidence is unusually high in some ethnic groups, including many Native-American groups and—perhaps—inner-city blacks (Gilbert et al., 1992; Sherry et al., 1992).

Obesity is a significant long-term health problem. Among adults, the obese have shorter life expectancies and higher risk of heart disease and high blood pressure. And fatness in childhood and obesity in adulthood are linked, albeit imperfectly. Only about a third to a fifth of obese preschoolers are still obese as adults, but about half of obese school-age children are still obese as adults (Serdula et al., 1993). Put another way, an obese child has three to five times the risk of being an obese adult. This does not mean, by the way, that all fat adults were fat children. More than half of obese adults were *not* fat as children. But being obese in childhood significantly increases the risk.

Obesity in childhood or adulthood appears to result from an interaction between a genetic predisposition and environmental factors that promote overeating or low levels of activity. The genetic component is clear from both twin and adoption studies. Adult identical twins, for example, have extremely similar adult weights even if they are reared apart, while fraternal twins differ much more (Stunkard et al., 1990). Similarly, adopted children reared by obese parents are less likely to be obese than are the natural children of obese parents (Stunkard et al., 1986).

Whether a child with a genetic propensity to fatness will actually become obese, however, depends on "energy balance"—the balance between the calories taken in and the number expended by exercise. On the "intake" side of this balance, the data are just plain confusing. Most studies of eating patterns show little or no difference in food intake between obese and nonobese children (Bandini & Dietz, 1992; Klesges, Shelton, & Klesges, 1993), although some newer studies suggest that obese children may take in higher proportions of dietary fat (Gazzaniga, 1993). On the "outgo" side, the evidence is somewhat clearer. There are various indications that obese children choose more sedentary activities or exercise somewhat less. In particular, recent studies show a link between amount of TV watching and obesity. One group of researchers, studying a national sample of more than 6000 children, estimates that the prevalence of obesity increases roughly 2 percent for each additional hour of television a child or teenager watches per day, even when prior weight, family influences, and other background variables are taken into account (Dietz & Gortmaker, 1985). These investigators are not arguing that watching TV makes you fat; they are suggesting that the more TV a child watches, the less exercise he or she is getting and the greater the likelihood that the youngster will eat high-fat junk food.

Obesity obviously affects a child's social experiences during the school years, which may have effects detectable into adulthood. At the same time, I should point out that *fear* of fatness may also become a significant problem for some children, leading to the disorders of bulimia and anorexia, which I'll talk about shortly. The balancing act required for the parents of an overweight child, then, is to try to help the child develop better eating

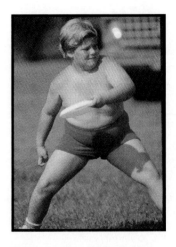

This overweight child not only has different kinds of encounters with his peers, but also is more likely to be fat as an adult, with accompanying increased health risks.

and exercise habits without so emphasizing the importance of thinness that the child develops pathological patterns of dieting. In either case, it is clear that both health habits and body images established in these early years will tend to persist into adolescence and adulthood, with potentially pervasive health consequences.

Health in Adolescence

Adolescents have fewer acute illnesses than do infants, toddlers, or school-age children, but teenagers engage in many forms of risky behavior, often described as sensation seeking, that lead to markedly increased rates of accidents, injuries, and illnesses in this age range. Indeed, Jeffrey Arnett (1992) proposes that, "Adolescence bears a heightened potential for recklessness compared to other developmental periods in every culture and in every time" (p. 339). The form this recklessness takes, and the extent to which it is allowed expression, varies from one culture and one historical time to the next. In the United States, at this time, the cultural mores allow—perhaps even encourage—a wide variety of risky behaviors. Adolescents engage in more unprotected sex, drive faster, tailgate more often, and use seat belts less than do adults (Arnett, 1992; Centers for Disease Control, 1994e). Rates of driving while intoxicated are also high among adolescents, although arrests for driving while intoxicated are actually at their peak among those in their middle twenties (U.S. Bureau of the Census, 1994).

Such high-risk behaviors, not surprisingly, lead to a variety of problems, especially for teenage males, in whom the tendency toward sensation seeking or risk taking is especially marked. Not only are auto accidents, homicide, and suicide the leading causes of death among teenage boys (U.S. Bureau of the Census, 1994), but 80 out of every 1000 teenage males in the U.S. were on the receiving end of some kind of violent crime, a rate nearly double that for teenage girls (Hammond & Yung, 1993). These figures are still higher among Hispanic, African-American, and Native-American teens.

Furthermore, 4 percent of adolescents in the U.S. contract a sexually transmitted disease each year, a rate that has been rising in the past decade, especially for syphilis (Panel on High Risk Youth, 1993). Unprotected sex among adolescents has also led to a marked rise in the risk of AIDS—a disease that is the fastest-growing cause of death among adolescents and young adults. As of April 1991, there were 8000 reported cases of AIDS among U.S. teens and young adults (ages 13 to 29). The Centers for Disease Control estimates that the total number of those infected is roughly 4.5 times as high, which means something on the order of 36,000 teens and young adults are infected with HIV. Those teens at greatest risk for infection are runaways, those with homosexual experiences, those engaged in prostitution, and intravenous drug users. But the disease has begun to spread beyond these risk groups within the adolescent population in the United States (Panel on High Risk Youth, 1993).

Alcohol and Drug Use in Adolescence. One major type of risk-taking behavior among teenagers is alcohol and drug use. National data suggest that many types of teenage drug use have been declining in the United States over the past several decades. For example, 23 percent of teenagers in 1974 reported that they had used marijuana, compared to only 10.6 percent in 1992. In the same years, the percentage of teenagers who had ever used cocaine also dropped by half, from 3.6 to 1.7 percent (U.S. Bureau of the Census, 1994).

The figures for alcohol use, however, have been moving in the opposite direction. In 1992, 65.6 percent of high school students said they had tried alcohol at least once, and 21 percent reported regular episodes of heavy drinking. These teenagers had had five or

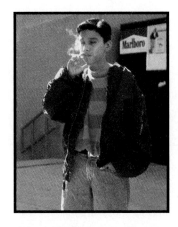 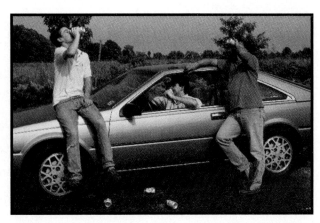

During adolescence, we see a rise in a whole range of high-risk behaviors, particularly those that involve sensation seeking, all of which have highly negative implications for the adolescent's health.

more drinks in a row at least once in the last month (Centers for Disease Control, 1994c). And a study of Oklahoma students revealed that 4.5 percent of middle-school and 19.2 percent of high school students used alcohol weekly (Novacek, Raskin, & Hogan, 1991).

Risky Behavior in Context. When the teenagers in the Oklahoma study were asked why they drank or took drugs, the most frequent reason given was that they were depressed. Other important reasons were a desire to escape from their problems and a wish to relax and have a good time. These answers suggest a more general point, one that Richard Jessor makes particularly clearly:

> *Adolescent risk behaviors are functional, purposive, instrumental, and goal-directed and . . . the goals involved are often those that are central in normal adolescent development. (Jessor, 1992, p. 378)*

The goals involved are peer acceptance or respect, establishing autonomy from parents and from other authority figures, coping with anxiety or fear of failure, and affirming maturity. Jessor argues that these are absolutely normal, central goals of adolescence. To the extent that some risky behavior, such as smoking, drinking, or early sexual activity, helps individual teenagers to meet those goals, such behaviors will be hard to change, *unless* alternative ways of meeting these same goals are available or encouraged.

Jessor's argument also implies that those teenagers who enter adolescence with few social skills and hence few alternative avenues for meeting these social and personal goals will be most likely to show risky behavior. And that is indeed what researchers have found. Those teens who showed behavior problems at earlier ages and have had poor school records, early rejection by peers, neglect at home, or a combination of these early problems are most likely to engage in high-risk behaviors (Robins & McEvoy, 1990). By default, such children or teens are drawn to peers who share their patterns and their internal models of the world, and for these adolescents, risky behaviors of various kinds provide an avenue for meeting some of the goals Jessor mentions.

Bulimia and Anorexia. Another growing health problem among adolescents—although in this case mostly among girls—is eating disorders, specifically bulimia and anorexia nervosa. What we are learning about the causes of these disorders underlines both the impact of cultural values and the importance of the child's internal working models.

The Real World

How to Get Your Teenager to Stop Smoking, or Not to Start

Nearly half of eighth graders think that smoking a pack or two of cigarettes a day carries no great risk. By senior year, only about 30 percent still believe this, but by then many have a well-established smoking habit. In fact, nearly all first tobacco use occurs before high school graduation; most of those who do not smoke in high school never develop the habit, while most of the 3 million adolescents who do smoke become addicted and are unable to quit, even when they try (Centers for Disease Control, 1994b). About a third of all high-school-age teens in the U.S. smoke or use smokeless tobacco, with smoking about equally likely among males and females. Across ethnic groups, however, there are wide disparities. Less than 5 percent of African-American high school seniors smoke daily, compared to about 12 percent of Hispanics and more than 20 percent of whites (Hilts, 1995).

The health risks linked to smoking are well established. What is not well established is how to prevent young people from taking up this habit. Among young blacks, family and peer pressure *against* smoking appears to be the crucial factor. Among white teens, there appears to be pressure in the other direction. So how can a parent change this? Reminding young people of the long-term health risks turns out not to be an especially effective strategy, at least not in isolation. Several other strategies are much more successful.

Stop Smoking Yourself. If you yourself are a smoker, and want your children not to smoke, the first step is for you to quit. There is clear evidence that children of parents who smoke are more likely to smoke themselves—a pattern that is especially clear for mothers and daughters (Kandel & Wu, 1995). It does no good to tell your child that he or she should do what you say and not what you do. Modeling does not work like that. Kids copy what you do.

Emphasize the Bad Breath. Tell them about all the negative *social* consequences of smoking. Their breath will smell bad, their teeth will turn yellow, their hair and clothes will smell like smoke all the time, and their ability to do well in athletics may be impaired. Tell them that

teenagers themselves say that they find smokers less attractive. And tell teenage girls that smoking will not help them lose weight (a major reason for smoking for nearly all teenage girls), at least not enough to counterbalance the social costs.

Encourage Your Schools to Adopt Antismoking Programs. All these messages are more effective if they come from other teenagers rather than from Mom and Dad, so lobby the local high school to organize systematic school-based prevention programs, with teens as models. Such programs work, especially if they are reinforced by community efforts and parent participation. A part of the school's program should be a complete ban on smoking on school premises. If the school your child attends has a designated smoking area, try to persuade the school board to abolish it. In schools that allow smoking, 25 percent more of the students become smokers than in schools that forbid it on the school grounds.

Focus on the Manipulation. Remind your child that the cigarette companies are trying to manipulate them through their advertising. You may want to get them to look at specific ads and talk about the particular forms of manipulation involved. In particular, you may want to try to counteract the common adolescent belief, fostered by advertising, that the majority of adults smoke.

Pay Attention to Your Child's Friends. Teenagers whose friends smoke are more likely to take up the habit. You need to start paying attention to this *very* early—certainly by junior high school, when you may still have enough influence over the child's choice of friends to help steer the child toward a different crowd of kids.

Do Not Call Smoking an "Adult Choice." Many tobacco company programs ostensibly aimed at reducing teenage smoking tell teenagers that they are too young to smoke. But because teenagers want to do anything defined as "adult," this message may encourage smoking rather than the reverse. Instead, tell teenagers that they are old enough to know better; they are old enough to decide *not* to smoke.

Bulimia (sometimes called *bulimia nervosa)* involves an intense concern about weight, combined with binge eating followed by purging, either through self-induced vomiting, excessive use of laxatives, or excessive exercise (Attie, Brooks-Gunn, & Petersen, 1990). Alternating periods of restrained and binge eating are common among individuals in all weight groups. Only when binge eating occurs as often as twice a week and is combined with repeated episodes of some kind of purging is the syndrome properly called bulimia. Bulimics are ordinarily not exceptionally thin, but they are obsessed with their weight, feel intense shame about their abnormal behavior, and often experience significant depression. There are also physical consequences, including marked tooth decay (from repeated vomiting), stomach irritation, lowered body temperature, disturbances of body chemistry, and loss of hair (Palla & Litt, 1988).

The incidence of bulimia appears to have been increasing in recent decades, particularly among adolescent girls, but just how common it may be has been hard to establish. Current estimates are that from 1.0 to 2.8 percent of adolescent girls and young adult women show the full syndrome of bulimia; as many as 20 percent of girls show at least some bulimic behaviors, such as occasional purging (Attie & Brooks-Gunn, 1995; Graber et al., 1994).

Anorexia nervosa is less common but potentially more deadly. It is characterized by extreme dieting, intense fear of gaining weight, and obsessive exercise. In girls or women, who are by far the most common sufferers, the weight loss eventually produces a variety of physical symptoms associated with starvation: sleep disturbance, cessation of menstruation, insensitivity to pain, loss of hair on the head, low blood pressure, a variety of cardiovascular problems, and reduced body temperature. Anorexics also typically develop thick, soft hair over their bodies. Their body image is so distorted that they can look in the mirror at a skeletally thin body and remain convinced that they are "too fat." Ten to 15 percent of anorexics literally starve themselves to death, and others die because of some type of cardiovascular dysfunction (Deter & Herzog, 1994).

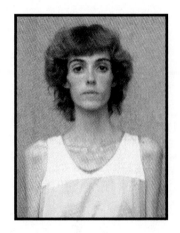

This 17-year-old has been hospitalized for anorexia. When she looks at herself in the mirror, chances are she sees herself as "too fat," despite her obvious emaciation.

In Western countries, where both these types of eating disorders are most common, perhaps one girl out of every 500 is anorexic (Graber et al., 1994); the rate is considerably higher among subgroups who are under pressure to maintain extreme thinness, such as ballet dancers and high-performance athletes in sports in which thinness is highly valued, such as gymnastics (Stoutjesdyk & Jevne, 1993).

The causes of both these eating disorders are unknown. Some theorists have proposed biological causes, such as some kind of brain dysfunction in the case of bulimics, who often show abnormal brain waves. Others argue for a psychoanalytic explanation, such as, in the case of anorexic patients, a fear of growing up. My own view is that the most promising explanation lies in the discrepancy between the young person's internal image of what kind or shape of body is desired and her (or his) perception of her own body. Both syndromes seem to be increasing in frequency because of the currently intense emphasis in many Western countries on a very slender, almost prepubescent body shape as the ideal for girls. Furthermore, from very early in life, girls (much more than boys) are taught both explicitly and implicitly that it matters if they are pretty or attractive and that thinness is one of the critical variables in attractiveness. Current research, for example, shows that roughly three-quarters of teenage girls have dieted or are dieting. If you look only at chronic dieters (those who have dieted at least 10 times in the past year), the figures are lower, but still striking, as you can see in Figure 4.11. These numbers come from a questionnaire study of all junior high and high school students in Minnesota in 1987 and 1988—a total of more than 36,000 teenagers (Story et al., 1991). You can see that chronic dieting is far less common among boys than among girls. Such dieting was also more common among Hispanic and white girls than among blacks.

Those girls who most fully accept and internalize this model of beauty are most prone to develop bulimia or anorexia. For example, Ruth Striegel-Moore and her colleagues

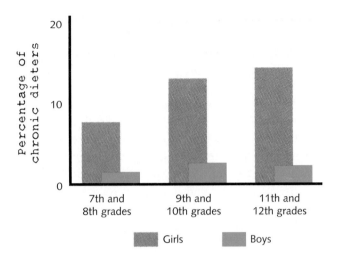

FIGURE 4.11 The percentage of junior high and high school students in Minnesota in 1987–1988 who reported having dieted at least 10 times in the previous year. (*Source:* Story et al., 1991, from Table 3, p. 995.)

(Striegel-Moore, Silberstein, & Rodin, 1986) have found that bulimic girls and women are more likely than are nonbulimics to agree with statements like "attractiveness increases the likelihood of professional success."

Both bulimia and anorexia seem to develop in adolescence, and not before that, precisely because one of the effects of puberty is to increase the amount of fat in the girl's body. This is particularly true of early-developing girls, who characteristically acquire and retain higher fat levels than do later-maturing girls. Indeed, early-developing girls are nearly twice as likely to have an eating disorder as are normal- or late-developing girls (Graber et al., 1994; Killen et al., 1992). Thus, an early-developing girl who deeply be-

Research Report

An Australian Study of Sex Differences in Body Image Among Adolescents

Susan Paxton's study of Australian high school students illustrates that the preoccupation with thinness among teenage girls is not restricted to the United States and shows what that preoccupation can do to girls' body images (Paxton et al., 1991).

A total of 562 teenagers in grades 7 through 11 reported on their current weight and height and their judgment of that weight as underweight, good weight, or overweight. They also responded to questions about the effect it might have on their lives if they were thinner and described their weight control behaviors, including dieting and exercise.

Paxton reports that among teenagers who were actually *normal* in weight for their height, 30.1 percent of the girls but only 6.8 percent of the boys described them-

selves as overweight. Thus, many girls *perceive* themselves as too fat when they are actually normal. Furthermore, the majority of girls thought that being thinner would make them happier; a few even thought that being thinner would make them more intelligent. Boys, in contrast, thought that being thinner would actually have some negative effects.

Not surprisingly, these differences in the perception of thinness were reflected in dieting behavior in this sample. Twenty-three percent of the girls reported that they went on a crash diet at least occasionally; 4 percent said they did so once or twice a week. The comparable percentages for boys were 9 and 1 percent, respectively. More girls than boys also reported using diet pills, laxatives, and vomiting, although the rates were low for both sexes.

lieves that thinness is essential for beauty and that beauty is essential for happiness, especially if she sees her own body as failing to meet her internalized standard, seems at particularly high risk for developing bulimia or anorexia (Attie & Brooks-Gunn, 1989; Rolls, Fedoroff, & Guthrie, 1991; Striegel-Moore et al., 1986).

Determinants of Growth: Explanations of Physical Development

In what I have said so far, I have mostly been dealing with description, with answering "what" questions. But "why" questions are equally important. Why does physical development occur as it does, and what can affect it?

Maturation

Maturational sequences certainly seem to be part of the explanation, especially for such central patterns as neuronal changes and changes in muscles, bones, and fat. In all these areas, while the *rate* of development varies from one child to the next, the *sequence* is virtually the same for all children, even those with marked physical or mental handicaps. Whenever we find such robust sequences, maturation of some kind seems an obvious explanation.

But Esther Thelen, one of the leading experts on motor development, points out that most of us have an overly simplistic view of the whole idea of maturation (Lockman & Thelen, 1993; Thelen, 1995). There is no "crawling gene" or "walking gene" that somehow "unfolds" in a sequence. Instead, she argues that any new movement or motor skill is a "final common pathway," a result of a complex system of forces operating together, including cognition, perception, and motivation, as well as underlying physical changes.

For example, for the toddler to learn to use a spoon to feed herself requires development of muscles in the hand and wrist, bone development in the wrist, eye-hand coordination skills that allow her to readjust the aim of the spoon as she moves it toward her mouth, and coordination of all these with properly timed mouth opening (Connolly & Dalgleish, 1989).

Obviously, Thelen is not denying the fundamental significance of the maturation of nerves and muscles. But she is saying that the concept of maturation alone does not *explain* the development of motor skills. In addition, of course, we should not forget the other elements in the explanatory equation.

Heredity

Our genetic heritage is individual as well as species-specific, so that each of us receives instructions for unique as well as shared growth tendencies. Both size and body shape seem to be heavily influenced by such specific inheritance. Parents and children are similar not only in such obvious characteristics as height, but also in hip width, arm length, and short or long trunk. (Some ancestor certainly passed on a gene for long arms to me!)

Rate or tempo of growth, as well as final shape or size, seems to be an inherited pattern as well. Parents who were themselves early developers, as measured by such things as bone hardening or age of menarche, tend to have children who are faster developers too (Garn, 1980).

If you had the power to change our culture in such a way that the rate of bulimia and anorexia would go way down, what changes would you want to make? Why and how?

Environmental Effects

There are potent external influences on physical growth as well. One of the clearest pieces of evidence pointing toward such environmental influences is the observation that children in different birth cohorts grow at different rates, a pattern of findings referred to as **secular trends.** For example, the age of menarche has decreased at the rate of about four months per decade over the past 100 years among European populations, shifting from an average age of roughly 17 in 1840 to roughly $12\frac{1}{2}$ or 13 today (Roche, 1979). Over the same decades, average final height and weight have increased, not only among European populations but also among the Japanese as well.

What could account for such changes over time? The most obvious possibility is that there have been changes in life-style and diet.

Diet. Differences in diet may not only help to explain such secular trends, but also contribute to the individual differences we see in rates of physical development in any one cohort. Most generally, we know that poorly nourished children grow more slowly and then don't end up as large (Malina, 1982). If their diet later improves, such children may show some catch-up in height or growth rate, but they are typically shorter and slower than their peers. In addition, of course, malnourished or undernourished children have less energy, which in turn can affect the nature of the interactions the child has with both the objects and the people around him. For example, in a recent study of schoolchildren in Kenya, Michael Espinosa and his colleagues (Espinosa et al., 1992) observed that undernourished kids were more solitary and less active on the playground than their well-nourished peers. The children in this study were not severely malnourished. They were taking in about 1500 calories per day, which is enough to sustain a child but not enough to provide the energy needed for play, perhaps for concentration in school over long periods.

Prenatal Environmental Influences. Prenatal environments can also have long-term effects on a child's physical development. One example is the impact of prenatal exposure to alcohol. Streissguth and her colleagues, whose work I described in Chapter 2, have found that 4-year-olds whose mothers drank while pregnant, compared to those whose mothers did not drink or drank less, had poorer balance and poorer fine motor skills, such as hand steadiness or the ability to tap rapidly with a finger (Barr et al., 1990). Caffeine ingestion and high use of aspirin during the pregnancy were also related to poorer fine motor skills among the 4-year-olds.

Practice. Both diet and prenatal exposures of various kinds are environmental variations that are external to the child. But we can also think of environmental influences on physical development in terms of the child's own practice of various physical activities. Does a baby who spends a lot of time in a toy called an infant walker, which holds up the baby while he moves around, learn independent walking any sooner than a baby who never has that practice? Does a toddler who has a chance to try to climb stairs learn to climb them sooner, or more skillfully, than a toddler who is rarely exposed to stairs? If you go back and look at Aslin's models of the possible role of early experience in Figure 1.1, you'll see that I am asking whether practice has a *facilitative* effect or even if it operates as what he calls *attunement.* Alternatively, perhaps practice has no effect at all on the emergence of basic skills.

The answer, as usual, is fairly complicated. Two conclusions are reasonably clear. First, the development of such universal, basic skills as crawling or walking requires some minimum amount of practice just to keep the system working as it should—what Aslin calls a *maintenance* effect of environment. Children who are deprived of such normal practice develop motor skills much more slowly, and not in the normal sequence. A classic early study by Wayne Dennis (1960) of children raised in Iranian orphanages is a good illustration. The babies in one of the institutions were routinely placed on their backs in cribs with very lumpy mattresses. They had little or no experience of lying or moving on their stomachs as a normal baby would and even had difficulty rolling over because of the hollows in the mattresses. These babies almost never went through the normal sequence of learning to walk—presumably because they didn't have enough opportunity to practice all the on-the-stomach parts of the skill. They did learn to walk eventually, but they were about a year late.

We also know that the development of really smooth, coordinated skill in virtually all complex motor tasks requires practice. The strength and coordination required to throw a basketball high enough to reach the basket may develop in predictable ways over the early years, assuming the environment is sufficiently rich to provide needed maintenance. But to develop the skill needed to get the ball through the hoop with regularity, from different angles and distances, requires endless practice.

Where we are still uncertain is about the role of practice in the acquisition of the basic component skills, such as sitting, walking up stairs, climbing, or catching objects. Early studies seemed to show that extra practice in such basic skills didn't speed up their development at all, perhaps because virtually all children have enough opportunity for minimal practice in their ordinary lives. But some recent studies contradict this conclusion, including one showing that very young babies who are given more practice sitting are able to sit upright longer than those without such practice (Zelazo et al., 1993). The jury is still out on this one.

As a final point about physical development, let me remind you of something I said at the very beginning of the chapter: The links between experience and physical development operate in both directions. Experience affects the child's skills, but the rate and pattern of the child's physical development also affect his self-image, his personality, his interactions with the world around him. So physical development influences experience as much as the reverse.

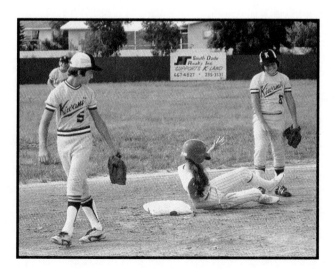

To acquire the basic skills needed to run, even to throw an object like a ball, a child probably doesn't need any special practice. But to be able to run and throw well enough to be a good baseball player requires an enormous amount of very specific practice.

Summary

1   It is important to know something about physical growth and development because specific new behaviors are triggered by physical changes, because physical skills affect the kinds of experiences the child can have, and because the child's feelings about her own body can affect self-concept and personality.

2   Changes in height and weight are rapid during the first year and then level off to a steady pace until adolescence, when a sharp "growth spurt" occurs.

3   Bones increase in number and harden slowly. Muscle tissue increases primarily in density and length of fibers, with a much larger increase at adolescence for boys than for girls.

4   Fat cells are added in the early years and then again rapidly at adolescence, in this case more for girls than for boys.

5   At birth the medulla and midbrain are most developed; the cortex develops primarily over the first two years. Major neural changes after birth are the growth of dendrites and of synapses as well as myelinization of axons.

6   Hormones are vital influences throughout growth, particularly during adolescence. The pituitary gland secretes triggering hormones at the beginning of puberty, which stimulate the development of sex hormones, which in turn trigger the development of primary and secondary sex characteristics.

7   Pubertal changes begin as early as 8 or 9 in girls and continue until the mid-teens. In boys, the changes begin somewhat later, with the growth spurt roughly two years later. In both sexes, the physical changes occur in reliable sequences, starting with changes in secondary sex characteristics, followed by the growth spurt, with reproductive maturity late in the sequence.

8   The collective changes in bone, muscle, fat, and nervous system make possible the emergence of the various motor skills. Most basic motor skills are present by about age 6.

9   At adolescence, pubertal changes make mature sexual behavior possible. Sexual activity among teens has increased in recent decades. Roughly half of all high school students in the U.S. are sexually active, and one in ten teenage girls becomes pregnant each year.

10   Children differ markedly in the rate with which all these changes take place. In general, rapidly developing children have advantages over slower-developing children in intellectual skill. Personality effects are more complex. In general, children whose physical development is markedly earlier or later than they expect or desire show more negative effects than do those whose development is "on time."

11   Some social class and racial differences can also be detected, with children from poverty-level environments developing more slowly. Both black and Asian children show more rapid tempo of development than do white children.

12   Illness is also a normal part of children's early lives. Young children have brief illnesses six to nine times each year. Chronic illness is less common. Repeated or frequent illness in childhood is associated with poorer health later on.

13   Adolescents have fewer acute illnesses than younger children but more deaths from accidents, particularly automobile accidents. In general, they show higher rates of various kinds of risky behavior.

14   Alcohol and drug use among teenagers has been declining in recent decades, but regular alcohol use may be on the rise. Those most likely to use or abuse drugs are those who also show other forms of deviant or problem behavior, including poor school achievement.

15   Eating disorders such as bulimia and anorexia are more common among teenage girls. Both appear to be a response to a major discrepancy between culturally defined body ideals and girls' perceptions of their own bodies.

16 Maturation is a key process underlying physical growth and development, but maturation alone cannot account for the patterns that we see. Some environmental support is required, and specific heredity, prenatal teratogens, and prenatal and postnatal diet affect both the rate and pattern of development in individual children.

17 The role of practice is complex. A minimum amount of practice is required to sustain development of basic physical skills; for more complex skills, specific practice is required for skill acquisition.

Key Terms

anorexia nervosa **(p. 121)**

bulimia **(p. 120)**

cephalocaudal **(p. 98)**

cortex **(p. 100)**

endocrine glands **(p. 102)**

estrogen **(p. 103)**

fontanels **(p. 98)**

gonadotropic hormones **(p. 103)**

medulla **(p. 100)**

menarche **(p. 104)**

midbrain **(p. 100)**

motor development **(p. 107)**

myelin **(p. 101)**

myelinization **(p. 101)**

ossification **(p. 98)**

proximodistal **(p. 98)**

puberty **(p. 104)**

secular trends **(p. 124)**

Suggested Readings

Gullotta, T. P., Adams, G. R., & Montemayor, R. (Eds.). (1993). *Adolescent sexuality.* Newbury Park, CA: Sage.

A first-rate volume of papers on all aspects of this important subject. Of particular interest are a paper by Dyk reviewing information on physical changes at adolescence and one by Miller et al. on sexual behavior in adolescents.

Malina, R. M. (1990). Physical growth and performance during the transitional years (9–16). In R. Montemayor, G. R. Adams, & T. P. Gullotta (Eds.), *From childhood to adolescence: A transitional period?* (pp. 41–62). Newbury Park, CA: Sage.

To some extent Malina has picked up where Tanner has left off, providing us with updated information on normal physical growth. This particular paper focuses on puberty, but it contains references to much of Malina's work on other ages as well.

Millstein, S. G., Petersen, A. C., & Nightingale, E. O. (Eds.). (1993). *Promoting the health of adolescents. New directions for the twenty-first century.* New York: Oxford University Press.

An excellent new volume covering all aspects of the important question of how we can promote better health and health habits in adolescence.

Tanner, J. M. (1978). *Fetus into man: Physical growth from conception to maturity.* Cambridge, MA: Harvard University Press.

I don't usually recommend a book published almost 20 years ago. But Tanner's book is a classic, providing a detailed but very thorough and remarkably understandable discussion of all but the most current information about physical growth.

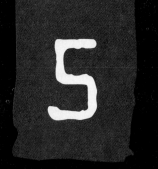

5

Perceptual Development

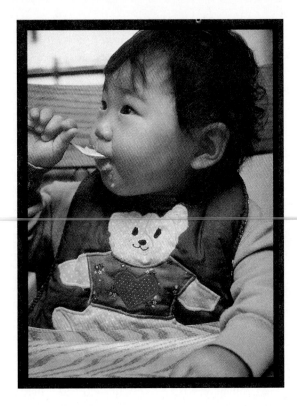

Have you ever seen a baby trying to feed herself something mushy and messy like chocolate pudding? It is a wonderful and fascinating sight—more charming, of course, if someone else has to clean up the child afterward! In the beginning, most babies don't have very good aim, so the chocolate pudding goes in the hair, all over the face, and down the front of the shirt. Most babies are not at all bothered by the mess and will look at you with delighted grins in the midst of the goo.

In fact, it is no small task for the toddler to get that spoon reliably into her mouth. It obviously involves motor skills, since she has to be able to grasp the spoon and move her hand and arm toward her mouth. But motor skills alone are not enough. She also has to use a wide range of *perceptual* information. She has to see the spoon and/or feel it in her hand, estimate the distance from the mouth and gauge the appropriate trajectory, meanwhile coordinating the visual and kinesthetic information as she goes along, so that she can change her aim if she needs to.

In the last chapter I tried hard to make the case that we cannot understand the development of the child's thinking, or of her emerging social relationships, without having some understanding of physical development. Here I want to make the same case for perceptual development. Perceptual processes form a part of virtually every task a child must perform, of every motor or cognitive skill that is developed. To identify Mom or Dad she has to discriminate among voices, faces, or even smells. To recognize faces, she must pay attention to (and remember) individual features or patterns of features. To learn to talk she must hear differences among sounds, focusing eventually on the repertoire of sounds used in the language spoken around her.

To understand a child's development, then, we have to understand what kinds of sense impressions are possible for her, both at birth and over the years of development. And we have to understand how the child comes to interpret those sense impressions—to discriminate among them, to recognize or understand patterns. In this sense the study of perceptual development forms a kind of bridge between the study of physiological changes, such as the changes in the nervous system I described in the last chapter, and the study of thinking, which I'll be turning to in Chapter 6.

The study of perceptual development has also been significant because it has been a key battleground for the dispute about nature versus nurture. Theorists who study perceptual development have always labeled this as the contrast between **nativism** and **empiricism,** rather than nature versus nurture, but the issue is precisely the same: How much of our basic perceptual understanding of the world is built in? How much is the product of experience? This issue has been so central in studies of perception that researchers have focused almost all their attention on young infants, because it is only among infants that we can observe the organism when it is relatively uninfluenced by specific experience. The early months are also the time of most rapid change in perceptual skills, and hence a time of greater interest to psychologists trying to understand the processes of development. For both these reasons, most of the information I'll be giving you in this chapter describes perceptual processes in very young children. But that age limitation makes the issues no less fascinating.

Ways of Studying Early Perceptual Skills

It took a while for psychologists to figure out how to study infants' perceptual skills. Babies can't talk, they can't respond to ordinary questions. So how were we to decipher just what they could see, hear, or discriminate? Eventually, clever researchers figured out three basic methods that allow us to "ask" a baby about what he experiences.

In the *preference technique,* devised by Robert Fantz (1956), the baby is simply shown two pictures or two objects, and the researcher keeps track of how long the baby looks at each one. If many infants shown the same pair of pictures consistently look longer at one picture than the other, it not only tells us that babies see some difference between the two, but also may reveal something about the kinds of objects or pictures that capture babies' attention.

Another strategy takes advantage of the processes of *habituation* and *dishabituation* that I described in Chapter 3. You first present the baby with a particular sight or sound over and over until he habituates, that is, until he stops looking at it or showing interest in it. Then you present another sight or sound or object that is slightly different from the original one and watch to see if the baby shows renewed interest (dishabituation). If the baby does show such renewed interest, you know he perceives the slightly changed sight or sound as "different" in some way from the original.

The third option is to use the principles of *operant conditioning* I described in Chapter 1. For example, an infant might be trained to turn her head when she hears a particular sound, using the sight of an interesting moving toy as a reinforcement. After the learned response is well established, the experimenter can vary the sound in some systematic way to see whether the baby still turns her head or not.

Research using variations on these three techniques has now yielded a rich array of information about young infants' perceptual capacities. To simplify the descriptive task, let me divide the information into two rough groups, which we might call "basic" and "more complex" skills. The distinction I am using here is similar to the distinction between sensation and perception given in most psychology texts. When we study *sensation,* we are asking just what information the sensory organs receive. Does the structure of the eye permit infants to see color? Is the structure of the ear and of the cortex such that a very young infant can discriminate among different pitches? When we study *perception* we are asking what the individual does with the sensory information, how it is interpreted or combined. So let me begin with the basic sensory capacities present in the newborn or developing over the first years of life.

Basic Sensory Skills

The common theme running through all of what I will say about basic sensory skills is that newborns and young infants have far more sensory capacity than physicians or psychologists thought even as recently as a few decades ago. Perhaps because babies' motor skills are so obviously poor, we assumed that their sensory skills were equally poor. But we were wrong. A newborn does not have all the sensory capacities of a 2-month-old, a 1-year-old, or an adult. But most of the basic skills are in place in at least rudimentary form.

Seeing

There are a great many basic visual skills, but let me focus on three that seem especially important: acuity, tracking moving objects, and color vision.

Acuity. Acuity refers to how well or how clearly you can perceive something. When you apply for a driver's license and take the eye test that involves reading the letters on one line of a large chart, you're being tested for visual acuity. The usual standard for visual acuity in adults is "20/20" vision. This means that you can see and identify something that is 20 feet away that the average person can also see at 20 feet. A person with 20/100

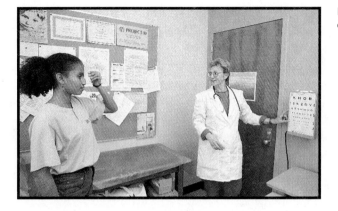

Eye tests like this one are measures of visual acuity.

vision, in contrast, has to be as close as 20 feet to see something that the ordinary person can see at 100 feet. In other words, the higher the second number, the poorer the person's visual acuity.

Until 25 or 30 years go, many medical texts stated that the newborn infant was blind. Now we know that the newborn has quite poor visual acuity but is quite definitely not blind. Findings from research using a variety of different techniques have converged on a virtually unanimous conclusion that at birth the infant's acuity is in the range of 20/200 to 20/400 and reaches roughly adult levels (20/20) by about one year of life (Haith, 1990).

The fact that the newborn sees so poorly is not so negative a thing as it might seem at first. Of course it does mean that a baby doesn't see faraway things very clearly; he probably can't see well enough to distinguish two people standing nearby. But he sees quite well close up, which is all that is necessary for most encounters with the people who care for him or with objects immediately at hand, such as breast, bottle, or mobiles hanging above his crib.

Tracking Objects in the Visual Field. When our young chocolate pudding eater tries to get the spoon in her mouth, one of the things she needs to do is keep her eyes on her hand or the spoon as she moves it toward herself. This process of following a moving object with your eyes is called **tracking,** and you do it every day in a variety of situations. You track the movement of other cars when you are driving; you track as you watch a friend walk toward you across the room; a baseball outfielder tracks the flight of the ball so that he can catch it. Because a newborn infant can't yet move independently, a lot of her experiences with objects are with things that move toward her or away from her. If she is to have any success in recognizing objects, she has to be able to keep her eyes on them as they move; she must be able to track.

Studies by Richard Aslin (1987a) and others show that tracking is initially fairly inefficient but improves quite rapidly. Infants younger than 2 months show some tracking for brief periods if the target is moving very slowly. But somewhere around 6 to 10 weeks a shift occurs, and babies' tracking becomes skillful rather quickly. You can see the change very graphically in Figure 5.1, taken from a study by Aslin.

Color Vision. The tale I can tell about color vision is similar. Researchers in this field have established that the types of cells in the eye (cones) necessary for perceiving red and

Can you think of other examples of tracking in your everyday life or examples of professions in which the ability to track well would be especially important?

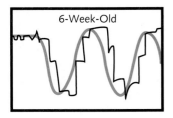

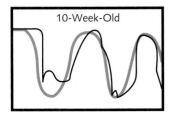

FIGURE 5.1 The blue line in each figure shows the trajectory of the moving line that each baby tried to follow with its eyes in Aslin's experiment. The black line represents one baby's eye movements at 6 weeks and again at 10 weeks. At 6 weeks, the baby more or less followed the line, but not smoothly. By 10 weeks the same baby's tracking skill was remarkably smooth and accurate. (*Sources:* Aslin, 1987a, p. 87; redrawn from Aslin, 1981b.)

Why is it important for an infant to be able to identify the direction of some sound?

green are clearly present by 1 month, perhaps at birth; those required for perceiving blue are probably present by then as well (Bornstein, 1992). Thus, infants can and do see and discriminate among various colors.

Taken together, these findings certainly do not support the notion that an infant is blind at birth! While it is true that the infant's acuity is initially poor, it improves rapidly, and other visual capacities are remarkably well developed early on. There are also some interesting hints here that there may be some kind of shift of gears at roughly 2 months, since a number of skills, including the scanning of objects as well as smooth pursuit, improve incrementally at about that age (Bronson, 1994). Whether such a change is the result of such neurological changes as the rapid proliferation of synapses and the growth of dendrites, or of changes in the eye itself, or perhaps of the child's experience, we don't yet know.

Hearing

Acuity. Although children's hearing improves up to adolescence, newborns' auditory acuity is actually better than their visual acuity. Current research evidence suggests that within the general range of pitch and loudness of the human voice, newborns hear nearly as well as adults do. They have somewhat more difficulty with high-pitched sounds; such a sound needs to be louder before the newborn can hear it than is true for older children or adults (Werner & Gillenwater, 1990).

Detecting Locations. Another basic auditory skill that exists at birth but improves with age is the ability to determine the location of a sound. Because your two ears are separated from one another, sounds arrive at one ear slightly before the other, which allows you to judge location. Only if a sound comes from a source equidistant from the two ears (the "midline") does this system fail. In this case, the sound arrives at the same time to the two ears and you know only that the sound is somewhere on your midline. We know that newborns can judge at least the general direction from which a sound has come because they will turn their heads in roughly the right direction toward some sound. But finer-grained location of sounds is not well developed at birth. For example, Barbara Morrongiello has observed babies' reactions to sounds played at the midline and then sounds coming from varying degrees away from the midline. Among infants 2 months old it takes a shift of about 27 degrees off of midline before the baby shows a changed response; among 6-month-olds only a 12-degree shift is needed, while by 18 months discrimination of a 4-degree shift is possible—nearly at the skill level seen in adults (Morrongiello, 1988; Morrongiello, Fenwick, & Chance, 1990).

Other Senses

Smelling and Tasting. The senses of smell and taste have been studied much less, but we do have some basic knowledge. As with adults, the two senses are intricately related—that is, if you cannot smell for some reason (like when you have a cold), your taste sensitivity is also significantly reduced. Taste is detected by the taste buds on the tongue, which register four basic tastes: sweet, sour, bitter, and salty. Smell is registered in the mucous membranes of the nose and has nearly unlimited variations.

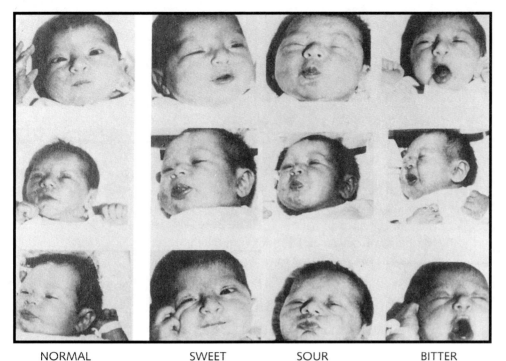

NORMAL   SWEET   SOUR   BITTER

FIGURE 5.2 These are three of the newborns Steiner observed in his experiments on taste response. The left-hand column shows each baby's normal expression; the remaining columns show the change in expression when they were given sweet, sour, and bitter tastes. What is striking is how similar the expressions are for each taste. (*Source:* J. E. Steiner, Human facial expressions in response to taste and smell stimulation. In H. W. Reese & L. P. Lipsett [Eds.], *Advances in child development and behavior,* Vol. 13. New York: Academic Press, 1979, Figure 1, p. 269.)

Newborns appear to respond differentially to all four of the basic flavors (Crook, 1987). Some of the clearest demonstrations of this come from an elegantly simple set of early studies by Jacob Steiner (Ganchrow, Steiner, & Daher, 1983; Steiner, 1979). Newborn infants who had never been fed were photographed before and after flavored water was put into their mouths. By varying the flavor, Steiner could determine whether the babies reacted differently to different tastes. As you can see in Figure 5.2, babies responded quite differently to sweet, sour, and bitter flavors.

Babies as young as a week old can also tell the difference between such complex smells as personal body odors. Specifically, they can discriminate between their mother's and other women's smells, although this seems to be true only for babies who are being breast-fed and who thus spend quite a lot of time with their noses against the mother's bare skin (Cernoch & Porter, 1985).

Senses of Touch and Motion. The infant's sense of touch and motion may well be the best developed of all. Certainly they are sufficiently well developed to get the baby fed. If you think back to the list of reflexes in the newborn I gave you in Chapter 3, you'll realize that the rooting reflex relies on a touch stimulus to the cheek, and the sucking reflex relies on touch in the mouth. Babies appear to be especially sensitive to touches on the mouth, the face, the hands, the soles of the feet, and the abdomen, with less sensitivity in other parts of the body (Reisman, 1987).

I am aware that all of what I have said about these sensory abilities is fairly dry and technical. The important point for you to remember is that, as Reisman puts it, "We think of infants as helpless but they are born with some exquisitely tuned sensory abilities" (1987, p. 265).

Complex Perceptual Skills: Preferences, Discriminations, and Patterns

When we turn to studies of more complex perceptual skills, such as perceiving depth, discriminating among faces, or noticing patterns, the abilities of very young infants seem even more remarkable. Let's begin, as we did in talking about the simple sensory abilities, with vision.

Looking

Depth Perception. One of the complex skills that has been most studied is depth perception. You need this ability any time you reach for something or decide whether you have room to make a left turn before an oncoming car gets to you. In these cases and many, many others, you need to judge distance or depth, just as our young pudding eater needs to do when she aims her spoon toward the bowl of pudding.

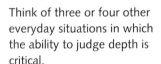

Think of three or four other everyday situations in which the ability to judge depth is critical.

It is possible to judge depth using any (or all) of three rather different kinds of information: First, *binocular* cues involve both eyes, each of which receives a slightly different visual image of an object; the closer the object is, the more different these two views are. In addition, of course, information from the muscles of the eyes also tells you something about how far away an object may be. Second, *pictorial* information, sometimes called *monocular* cues, requires input from only one eye. For example, when one object is partially in front of another one, you know that the partially hidden object is further away—a cue called *interposition*. The relative size of two similar objects, such as telephone poles or two people you see in the distance, may also indicate that the smaller-appearing one is further away. Linear perspective (like railroad lines that seem to get closer together as they are further away) is another monocular cue. Third, *kinetic* cues come from either your own motion or the motion of some object: If you move your head, objects near you seem to move more than objects further away (a phenomenon called *motion parallax*). Similarly, if you see some object moving, such as a person walking across a street or a train moving along a track, closer objects appear to move over larger distances in a given space of time.

How early can an infant judge depth, and which of these cues does he use? This is still an active area of research, so the answer I can give you is not final. The best conclusion at the moment seems to be that kinetic information is used first, perhaps by about 3 months of age; binocular cues are used beginning at roughly 4 months; and pictorial (monocular) cues are used last, perhaps at 5 to 7 months (Bornstein, 1992).

I don't have enough room to talk about the research on each of these three types of cues, so let me concentrate on the most extensive and most fascinating line of research, which has involved the use of kinetic cues. In a remarkably clever early study, Eleanor Gibson and Richard Walk (1960) devised an apparatus called a *visual cliff*. You can see from the picture in Figure 5.3 that it consists of a large glass table with a sort of runway in the middle. On one side of the runway is a checkerboard pattern immediately below the glass; on the other side—the "cliff" side—the checkerboard is several feet below the glass. The baby could judge depth here by several means, but it is primarily kinetic information that is useful, since the baby in motion would see the nearer surface move more than the further surface. If a baby has no depth perception, she should be equally willing to crawl

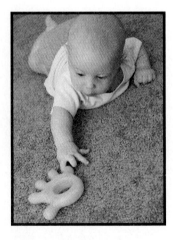

One of the many skills 5-month-old Shina-Mira has to have to reach for and grasp her toy is the ability to judge depth. How far away is the toy? Is it near enough for her to reach with her hand?

on either side of the runway, but if she can judge depth, she should be reluctant to crawl out on the "cliff" side.

Since an infant had to be able to crawl in order to be tested in the Gibson and Walk procedure, the original subjects were all 6 months old or older. Most of these infants did *not* crawl out on the cliff side but were quite willing to crawl out on the shallow side. In other words, 6-month-old babies have depth perception.

But what about younger infants? The traditional visual cliff procedure can't give us the answer, since the baby must be able to crawl in order to "tell us" whether he can judge depth. With younger babies, researchers have studied kinetic cues by watching babies react to apparently looming objects. Most often the baby observes a film of an object moving toward him, apparently on a collision course. If the infant has some depth perception, he should flinch, move to one side, or blink as the object appears to come very close. Such flinching has been consistently observed in 3-month-olds (Yonas & Owsley, 1987). Most experts now agree that this is about the lower age limit of depth perception.

What Babies Look At. Even though a baby cannot judge depth right away, her behavior is governed by visual information from the very first minutes of life. We know that from the beginning, babies look at the world around them in a nonrandom way. In Marshall Haith's phrase (1980), there are "rules babies look by." Furthermore, those rules seem to change with age.

In the first two months, a baby's visual attention is focused on *where* objects are in his world (Bronson, 1991). Babies scan the world around them—not very smoothly or skillfully, to be sure, but nonetheless regularly, even in the dark. This general scanning continues until they come to a sharp light/dark contrast, which typically signals the edge of some object. Once he finds such an edge, a baby stops searching and moves his eyes back and forth across and around the edge. Thus, the initial rules seem to be: Scan till you find an edge and then examine the edge. Motion also captures a baby's attention at this same age, so he will look at things that move as well as things with large light/dark contrast.

These rules seem to change between 2 and 3 months, perhaps because the cortex has then developed more fully. At about this time the baby's attention seems to shift from *where* an object is to *what* an object is. Put another way, the baby seems to move from a strategy designed primarily to *find things* to a strategy designed primarily to *identify* things. Babies this age begin to scan rapidly across an entire figure, rather than getting stuck on edges. As a result, they spend more time looking at the internal features of some object or array of objects and are thus better able to identify the objects.

What is amazing about this shift is the degree of detail infants now seem to be able to take in and respond to. They notice whether two pictures are placed horizontally or vertically, they can tell the difference between pictures with two things in them and pictures with three things in them, and they clearly notice patterns, even such apparently abstract patterns as "big-thing-over-small-thing."

One early study that illustrates this point particularly well comes from the work of Albert and Rose Caron (1981), who used stimuli like those in Figure 5.4 in a habituation procedure. The babies were first shown a series of pictures, like those on the left in Figure 5.4, that shared some particular relationship. The example I've shown in the figure is "small over big." After the baby stopped being interested in these training pictures (that is, after he habituated), the Carons showed him another figure (the "test

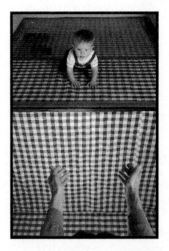

FIGURE 5.3 In this "visual cliff" apparatus, like the one used by Gibson and Walk, Mom tries to entice her baby out onto the "cliff" side. But because the infant can perceive depth, he thinks he will fall if he comes toward her, so he stays put, looking concerned.

Training stimuli

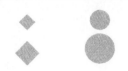

Test stimuli

A   B

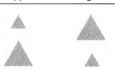

FIGURE 5.4 In the Carons' study, the researchers first habituated each baby to a set of training stimuli (all "small over large" in this case), then showed each baby two test stimuli: one that had the same pattern as the training stimuli (A) and one that had a different pattern (B). Three- and 4-month-old babies showed renewed interest in the B stimulus but not in the A stimulus, showing that they pay attention to the pattern and not just to specific stimuli. (*Source:* Caron & Caron, 1981, p. 227.)

Does this mean that researchers ought to believe mothers and fathers more often when they describe their infants and what the babies can do? How should scientists weigh anecdotal evidence against research evidence?

stimulus") that either followed the same pattern or followed some other pattern, such as those you can see on the bottom right-hand side of Figure 5.4. If the baby had really habituated to the *pattern* of the original pictures (small-over-large), he should show little interest in stimuli like the A test stimulus (ho hum, same old boring small over large thing), but he should show renewed interest in test stimulus B (hey, here's something new!). Caron and Caron found that 3- and 4-month-old children did precisely that. So even at this early age, babies find and pay attention to patterns, not just to specific stimuli.

Faces: An Example of Responding to a Complex Pattern. From the beginning of this new era of research on infant perception, researchers have been especially interested in babies' perception of faces, not only because of the obvious relevance for parent-infant relationships, but also because of the possibility that there might be a built-in preference for faces or facelike arrangements—a variant of the now familiar nativism/empiricism issue. After 30 years of research, we do not have all the answers. In fact, research brings new surprises all the time. Here is a sample of what we think we know at this point.

First, there is little indication that faces are uniquely interesting to infants, which fails to support one of the early assumptions of many nativists. That is, babies do not systematically choose to look at faces rather than at other complex pictures.

On the other hand, among faces, babies clearly prefer some to others. They prefer *attractive* faces (an intriguing result that I've discussed in the *Research Report* on the facing page), and it now looks as if they prefer their *mother's* face from the earliest hours of life, a finding that has greatly surprised psychologists, although it may not surprise you.

For years I have been telling my friends and relatives that there was clear research showing that babies can't recognize their mothers' faces until at least 1 or 2 months of age but that they can recognize the mother by sound or smell immediately. None of my friends or relatives believed me; they all said, "I don't care what the research says; I know my baby could recognize my face right away." Well, it looks like they were right and the older research (and I) was wrong.

Several new studies show this, but the clearest and cleanest is one by Gail Walton and her colleagues (Walton, Bower, & Bower, 1992). Walton videotaped the faces of 12 mothers of newborns and then matched each of these faces with the face of another woman whose hair color, eye color, complexion, and hairstyle were the same as Mom's. Each baby was then tested with one picture at a time in a modification of the preference technique. The babies could keep the picture turned on by sucking on a pacifier. The experimenters could then count how often the babies sucked in order to keep Mom's picture available, compared to their sucking rate for the non-Mom photo. These babies, who were only a day or two old at the time of the testing, clearly preferred to look at their Moms, as you can see in Figure 5.5 (p. 138). Walton also has some preliminary information that babies do *not* discriminate, or do not prefer, their fathers' faces as early as this, even in cases in which the father had spent more time with the baby than the mother had.

This is a fascinating result. Clearly, the baby has to *learn* the mother's features in those first hours after birth. But how is this possible? Is there some kind of imprinting going on here to the first face the baby sees after it is born? If so, then the process should be affected by birth practices or by the amount of contact the baby had had with various individuals. In the particular hospital where Walton's subjects

Research Report

Langlois' Studies of Babies' Preferences for Attractive Faces

Among all the current studies on infant perception that seem to point toward the conclusion that many more abilities and preferences are built in than we had supposed, Judith Langlois' studies of infant preferences for attractive faces rank as some of the most surprising and intriguing. Langlois has found that babies as young as 2 months old will look longer at a face that adults rate as attractive than at one adults judge to be less attractive.

In the first study in this series, Langlois and her colleagues (Langlois et al., 1987) tested 2- to 3-month-olds and 6- to 8-month-olds. Each baby, while seated on Mom's lap, was shown pairs of color slides of 16 adult Caucasian women, half rated by adult judges as attractive, half rated as unattractive. On each trial, the baby saw two slides simultaneously shown on a screen in front of him/her, with each face approximately life size, while the experimenter peeked through a hole in the screen to count the number of seconds the baby looked at each picture. Each baby saw some attractive/attractive pairs, some unattractive/unattractive pairs, and some mixed pairs.

The crucial trials are obviously those in which there was one attractive and one unattractive face. The results, which are on the left side of the table below, show that even the 2- to 3-month-olds preferred to look at the attractive faces.

One of the nice features of this study is that they used a variety of attractive and unattractive faces, which makes the conclusion clearer. But because Langlois used only Caucasian female faces in this first study, generality of the result was in question. In a later study (Langlois et al., 1991), Langlois used the same procedure but showed some 6-month-old infants pictures of (1) both unattractive and attractive men and women, (2) attractive and unattractive black women's faces, or (3) baby faces varying in attractiveness, all with neutral expressions. You can see the results on the right half of the table.

Once again the results are consistent: In every case babies look significantly longer at the attractive than at the unattractive faces.

In another exploration of this same issue, Langlois, Roggman, and Rieser-Danner (1990) observed 1-year-old babies interacting with an adult wearing either an attractive or an unattractive mask. They found that the toddlers showed more positive affective tone, less withdrawal, and more play involvement with the stranger in the attractive mask. These 1-year-olds also played more with an attractive than with an unattractive doll.

It is hard to imagine what sort of learning experiences could account for such a preference in a 2-month-old. Instead, these findings raise the possibility that there is some inborn template for the "correct" or "most desired" shape and configuration for members of our species and that we simply prefer those who match this template better. If that's true, what kind of consequences might it have for child and adult development, especially the development of the less attractive baby, child, or adult?

Average Looking Time (in Seconds)

	2–3-month-olds	6–8-month-olds	Male and Female	Black Women	Baby Faces
Attractive faces	9.22[a]	7.24[a]	7.82[a]	7.05[a]	7.16[a]
Unattractive faces	8.01	6.59	7.57	6.52	6.62

[a]Contrast between attractive and unattractive faces is statistically significant.

Sources: Langlois et al., 1987, from Table 1, p. 365; Langlois et al., 1991, Table 1, p. 81.

were born, babies spend as much as an hour with their mothers immediately after birth—even when the birth is by cesarean section—so the mother's face is normally the first one the baby sees. It would be very interesting to see if Walton's result would be replicated when someone else was the first face or when the mother and

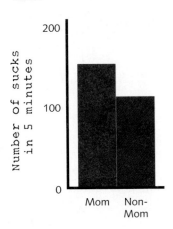

FIGURE 5.5 The babies in this study were 12 to 36 hours old at the time they were tested. They sucked more to see a picture of Mom than a picture of another woman who looked very like the mom. (*Source:* Walton, Bower, & Bower, 1992, p. 267.)

infant spent only a moment together after delivery. A⟨...⟩ the case, this one study seems to settle one question but raise many more.

Beyond the issue of preference, we also have to answer the question of just what it is that babies are looking at when they scan a face. Before about 2 months of age, babies seem to look mostly at the edges of the faces (the hairline and the chin); after 2 months they seem to look more at the internal features, particularly the eyes—yet another example of the basic shift in rules at 2 months that I already described.

Discriminating Emotional Expressions. At about the same time—2 to 3 months of age—babies begin to respond differently to various emotional expressions as well as to facial features. For example, Haviland and Lelwica (1987) found that when mothers expressed happiness, 10-week-old babies looked happy and interested and gazed at the mother; when the mother expressed sadness, babies showed increased mouth movements or looked away; when the mother expressed anger, some babies cried vigorously, while others showed a kind of still or "frozen" look. These responses did not seem to be merely imitation, but rather responses to the parent's specific emotions.

By 5 or 6 months, babies respond differently to strangers' faces displaying different emotions (Balaban, 1995) as well as to voices speaking with varying emotional tones. They can tell the difference between happy and sad voices (Walker-Andrews & Lennon, 1991) and between happy, surprised, and fearful faces (Nelson, 1987). By roughly 10 to 12 months, infants sometimes use such emotional cues to help them figure out what to do in novel situations, such as when a stranger comes to visit, in the doctor's office, or even when a new toy is put in front of them. Babies this age will first look at Mom's or Dad's face to check for the adult's emotional expression. If Mom looks pleased or happy the baby is likely to explore the new toy with more ease or to accept the stranger with less fuss. If Mom looks concerned or frightened, the baby responds to those cues and reacts to the novel situation with equivalent fear or concern. Researchers have described this as a process of **social referencing** (Walden, 1991).

Listening

When we turn from looking to listening we find similarly intriguing indications that very young infants not only make remarkably fine discriminations among individual sounds, but also pay attention to patterns.

A baby this age can already discriminate his mom's face from the face of another woman; he can also recognize his mom's voice and smell.

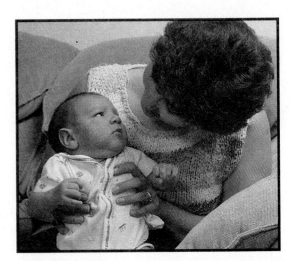

Discriminating Speech Sounds. One of the central questions has to do with how early a baby can make discriminations among different speech sounds. This has obvious relevance for the psychologists interested in language development, since a baby cannot learn language until he can hear the individual sounds as distinct. But perception researchers have also been interested in this question because the answers may tell us some very interesting things about what may be built into the neurological system. Much of this research is quite technical, but I will do my best to try to convey to you why psychologists have found the results so remarkable.

For starters, researchers have established that as early as 1 month, babies can discriminate between speech sounds like *pa* and *ba* (Trehub & Rabinovitch, 1972). Studies using conditioned head-turning responses have shown that by perhaps 6 months of age, they can discriminate between two-syllable "words" like *bada* and *baga* and can even respond to a syllable that is hidden inside a string of other syllables, (like ti*bati* or ko*ba*ko) (Fernald & Kuhl, 1987; Goodsitt et al., 1984; Morse & Cowan, 1982). Even more remarkable, it doesn't seem to matter what voice quality the sound is said in. By 2 or 3 months of age, babies respond to individual sounds as the same whether they are spoken by male or female voices, or a child's voice (Marean, Werner, & Kuhl, 1992).

That's already pretty impressive evidence that infants listen to quite fine variations in speech sounds, not just at the beginnings of words but in other vocal positions as well. But that is not the end of the story. It also turns out that infants can accurately discriminate among sound contrasts that appear in *any* language, not just sounds that they are actually hearing in the language being spoken around them. Babies in an English-speaking environment can discriminate pairs of sounds that occur in Hindi (a language of India) but not in English; babies in Spanish-speaking environments can discriminate pairs of sounds that are relevant in English but not in Spanish. Japanese babies can discriminate between the *l* and *r* sounds that occur in English but not in Japanese. But by about 6 months of age, babies begin to lose the ability to distinguish pairs of vowels that do not occur in the language they are hearing; by 1 year, the ability to discriminate pairs of nonheard consonant contrasts begins to fade (Polka & Werker, 1994), although such an ability does not disappear altogether. Adults can learn to "hear" such sound variations if they work very hard at it, such as when trying to learn to speak a foreign language without an accent. But the infant appears to hear all these distinctions naturally.

An unusually complete study by Janet Werker and Richard Tees (1984) illustrates the point. Combining cross-sectional and longitudinal designs, they first studied separate groups of 6- to 8-month-olds, 8- to 10-month-olds, and 10- to 12-month-olds being raised in English-speaking homes. Each baby was tested on three sound pairs, one heard in English (*ba* versus *da*); one from a North-American Indian language, Salish (*ki* versus *qi*); and one from Hindi, a language from the Indian subcontinent (*ṭa* versus *ta*) You can see in Figure 5.6 that the 6- to 8-month-old English-environment babies could easily hear and respond to both the Hindi and Salish contrasts, but very few of the 10- to 12-month-olds could do so. When Werker and Tees later retested some of the 6-month-olds at 9 and 12 months, they found that these babies had *lost* the ability to make these discriminations. In separate tests, Werker and Tees also tested Hindi- and Salish-environment infants and found that 12-month-old Hindi infants could easily discriminate the Hindi contrast and Salish toddlers could still hear the Salish contrast.

FIGURE 5.6 In these studies, babies growing up in English-speaking environments were tested for their ability to make two discriminations: between two speech sounds that are used differently in Hindi but that are treated the same in English and between a pair of sounds used differently in Salish but treated as the same in English. The upper part of the figure shows a cross-sectional comparison, with 12 babies in each age group. The lower part of the figure shows what happened to the discrimination ability of six babies studied longitudinally. You can see that virtually all the babies could make these discriminations at 8 months but that this ability rapidly disappeared. (*Source:* Werker & Tees, 1984, Figure 4, p. 61.)

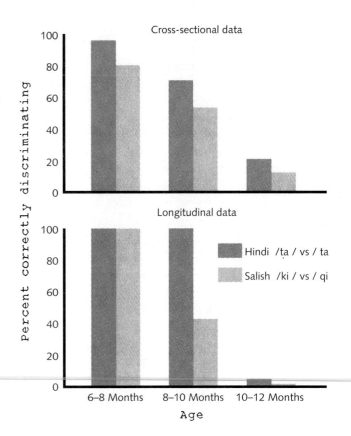

It seems to me that these findings are consistent with what we now know about the pattern of rapid, apparently preprogrammed, growth of synapses in the early months of life, followed by synaptic pruning. Many connections are initially created, permitting discriminations along all possible sound continua. But only those pathways that are actually used in the language the child hears are retained.

Discriminating Individual Voices. Newborns also seem to be able to discriminate between individual voices. DeCasper and Fifer (1980) have found that newborns can tell their mother's voice from another female voice (but not their father's voice from another male voice) and prefer the mother's. This is easier to account for than is the newborn's preferences for the mother's face, since the baby could learn the sound of the mother's voice while still *in utero*. But it is still a striking finding.

By 6 months, babies even know which voice is supposed to go with which face. If you put an infant of this age in a situation where she can see both her father and mother and can hear a tape-recorded voice of one of them, she will look toward the parent whose voice she hears (Spelke & Owsley, 1979).

Other Sound Patterns. As was true with studies of looking, there is also evidence that infants pay attention to *patterns* of sounds from the very beginning. Two other studies by DeCasper demonstrate the point strikingly. In the first study (DeCasper & Spence, 1986), he had pregnant women read a particular children's story (such as Dr. Seuss's *The Cat in the Hat*) out loud each day for the final six weeks of the pregnancy. After the infants were born, he played recordings of the mother reading this same story, or another previously unheard story, to see which the infant preferred. The newborns clearly preferred the sound of the story they had heard *in utero.* In the more recent study (DeCasper et al., 1994), done in France, he had pregnant women recite a short children's rhyme out loud each day between the thirty-third and thirty-seventh weeks of their pregnancy. In the thirty-eighth week he played a recording either of the same rhyme the mother had been reading or of another rhyme, and measured the fetal heart rate. He found that fetal heart rates dropped during the recording of the familiar rhyme, but not during the unfamiliar rhyme. These studies obviously tell us that key features of the auditory system are well developed some weeks before birth. But they also tell us that even in the last weeks of gestation the fetus is already paying attention to and discriminating among complex patterns of sounds.

Further evidence for the same point comes from the observation that babies as young as 6 months listen to melodies and recognize the patterns. Sandra Trehub and her colleagues (Trehub, Bull, & Thorpe, 1984; Trehub, Thorpe, & Morrongiello, 1985) trained 6-month-old babies to turn their heads toward a loudspeaker for a particular six-tone melody and then tested the babies with melodies that varied in a number of ways. Babies continued to turn their heads to new melodies if the melody had the same contour (notes going up and down in the same sequence) and were in approximately the same range. They responded to them as different if the contour changed or if the notes were much higher or much lower. Thus, as is true with patterns of looking, within the first few months of life babies appear to pay attention to and respond to pattern and not just the specific sounds. Whether such pattern perception skills are built into the neurological system as it develops or whether they are the result of the child's learning after birth is still a matter of fairly hot debate. But the fact that such skills are present very early in life is no longer in dispute.

Combining Information from Several Senses

I have been talking about each sense separately, as if we experience the world through only one sense at a time. But think about the way you receive and use perceptual information; you rarely have information from only one sense at a time. Ordinarily, you have *both* sound and sight, touch and sight, or still more complex combinations of smell, sight, touch, and sound. Psychologists have been interested in knowing how early an infant can combine such information. For example, how early can an infant integrate information from several senses, such as knowing which mouth movements go with which sounds? Even more complex, how early can a baby learn something via one sense and transfer that information to another sense? For example, at what age can a child recognize solely by feel a toy he has seen but never felt before? The first of these two skills is usually called *intersensory integration,* while the latter is called **cross-modal** (or intermodal) **transfer.**

Piaget believed that both these skills were simply not present until quite late in the first year of life, after the infant had accumulated many experiences with specific objects and how they simultaneously looked, sounded, and felt. Other theorists, including James and Eleanor Gibson, have argued that some intersensory integration or even transfer is built in from birth. The baby then builds on that inborn set of skills with specific experience with objects. Research favors the Gibsonian view: Empirical findings show that cross-modal transfer is possible as early as 1 month and becomes common by 6 months (Rose & Ruff, 1987).

For example, if you attach a nubby or a smooth sphere to a pacifier and give one or the other to each of several babies to suck, you can test for cross-modal transfer using

What might be some practical implications of the fact that fetuses can hear clearly enough to distinguish the pattern of a story read to them *in utero?*

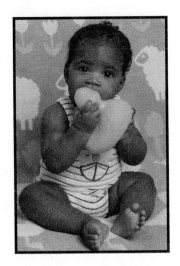

Even though 7-month-old Leslie is not looking at this toy while she chews on it, she is nonetheless learning something about how it *ought* to look, just based on how it feels in her mouth and in her hands—an example of cross-modal transfer.

Fantz's preference technique: You show the babies pictures of the two spheres to see if infants look longer at one than at the other. In one early study following this method, Meltzoff and Borton (1979) found that 1-month-old babies preferred to look at the picture of the object they had sucked on earlier. In a similar recent study, Kaye and Bower have demonstrated such transfer in infants 12 *hours* old (1994). Both Bower and Meltzoff have argued that babies this age are not really transferring information from one sense to another but instead are paying attention to features of objects that are relevant in any sense modality. For example, identifying an object as being "flat on one side" is useful whether one is later trying to identify the object by feel or by sight. Whether this explanation is correct or not remains a matter of debate. But the very fact that it can be demonstrated at all is a strong argument for the nativist side of the ancient argument.

In older children, intersensory integration and transfer can be readily demonstrated, not only between touch and sight, but also between other modalities such as sound and sight. For instance, in several delightfully clever experiments, Elizabeth Spelke showed that 4-month-old infants can connect sound rhythms with movement (1979). She showed babies two films simultaneously, one showing a toy kangaroo bouncing up and down, the other a donkey bouncing up and down, with one of the animals bouncing at a faster rate. Out of a speaker located between the two films the infant heard a tape recording of a rhythmic bouncing sound that matched the bounce pattern of one of the two animals. In this situation, babies showed a preference for looking at the film showing the bounce rate that matched the sound. A recent extension of this by Jeffery Pickens (1994) is even more striking. He showed 5-month old babies two films side by side, each displaying a train moving along a track. Then out of a loudspeaker he played engine sounds of various types, such as getting gradually louder (thus appearing to come closer) or getting gradually fainter (thus appearing to be moving away). The babies in this experiment looked longer at a picture of a train whose movement matched the pattern of engine sounds. That is, they appeared to have some understanding of the link between the pattern of sound and the pattern of movement—knowledge that demonstrates not only intersensory integration, but also surprisingly sophisticated understanding of the accompaniments of motion.

In the same vein, researchers have shown that 4- to 5-month-old babies will look longer at a face of a person mouthing a vowel that the baby hears spoken over a loudspeaker than at the face of a person mouthing another vowel (Kuhl & Meltzoff, 1984; Walton & Bower, 1993). Similarly, somewhat older infants shown a photo of a male and one of a female will look longer at the face that matches the gender of a voice heard over a loudspeaker—although only when the photo/voice match is female (Poulin-Dubois et al., 1994). Even more remarkable is a study in which 7-month-olds saw pairs of faces displaying happy and angry expressions, while listening to words spoken in either a happy or an angry voice. The babies looked longer at the face that matched the *emotion* in the speaking voice—a finding that suggests remarkable sophistication of intermodal transfer by age 7 or 8 months (Soken & Pick, 1992).

I do not want to leave you with the impression that intermodal integration or transfer is a completely automatic process in young infants. It isn't. In 4- and 5-month-olds, it often doesn't occur at all, or only under special circumstances (Lewkowicz, 1994). But it is clear that young infants have at least some ability to link simultaneous information from several senses, a conclusion that raises several interesting theoretical issues. For one thing it is now perfectly clear that a baby or child does not need language to transfer information from one mode to another. And the fact that at least some transfer is possible within the first few weeks of life certainly points rather strongly to the possibility that *some* connections may be built in, although experience with specific objects and combinations clearly makes a difference as well. So this body of information enriches but does not settle the nativism/empiricism debate.

Ignoring Perceptual Information: The Perceptual Constancies

All of what I have said so far has been aimed at persuading you that from early in life, babies are remarkably skillful at making perceptual discriminations of various kinds. But there is another, very different kind of perceptual skill the infant must also acquire—the ability to *ignore* some kinds of perceptual data. Specifically, the child must acquire a set of rules we call **perceptual constancies.**

When you see someone walking away from you, the image of the person on your retina actually becomes smaller. But you don't see the person getting smaller. You see him as the same size but moving farther away. When you do this, you are demonstrating **size constancy;** you are able to see the size as constant even though the retinal image has changed.

Other constancies include the ability to recognize that shapes of objects are the same even though you are looking at them from different angles, called (logically enough) **shape constancy,** and the ability to recognize that colors are constant even though the amount of light or shadow on them changes, called **color constancy.**

Taken together, the several specific constancies add up to the larger concept of **object constancy,** which is the recognition that objects remain the same even when the sensory information you have about them has changed in some way. Babies begin to show signs of these constancies at 3 or 4 months of age and become more skilled over the first several years. Let me use shape constancy as an illustration.

Shape constancy has perhaps the most obvious day-to-day relevance for the baby. She has to realize that her bottle is still her bottle even though it is turned slightly and thus presents a different shape; she has to figure out that her toys are the same when they are in different positions. The beginnings of this understanding seem to be present by about 2 or 3 months of age. The classic study was done by Thomas Bower (1966), who first trained 2-month-old babies to turn their heads when they saw a particular rectangle. He then showed them tilted or slightly turned images of the same rectangle to see if the babies would respond to these as "the same," even though the retinal image cast by these tilted rectangles was actually a trapezoid and not a rectangle at all. Two-month-olds did indeed continue to turn their heads to these tilted and turned rectangles, showing that they have some shape constancy.

One of the ironies about perceptual development is that at a later age, when learning to read, a child has to *unlearn* some of these shape constancies. Pairs of letters like *b* and *d*, *p* and *q*, or *p* and *b* are the same shape, except with the direction reversed or one upside down. So to learn to read (at least the Latin alphabet) the child must now learn to pay attention to something she has learned to ignore—namely, the rotation of the letter in space.

Of course learning to read involves a good deal more than simply ignoring shape constancy (and I'll have more to say about it in Chapter 8, when I talk about language development). But we do know that among 5-year-olds, those who have difficulty discriminating between mirror images of shapes also have more difficulty learning to read (Casey, 1986).

The Object Concept

Grasping the various object constancies is only part of a larger task facing the child; he must also figure out the nature of objects themselves. First of all, an infant must somehow learn to treat some combinations of stimuli as "objects" and others not, a process usually referred to now as *object perception.* For example, if a baby sees a heap of blocks on a carpet, does she "know" that each block is a separate object? Does she treat the carpet as an object as well? What makes an object an object? A still more sophisticated aspect of the infant's emerging concept of objects is the understanding that objects continue to exist even when they are out of view. I know that my computer is still sitting here even when I am not in the room. Does a baby know that Mom continues to exist when she leaves the room or that her bottle still exists when she drops it over the edge of the crib? Such an understanding is usually referred to as **object permanence.**

Object Perception

The most thorough and clever work on object perception in infants has been done by Elizabeth Spelke and her colleagues (1982; 1985; Spelke, von Hofsten, & Kestenbaum, 1989). Spelke believes that babies are born with certain built-in assumptions about the nature of objects. One of these is the assumption that when two surfaces are connected to one another they belong to the same object, which Spelke calls the *connected surface principle.* To study this (1982), she first habituated some 3-month-old babies to a series of displays of two objects; other babies were habituated to the sight of one-object displays. Then the babies were shown two objects touching each other, such as two square blocks placed next to each other so that they created a rectangle. Under these conditions the babies who had been habituated on two-object displays showed renewed interest, clearly indicating that they "saw" this as different, presumably as a single object. Babies who had seen the one-object displays during habituation showed no renewed interest. Spelke has also shown that babies as young as 2 and 3 months old are remarkably aware of what kinds of movements objects are capable of, even when the objects are out of sight. They expect objects to continue to move on their initial trajectory, and they show surprise if the object's movement violates this expectancy. They also seem to have some awareness that solid objects cannot pass through other solid objects.

In one experiment, Spelke (1991) used the procedure shown schematically in the upper part of Figure 5.7. Two-month-old babies were repeatedly shown a series of events like that in the "familiarization" section of the figure: A ball starting on the left-hand side was rolled to the right and disappeared behind a screen. The screen was then taken away and the baby could see that the ball was stopped against the wall on the right. After the baby got bored looking at this sequence (habituated), he or she was tested with two variations, one "consistent" and one "inconsistent." In the consistent variation, a second wall was placed behind the screen and the sequence run as before, except now when the screen was removed, the ball could be seen resting up against the

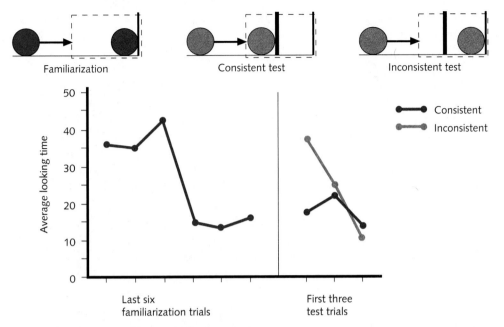

FIGURE 5.7 The top part of the figure shows a schematic version of the three conditions Spelke used. The bottom half shows the actual results. You can see that the babies stopped looking at the ball and screen after a number of familiarization trials but showed renewed interest in the inconsistent version—a sign that the babies saw this as somehow different or surprising. The very fact that the babies found the inconsistent trial surprising is itself evidence that infants as young as 2 months have far more knowledge of objects and their behavior than most of us had thought. (*Source:* Spelke, 1991, Figures 5.3 and 5.4.)

nearer wall. In the inconsistent variation, the ball was surreptitiously placed on the *far* side of the new wall. When the screen was removed the ball was visible in this presumably impossible place. Babies in this experiment were quite uninterested in the consistent condition but showed sharply renewed interest in the inconsistent condition, as you can see in the lower part of Figure 5.7, which shows the actual results of this experiment.

Spelke is not suggesting that all the child's knowledge of objects is built in; she is suggesting that *some* rules are built in and that others are learned through experience. Others, such as Renée Baillargeon, argue that basic knowledge is not built in, but that strategies for learning are innate. According to this view, infants initially develop basic hypotheses about the way objects function—how they move, how they connect to one another. Then these early basic hypotheses are quite rapidly modified, based on the baby's experience with objects. For example, Baillargeon finds that 2- to 3-month-old infants are already operating with a basic hypothesis that an object will fall if it isn't supported by something. But they have no notion of how much support is required. By about 5 months of age this basic hypothesis has been refined, so that they understand that the smiling-face block in the arrangement on the top of Figure 5.8 (A) will stay supported, but the block in the arrangement on the bottom (B) will not (Baillargeon, 1994). At this point, I can't tell whether Spelke or Baillargeon will ultimately turn out to be correct about the extent to

I find it astonishing that a 2-month-old baby can have enough understanding of the physical world to "know" in some fashion that it is unexpected for the ball to be on the other side of the middle wall in this experiment. Are you also astonished by this result?

which these forms of knowledge are built in. But in either case, it is striking to see just how early babies know such complex things about the physical world.

Object Permanence

The study of object perception is a rather new area of research. In contrast, object permanence has been extensively explored, in large part because this particular understanding was strongly emphasized in Piaget's theory of infant development. According to his observations, replicated frequently by later researchers, understanding of object permanence emerges in a series of steps.

The first sign that the baby is developing object permanence comes at about 2 months of age. Suppose you show a toy to a child of this age and then put a screen in front of the toy and remove the toy. When you then remove the screen, the baby shows some indication of surprise, as if she knew that something should still be there. The child thus seems to have a rudimentary schema or expectation about the permanence of an object. But infants of this age show no signs of searching for a toy they may have dropped over the edge of the crib or that has disappeared beneath a blanket or behind a screen.

Six- or 8-month-old babies, however, *will* look over the edge of the crib for the dropped toys or for food that was spilled. (In fact, babies of this age may drive their parents nuts playing "dropsy" in the high chair.) Infants this age will also search for partially hidden objects. If you put a favorite toy under a cloth but leave part of it sticking out, the infant will reach for the toy, which suggests that in some sense the infant "recognizes" that the whole object is there even though she can see only part of it. But if you cover the toy completely with the cloth or put it behind a screen, the infant will stop looking at it and will not reach for it, even if she has seen you put the cloth over it—a pattern shown in the photos in Figure 5.9.

This changes again somewhere between 8 and 12 months; infants this age will reach for or search for a toy that has been covered completely by a cloth or hidden by a screen. Thus, by 12 months, most infants appear to grasp the basic fact that objects continue to exist even when they are no longer visible.

Object constancy has intrigued researchers and theorists in part because it forms one kind of bridge between studies of perception and early cognitive development. Many

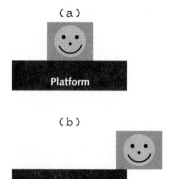

(a)

(b)

FIGURE 5.8 Renée Baillargeon's research suggests that 2- and 3-month-old babies think that the clown-face block will not fall under either of these conditions, but by 5 months, they realize that only the top (a) condition is stable. In the lower (b) condition, the block will fall. (*Source:* Baillargeon, 1994, adapted from Figure 1, p. 134.)

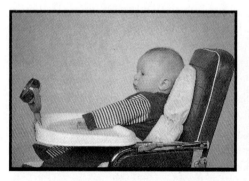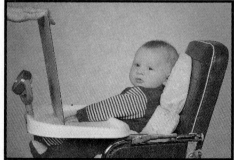

FIGURE 5.9 These photos show very graphically the response of a 6- or 7-month-old infant in an object permanence test. The baby stops reaching for or searching for the toy when it is hidden from him. An older baby would keep searching or push the screen aside to reach for the toy.

Cultures and Contexts

Object Permanence in Zambian Infants

Piaget believed that the emergence of the child's understanding of object permanence followed a universal sequence. One way to test this assumption, of course, is to observe or test children in non-Western societies, particularly infants or children whose early experiences are different from what we see in the U.S. or Europe. Susan Goldberg's longitudinal study of 38 Zambian infants (1972) gives us one such cross-cultural look.

Goldberg's two years of observations in Zambia made clear that the typical experience of a Zambian baby was quite different in a number of respects from that of most Western infants. From shortly after birth, Zambian babies are carried about in a sling on their mother's back. They spend very little time on the floor or in any position in which they have much chance of independent movement until they are able to sit up at about 6 months. At that point they are usually placed on a mat in the yard of the house. From this vantage the baby can watch all the activity around the house and in the neighborhood, but he has few objects to play with. Goldberg noted that the Zambian mothers did not see it as their task to provide play objects for their infants or to structure the child's play in any way. Indeed, Goldberg says she rarely saw the babies playing with objects, even those that might have been available in the yards.

Despite this very limited experience manipulating objects, tests of object permanence showed that the Zambian babies were *ahead* of the American averages on a measure of the object concept at 6 months of age. At 9 and 12 months of age, the Zambian babies were slightly behind the U.S. norms, but Goldberg believes this difference is due not to any cognitive failure but to the fact that at these ages the Zambian babies were quite unresponsive and passive toward objects, and thus very difficult to test. One possible explanation of this is that in Zambian culture, at least as Goldberg observed it, obedience is a highly valued quality in a child. The babies are trained from very early on to be particularly obedient to prohibitions of various kinds. When the baby plays with some object that he is forbidden to touch, the object is taken away. Perhaps, then, the infant learns that when an object is removed, it means "don't play with that" and he makes no further move to reach for the toy during the object permanence test. This does not necessarily mean that the baby has not understood these later stages of object permanence; it could also mean that our traditional ways of measuring this understanding would need to be modified for these children.

Goldberg's observations thus illustrate both the robustness of some basic developmental patterns *and* the impact of culture on the ways those patterns are displayed by children. Babies in Zambia appear to develop the early steps of the understanding of object permanence even though they have little chance to manipulate objects. But their response to objects is also affected by their training and experience.

have also been struck by a possible link between the emergence of object constancy and the infant's earliest attachment. It seems reasonable to assume that some kind of object permanence is required before the baby can become attached to an individual person, such as his mother or father. Since we know that clear single attachments don't appear much before 5 months, right about the time that the baby is showing signs of object permanence, the connection seems very reasonable. Interestingly, and surprisingly to a lot of us, most direct tests of this hypothesis have not shown much sign of such a causal link. Still, the problem may be with our research techniques rather than the hypothesis. As John Flavell says,

How ever could a child persistently yearn and search for a specific other person if the child were still cognitively incapable of mentally representing that person in the person's absence? (1985, p. 135)

I find Flavell's logic persuasive, but as usual we will have to wait for further research evidence to be sure.

Individual Differences in Perception: Speed and Efficiency

I pointed out in the last chapter that the shared patterns of physical development are extremely robust. Highly similar sequences are seen in all children. The same is clearly true for many of the patterns of perceptual development I've been describing here. But as with physical development, there are nonetheless some individual variations in the process, of which the most interesting are the indications that babies may differ in the efficiency with which they are able to deal with perceptual information.

The most extensive body of research has dealt with variations in "recognition memory" among infants—the ability to recognize that one has seen or experienced some object or person before. One way to measure this is with a standard habituation test. That is, we can count how many repeated exposures it takes before a baby stops responding with interest to some stimulus. The speed with which such habituation takes place may tell us something about the efficiency of the perceptual/cognitive system and its neurological underpinnings. And if such efficiency lies behind some of the characteristics we normally call "intelligence," then it is possible that individual differences in rate of habituation in the early months of life may predict later intelligence test scores.

What do you think this finding—that babies who habituate faster later have higher IQs—means in practical terms? Could it mean that babies who have had more stimulation in the early months develop more quickly? Could it mean that what we measure with IQ is really all just wiring? What other possibilities can you think of?

This is exactly what researchers have found in studies over the past 15 years. The rate of habituation shown by 4- to 5-month-old babies is correlated positively with IQ and language development at 3 or 4 years of age or older. That is, slower habituation is associated with lower IQ and poorer language. The average correlation in studies in both the U.S. and England is in the range of .45 to .50 (Slater, 1995). This is certainly not perfect, but it is remarkably high, given the difficulties involved in measuring habituation rate in babies.

Certainly these correlations do not prove that intelligence, as we measure it on an IQ test, is *only* a reflection of some kind of "speed of basic processing." But results like these underline the potential importance of individual differences in perceptual efficiency in early infancy.

Explanations of Perceptual Development

I pointed out at the beginning of this chapter that the study of perception, more than any other topic in developmental psychology except perhaps intelligence, has been dominated by questions of nature versus nurture, nativism versus empiricism. Certainly there are now other theoretical approaches or issues to choose from, but given the importance of the historical argument between the nativists and the empiricists, it's worthwhile to take a look at just where we stand on this question in our current understanding of perceptual development.

Nativism Versus Empiricism

Arguments for Nativism. It is certainly not hard to find strong arguments for a nativist position on perceptual development. As researchers have become more and more clever in devising ways to test infants' perceptual skills, they have found more and more skills already present in newborns or very young infants: Newborns have good auditory acuity, poor but adequate visual acuity, excellent tactual and taste perception. They have at least some color vision and at least rudimentary ability to locate the source of sounds around them.

More important, babies do not have to be taught what to look at. There are "rules" for looking, listening, and touching that can be detected at birth. As Kagan puts it: "Nature has apparently equipped the newborn with an initial bias in the processing of experience. He does not, as the nineteenth-century empiricists believed, have to learn what he should examine" (Kagan, 1971, p. 60). Furthermore, studies like Spelke's on babies' object understanding points to the strong possibility that other "assumptions" or biases about the way the world is organized may also be built in.

The fact that the "rules" seem to change with age can also be explained in nativist terms, since we know that the nervous system is undergoing rapid maturation during the early months of life, much of it apparently in an automatic way, as synapses are formed rapidly. Furthermore, these "rule changes" seem to occur in bursts. One such set of changes seems to occur at about 2 to 3 months, when infants appear to shift away from fixation on contours or edges and toward more detailed analysis of objects or figures. At about the same age, the baby becomes able to track objects smoothly. Another shift seems to occur at about 4 months, when we see a whole host of discrimination skills for the first time, including depth perception based on kinetic cues and consistent evidence of cross-modal transfer, especially coordination of auditory and visual information.

Of course it is possible that this apparent pileup of changes at 4 months reflects the accidental fact that many researchers have chosen to study babies of this age rather than younger babies, so we simply know a great deal more about 4-month-olds. But one major reason that researchers choose this age to study is that babies this age are significantly easier to test—perhaps because there has now been some underlying maturational shift that makes them more attentive, more able to focus, more stable in state.

Finally, we can find support for a nativist position in comparisons of the perceptual development of babies born *after* the normal gestational period versus those born preterm or postterm. In one such study, Yonas (1981) compared the response of two groups of 6-week-old babies: normal-term babies and a group of babies born 3 to 4 weeks late (postterm). Both sets of infants were tested for depth perception using the method of looming objects. Yonas found that the postterm infants showed more consistent reactions to the looming objects even though both groups had had precisely the same number of weeks of experience with objects since birth. Thus, it looks as if it is maturational age, not experience, that matters in this case, which strengthens a nativist or biological position.

Arguments for Empiricism. On the other side of the ledger, however, we can find a great deal of evidence from research with other species that some *minimum level* of experience is necessary to support the development of the perceptual systems—the pattern of environmental effect Aslin calls maintenance. For example, animals deprived of light show deterioration of the whole visual system and a consequent decrease in perceptual abilities (Hubel & Weisel, 1963).

It is also possible to find support for the negative version of Aslin's facilitation effect: Infants lacking sufficient perceptual stimulation may develop more slowly. Wayne

Dennis's study of orphanage babies in Iran, which I described in Chapter 4, illustrates this possibility. The infants who didn't have a chance to look at things, to explore objects with hands and eyes and tongue, and who were deprived of the opportunity to move around freely were retarded in the development of both perceptual and motor skills.

Attunement may also occur. Evidence from studies of other species suggests that those who are completely deprived of visual experiences in the early months of life never develop the same degree of depth perception as do those with full visual experience (Gottlieb, 1976).

The relationship between the built-in process and the role of the environment is a little like the difference between computer hardware and software. The perceptual hardware—specific neural pathways, rules for examining the world, a bias toward searching for patterns, and the like—may be preprogrammed. But the software—the specific program that governs the child's response to a particular real environment—depends on specific experience. A child is *able* to make visual discriminations between people or among objects within the first few days or weeks of life. That's built into the hardware. But the specific discriminations she learns and the number of separate objects she learns to recognize will depend on her experience. She is initially able to discriminate all the sound contrasts that exist in any spoken language, but the specific sound contrasts she eventually focuses on and the actual language she learns depend on the language she hears. The basic system is thus adapted to the specific environment in which the child finds herself. A perfect example of this, of course, is the newborn's ability to discriminate her mother's face from that of a very similar woman's face. Such discrimination *must* be the result of experience, yet the capacity to do so must be built in.

Thus, as is true of virtually all dichotomous theoretical disputes, both sides are correct. Both nature and nurture are involved. No doubt this particular dichotomy will continue to be part of the theoretical vocabulary in studies of perception for a long time to come. But in the past decade or so, theorists have begun to move away from the either/or, yes/no approach to studying perception in young infants and have begun to ask a different set of questions: What are the systematic patterns of *change* in perceptual skills or preferences with age? What are the roles of context and specific experience in those changes? How are the basic sensory skills and the basic perceptual discrimination abilities combined into higher-order perceptual skills, such as judging "objectness" or patterns of sounds or sights? Eleanor Gibson has been one of the key figures in this newer view, so let me sample some of her ideas very briefly, to give you some of the flavor.

An Alternative Theoretical Approach: Eleanor Gibson's Views

Setting aside the nativism/empiricism issue, Gibson turns to a search for systematic patterns or dimensions of change in perceptual skills or strategies. She identifies a number of such dimensions (1969; Gibson & Spelke, 1983), four of which are particularly interesting for this discussion.

Purposefulness of Perceptual Activity. Even as recently as a decade ago, many psychologists thought that the young infant was "captured" by stimulation—that the baby was a relatively passive recipient of stimulation. William James proposed a version of this view more than 100 years ago when he suggested that for the baby, the world was a "blooming, buzzing confusion." Now we know that even the newborn explores the world around herself in an apparently nonrandom way, using some rules, some strategies.

Nonetheless, as the child gets older, her rules become more flexibly applied, more intentional, more adapted to the setting.

For example, Brian Vandenberg (1984) gave children ages 4 through 12 years a series of toys to play with, including many novel toys. The younger children were more likely to have their attention "captured" by one particular toy and to stay with that toy for most of the session. The older children typically looked at and explored all the toys first and then went back to the ones of special interest. Thus, as the child gets older, he not only explores more systematically, but does so more intentionally, less controlled by some dominant stimulus.

Awareness of the Meaning of Perceptual Information. If you see a ball that reflects back the light, you would guess that the ball would feel smooth; you also recognize that round things of a certain size can be held easily in the hand and thrown. Gibson calls these qualities of objects *affordances:* An object affords the opportunity for certain actions. With development, the infant and the child gradually learn the links between how objects appear and what those objects can do or be used for.

What has been striking in the recent research is the demonstration that almost from the first day of life, babies do pay attention to some such affordances. They notice the underlying pattern, the *information* given in some object or stimulus (Pick, 1986). Over the years of toddlerhood and early childhood they discover more subtle, more complex, or more superordinate meanings or affordances. This development is especially hastened when the baby is able to move more freely on his own, since that enables him to explore objects in new ways.

Degree of Differentiation. Gibson suggests that initially the baby focuses on fairly big chunks or prominent features. With development, the child focuses on more and more detail, on finer gradations, on more difficult discriminations. Newborns pay attention to only a few features, such as the edges of things or movement; older babies attend to many more properties of objects, including their texture, their color, shape, density, flexibility, and the like. In each of these areas, the child's discriminations become still more subtle in the preschool and later years—although there are some interesting exceptions here, such as the *loss* of discriminability of speech sounds not heard in child's language environment.

Ignoring the Irrelevant. The fourth dimension Gibson suggests is a gradually improving ability to ignore the irrelevant. This ability is obviously part of what is needed for the child to acquire the various perceptual constancies. But more generally, the child becomes slowly more efficient at focusing on the essentials in some situation and ignoring everything else. If you're taking an exam, you have to be able to focus your attention on the questions and on your thinking, and not be distracted by the snuffling of the person next to you, the discomfort of the chair, or even your own anxiety. Similarly, a child in a noisy classroom must learn to focus his attention on the teacher's voice and ignore the voices of the children around him. Children become steadily better at identifying what is irrelevant and then ignoring it. In one study, for example, Higgins and Turnure (1984) gave preschoolers, second graders, and sixth graders easy and difficult learning tasks to do, with music playing in the background. Preschoolers were much more disrupted by the sound than were older children. In fact, the sixth graders actually performed better when there was music playing, as if the distractor forced them to focus their attention more fully on the task.

Do you think there might be some individual differences here too? That is, at any age might there be some children who would be more likely to have their attention captured by something and others who would scan carefully first? Would such a difference be important in a classroom?

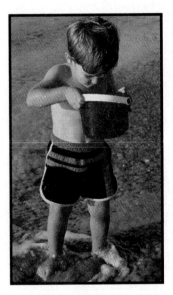

This little guy has clearly learned one of the "affordances" of a bucket: It can carry things.

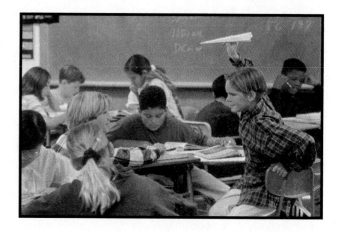

By school age, children have become considerably less distractible, which is a good thing, because most classrooms are full of noises and activity.

This sample of Gibson's ideas does not begin to convey the richness of her thinking or the extent of her influence on current researchers, such as Elizabeth Spelke. Whether Gibson's views will form the framework for a dominant future theory of perceptual development is not yet clear. But she has at least helped to turn the field away from a preoccupation with answering questions about whether newborns can do X or Y toward what may be a much more fruitful search for underlying patterns of change or continuity.

Perceptual Development: A Summing Up

The research on perceptual development in the early years of life has called into question a whole series of previously cherished beliefs about infants and their abilities. Despite their many limitations, infants seem to approach and respond to the world around them in a much more organized and sophisticated way than most psychologists thought 20 or 30 years ago. And the fact that babies respond to *patterns* of stimulation, to underlying information, and not just to the surface sensory input means that the infant is capable of far more complex cognitive processes than we had given her credit for—which takes us directly to the next subject for study: cognitive development.

Summary

1 A central issue in the study of perceptual development continues to be the nativism/empiricism controversy: Are sensory and perceptual skills built in at birth? If not, how early do they develop?

2 Studies of perceptual development have been greatly aided by methodological advances, such as Fantz's preference technique and the use of habituation or operant conditioning paradigms with very young infants.

3 Most basic sensory capacities are present in at least rudimentary form at birth or develop soon thereafter.

4 Color vision is present at birth, but visual acuity and visual tracking skill are relatively poor at birth and then develop rapidly during the first few months.

5   Basic auditory skills are more fully developed at birth; acuity is good for the range of the human voice, and the newborn can locate at least the approximate direction of sounds. The sensory capacities for smelling, tasting, and the senses of touch and motion are also well developed at birth.

6   Depth perception is not present at birth; it is present in at least rudimentary form by 3 months, initially using kinetic cues, then binocular cues, and finally pictorial cues by about 5 to 7 months.

7   Visual attention appears to follow definite rules, even in the first hours of life. Newborns search for objects and focus on the edges, on points of dark/light contrast, or on movement. At about 2 months of life, babies' focus shifts toward examining the middle as well as the edges and attending to more complex relationships and patterns.

8   Babies can discriminate the mother's face from other faces, and the mother's voice from other voices, almost immediately after birth.

9   From the beginning, babies appear to attend to and discriminate among speech contrasts present in all possible languages; by the age of 1 year, the infant makes fine discriminations only among speech sounds salient in the language he is actually hearing.

10 From early in life, certainly by 4 months, babies also attend to and discriminate among different patterns of sounds, such as melodies or speech inflections.

11 Touch/sight and sound/sight cross-modal transfers have been demonstrated as early as 1 month, reliably by 4 months.

12 Perceptual constancies such as size constancy, brightness constancy, and shape constancy are all present in at least rudimentary form by 4 months, perhaps earlier.

13 Young babies also have quite complex understanding of objects, their properties, and their possible movements. The understanding of object permanence (the realization that objects exist even when they are out of sight) begins at 2 or 3 months of age and is quite well developed by 10 months.

14 Babies differ in the apparent speed or efficiency of perceptual processes, such as habituation to a repeated stimulus. Such variations in habituation rate are correlated with later measures of IQ and language skill.

15 Both the empiricists and the nativists appear to be partially correct about the origin of perceptual skills. Many basic perceptual abilities, including strategies for examining objects, appear to be built into the system at birth or to develop as the brain develops over the early years. But specific experience is required both to maintain the underlying system and to learn fundamental discriminations and patterns.

16 Gibson's theoretical approach focuses more on dimensions of change than on the either/or approach common to earlier studies of perceptual skills in infancy. She identifies four dimensions of increase from early infancy through childhood: purposefulness of activity, awareness of meaning, degree of differentiation of features of a stimulus, and ability to ignore the irrelevant.

Key Terms

acuity (p. 130)

color constancy (p. 143)

cross-modal transfer (p. 141)

empiricism (p. 129)

nativism (p. 129)

object constancy (p. 143)

object permanence (p. 144)

perceptual constancies (p. 143)

shape constancy (p. 143)

size constancy (p. 143)

social referencing (p. 138)

tracking (p. 131)

Suggested Readings

Aslin, R. N. (1987b). Visual and auditory development in infancy. In J. D. Osofsky (Ed.), *Handbook of infant development* (2nd ed.). New York: Wiley-Interscience.

Aslin has written a number of summaries and reviews of the research on early perceptual development, of which this is perhaps the most easily understood by a nonexpert. Even so, this is quite technical and considerably more detailed than I have been in this chapter.

Baillargeon, R. (1994). How do infants learn about the physical world? *Current Directions in Psychological Science, 3,* 133–140.

This is a wonderful brief paper describing some of Baillargeon's fascinating work on young infants' understanding of objects and the physical world. The paper was written for a general audience of fellow psychologists rather than for experts in perception, so with a little effort it should be comprehensible to an undergraduate student.

Bower, T. G. R. (1989). *The rational infant.* New York: Freeman.

Bower has been one of the major researchers and theorists in the area of perceptual development. In this book he lays out the current evidence and his interpretation of it.

Haith, M. M. (1990). Progress in the understanding of sensory and perceptual processes in early infancy. *Merrill-Palmer Quarterly, 36,* 1–26.

In this relatively brief paper Haith looks back on the last 25 years of research on perceptual development. He comments not only on the knowledge gained but on the processes by which scientific progress has been made and the tasks still facing the field. Very interesting reading.

Cognitive Development I: Cognitive Power

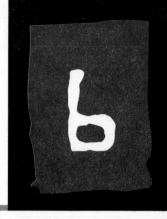

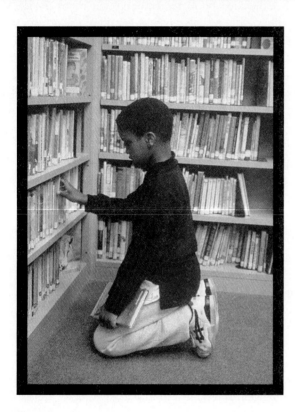

Two years ago, my husband and I lived in Germany for eight months. Because he was born in Germany and has many relatives there who speak no English, it seemed like a good idea for me to learn enough German to be able to speak to his family. So I took intensive German classes and struggled to learn new vocabulary and complex grammar. The entire process turned out to be a lot harder than I had expected, but it certainly gave me a chance to observe the ways I go about learning, remembering, and using new information. I had, throughout, an almost physical sense of my brain at work, struggling to create order and sense out of a mass of new information. (Periodically my brain would simply go on strike and refuse to take in anything more—at which point I would announce to the assembled group [in German, of course] that "my German window is now closed for 10 minutes." My various in-laws found this hilarious.)

In our everyday lives, each of us faces myriad tasks that call for the same kinds of skills I had to use in learning a new language. We study for exams, try to remember what to buy at the grocery store, balance the checkbook, remember phone numbers, use a map. Not all of us do these things equally well or equally quickly. But all of us perform such activities every day of our lives.

These activities are all part of what we normally describe as *cognitive functioning* or "intelligence." What I will be exploring in this and the next chapter is how we have all acquired the ability to do all these things. One-year-olds cannot use maps or balance a checkbook. How do they come to be able to do so? And how do we explain the fact that not all children learn these things at the same rate or become equally skilled?

Answering questions like these has been complicated by the fact that there are three distinctly different views of cognition or intelligence, each of which has led to a separate body of research and commentary. Blending the three turns out to be a tricky task—one that I don't want to attempt until I have first presented each view separately.

Three Views of Intelligence

Historically, the first approach to studying cognitive development or intelligence was focused on the basic observation that people clearly differ in their intellectual skill—their ability to remember lists for the grocery store, the speed with which they solve problems or learn new words, their ability to analyze complex situations. When we say someone is "bright" or "very intelligent," it is just such skills we mean, and our label is based on the assumption that we can rank-order people in their degree of "brightness." It was precisely this assumption that led to the development of intelligence tests, which were designed simply to give us a way of measuring such individual differences in intellectual *power*.

This "power" definition of intelligence, also referred to as a *psychometric* approach, held sway for many years. But it has one great weakness: It does not deal with the equally compelling fact that intelligence develops. As children grow, their thinking becomes more and more abstract and complex. If you give a 5-year-old a mental list of things to remember to buy at the grocery store, she will have trouble remembering more than a few items. She is also very unlikely to use good strategies to aid her memory, such as rehearsing the list or organizing the items into groups. An 8-year-old would remember more things and probably would rehearse the list under his breath, or in his head, as he was walking to the store.

The fact that intelligence develops in this way forms the foundation of the second great tradition in the study of cognitive development, the *cognitive developmental* approach of Jean Piaget and his many followers. Piaget's focus was on the development of cognitive *structures* rather than on intellectual power, on patterns of development that are *common* to all children rather than on individual differences.

These two traditions have lived side by side for several decades, rather like not very friendly neighbors who smile vaguely at one another when they meet but never get together for coffee. In the past few years, though, the two have developed a mutual friend—a third view, called the *information-processing approach,* that at least partially integrates the first two. Proponents of this third view argue that what is needed is an understanding of

Is this what you mean when you say someone is "bright" or "intelligent"? What else do you mean by these terms?

the *underlying processes* or strategies that make up all cognitive activity. Joseph Fagan (1992) puts it this way:

> Intelligence is not a faculty or trait of the mind. Intelligence is not mental content. Intelligence is *processing. Knowledge is gained as the result of the assimilation, over time, of information by the intellectual processes. (p. 82, emphasis in original)*

Researchers in this tradition obviously ask a different kind of question: What are the basic intellectual processes and how should we measure them? One of the strengths of this approach is that once we have identified such basic processes, we can ask *both* developmental and individual-differences questions: Do these basic processes change with age? Do people differ in their speed or skill in using the basic processes? The research on individual differences in infants' speed of habituation or "recognition memory," which I described briefly in Chapter 5, is an example of one body of research that has emerged from this new theoretical model.

Each of these three views tells us something useful and different about intelligence, so we need to look at all three. In other chapters I usually begin by talking about developmental changes and then turn to a discussion of individual differences. But in this case, I will follow the historical pattern and begin in this chapter by describing the oldest of these three traditions—the measurement of individual differences in intellectual skill. In the next chapter I'll talk about developmental changes in intellectual structure and about information processing.

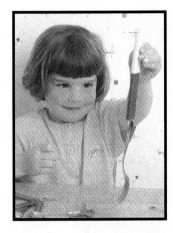

Three-year-old Anna is having a fine time figuring out how to lift the spoon with a magnet. How might you describe the "intelligence" of her behavior from each of the three different perspectives?

Measuring Intellectual Power: IQ Tests and Other Measures

Intelligence tests have a certain mystique about them, and most of us have a greatly inflated notion of the permanence or importance of an IQ score. If you are going to acquire a more realistic view, it's important for you to know something about what such tests were designed to do and something about the beliefs and values of the men and women who devised them.

The First IQ Tests

The first modern intelligence test was published in 1905 by two Frenchmen, Alfred Binet and Theodore Simon. From the beginning, the test was based on the assumption that individuals differed in mental ability. Equally important, the test had a practical purpose, which was to identify those children who would have difficulty in school. For this reason, the tests Binet and Simon devised were school-like tasks, such as measures of vocabulary, comprehension of facts and relationships, and mathematical and verbal reasoning. For example, can the child describe the difference between wood and glass? Can the young child touch his nose, his ear, his head? Can the child tell which of two weights is heavier?

Lewis Terman and his associates at Stanford University (Terman, 1916; Terman & Merrill, 1937) modified and extended many of Binet's original tests when they translated and revised the test for use in the U.S. The several Terman revisions, called the **Stanford-Binet,** consist of a series of individual tests for children of each age. There are six tests for 4-year-olds, six tests for 5-year-olds, and so on. When a child takes the test, he is first given the tests for the year below his actual age, then the tests for his own age, moving upward in age until a level is reached at which he fails them all.

Terman initially described a child's performance in terms of a score called an **intelligence quotient,** later shortened to **IQ.** This score was computed by comparing the child's chronological age with his *mental age* (the level of questions he could answer correctly). For example, a child who could solve the problems for a 6-year-old and half of those for a 7-year-old would have a mental age of 6.5. The formula used to calculate the IQ was

$$\text{Mental age/Chronological age} \times 100 = \text{IQ}$$

This formula results in an IQ above 100 for children whose mental age is higher than their chronological age and an IQ below 100 for children whose mental age is below their chronological age.

This old system for calculating the IQ is not used any longer, even in the modern revisions of the Stanford-Binet. Nowadays IQs from any type of test are calculated by a direct comparison of a child's performance with those of a large group of other children his own age. But an IQ of 100 is still average, and higher and lower scores still mean above- and below-average performance. The majority of children achieve scores that are right around the average of 100, with a smaller number scoring very high or very low. Figure 6.1 shows the distribution of IQ scores that we would see if we gave the test to thousands of children. You can see that two-thirds of all children will achieve scores between 85 and 115, while 96 percent will achieve scores between 70 and 130. The groups we refer to as *gifted* or *retarded*, both of which I'll discuss in some detail in Chapter 15, clearly represent only very small fractions of the distribution.

Modern IQ Tests

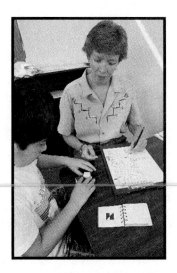

This second grader is working on one of the subtests of the WISC, in which he must use a set of blocks to try to copy the design shown in the book.

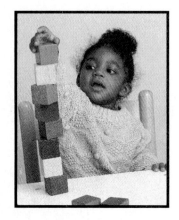

Salma, at 21 months, would clearly pass the 17-month item on the Bayley Scales of Infant Development that calls for the child to build a tower of three blocks.

The tests used most frequently by psychologists today are the Revised Stanford-Binet and the third revision of the Wechsler Intelligence Scales for Children, called the **WISC-III,** a test originally developed by David Wechsler (1974). On all the WISC tests, the child is tested with 10 different types of problems, each ranging from very easy to very hard. The 10 tests are divided into two subgroups, one calling strongly on verbal skills (e.g., vocabulary, describing similarities between objects, general information) and the other involving less-verbal types of thinking, collectively called *performance* tests, such as arranging pictures in an order that tells a story or copying a pattern using a set of colored blocks. Many psychologists find this distinction between verbal and performance tests helpful, because significant unevenness in a child's test skill may indicate particular kinds of learning problems.

Infant Tests. Neither the Binet nor the WISC-III can be used with infants much younger than about 3. Infants and toddlers don't talk well, if at all, and the usual childhood tests rely heavily on language. So how do we measure "intelligence" in an infant? This becomes an important question if we want to be able to identify, during infancy, those children who are not developing normally or if we want to predict later intelligence or school performance.

Most "infant IQ tests," such as the **Bayley Scales of Infant Development** (Bayley, 1969, revised 1993), were constructed rather like IQ tests for older children in that they included series of items of increasing difficulty. But instead of testing school-like skills— skills an infant does not yet have—the items measure primarily sensory and motor skills, such as reaching for a dangling ring (an item for a typical 3-month-old), putting cubes in a cup on request (9 months), or building a tower of three cubes (17 months). Some more clearly cognitive items are also included, such as uncovering a toy hidden by a cloth, an item used with 8-month-old infants to measure an aspect of object permanence.

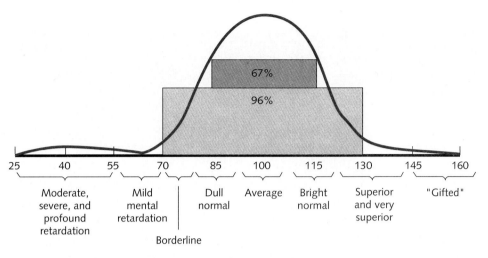

IQ test scores

FIGURE 6.1 The approximate distribution of scores on most modern IQ tests, along with the labels typically used for scores at various levels. The tests are designed so that the average score is 100 and that two-thirds of the scores fall between 85 and 115. Because of brain damage and genetic anomalies, there are slightly more low-IQ children than there are very-high-IQ children.

Bayley's test and others like it, such as the Denver Developmental Screening Test, have proven to be helpful in identifying infants and toddlers with serious developmental delays (Lewis & Sullivan, 1985). But as a more general predictive tool to forecast later IQ or school performance, such tests have not been nearly as useful as many had hoped. On the whole, it looks as if what is being measured on typical infant tests is not the same as what is tapped by the common childhood or adult intelligence tests (Colombo, 1993).

Achievement Tests

Another kind of test of intellectual skill with which you are probably more personally familiar is the **achievement test,** which nearly all of you have taken in elementary and high school. Achievement tests are designed to test *specific* information learned in school, using items like those in Table 6.1. The child taking an achievement test doesn't end up with an IQ score, but his performance is still compared to that of other children in the same grade across the country.

How are these tests different from an IQ test? IQ tests are intended to tell us something about how well a child *can* think and learn, while an achievement test tells us something about what a child *has* learned. Or to put it another way, the designers of IQ tests thought they were measuring the child's basic capacity (her underlying **competence,)** while an achievement test is intended to measure what the child has actually learned (her **performance**). This is an important distinction. Each of us presumably has some upper limit of ability—what we could do under ideal conditions, when we are maximally motivated, well, and rested. But since everyday conditions are rarely ideal we typically perform below our hypothetical ability.

In fact, it is not possible to measure competence. We can never be sure that we are assessing any ability under the best of all possible circumstances. We *always* measure performance. The authors of the famous IQ tests believed that by standardizing the procedures

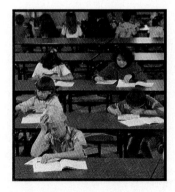

In the United States, virtually all fourth graders—like these in Austin, Texas—are given achievement tests, so as to allow schools to compare their students' performance against national norms.

Table 6.1

Some Sample Items from a Fourth-Grade Achievement Test

Vocabulary

jolly old man
1. angry
2. fat
3. merry
4. sorry

Reference Skills

Which of these words would be first in ABC order?
1. pair
2. point
3. paint
4. polish

Language Expression

Who wants ___ books?
1. that
2. these
3. them
4. this

Spelling

Jason took the *cleanest* glass.
right ___ wrong ___

Mathematics

What does the "3" in 13 stand for?
1. 3 ones
2. 13 ones
3. 3 tens
4. 13 tens

Mathematics Computation

79	149	62
+14	−87	×3

Source: From *Comprehensive Tests of Basic Skills, Form S.* Reprinted by permission of the publisher, CTB/McGraw-Hill, Del Monte Research Park, Monterey, CA 93940. Copyright © 1973 by McGraw-Hill, Inc. All rights reserved. Printed in the U.S.A.

for administering and scoring the tests they could come close to measuring competence. Certainly it is good practice to design the best possible test and to administer it carefully. But it is important to understand that no test really measures "underlying" competence, only performance when the test is taken.

If you follow this logic to the end, you realize that all IQ tests are really achievement tests. The difference between tests called IQ tests and those called achievement tests is really a matter of degree. IQ tests include items that are designed to tap fairly fundamental intellectual processes like comparison or analysis; achievement tests call for specific information the child has learned in school or elsewhere. College entrance tests, such as the Scholastic Aptitude Tests (SATs, which many of you have probably taken recently), fall somewhere in between. They are designed to measure basic "developed abilities," such as the ability to reason with words, rather than just specific knowledge. All three types of tests, though, measure aspects of a child's or young person's performance and not competence.

Stability and Predictive Value of IQ Tests

For most psychologists, the critical question about IQ tests is not whether they measure intellectual competence, but whether the scores are stable and whether they predict anything interesting or useful.

The Real World

Performance Tests: A New Way to Measure School Achievement

Traditional achievement tests, like IQ tests, are designed to show how well a given child, or a classroom of children, performs against some average or norm. Hence, both achievement and IQ tests are sometimes referred to as *norm-referenced.* In both cases the norm is the performance of the average child of a given age. An alternative way to think about testing is to define some criterion, some absolute standard that you think all children should meet, and to compare each child's performance to that criterion. Many educators today are advocating exactly such *criterion-referenced* tests, especially the form of criterion-referenced test called a **performance test.**

For example, suppose that one of the goals of an educational system is that each student be able to write clearly and persuasively, using complete sentences and correct grammar. Such a skill can only be assessed with a test that actually asks the students to write something. Then each student's writing can be evaluated as acceptable or not acceptable against some absolute standard. Similarly, a performance test in science or mathematics might involve an actual science experiment. Children would complete the experiment on their own and would describe and explain the results in writing.

An example would probably help. In one reading/writing test devised as part of the Maryland School Performance Assessment Program, eighth graders are asked to read and write about the intense cold of the winter in the Yukon Territory of Canada. They read a story by Jack London called "To Build a Fire," about a man who dies of the cold. Later they also read a brief excerpt entitled "Hypothermia: Causes, Effects, Prevention." Over several days, the students answer questions in test booklets about these readings and discuss some of the material in class. At the end, they must write some form of commentary, such as a piece giving advice to a group of friends about what they would need to do to stay safe on a winter hiking trip; a story, play, or poem expressing their feelings about extreme states; or a speech intended to persuade people not to travel in the Yukon (Mitchell, 1992).

Here's another example, this time from a mathematics performance test for junior high school students:

Five students have test scores of 62, 75, 80, 86, and 92. Find the average score. How much is the average score increased if each student's score is increased by 1, 5, 8, or X points? Write a statement about how much the average score is increased if each individual score is increased X points, and write an argument to convince another student that the statement is true. (Mitchell, 1992, p. 67)

The students' performance on both the writing and mathematics tests are normally scored (by experts, usually on a statewide basis) on a 4-point or 6-point scale, with the top one or two points reserved for those performances that meet the criterion, and lower scores for unacceptably poor responses. Thus, the issue is not whether the students in some class or school do better or worse than other children, but whether each one individually meets some absolute standard.

Tests like these are now in use in a number of states in the United States, as well as in England and Wales, where many of the performance tests of science and mathematics were first devised. They are more complicated (and more expensive) to administer and score than are norm-referenced achievement tests, but they are growing in popularity not only because they assess the actual behaviors or skills educators are interested in, but also because the very existence of such tests shapes the way in which reading, writing, science, and mathematics are taught in the classroom. Just as teachers who know their students will be tested with standard achievement tests inevitably "teach to the test," so teachers who know their students will be tested with performance tests of reading, writing, math, or science must change the way they teach these subjects to be sure that their students acquire the needed reasoning and communication skills. Since these are precisely the skills that most educators believe should be taught in schools, performance tests may prove to be a vehicle for educational reform.

Stability of Test Scores

One of the bits of folklore about IQ tests is that a particular IQ score is something you "have," like blue eyes or red hair—that a child who achieves a score of, say, 115 at 3 years of age will continue to score in about the same range at age 6 or 12 or 20.

IQ scores are, in fact, very stable, but there are also some exceptions to this general statement. First of all, as I pointed out earlier, scores on infant IQ tests like the Bayley are not strongly related to later IQs. The typical correlation between a 12-month-old Bayley mental test score and a 4-year-old Binet IQ is only about .20 to .30 (Bee et al., 1982)—significant but not robust. Newer tests of infant intelligence, such as those based on habituation rates or other basic processes, may ultimately prove to be more helpful predictors (Colombo, 1993). But at the moment, there is no widely used method of reliably predicting which 1-year-olds will later have high or low IQ scores.

Beginning at about age 3, consistency in IQ test performance on tests like the Binet or WISC-III increases markedly. If two tests are given a few months or a few years apart, the scores are likely to be very similar. The correlations between adjacent-year IQ scores in middle childhood, for example, are typically in the range of .80 (Honzik, 1986). This high level of predictability, however, masks an interesting fact: Many children show quite wide fluctuations in their scores. Robert McCall, analyzing several longitudinal studies in which children have been given IQ tests repeatedly over many years, concludes that about half of children show little or no significant fluctuation in their scores. The remaining half, however, show changes from one test to another and over time (McCall, 1993). Some show steadily rising scores, some declining, and some a peak in middle childhood followed by a decline in adolescence. In individual cases, the shifts may cover a range as large as 40 points.

Such wide fluctuations are more common in young children. The general rule of thumb is that the older the child, the more stable the IQ score becomes. Older children may show some fluctuation in scores in response to major stresses such as parental divorce, a change in schools, or the birth of a sibling, but by age 10 or so, IQ scores are normally highly stable.

Given the degree of variability I have described, does it make sense to select children for special classes, such as classes for the gifted, on the basis of a single test score? How else could you go about it?

What IQ Tests Predict

The information on long-term stability of IQ tests tells us something about the *reliability* of the tests. But what about *validity?* Validity, as you'll recall from introductory psychology, has to do with whether a test is measuring what it is intended to measure. One way to measure validity is to see whether scores on a particular test predict real behavior in a way that makes sense. In the case of IQ tests, the most central question is whether IQ tests predict school performance. That was what Binet originally intended the test to do; that is what all subsequent tests were designed to do. The research findings on this point are quite consistent: The correlation between a child's test score and her grades in school or performance on other school tests is about .60 (Carver, 1990; Sattler, 1988). This is a strong but by no means perfect correlation. It tells us that on the whole, children with top IQ scores will also be among the high achievers in school, and those who score low will be among the low achievers. Still, some children with high IQ scores don't shine in school while some lower-IQ children do.

IQ scores also predict future grades as well as current grades. Preschool children with high IQ scores tend to do better when they enter school than those with lower scores; elementary school-age children with higher IQs later do better in high school as well.

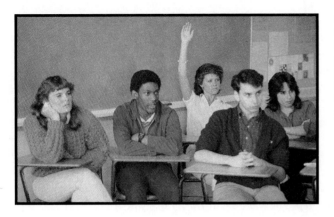

Among these high school students, those with higher IQ are not only more likely to get good grades but are also more likely to go on to college. Intelligence also adds to the child's resilience—his ability to survive stress, including poverty.

It is important to point out that this relationship holds *within* each social class and racial group in the United States. Among the poor, and among African-Americans and Hispanics, as well as among middle-class Anglos, those children with higher IQs are most likely to get good grades, complete high school, and go on to college (Brody, 1992). Such findings have led a number of theorists to argue that intelligence adds to the child's *resilience*—a concept I talked about in Chapter 1. Numerous studies now show that poor children, be they white, Hispanic, African-American, or from another minority group, are far more likely to develop the kind of self-confidence and personal competence it takes to move out of poverty if they have higher IQ (Luthar & Zigler, 1992; Werner & Smith, 1992).

At the other end of the scale, low intelligence is associated with a number of negative long-term outcomes, including adult illiteracy, delinquency in adolescence, and criminal behavior in adulthood (Stattin & Klackenberg-Larsson, 1993). For example, in a 20-year longitudinal study of a group of children born to black teenage mothers in Baltimore, Nazli Baydar (Baydar, Brooks-Gunn, & Furstenberg, 1993) has found that the best single predictor of adult literacy or illiteracy was each subject's childhood IQ score. This is not to say that all lower-IQ individuals are illiterate or criminals. That is clearly not the case. But low IQ makes a child more vulnerable, just as high IQ increases the child's resilience.

How or why do you think having a higher IQ makes a child more resilient? For example, in what specific ways might the life of a brighter child living in a slum be different from the life of a less-bright child in the same environment?

Limitations of Traditional IQ Tests

Judging from the evidence I've just presented, we can argue that IQ tests are valid: They measure what they purport to measure. But they do not measure everything. Most important, they do not measure underlying competence. An IQ score cannot tell you (or a teacher, or anyone else) that your child has some specific, fixed, underlying intellectual capacity.

Traditional IQ tests also do not measure a whole host of skills that are likely to be highly significant for getting along in the world. IQ tests were originally designed to measure only the specific range of skills that are needed for success in school. They do this reasonably well. But these tests do not tell us how well a particular person may perform other cognitive tasks requiring skills such as creativity, insight, street smarts, ability to read social cues, or understanding of spatial relationships.

Finally, it is worth pointing out yet again that IQ scores are not etched on a child's forehead at birth. Such scores become quite stable in late childhood, but individual children can and do shift, in response to especially rich or especially impoverished environments, or in response to any stress in their lives (McCall, 1993; Pianta & Egeland, 1994).

In the past decade, a number of psychologists have been particularly struck by these limitations in the traditional ways of thinking about intelligence. Howard Gardner (1983), for example, proposes six separate types of intelligence (linguistic, musical, logical-mathematical, spatial, bodily-kinesthetic, and personal), only two of which are actually measured on traditional IQ tests. Another current view, which I find even more intriguing because it has some obvious practical implications, is Robert Sternberg's **triarchic theory of intelligence.**

An Alternative View: Sternberg's Triarchic Theory of Intelligence

Sternberg argues that there are three aspects or types of intelligence. The first, which he calls **componential intelligence,** includes what we normally measure on IQ and achievement tests. Planning, organizing, remembering facts, and applying them to new situations are all part of componential intelligence.

The second aspect he calls **experiential intelligence.** A person with well-developed experiential intelligence is creative, can see new connections between things, can relate to experiences in insightful ways. A graduate student who can come up with good ideas for experiments, who can see how a theory could be applied to a totally different situation, or who can synthesize a great many facts into a new organization would be high in experiential intelligence. You might like to try your hand at some of the kinds of tests Sternberg has devised to measure this kind of ability, shown in Table 6.2. The answers are at the bottom in case you are stumped—as many people are.

The third aspect Sternberg calls **contextual intelligence,** sometimes also called "street smarts." People who are skilled in this are able to manipulate their environments, to see how they can fit in best, to know which people to cultivate and how to cultivate them, to adapt themselves to their setting or the setting to themselves. In college we would see this form of intelligence in a student who was particularly good at figuring out what the professor wanted in any given course, who went regularly to office hours to talk to the professor, who chose paper topics he knew the professor preferred. This is not just manipulation. It requires being attuned to a variety of fairly subtle signals and then acting on the information. Good salespeople, for example, would have to have a high level of contextual intelligence in order to tailor their sales pitch on the basis of subtle cues from each customer.

Can you think of a nonacademic job or task situation in which experiential intelligence would be helpful?

Car salesmen, to be successful, probably need a good deal of what Sternberg calls contextual intelligence, or "street smarts."

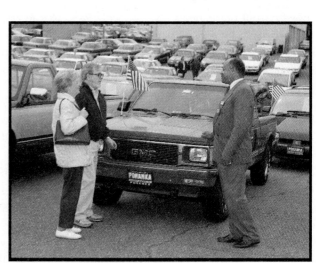

Table 6.2
Insight Questions from Sternberg's Tests of Experiential Intelligence

1. Aeronautical engineers have made it possible for a supersonic jet fighter to catch up with the bullets fired from its own guns with sufficient speed to shoot itself down. If a plane flying at 1000 miles an hour fires a burst, the rounds leave the plane with an initial velocity of about 3000 miles an hour. Why won't a plane that continues to fly straight ahead overtake and fly into its own bullets?

2. If you have black socks and brown socks in your drawer, mixed in a ratio of 4 to 5, how many socks will you have to take out to make sure of having a pair of the same color?

3. In the Thompson family, there are five brothers, and each brother has one sister. If you count Mrs. Thompson, how many females are there in the Thompson family?

In solving the following analogies, assume that the statement given before the analogy is true, whether it actually is true or not, and use that assumption to solve the analogy.

4. LAKES are dry.
   TRAIL is to HIKE as LAKE is to:
   a. swim
   b. dust
   c. water
   d. walk

5. DEER attack tigers.
   LION is to COURAGEOUS as DEER is to:
   a. timid
   b. aggressive
   c. cougar
   d. elk

Answers:

1. Gravity pulls the bullets down. If the plane continues to fly a level course, it cannot shoot itself. 2. Three (the proportion of black and brown socks is irrelevant). 3. Two, the mother and her daughter, who is sister to each brother. 4. d.   5. b.

Source: From *Intelligence applied* by R. J. Sternberg. Copyright © 1986 by Harcourt Brace Jovanovich, Inc. Reprinted by permission of the publisher.

Sternberg's point is not just that standard IQ tests have omitted many of these kinds of items, but that in the world beyond the school walls, experiential or contextual intelligence may be required as much or more than the type of skill measured on an IQ test (Sternberg & Wagner, 1993). These are important points to keep in mind as we move on to questions about the origins of individual differences in IQ. What we know about "intelligence" is almost entirely restricted to information about componential intelligence—the kind of intelligence demanded in school. We know almost nothing about the origins or long-term consequences of variations in experiential or contextual intelligence.

Explaining Differences in IQ

You will not be surprised to discover that the arguments about the origins of differences in IQ nearly always boil down to a dispute about nature versus nurture. When Binet and Simon wrote the first IQ test, they did not assume that intelligence as measured on an IQ test was fixed or inborn. But many of the American psychologists who revised and promoted the use of the tests *did* believe that intellectual capacity is inherited and largely fixed at birth. Those who took this view and those who believe that the environment plays a crucial role in shaping a child's intellectual performance have been arguing for at least 60 years. Let me walk you through some of the major points.

Evidence for the Importance of Heredity

Both the twin studies and studies of adopted children show strong hereditary influences on IQ, as you already know from Chapter 1. Identical twins are more like one another in IQ than are fraternal twins, and the IQs of adopted children are better predicted from the IQs of their natural parents than from those of their adoptive parents (Brody, 1992; Loehlin, Horn, & Willerman, 1994; Scarr, Weinberg, & Waldman, 1993). This is precisely the pattern of correlations we would expect if there were a strong genetic element at work.

Evidence for the Importance of Environment

Adoption studies also provide some strong support for an environmental influence on IQ scores, because the actual *level* of IQ scores of adopted children is clearly affected by the environment in which they have grown up. Early studies of adopted children involved mostly children born to poverty-level parents who were adopted into middle-class families. Such children typically have IQs that are 10 to 15 points higher than that of their birth mother (Scarr & Kidd, 1983), suggesting that the effect of the middle-class adoptive family was to raise the child's IQ. But this doesn't tell us whether a *less*-stimulating adoptive family would *lower* the IQ of a child born to average- or above-average-IQ parents. That piece of information is now available from a French study by Christiane Capron and Michel Duyme (1989). They identified a group of 38 children, all adopted in infancy, who represent all possible combinations of high and low social class and education in the birth parents and the adoptive parents. Table 6.3 shows the children's IQ scores in adolescence. If you look across both rows, you can see a difference of 11 or 12 points between the IQs of children reared in upper-class homes and those reared in lower-class families, no matter what the social class level or education of the birth parents. At the same time, the data also show a genetic effect, because the children *born to* upper-class parents have higher IQs than do those from lower-class families, no matter what kind of rearing environment they encountered.

    Social Class Differences. This relationship between social class and IQ, so clear in the Capron and Duyme study, is echoed in a great deal of other research. But just what is meant by "social class"?

    Every society is divided into social strata of some kind. In Western societies, an individual's social status or **social class** is typically defined or measured in terms of three di-

Table 6.3
IQ Scores at Adolescence for Capron and Duyme's Adopted Children

		Social Class of Adoptive Parents	
		High	**Low**
Social Class of Biological Parents	**High**	119.60	107.50
	Low	103.60	92.40

Source: Capron & Duyme, 1989, Table 2, p. 553.

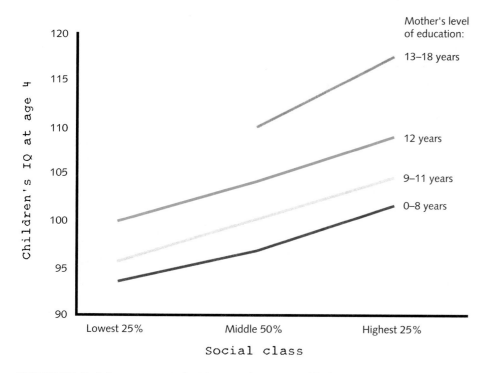

FIGURE 6.2 Each line represents the IQ scores for 4-year-old white children whose mothers had a particular level of education and whose families were classed in one of three broad social-class levels. Both elements are obviously related to the childrens' IQs. (*Source:* Broman, Nichols, & Kennedy, 1975, p. 47.)

mensions: education, income, and occupation. Thus, a person with higher status is one with more education, higher income, and a more prestigious occupation. In other societies, the dimensions of status might be different, but some status differences exist in every society. Distinctions between "blue collar" and "white collar," or "middle class" and "working class," are fundamentally status distinctions.

Dozens of research studies tell us that children from poor or working-class families, or from families in which the parents are relatively uneducated, have lower average IQs than do children from middle-class families. You can see this effect particularly vividly in Figure 6.2, which is based on data from a huge national study of more than 50,000 children born in 12 different hospitals around the U.S. between 1959 and 1966 (Broman, Nichols, & Kennedy, 1975). In this figure, in order to make sure that we are not confounding social class and ethnic differences, I have given only the results for white children who were tested with the Stanford-Binet at age 4, a total sample of more than 11,800 children. As you can see in the figure, the average IQ of the children rises as the family overall social class rises and as the mother's education rises.

These differences are *not* found on standardized tests of infant IQ such as the Bayley (Golden & Birns, 1983). But after age 2½ or 3, social class differences appear to widen steadily with age (Farran, Haskins, & Gallagher, 1980), producing what is sometimes called a **cumulative deficit.** That is, the longer the child lives in poverty, the more negative the effect on IQ and other measures of cognitive functioning becomes (Duncan, 1993). These cumulative effects are especially large on *verbal* tests (Jordan, Huttenlocher, & Levine, 1992).

Genetic differences are obviously contributing to the pattern in Figure 6.2, since brighter parents typically have more education and better jobs, and also pass on their "bright" genes to their children. The results could also be due to differences in prenatal risks, diet, or general health. We know, for example, that poor children are likely to be exposed to higher levels of lead and that this is causally linked to lower IQs (Tesman & Hills, 1994); we know that when children living in poverty in developing countries are given high-quality nutritional supplements in infancy and early childhood, they later have higher IQs or vocabularies (Pollitt & Gorman, 1994). In addition, real differences exist in the ways infants and children are treated in poor versus middle-class families that are independently important in cognitive development. It is these differences in early experiences that have been the focus of most of the research on environmental effects on IQ.

Specific Family Characteristics and IQ. When we watch the ways individual families interact with their infants or young children and then follow the children over time to see which ones later have high or low IQs, we can begin to get some sense of the kinds of specific family interactions that foster higher scores. At least five dimensions of family interaction or stimulation seem to make a difference. Parents of higher-IQ children, or of children whose IQs show a rising pattern over age, tend to do the following:

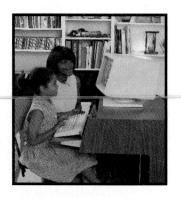

This kind of rich, complex, stimulating environment is consistently linked to higher IQs in children.

1. They provide an *interesting and complex physical environment* for the child, including play materials that are appropriate for the child's age and developmental level (Bradley et al., 1989; Pianta & Egeland, 1994).

2. They are *emotionally responsive* to and *involved* with their child. They respond warmly and contingently to the child's behavior, smiling when the child smiles, talking when the child speaks, answering the child's questions, and in myriad ways responding to the child's cues (Barnard et al., 1989; Lewis, 1993).

3. They *talk to their child* often, using language that is diverse, descriptively rich, and accurate (Hart & Risley, 1995; Sigman et al., 1988).

4. They *avoid excessive restrictiveness,* punitiveness, or control, instead giving the child room to explore, even opportunities to make mistakes (Bradley et al., 1989; Olson, Bates, & Kaskie, 1992). In a similar vein, they ask questions rather than giving commands (Hart & Risley, 1995).

5. They *expect* their child to do well and to develop rapidly. They emphasize and press for school achievement (Entwisle & Alexander, 1990).

You may have figured out the methodological problem in research of this type—the same problem that exists in comparisons of the IQs of children in families that differ in social class. Because parents provide *both* the genes and the environment, we can't be sure that these environmental characteristics are really causally important. Perhaps these are simply the environmental features provided by brighter parents, and it is the genes and not the environment that cause the higher IQs in their children. The way around this problem is to look at the link between environmental features and IQ in adopted children. Fortunately, we have a few studies of this type, and they point to the same critical environmental features. That is, among adoptive families, those that behave in the ways listed earlier have adopted children who score higher on IQ tests (Plomin, Loehlin, & DeFries, 1985).

Cultures and Contexts

Maternal "Responsiveness" in Different Cultures

Many studies in the U.S. and other Western countries have pointed to the central importance of parental *responsiveness* for the child's intellectual and social development. Mothers and fathers who respond to their infant's noises by talking to the baby, who smile when the baby smiles, who pick up on the baby's other signals have children who later turn out to have higher IQs, better language, and more secure attachments.

Since this aspect of the parent–infant interaction appears to be so significant, it seems especially important for us to discover if the same relationship holds in other cultures and contexts. Amy Richman and her colleagues (Richman, Miller, & LeVine, 1992) have taken a first step toward answering this question with two studies in other cultures. They compared responsiveness among American and Kenyan mothers, and they observed the responsiveness of Mexican mothers who varied in level of education.

In the Kenyan/American comparison, Richman observed marked differences in the ways mothers responded to their babies. When the Kenyan babies vocalized, cried, or looked at the mothers, their mothers were most likely to pick them up and hold them. Mothers in Boston were far more likely to talk to or look at their babies in response to the same baby signals.

Profound cultural differences are at work here. The Kenyan mothers, all from the Gusii tribe, said that they thought it was ridiculous to talk to a baby before the baby is capable of speech. This culture also has different social conventions about eye contact during speech: Mutual gaze is much less common than in the U.S. and other Western cultures. Thus, the ways the mothers behave with their babies is entirely consistent with cultural beliefs and interaction patterns.

It is also important to note that the two groups did not differ in their absolute amount of responsiveness. Thus, both groups of mothers are "responsive" to their babies. But they respond in very different ways. The Gusii mothers "show a pattern of responsiveness that is strikingly designed to reduce distress and maintain calm in the infant during the 1st year of life" (p. 620). In contrast, the responsiveness of the Boston mothers seems designed to stimulate the baby and encourage further interaction.

The Mexican mothers, as a group, showed yet another pattern. They were most likely to look at the baby when the infant vocalized or looked at them and less likely to pick the baby up than were the Gusii mothers. But they responded to the baby's signals with speech about as often as the Boston mothers did. What is especially interesting here is that Richman found that the amount of formal education the Mexican mothers had received was related to their pattern of responsiveness. The more formal education they had (and the maximum was only about 8 or 9 years), the more their pattern of responsiveness was like the Boston mothers'. Studies in the U.S. also show that the mother's education is linked in this same way to her manner of interacting with her baby. This does not mean that the Gusii mothers behave as they do because they have little formal education. We don't know if that is the case, and we do know that other cultural values and beliefs among the Gusii contribute to the pattern of responsiveness these mothers show. But the results from the Mexican women show at least that the link between education and patterns of responsiveness is not unique to U.S. samples.

What Richman's study does not tell us is whether these varying styles of responsiveness have differential effects on the child's cognitive development. That piece of the puzzle will have to await further cross-cultural research.

Differences in Environments Within Families. Within families the experiences of individual children also differ in ways that affect IQ. Being the oldest of a large family, for example, is a very different experience from being the youngest or being in the middle; being the only girl in a family of boys is different from being a girl with only sisters. Psychologists are just beginning to study these within-family variables. Thus far, we have been looking mostly at fairly obvious differences, like how many children are in a family, or the child's position within the family, both of which seem to be at least slightly related to the child's IQ. On average, the more children in the family, the lower the average IQ of the children. And on average, firstborn children have the highest IQs, with average IQs declining steadily as you go down the birth order (Zajonc, 1983; Zajonc & Marcus, 1975). Children who are born very close together also have slightly lower IQs on average than do those born further apart (Storfer, 1990). One fairly typical set of data is in Figure 6.3, based on scores of nearly 800,000 students who took the National Merit Scholarship Examination in 1965, with the scores converted to the equivalent of IQ scores.

Please notice that the differences shown in this figure are not huge. Yet this pattern has been observed repeatedly, in European samples as well as those in the U.S., leaving us with a puzzle. Why would such a pattern occur? Robert Zajonc's hypothesis is that the birth of each succeeding child "dilutes" the intellectual climate of the home. The oldest child initially interacts only with his parents and thus has a maximally complex and enriching environment. Second- or later-born children, in contrast, experience a lower average intellectual level in the family simply because they interact with both other children and adults. A later-born child *may* have an advantage if the children are very widely spaced, since then he is interacting entirely with others who are intellectually advanced, including both parents and much older siblings.

This hypothesis has prompted a good deal of debate and criticism (Rogers, 1984); most researchers have concluded that it is probably not the right way to conceptualize what is going on, because the data do not always fit the predictions. But no one has yet offered a better explanation. To solve this puzzle, we will need to know a good deal more about the actual experiences of children in different birth-order positions and in large versus small families.

School Experience and Special Interventions. Home environments and family interactions are not the only source of environmental influence. Many young children also spend a very large amount of time in group care settings, including day care, special programs like Head Start, or regular preschools. How much effect do these environments have on the child's intellectual performance?

On a theoretical level, this question is of interest because it may tell us something about early experience in general and about the resilience of children. Are the effects of an initially impoverished environment permanent, or can they be offset by an enriched expe-

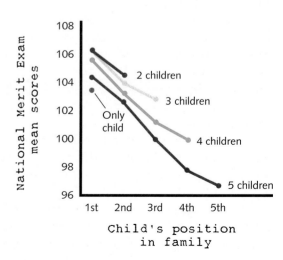

FIGURE 6.3 These data from the 1965 National Merit Scholarship Qualifying Test show the commonly found relationship between test scores and family size and birth order. Within each family size, the average score is highest for the firstborn and declines with each position in the birth order sequence. (*Sources:* Data from Breland, 1974, recalculated by Storfer, 1990, Table 7, p. 32.)

rience, such as a special preschool? In Aslin's terms (Figure 1.1), the question is whether special programs can produce *attunement*—a permanent gain over the level of performance the child would have shown without the added enrichment. Programs like Head Start are based squarely on the assumption that it *is* possible to modify the trajectory of a child's intellectual development, especially if you intervene early.

Attempts to test this assumption have led to a messy body of research. In particular, children are rarely assigned randomly to Head Start or non-Head Start groups, which makes interpretation difficult. Still, researchers agree generally on the effects. Children enrolled in Head Start or other enriched preschool programs, compared to similar children without such preschool, normally show a gain of about 10 IQ points during the year of the Head Start experience. This IQ gain typically fades and then disappears within the first few years of elementary school (Zigler & Styfco, 1993), but on other measures, a clear residual effect can be seen. Children with Head Start or other quality preschool experience are less likely to be placed in special education classes, somewhat less likely to repeat a grade, and somewhat more likely to graduate from high school (Darlington, 1991; Haskins, 1989). They also have better health, better immunization rates, and better school adjustment than their peers (Zigler & Styfco, 1993). So although poor children with preschool experience do not typically *test* much higher than their non-preschool-attending peers (and do *not* differ in IQ), they *function* better in school. And when some kind of supportive intervention continues into the early years of elementary school, the beneficial effects on school performance are even clearer (Reynolds, 1994; Zigler & Styfco, 1993). Furthermore, the only study that has looked at adult outcomes of such preschool attendance suggests lasting effects. Young adults who had attended a particularly good experimental preschool program, the Perry Preschool Project in Milwaukee, had higher rates of high school graduation, lower rates of criminal behavior, lower rates of unemployment, and less likelihood of being on welfare (Barnett, 1993). Thus, the potential effects of such early education programs may be broad—even though the programs appear to have no lasting effect on standardized IQ test scores.

But when the enrichment program is begun in infancy, rather than at age 3 or 4, IQ scores do show an attunement effect: The IQ scores remain elevated even after the intervention has ended. The best-designed and most meticulously reported of the infancy interventions has been carried out by Craig Ramey and his colleagues at North Carolina (Campbell & Ramey, 1994; Ramey, 1993; Ramey & Campbell, 1987). Infants from poverty-level families, whose mothers had low IQs, were randomly assigned either to a special day-care program, eight hours a day, five days a week, or to a control group, which received nutritional supplements and medical care but no special enriched day care. The special care program, which began when the infants were 6 to 12 weeks of age and lasted until they began kindergarten, involved very much the kinds of "optimum" stimulation I just described. When they reached kindergarten age, half the children in each group were enrolled in a special supplemental, supportive program that focused on family support and increasing educational activities at home. The remaining children had only the normal school experience.

The average IQ scores of the children at various ages are shown in Figure 6.4. You can see that the IQs of the children who had been enrolled in the special program were higher at every age, whether they had the school-age supplementary program or not,

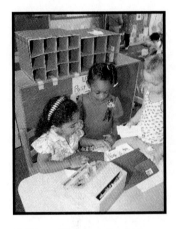

Children who have attended Head Start programs like this one don't show permanent increases in IQ, but they are less likely to repeat a grade or to be assigned to special education classes.

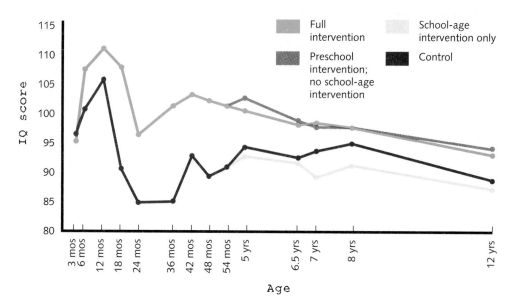

FIGURE 6.4 In the Ramey study, children were randomly assigned in infancy to an experimental group with special day care (the "intervention" group) or to a control group. From kindergarten through third grade, half of each group received supplementary family support, while the other half received none. Thus, the "school-age control" group had the intervention for five years, but nothing beyond that; the "school-age intervention" group had no intervention before school age but did have assistance in early elementary school. The difference in IQ between the intervention and control groups remained statistically significant even at age 12. (*Source:* Campbell & Ramey, 1994, Fig. 1, p. 690.)

Considering the results of Ramey's study, would you be in favor of providing such enriched day care to all infants from high-risk or poverty-level families? What are the arguments, pro and con?

although the scores for both groups declined in the elementary school years. What is perhaps more important is the observation that fully 44 percent of the control group children had IQ scores classified as borderline or retarded (scores below 85), compared to only 12.8 percent of the children who had been in the special program. In addition, the enriched infant care group had significantly higher scores on both reading and mathematics achievement tests at age 12 and were only half as likely to have repeated a grade (Campbell & Ramey, 1994).

Ramey found additional insights in the varying experiences of the control group children. Some of them had been reared primarily at home, but others had spent periods of time in other types of day-care or preschool programs. When he compared the IQ scores of these two groups with those in the special intervention program, he found a consistent rank order: Children in the special program were highest, followed by those who had had some kind of day-care experience, with those reared wholly at home the lowest. The IQs at age 4 for these three groups were 101.1, 94.0, and 84.2, respectively (Burchinal, Lee, & Ramey, 1989). So the length and quality of the intervention appeared to be directly related to the size of the effect.

These results do *not* mean that all mental retardation could be "cured" by providing children with heavy doses of special education in infancy. What they do show is that the intellectual power (componential intelligence, at least) of those children who begin life with few advantages can be significantly increased if richer stimulation is provided early in life.

Interaction of Heredity and Environment

When we put together all the information about the role of heredity and environment in influencing IQ, it is clear that both factors are highly significant. Studies around the world consistently yield estimates that roughly half of the variation in IQ within the population is due to heredity (Plomin, 1989; Plomin & Rende, 1991; Rogers, Rowe, & May, 1994). The remaining half is clearly due to environment or to interactions between environment and heredity.

One useful way to conceptualize this interaction is with the concept of *reaction range*. The basic idea is that genes establish some range, some upper and lower boundaries, of possible functioning. Where a child's IQ score will fall within those boundaries will be determined by environment. Richard Weinberg (1989) estimates that the reaction range for IQ is about 20 to 25 points. That is, given some specific genetic heritage, each child's actual IQ test performance may vary as much as 20 or 25 points, depending on the richness or poverty of the environment in which he grows up. When we change the child's environment for the better, the child moves closer to the upper end of his reaction range. When we change the environment for the worse, the child's effective intellectual performance falls toward the lower end of his reaction range. Thus, even though intelligence as measured on an IQ test is highly heritable, the absolute score within the reaction range is determined by environment.

We could also think about the interaction between heredity and environment in terms rather like Horowitz's model (recall Figure 1.3), or we could use Aslin's concept of maintenance. Some theorists (Turkheimer & Gottesman, 1991) have argued that *within the normal range of environments*, IQ scores may be largely a function of heredity, not because environment is unimportant, but simply because most environments are sufficiently rich to support or maintain normal intellectual development. It is only when environmental quality falls below some crucial threshold that it has a major effect on the level of measured IQ, such as might be true for children reared in an orphanage or in a severely impoverished environment. This view does not necessarily contradict the concept of reaction range. Rather, the argument is that the lower end of any given child's reaction range is likely to be manifested only if the child is reared in an environment that falls below the critical threshold. If we think about it in this way, then it makes sense that special education programs like Ramey's would be effective for children from poverty-level environments, since the program brings the child's experience up into the sufficiently supportive range and thus adequately supports normal intellectual development. The same program provided to a child from a more enriched family environment, however, should have little or no effect on IQ—which is essentially what researchers have found.

Group Differences in IQ

So far I have sidestepped two difficult issues, namely, racial and sex differences in IQ or cognitive power. Because these issues have powerful personal and political ramifications and can easily be blown out of proportion, I do not want to place too much emphasis on either topic. But you need to see what we know, what we don't know, and how we are trying to explain both kinds of differences.

The Real World

IQ Testing of Blacks in the Schools

One of the primary uses for IQ tests in schools has been to identify children with special needs, so that they can be placed in appropriate special classes. Children whose speed of learning seems to be much faster or slower than normal may be given an IQ test to see if they might be retarded or gifted. The test score is then used along with other data, such as teacher comments and recommendations, to decide if the child should be in a special class.

This use of IQ tests has been the center of a great deal of controversy, largely because when the tests are used in this way, proportionately many more African-American children end up being classified as slow or retarded than is true for whites. Many parents, educators, and psychologists have argued that such a pattern of results occurs because the tests are culturally biased. The tests may contain items that are not equally accessible to blacks and whites. Taking such tests and doing well may also require certain test-taking skills, motivations, or attitudes less common among African-American children.

Assertions of such bias have led to careful reexamination of individual test items, and all obvious types of bias have been eliminated from recent revisions. Despite such changes, however, proportionately more black than white children continue to be diagnosed as retarded or slow. This fact has led to a number of lawsuits, including *Larry P. v. Riles,* in which a group of parents of black children sued the California school system for bias in labeling a disproportionately large number of black children as retarded and assigning them to special classes. The parents argued that there was no underlying difference in *competence* between black and white children, so if the tests showed a difference the tests must clearly be biased. The school system argued that IQ tests don't measure underlying capacity or competence but only a child's existing repertoire of basic intellectual skills. By school age, that repertoire has already been affected by such environmental factors as prenatal care, diet, health, and family stability—all of which tend to be less optimal among blacks. Thus, the test accurately reflects a child's current abilities and is a proper basis for assigning the child to a special program, even though that child might have far greater underlying capacity or competence that could have been expressed under more ideal life circumstances.

The judge in the *Larry P. v. Riles* case ruled in favor of the parents and prohibited the use of standardized IQ test scores for placement in special classes in California. Other legal decisions have gone the other way (Elliott, 1988), so the legal question is not settled, although there are now many places in the U.S. in which the use of IQ tests for diagnosis and placement of African-American or other minority children is forbidden. One unintended consequence of this is that since placement decisions must still be made, they are now being made on the basis of evidence that may be even more culturally biased, such as less-standardized tests and teacher evaluations.

I have no quick or easy solution to this dilemma. It is certainly true that schools in the United States reflect the dominant middle-class white culture, with all its values and assumptions. But it is also true that succeeding in these schools is essential if the child is to acquire the basic skills needed to cope with the complexities of life in an industrialized country. For a host of reasons, including poorer prenatal care, greater poverty, and different familial patterns, more African-American children appear to *need* special classes in order to acquire the skills they lack. Yet I am well aware of the self-fulfilling prophecy when a child is placed in a special class. Expectations are typically lower in such classes, so the children—who were already learning more slowly—are challenged still less and so proceed even more slowly. Yet to offer no special help to children who come to school lacking the skills needed to succeed there seems equally unacceptable to me. What do you think?

Racial Differences

Debates about racial differences in IQ, which had been highly volatile for some decades, had largely died down in recent years. But the publication in 1994 of a controversial book, *The Bell Curve* (Herrnstein & Murray, 1994), has reopened the debate.

A number of different racial differences in intellectual performance have been found, including consistently higher performance on achievement tests—particularly math and science tests—by Chinese and Japanese children (Geary, et al., 1993; Stevenson et al.,

1990; Sue & Okazaki, 1990). But the basic finding that has given researchers and theorists the most difficulty is that in the United States, black children consistently score lower than white children on measures of IQ. This difference, which is on the order of 12 IQ points, is *not* found on infant tests of intelligence or on measures of infant habituation rate (Fagan & Singer, 1983), but it becomes apparent by the time children are 2 or 3 years old (Brody, 1992). There is some evidence that the size of this difference has been declining in the past several decades and is now closer to 10 points. But a noticeable difference persists (Herrnstein & Murray, 1994).

Some scientists, including the authors of *The Bell Curve,* even while acknowledging that the environments of the two groups are, on average, substantially different, argue that the IQ difference must nonetheless reflect—at least in part—basic genetic differences between the races (Jensen, 1980). Other scientists, even granting that IQ is highly heritable, point out that the 12-point difference falls well within the presumed reaction range of IQ. They emphasize that there are sufficiently large differences in the environments in which black and white children are typically reared to account for the average difference in score (Brody, 1992). Black children in the U.S. are more likely to be born with low birth weight, more likely to suffer from subnutrition, more likely to have high blood levels of lead, less likely to be read to or provided with a wide range of intellectual stimulation. And each of these environmental variations is known to be linked to lower IQ scores.

Cultural differences are clearly also at work, as black psychologists have long pointed out (e.g., Ogbu, 1994). We can see such differences at work in the way children from different cultures respond to the testing situation itself. For example, in a study of adopted black children, Moore (1986) found that those who had been reared in white families (and thus imbued with the majority culture) not only had higher IQ scores than those adopted into black families (117 versus 103), but also approached the IQ-testing situation quite differently. They stayed more focused on the task and were more likely to try some task even if they didn't think they could do it. Black children adopted into middle-class black families did not show this pattern of persistence and effort. They asked for help more often and gave up more easily when faced with a difficult task. When Moore then observed each adoptive mother teaching her child several tasks, he could see parallel differences. The white mothers were more encouraging and less likely to give the child the answer than were the black mothers.

Findings like these persuade me that the IQ difference we see is primarily a reflection of the fact that the tests, and the schools, are designed by the majority culture to promote a particular form of intellectual activity (Sternberg's componential intelligence) and that many black or other minority families rear their children in ways that do not promote or emphasize this particular set of skills. In fact, Sternberg has argued that in some black subcultures it is contextual intelligence that is particularly emphasized and trained (Sternberg & Suben, 1986).

In a similar vein, Harold Stevenson and others have argued that the differences between Asian and American children in performance on mathematics achievement tests result not from genetic differences in capacity, but from differences in cultural emphasis on the importance of academic achievement, number of hours spent on homework, and differences in the quality of the math instruction in the schools (Chang & Murray, 1995; Schneider et al., 1994; Stevenson & Lee, 1990; Stigler, Lee, & Stevenson, 1987)—a possibility I've explored in the *Cultures and Contexts* box on page 176.

Some psychologists have argued that IQ tests and achievement tests are biased against blacks and other minority group members. What kind of research results would demonstrate such bias? What kind would argue against it?

Cultures and Contexts
How Asian Teachers Teach Math and Science So Effectively

One highly significant contributor to the observed Asian/U.S. differences in science and mathematics achievement may be the different ways school is taught in these several cultures. The clearest information comes from research by James Stigler and Harold Stevenson (Stevenson, 1994; Stigler & Stevenson, 1991). They observed in 120 classrooms in Japan, Taiwan, and the United States, and are convinced that Asian teachers have devised a particularly effective mode of teaching both mathematics and science.

Japanese and Chinese teachers approach mathematics and science by crafting a series of "master lessons," each organized around a single theme or idea. These lessons are like good stories, with a beginning, a middle, and an end. They frequently begin with a problem posed for the students. Here is one example from a fifth-grade class in Japan:

> The teacher walks in carrying a large paper bag full of clinking glass. . . . She begins to pull items out of the bag, placing them, one-by-one, on her desk. She removes a pitcher and a vase. A beer bottle evokes laughter and surprise. She soon has six containers lined up on her desk. . . . The teacher, looking thoughtfully at the containers, poses a question: "I wonder which one would hold the most water?" . . . the teacher calls on different students to give their guesses: "the pitcher," . . . "the teapot." The teacher stands aside and ponders: "Some of you said one thing, others said something different. . . . How can we know who is correct?" (Stigler & Stevenson, 1991, p. 14)

The lesson continues as the students agree on a plan for determining which container will hold the most. In such lessons, students are frequently divided into small groups, each assigned to part of the problem. These small groups then report back to the class as a whole. At the end of the lesson, the teacher reviews the original problem and what they have learned. In this particular case, the children have learned not only something about measurement but also something about the process of hypothesis testing.

In United States classrooms, in contrast, it is extremely uncommon for a teacher to spend 30 or 60 minutes on a single coherent math or science lesson involving the whole class of children and a single topic. Instead, they shift often from one topic to another during a single math or science "lesson." They might do a brief bit on addition, then talk about measurement, then about telling time, and back to addition. Asian teachers shift *activities* in order to provide variety, such as shifting from lecture format to small-group work; American teachers shift *topics* for the same apparent purpose.

Stigler and Stevenson also found striking differences in the amount of time teachers actually spend leading instruction for the whole class. In the United States classrooms they observed, this occurred only 49 percent of the time; group instruction occurred 74 percent of the time in Japan and 91 percent in Taiwan.

Stigler and Stevenson point out that the Asian type of teaching is not new to Western teachers. American educators frequently recommend precisely such techniques. "What the Japanese and Chinese examples demonstrate so compellingly is that when widely implemented, such practices can produce extraordinary outcomes" (p. 45).

The fact that we may be able to account for such racial differences in IQ or achievement test performance by appealing to the concept of reaction range and to cultural or subcultural variations does not make the differences disappear, nor does it make them trivial. But it may put such findings into a less explosive framework.

Sex Differences

In contrast, comparisons of total IQ test scores for boys and girls do *not* reveal consistent differences. It is only when we break down the total score into several separate skills that some patterns of sex differences emerge. On average, studies in the U.S. show girls are slightly better on verbal tasks and at arithmetic computation and that boys are slightly better at numerical reasoning. For example, on the math portion of the Scholastic Aptitude Tests (SATs), the average score for boys is consistently higher than the average score for girls. Many of these differences have been getting smaller in recent years, although this is not true for the SAT mathematics score difference, which has persisted over the past three decades among students in the U.S. (Brody, 1992; Byrnes & Takahira, 1993; Jacklin, 1989).

Two other differences are also still found regularly. First, among children who test as gifted in mathematics, boys are considerably more common (Benbow, 1988; Lubinski & Benbow, 1992). Second, on tests of spatial visualization, like the ones illustrated in Figure 6.5, boys have slightly higher average scores. On measures of mental rotation (illustrated by item *c* in the figure) the sex difference is quite large, and in both cases the size of the difference becomes larger with age (Voyer, Voyer, & Bryden, 1995).

I want to point out that even on tests of mental rotation, the two distributions overlap. That is, some girls and women are good at this type of task, and some boys and men are not. But the average difference is fairly large. The fact that girls score lower on such tests does not mean that no women are qualified for occupations that demand such skill; it does mean that fewer girls or young women will be able to pass the entrance requirements for such jobs.

Where might such differences come from? The explanatory options should be familiar by now. Biological influences have been most often argued in the case of sex differences in

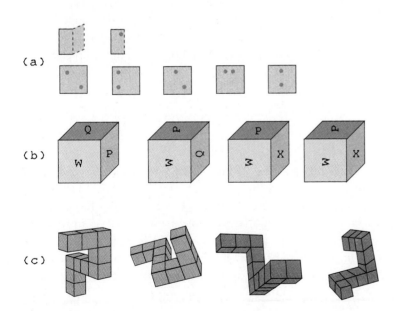

FIGURE 6.5 Three illustrations of spatial ability tests: (a) *Spatial visualization.* The figure at the top represents a square piece of paper being folded. A hole is punched through all the thicknesses of the folded paper. Which figure shows what the paper looks like when it is unfolded? (b) *Spatial orientation.* Compare the three cubes on the right with the one on the left. No letter appears on more than one face of a given cube. Which of the three cubes on the right could be a different view of the cube on the left? (c) *Mental rotation.* In each pair, can the three-dimensional objects be made congruent by rotation? (*Sources:* Halpern, 1986, Figure 3.1, p. 50, and Figure 3.2, p. 52.)

spatial abilities, where there may be both genetic differences and—more speculatively—differences in brain functioning resulting from prenatal variations in hormones (Newcombe & Baenninger, 1989).

In contrast, environmental explanations have been prominent in discussions of the sex differences in mathematical or verbal reasoning. Especially in the case of mathematics there is considerable evidence that girls' and boys' skills are systematically shaped by a series of environmental factors:

- Boys take more math courses than girls do. When the amount of math exposure is held constant, the sex difference becomes much smaller.

- Parental attitudes about mathematics are markedly different for boys and girls. Parents are more likely to attribute a daughter's success in mathematics to effort or good teaching; poor performance by a girl is attributed to lack of ability. In contrast, parents attribute a boy's success to ability and his failure to lack of application (Holloway & Hess, 1985; Parsons, Adler, & Daczala, 1982).

- Girls and boys have different experiences in math classes. In elementary school, teachers pay more attention to boys during math instruction (and more attention to girls during reading instruction), and in high school, math teachers direct more of their questions and comments to boys, even when girls are outspoken in class.

As you can see, a lot of effort has been spent trying to discover or explain possible sex differences in mathematical ability. What are the practical implications either way?

The cumulative effect of these differences in expectation and treatment show up in high school, when sex differences on standardized math tests usually become evident. In part, then, the sex differences in math achievement test scores appear to be perpetuated by subtle family and school influences on children's attitudes. Whether these differences can explain the greater percentage of boys than girls who show real giftedness in mathematics is not so clear—an issue that continues to be debated rather heatedly.

The Measurement of Intelligence: A Last Look

One of the questions that students often ask at about this point is whether, given all the factors that can affect a test score, it is worth bothering with IQ tests at all. I think that these tests do assess some important aspects of children's intellectual performance and that they can be helpful in identifying children who may have difficulties in school or gifted children who would benefit from special programs. But it is worth emphasizing again that IQ tests do *not* measure a lot of other things we may be interested in, including all the facets of intelligence Sternberg describes. An IQ test is a specialized tool, and like many such tools, it has a fairly narrow range of appropriate use. I don't want to throw out this tool, but you have to keep its limitations very firmly in mind when you use it.

You also have to keep in mind that the study of IQ is only one facet of the study of cognitive development. In the next chapter we'll look at the equally significant changes with age in children's understanding of the world around them.

Summary

1   When we study the development of "intelligence," we need to distinguish between measures of intellectual power and measures of intellectual structure. IQ tests tap individual differences in intellectual power.

2   The most commonly used individually administered tests are the current revisions of the Stanford-Binet and the Wechsler Intelligence Scales for Children (WISC).

3   All current IQ tests compare a child's performance to that of others her or his age. Scores above 100 represent better-than-average performance; scores below 100 represent poorer-than-average performance.

4   Both IQ tests and school achievement tests measure a child's performance, not capacity or underlying competence. Achievement tests, however, test much more specific school-related information than do IQ tests.

5   Criterion-referenced tests, which compare a student's performance against some specific criterion such as the ability to write clearly, have become more common lately.

6   IQ scores are quite stable from one testing to the next, and this becomes more and more true the older the child gets. But individual children's scores still may fluctuate or shift 20 or 30 points or more over the course of childhood.

7   IQ test scores are quite good predictors of school performance and years of education, which is one measure of the validity of the tests.

8   IQ tests do not measure many other facets of intellectual functioning in which we might be interested, including what Sternberg calls experiential and contextual intelligence.

9   Studies of identical twins and of adopted children clearly show a substantial genetic influence on measured IQ. Most psychologists agree that approximately half of the variation in individual IQs may be attributed to heredity.

10   The remaining half is attributed to environmental variation: Poor children consistently test lower than do children from middle-class families; children whose families provide appropriate play materials and encourage the child's intellectual development test higher on IQ tests.

11   Environmental influence is also shown by increases in test performance or school success among children who have been in special, enriched preschool or infant day-care programs.

12   One way to understand the interaction of heredity and environment is with the concept of reaction range. Heredity determines some range of potential; environment determines the level of performance within that range.

13   A consistent difference of about 12 points on IQ tests is found between African-American and Caucasian children in the U.S. It seems most likely that this difference is due to environmental and cultural differences between the two groups, such as differences in health and prenatal care, and in the type of intellectual skills trained and emphasized at home.

14   Males and females do not differ on total IQ test scores, but they do differ in some subskills. The largest differences are on measures of spatial reasoning, on which males are consistently better.

Key Terms

achievement test **(p. 159)**

Bayley Scales of Infant Development **(p. 158)**

competence **(p. 159)**

componential intelligence **(p. 164)**

contextual intelligence **(p. 164)**

cumulative deficit **(p. 167)**

experiential intelligence **(p. 164)**

intelligence quotient (IQ) **(p. 157)**

performance **(p. 159)**

performance tests **(p. 161)**

social class **(p. 166)**

Stanford-Binet **(p. 157)**

triarchic theory of intelligence **(p. 164)**

WISC-III **(p. 158)**

Suggested Readings

Brody, N. (1992). *Intelligence* (2nd ed.). San Diego: Academic Press.

Dense and detailed, but the best current source I know for further information about all aspects of this subject.

Elliott, R. (1988). Tests, abilities, race, and conflict. *Intelligence, 12,* 333–350.

An especially clear and fascinating discussion of the several lawsuits about the use of IQ tests in the schools.

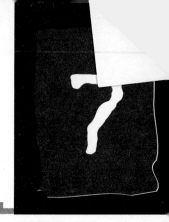

Cognitive Development II: Structure and Process

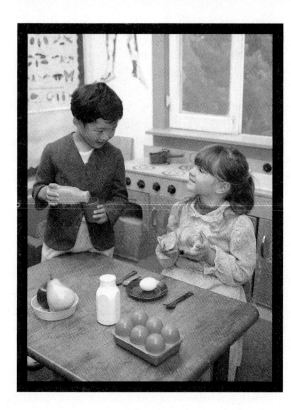

I magine the following scene: Your 5-year-old, John, and your 8-year-old, Anne, come into the kitchen after playing outside, both asking for juice. With both children watching, you take two identical small cans of juice from the refrigerator and pour them into two nonidentical glasses. One glass is narrower than the other, so the juice rises higher in that glass. The 5-year-old, having been given the fatter glass, complains: "Anne got more than I did!" To which Anne replies (with the wonderful grace of the 8-year-old to her sibling):

"I did not, you dummy. We both got the same amount. The two cans were just alike." To restore family harmony, you get out another glass identical to Anne's and pour John's juice into this new glass. The level of the liquid is now the same and John is satisfied.

If this were an item on an IQ test, we'd say that Anne was "right" and John was "wrong." But such an emphasis on rightness or wrongness misses an essential point about this interchange: There seems also to be a *developmental* change, a shift in the way the child sees or understands the world and the relationships of objects. John is not being pigheaded or "dumb." He is merely operating with a different kind of reasoning than Anne's. In a year or two, John will sound like Anne does now.

If we are to understand how children think, we need to understand such changes in the *form* or *structure* of their thinking as well as differences in *power*. How do children come to understand the world around them? What kind of logic do they use, and how does it change over time?

These were precisely the kinds of questions that Jean Piaget asked in his many years of research on children's thinking. Despite the fact that many aspects of his theory have been called into question by later research, his theory set the agenda for most research in this area for the past 30 years, and it still serves as a kind of scaffolding for much of our thinking about thinking. So let me begin by giving you a fairly detailed description of Piaget's original ideas before going on to talk about more current research and theory, including information processing.

Piaget's Basic Ideas

I mentioned in Chapter 1 that Piaget began with the observation that children seem to follow very regular sequences in their development of certain ideas, certain understandings. They make the same kinds of mistakes at similar ages and seem to arrive at similar solutions. Where could such shared mistakes come from? More broadly, how does a child's knowledge of the world develop?

In answering this question, Piaget's most central assumption was that the child is an active participant in the development of knowledge, *constructing* his own understanding. This idea, perhaps more than any other, has influenced the thinking of all those who have followed Piaget. The modern metaphor is that of the child as a "little scientist," engaged in active exploration, seeking understanding and knowledge.

In constructing such an understanding, Piaget thought that the child tries to *adapt* to the world around himself in ever more satisfactory ways. In Piaget's theory, this process of adaptation is in turn made up of several vital subprocesses.

The Processes of Adaptation

Schemes. A pivotal concept—and one of the hardest to grasp—is that of a **scheme** (sometimes written as *schema*). This term is often used as roughly analogous to the word *concept* or the phrases "mental category" or "complex of ideas." But Piaget used it even more broadly than that. He saw knowledge not as merely passive mental categories, but as *actions,* either mental or physical, and each of these actions is what he means by a scheme. So a scheme is not really a category, but the *action of categorizing* in some particular fashion. Some purely physical or sensory actions are also schemes. If you pick up and look at a ball, you are using your "looking scheme," your "picking-up scheme," and your "holding scheme." Piaget proposed that each baby begins life with a small reper-

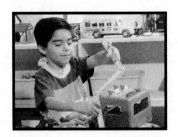

The metaphor of the child as a "little scientist," constructing his understanding of the world, comes directly from Piaget's theory.

toire of simple sensory or motor schemes, such as looking, tasting, touching, hearing, reaching. For the baby, an object *is* a thing that tastes a certain way, feels a certain way when it is touched, or has a particular color. Later, the toddler and child develops mental schemes as well, such as categorizing or comparing one object to another. Over development, the child gradually adds extremely complex mental schemes, such as deductive analysis or systematic reasoning. According to Piaget, the shift from the simple sensorimotor schemes of infancy to the increasingly complex mental schemes of later childhood is achieved through the operation of three basic processes: **assimilation, accommodation,** and **equilibration.**

Assimilation. Assimilation is the process of *taking in,* of absorbing some event or experience to some scheme. When a baby looks at and then reaches for a mobile above his crib, Piaget would say that the baby has assimilated the mobile to the looking and reaching schemes; when an older child sees a dog and labels it "dog," she is assimilating that animal to her dog category or scheme. When you read this paragraph you are assimilating the information, hooking the concept onto whatever other concepts (schemes) you have that may be similar.

The key here is that assimilation is an *active* process. For one thing, we assimilate information selectively. Two years ago, when I was struggling to learn German and listened to my instructor speak, I could only assimilate a portion of what she said—the parts for which I already had schemes—and could only imitate or use the parts that I had assimilated. In addition, the very act of assimilating changes the information that is assimilated, because each assimilated event or experience takes on some of the characteristics of the scheme to which it was assimilated. If I label your new sweater as green (that is, if I assimilate it to my green scheme) even though it is really chartreuse or some other more unusual color, I will remember it as more green and less yellow than it really is.

Accommodation. The complementary process is accommodation, which involves *changing the scheme* as a result of the new information you have taken in by assimilation. As I assimilated new German words and grammar, I gradually changed (accommodated) my concepts and categories, so that I had mental categories for several forms of past tense instead of only one, or mental groupings of words with a given prefix. The baby who sees and grasps a square object for the first time will accommodate her grasping scheme, so that next time she reaches for an object of that shape her hand will be more appropriately bent to grasp it. Thus, in Piaget's theory, the process of accommodation is the key to developmental change. Through accommodation, we reorganize our thoughts, improve our skills, change our strategies.

Equilibration. The third aspect of adaptation is equilibration. Piaget assumed that in the process of adaptation, the child is always striving for coherence, to stay "in balance," to have an understanding of the world that makes overall sense. This is not unlike what a scientist does when she develops a theory about some body of information (and hence the metaphor of the child as a "little scientist"). The scientist wants to have a theory that will make sense out of every observation, that has internal coherence. When new research findings come along, she assimilates them to the existing theory; if they don't fit perfectly, she might simply set aside the deviant data, or she may make minor modifications in her theory. But if enough nonconfirming evidence accumulates, the scientist either may have to throw out her theory altogether and start over or may need to change some basic theoretical assumptions, either of which would be a form of equilibration.

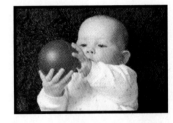

Piaget would say that baby Eleanor is assimilating this ball to her looking and grasping schemes. As she adapts her way of holding, she is also accommodating.

Piaget thought that a child operated in a similar way, creating coherent, more or less internally consistent models or theories. But since the infant starts with a very limited repertoire of schemes, the early "theories" or structures the child creates are simply not going to be adequate. Such inadequacies, so Piaget thought, force the child to make periodic major changes in her internal structure.

Piaget saw three particularly significant reorganization or equilibration points, each ushering in a new stage of development. The first is at roughly 18 months, when the toddler shifts from the dominance of simple sensory and motor schemes to the use of the first symbols. The second is at roughly ages 5 to 7, when the child adds a whole new set of powerful schemes Piaget calls **operations.** These are far more abstract and general mental actions, such as mental addition or subtraction. The third major equilibration is at adolescence, when the child figures out how to "operate on" ideas as well as events or objects. These three major equilibrations create four stages:

The **sensorimotor stage,** from birth to 18 months

The **preoperational stage,** from 18 months to about age 6

The **concrete operational stage,** from 6 to about 12, and

The **formal operational stage,** from age 12 onward.

The Four Stages

Sensorimotor Stage. According to Piaget, during the sensorimotor stage the infant (1) responds to the world almost entirely through sensory and motor schemes; (2) functions in the immediate present, responding to whatever stimuli present themselves; (3) does not plan or intend; and (4) has no internal representation of objects—mental pictures, or words, that stand for objects and that can be manipulated mentally. Piaget thought that such internal representations did not develop until about 18 to 24 months.

John Flavell (1985) summarizes this very nicely, pointing out that the infant

> exhibits a wholly practical, perceiving-and-doing, action-bound kind of intellectual functioning; she does not exhibit the more contemplative, reflective, symbol-manipulating kind we usually think of in connection with cognition. The infant "knows" in the sense of recognizing or anticipating familiar, recurring objects and happenings, and "thinks" in the sense of behaving toward them with mouth, hand, eye, and other sensory-motor instruments in predictable, organized, and often adaptive ways. . . . It is the kind of noncontemplative intelligence that your dog relies on to make its way in the world. (p. 13)

Piaget proposed that the infant moved through a series of substages, gradually building toward the development of internal representation at about 18 months. Only then, he thought, can the child both form and manipulate mental images and use symbols. That is, he can have images or words or actions *stand for* something else, a shift that Flavell rightly describes as "radically, drastically, qualitatively different" (1985, p. 82) from what came before. And it is precisely this shift that Piaget saw as the beginning point of the next stage.

Preoperational Stage. During the years from 2 to 6, Piaget saw the evidence of symbol use in many aspects of the child's behavior. Children this age begin to pretend in their play, for example (a development I've talked about in the *Real World* box on the facing page. At age 2 or 3 or 4 a broom may become a horsie, or a block may become a train. We can also see such symbol use in the emergence of language at about the same time (which

Think back to everything I said about perceptual skills in infancy in Chapter 5. Does Flavell's description of the sensorimotor infant match what you already know?

The Real World

Young Children's Play

If you watch young children during their unstructured time, you'll see them building towers out of blocks, talking to or feeding their dolls, making "tea" with the tea set, racing toy trucks across the floor, dressing up in grown-up clothes. They are, in a word, *playing.* This is not trivial or empty activity; it is the stuff of which much of cognitive development seems to be built.

The form of this play changes in very obvious ways during the years from 1 to 6, following a sequence that matches Piaget's stages rather well (Rubin, Fein, & Vandenberg, 1983).

Sensorimotor Play. The child of 12 months or so spends most of her playtime exploring and manipulating objects using all the sensorimotor schemes in her repertoire. She puts things in her mouth, shakes them, moves them along the floor.

Constructive Play. Such exploratory play with objects does continue past 12 months, especially with some totally new object, but by age 2 or so children also begin to use objects to build or construct things—creating a block tower, putting together a puzzle, making something out of clay or with Tinkertoys. Such "constructive" play makes up nearly half of the play of children aged 3 to 6 (Rubin et al., 1983).

First Pretend Play. Pretend play also begins at about the same time. The first sign of such pretending is usually something like a child using a toy spoon to "feed" himself or a toy comb to comb his hair. The toys are still used for their actual or typical purposes (spoon for feeding) and the actions are still oriented to the *self,* but pretending is involved. Between 15 and 21 months, a shift occurs: The recipient of the pretend action now becomes another person or a toy, most often a doll. The child is still using objects for their usual purposes (such as drinking from a cup), but now she is using the toy cup with a doll instead of herself. Dolls are especially good toys for this kind of pretending, because it is not a very large leap from doing things to yourself to doing things with a doll. So children feed dolls imaginary food, comb their hair, soothe them.

Substitute Pretend Play. Between 2 and 3 years of age children begin to use objects to stand for something altogether different. They may comb the doll's hair with a baby bottle while saying that it is a comb, use a broom to be a horsie, or make "trucks" out of blocks. By age 4 or 5, children spend as much as 20 percent of their playtime in this new, complicated kind of pretending (Field, De Stefano, & Koewler, 1982).

Sociodramatic Play. Somewhere in the preschool years children also begin to play parts or take roles. This is really still a form of pretending, except that now several children create a mutual pretense. They play "daddy and mommy," "cowboys and Indians," "doctor and patient," and the like. At first, children simply take up these roles; later, they name the roles to one another and may give each other explicit instructions about the right way to pretend a particular role. You can begin to see this form of play in some 2-year-olds; by age 4 virtually all children engage in some play of this type (Howes & Matheson, 1992). Interestingly, at about the same ages a great many children seem to create imaginary companions (Taylor, Cartwright, & Carlson, 1993). For many years psychologists believed that the existence of such an imaginary companion was a sign of disturbance in a child; now it is clear that such a creation is a normal part of the development of pretense in many children.

Children clearly get great delight out of all these often elaborate fantasies. Equally important, by playing roles, pretending to be someone else, they also become more and more aware of how things may look or feel to someone else, and their egocentric approach to the world declines.

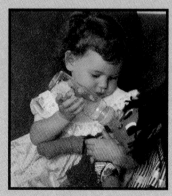

First pretend play.

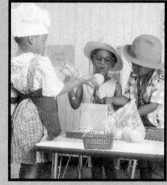

Sociodramatic play.

I'll describe in the next chapter). And we see the child's improving ability to manipulate these symbols internally in such things as her ability to search more systematically for lost or hidden objects.

Beyond the accomplishment of symbol use, Piaget focused mostly on all the things the preschool-age child still *cannot* do, which gives an oddly negative tone to his description of this period. Even the label he used for this stage conveys some of this tone: It is *pre*operational.

For example, Piaget described the preoperational child as one who looks at things entirely from his own perspective, his own frame of reference, a characteristic Piaget called **egocentrism** (1954). The child is not being selfish; rather, she simply thinks (assumes) that everyone sees the world as she does.

Figure 7.1 is a photo of a classic experiment illustrating this kind of egocentrism. The child is shown a three-dimensional scene with mountains of different sizes and colors. From a set of drawings, he picks out the one that shows the scene the way he sees it. Most preschoolers can do this without much difficulty. Then the examiner asks the child to pick out the drawing that shows how someone *else* sees the scene, such as the little clay man or the examiner. At this point preschool children have difficulty. Most often they again pick the drawing that shows their *own* view of the mountains (Gzesh & Surber, 1985). In Piaget's view, for the child to be able to succeed at this task she must "decenter"—she must shift from using herself as the only frame of reference. He thought that preschool children had not yet achieved this.

Piaget also pointed out that the preschool-age child was captured by the appearance of objects—a theme that still dominates the research on children of this age. In Piaget's work, this theme is evident in his famous studies on **conservation.**

It was a problem of conservation that confronted Anne and John and their juice glasses; to understand that both glasses of juice held the same amount, John would have to ignore the *appearance* of difference and understand that the amount of juice is "conserved"—remains the same—despite variations in the shape of the container. This is an example of conservation of quantity, one of six different conservations Piaget studied—listed in Table 7.1. In every case, his measurement technique involved first showing the child two equal sets or objects, getting the child to agree they were equal in some key respect such as weight or quantity or length or number, and then shifting or deforming one of the objects and asking the child if they were still equal. Children rarely show any of

Can you think of any examples of egocentrism in your own behavior? What about buying someone else the gift you were hoping to receive yourself? Other examples?

FIGURE 7.1 One of the types of experimental arrangements used to study egocentrism in children.

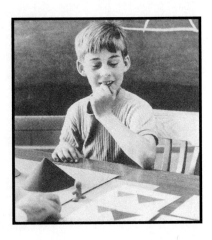

Table 7.1
Different Types of Conservation Studied by Piaget

Number	Two rows with equal numbers of pennies or buttons are laid out parallel to one another with the items matching. Then one row is stretched out longer or squeezed together, or rearranged in some other way and the child is asked, "Are there the same number?"
Length	Two pencils of identical length are laid one above the other so that they match perfectly. Then one is displaced to the right or left so that one pencil's point sticks out further than the other, and the child is asked if they are now the same length.
Quantity	Two equal beakers are filled with equal amounts of water: One is then poured into a differently shaped glass (tall and thin or short and squat), and the child is asked if there is still the same amount to drink in each.
Substance or mass	Two equal balls of clay are shown to the child. One is then squished into another shape, such as a sausage or a pancake. The child is asked if there is now the same amount of clay in each.
Weight	Two equal balls of clay are weighed on a balance scale so that the child sees that they weigh the same. One is then deformed into another shape, and the child is asked if they still weigh the same or "have the same amount of weight."
Volume	Two balls of clay are placed in two equal beakers of water so that the child sees that they each displace the same amount of water. Then one ball is deformed, and the child is asked if they will still "take up the same amount of space."

these forms of conservation before age 5, which Piaget took to be a sign that they were still captured by the appearance of change and did not focus on the underlying unchanging aspect.

Notice that the understanding of conservation is part of a chain of development that begins with the various object constancies and object permanence in infancy. The sensorimotor infant eventually figures out that objects remain the same even though they appear to change in some respects, and he understands that objects continue to exist even when they are out of sight. Now in the preschool years, he must come to understand that other, more abstract, aspects of objects also remain constant despite apparent changes, such as their mass or weight.

A third limitation Piaget saw in the preoperational child's thinking was in her ability to classify—to put things together that go together. His observations led him to believe that only at about age 4 does a child begin to group objects consistently into categories or classes, at first using only one dimension (e.g., shape, such as round things versus square things) and later two or more dimensions at once (e.g., size *and* shape: small round things versus small square things and large round things versus large square things).

Concrete Operations Stage. The next great leap forward, according to Piaget, comes somewhere between ages 5 and 7, when the child discovers a set of immensely powerful, abstract, general "rules" or "strategies" for examining and interacting with the world, which Piaget called *concrete operations.* The term *operation* refers specifically to powerful, *internal* schemes, such as addition, subtraction, multiplication, division, reversibility (reversing an action, thus reproducing the original state), and serial ordering (putting things in order of size or some other feature). The child now understands the *rule* that adding to something makes it more and that subtracting makes it less, which means that she can now understand the principle of conservation. She understands that objects can belong to more than one category at once and that categories have logical relationships, which is a great advance over the simple classifications of the preoperational period. The 7-year-old not only can group critters into classes of cats and dogs, but she can also understand that both cats and dogs, are *included in* the class of animals. And by understanding reversibility, she grasps a great many features about her own actions—that the opposite of adding is taking away, for example.

Piaget also proposed that during this third stage the child develops the ability to use **inductive logic.** He can go from his own experience to a general principle—for example, from the observation that when you add another toy to a set and then count the set, it has one more than it did before, he can form a general principle that adding to something always makes it more.

Elementary school children are pretty good observational scientists and will enjoy cataloging, counting species of trees or birds, or figuring out the nesting habits of guinea pigs. But they are not yet good at **deductive logic,** which requires starting with a general principle and then predicting some outcome or observation, like going from a theory to a hypothesis. Suppose, for example, that I asked you to think of all the ways human relationships would be different if women were physically as strong as men. Coming up with answers requires deductive and not inductive logic, and it is hard because you must imagine things that you have not experienced. The concrete operations child is good at dealing with things he knows or can see and manipulate; he does not do well with manipulating ideas or possibilities. Piaget thought that deductive reasoning did not develop until the period of formal operations in junior high or high school.

An important practical application of this difference in the child's logic is that elementary school children ought to be able to learn science (and other subjects) more easily if the material is presented "concretely," with plenty of opportunity for hands-on experience and inductive experimentation. They ought to learn less well when scientific concepts or theories are presented in a deductive fashion, which is precisely what research on science instruction has shown (Saunders & Shepardson, 1987).

In your everyday life, when do you use inductive logic? When was the last time you think you used deductive logic?

Because elementary school students are good at observational science and inductive reasoning, nature trips like this one are a particularly effective way of teaching.

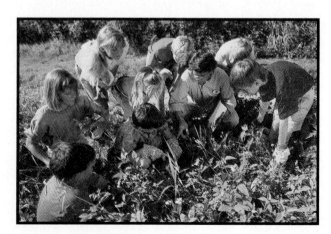

Formal Operational Stage. Piaget proposed a final step of cognitive development, beginning at about age 12 and continuing to emerge through the teenage years. The most important shift is that the teenager is now able to apply complex mental operations not just to objects or experiences, but to ideas and thoughts. One of the first steps in this process is for the child to extend her reasoning abilities to objects and situations that she has not seen or experienced firsthand or that she cannot see or manipulate directly. Instead of thinking only about real things and actual occurrences, she must start to think about possible occurrences. The preschool child plays "dress up" by putting on real clothes. The teenager *thinks* about options and possibilities, imagining herself in different roles, going to college or not going to college, marrying or not marrying, having children or not.

Using formal operational thought, the teenager can also search systematically and methodically for the answer to a problem. To study this, Piaget and his colleague Barbel Inhelder (Inhelder & Piaget, 1958) presented adolescents with complex tasks, mostly drawn from the physical sciences. In one of these tasks, the youngsters were given varying lengths of string and a set of objects of various weights that could be tied to the strings to make a swinging pendulum. They were shown how to start the pendulum by pushing the weight with differing amounts of force and by holding the weight at different heights. The subject had to figure out which one or combination of these four factors (length of string, weight of object, force of push, or height of push) determines the "period" of the pendulum (the amount of time for one swing). (In case you have forgotten your high school physics, the answer is that only the length of the string affects the period of the pendulum.)

If you give this task to a concrete operational child, she will usually try out many different combinations of length and weight and force and height in an inefficient way. She might try a heavy weight on a long string and then a light weight on a short string. Since both string length and weight have changed, it is impossible to draw a clear conclusion about either factor. An adolescent, in contrast, is likely to try a much more organized approach, attempting to vary just one of the four factors at a time.

Finally, Piaget argued that another facet of this shift is the appearance of deductive logic in the child's repertoire of skills. A great deal of the logic of science is of this deductive type. We begin with a theory and propose, "If this theory is correct, then I should observe such and such." In doing this, we are going well beyond our observations. We are conceiving things that we have never seen but that *ought* to be true or observable. We can think of this change as being part of a general "decentering" process that began earlier. The preoperational child gradually moves away from his egocentrism and comes to be able to take the physical perspective of others. During formal operations, the child takes another step by freeing himself even from his reliance on specific experiences.

Lasting Influences from Piaget's Ideas

As you will soon see, quite a few of the specifics of Piaget's theory have been called into question. He was wrong about the timing of development of many of the cognitive skills he described, and he was probably wrong about the breadth and generality of the stages themselves. Nevertheless, a number of aspects of his theory remain strongly influential, including the following:

Constructivism. The most pervasively influential idea to come from Piaget's theory is that the child is *constructing* her understanding of the world. She is not passive; she

Research Report
Piaget's Clever Research

Piaget had an enormous impact on developmental psychologists not only because he proposed a novel and provocative theory, but also because of the cleverness of many of the strategies he devised for testing children's understanding. These strategies often showed children doing or saying very unexpected things—results that other theorists found hard to assimilate into their models.

The most famous of all Piaget's clever techniques is probably his method for studying *conservation*. Piaget would begin with two equal balls of clay, show them to the child, and let the child hold and manipulate the clay until she agreed that they had the same amount. Then in full view of the child, Piaget would squish one of the balls into a pancake or roll it into a sausage. Then he'd ask the child whether there was still the same amount or whether the pancake or the ball had more. Children of 4 and 5 consistently said that the ball had more; children of 6 and 7 consistently said that they were still the same, indicating that they had grasped the concept of conservation—that the quantity of clay is *conserved* even though it is changed in some other dimension.

In another study, Piaget explored the concept of *class inclusion*—the understanding that a given object can belong simultaneously to more than one category. Fido is *both* a dog and an animal; a high chair is both a chair and furniture. Piaget usually studied this by having children first create their own classes and subclasses and then asking them questions about them. One 5½-year-old child, for example, had been playing with a set of flowers and

had made two heaps, one large group of primroses and a smaller group of other mixed flowers. Piaget then had this conversation with the child (Piaget & Inhelder, 1959, p. 108):

> *Piaget:* "If I make a bouquet of all the primroses and you make one of all the flowers, which will be bigger?"
> *Child:* "Yours."
> *Piaget:* "If I gather all the primroses in a meadow, will any flowers remain?"
> *Child:* "Yes."

The child understood that there are other flowers than primroses but did *not* yet understand that all primroses are flowers—that the smaller, subordinate class is *included in* the larger class.

In these conversations with children, Piaget was always trying to understand how the child thought rather than whether the child could come up with the right answer. So he used a "clinical method" in which he followed the child's lead, asking probing questions or creating special exploratory tests to try to discover the child's logic. In the early days of Piaget's work, many American researchers were critical of this method, since Piaget did not ask precisely the same questions of each child. Still, the results were so striking, and often so surprising, that they couldn't be ignored. And when stricter research techniques were devised, investigators often discovered that Piaget's observations and insights were accurate.

actively seeks to understand. A majority of developmentalists have accepted this proposition as a starting point (Flavell, 1992).

Qualitative Change. Piaget's emphasis on qualitative change has also been highly significant. The descriptions of and discussions about the nature of the qualitative changes have shifted, as we have learned more about children's knowledge at various ages. But virtually all would agree that a 15-year-old approaches problems and tasks in a way that is not just faster but qualitatively different from the way a 3-year-old approaches the same tasks.

Stages. Piaget's concept of stages has been perhaps the most controversial of his ideas, but it has nonetheless had a profound impact, still seen today. He argued that each stage was a coherent whole, that a child was "in" a given stage or another, and that all the child's thinking was affected by the basic properties of that stage. By the end of this chapter I think I will have persuaded you that this view of stages is not correct, but the idea that there are sequential changes in the *form* of a child's thinking continues to be the basis for an enormous amount of our research and thinking. In addition, the four-part stage division that Piaget described has shaped the very way we talk about childhood—as well as the way we organize our textbooks. We speak of infants, preschoolers, schoolchildren, and adolescents, almost as if these were four different species. In fact, I will use his four-stage division of ages/stages as the structure of my description, not only because it is convenient, but because so many researchers—influenced by Piaget—have studied children in only one age period.

Other Specific Concepts and Terms. Finally, of course, Piaget has left us with a legacy of terminology and concepts that are widely used. These include *scheme, assimilation, accommodation, egocentrism, conservation,* and the *object concept.*

All these influences will be apparent in my descriptions of our current understanding of the development of children's thinking. Let us begin with what we now know about cognition in infancy.

Cognitive Development in Infancy

The focus of a great deal of modern research in cognition in infancy has been on showing that Piaget greatly underestimated the cognitive skill of babies. This same point emerged clearly from all the research on infant perception that I described in some detail in Chapter 5, so this is not news to you. But let me give you several further examples.

Imitation

One active area of study has been the ability of an infant to imitate. This is an important issue not only because Piaget proposed a series of quite specific hypotheses about imitation in the early months, but also because it may tell us what and how soon a baby can learn from modeling—a major form of learning proposed by social-cognitive theorists like Bandura.

Piaget thought that as early as the first few months of life, infants could imitate actions they could see themselves make, such as hand gestures. But he thought they could *not* imitate other people's facial gestures until late in the first year. This form of imitation seems to require some kind of cross-modal transfer, combining the visual cues from seeing the other's face with the kinesthetic cues from one's own facial movements. Piaget did not think that cross-modal transfer was possible until at least 8 months, so he didn't think this form of imitation could occur until then either. He further argued that imitation of any action that wasn't already in the child's repertoire did not occur until about 1 year and that *deferred* imitation, in which a child sees some action and then imitates it at a later point, was possible only at the end of the sensorimotor period, since deferred imitation requires some kind of internal representation.

In broad terms, Piaget's proposed sequence has been supported. Imitation of someone else's hand movements or their actions with objects seems to improve steadily during the months of infancy, starting at 1 or 2 months of age; imitation of two-part actions develops much later, perhaps at 15 to 18 months (Poulson, Nunes, & Warren, 1989). Yet there are also two important exceptions to this general confirmation of Piaget's theory: Infants imitate some facial gestures in the first weeks of life, and deferred imitation seems to occur earlier than Piaget proposed.

Several researchers have found that newborn babies will imitate certain facial gestures, particularly tongue protrusion (Anisfeld, 1991). This only seems to work if the model sits there with his tongue out looking at the baby for a fairly long period of time, perhaps as long as a minute. But the fact that newborns imitate at all is striking—although it is entirely consistent with the observation that quite young babies are capable of tactual/visual cross-modal transfer.

Studies of deferred imitation are not so strikingly discordant with Piaget's description, but at least one study (Meltzoff, 1988) shows that babies as young as 9 months can defer their imitation over as long as 24 hours. By 14 months, toddlers recall others' actions over periods of two days. In one study, Elizabeth Hanna and Andrew Meltzoff (1993) trained a 14-month-old to play with five particular toys in distinctive ways, such as collapsing a collapsible cup or picking up a string of beads and placing it a cup. Other babies watched these play behaviors in a laboratory setting. Two days later, an unfamiliar adult took the special set of toys to the baby's home and gave them to the child one at a time, to see if the child would imitate the actions he had seen the other child perform two days earlier. The majority of the 14-month-olds imitated at least two of these behaviors, while a control group who were given the toys but had not seen the model typically did not use the toys in these particular ways.

These findings are significant for several reasons. First, they make it clear that children of this age can and do learn specific behaviors through modeling, even when they have no chance to imitate the behavior immediately. Second, deferred imitation clearly requires that the baby remember what he saw and connect that memory to the object, all of which seems to require internal representation—which Piaget did not think was present this early. The fact that they are present in children as young as 14 months and that the children were even able to imitate the action when the imitation occurred in a different setting from the setting in which the observation occurred suggests that Piaget was simply wrong about when we are first able to use some kind of internal representation to remember actions and events.

Memory

The same point emerges from Carolyn Rovee-Collier's fascinating studies of memory in very young infants (1993). She has used an ingenious variation of an operant conditioning procedure to demonstrate that babies as young as 3 months of age can remember particular objects and their actions with those objects over periods of as long as a week. And if you "remind" them in between times, they can remember their earlier actions over six weeks.

Rovee-Collier first hangs an attractive mobile over the baby's crib and watches to see how the baby responds. In particular, she is interested in how often the baby normally kicks his legs while looking at the mobile. After three minutes of this "baseline" observation, she attaches a string from the mobile to the baby's leg, as you can see in Figure 7.2, so that each time the baby kicks his leg, the mobile moves. Babies quickly learn to kick repeatedly in order to make this interesting new thing happen. Within three to six minutes, 3-month-olds double or triple their kick rates, showing that learning clearly occurred. She then tests the baby's memory of this learning by coming back some days later, hanging the same mobile over the crib, and counting the rate of the baby's kicks without attaching the string to his foot. If the baby remembers the previous occasion, he should kick at a higher rate than he did when he first saw the mobile, which is precisely what 3-month-old babies do, even after a delay as long as a week.

In some experiments, Rovee-Collier also "reminds" the baby of the original learning by coming back some time after the first training, hanging the mobile over the crib, and

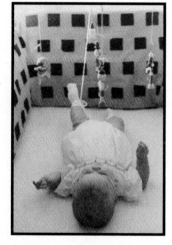

FIGURE 7.2 This 3-month-old baby in one of Rovee-Collier's memory experiments will quickly learn to kick her foot in order to make the mobile move. And she will remember this connection between kicking and the mobile several days later. (*Source:* Rovee-Collier, 1993, p. 131.)

tugging on the string herself at the same rate that the baby had learned to kick. So the baby sees the mobile moving in a rhythmic pattern. Then she comes back a third time to check if the baby still kicks at a higher rate when he sees this particular mobile. With the reminder in between, babies as young as 3 months old remember the original learned connection between kicking and the mobile over several weeks.

Why is this so interesting? Primarily because it contradicts Piaget's view of the sensorimotor infant, whom he saw functioning pretty much in the here and now. It shows us, once again, that the young infant is cognitively a whole lot more sophisticated than we had supposed. At the same time, Rovee-Collier's work offers some support for Piaget's views, since she finds systematic gains in the baby's ability to remember over the months of infancy. Two-month-olds can remember their kicking action for only one day; 3-month-olds can remember over a week, and by 6 months the baby can remember over two weeks. Similarly, reminders work better and better as the baby gets older. But all these early infant memories are *strongly* tied to the specific context in which the original experience occurred. Even 6-month-olds do not recognize or remember the mobile if you change the context even slightly, such as hanging a different-colored cloth around the playpen in which the child was originally tested. Thus, babies do remember—far more than Piaget believed—but their memories are highly specific. With age, their memories become less and less tied to specific cues or contexts.

Both Meltzoff's studies of imitation and Rovee-Collier's studies of memory raise the more general question of whether infants may be capable of some forms of internal representation well before Piaget thought that they were. The same point arises from much of the research on early perception that I talked about in Chapter 5, including the findings that cross-modal transfer occurs as early as 1 month and the research on children's responses to patterns like "big over little." All these accomplishments seem to require that the baby create a fairly complex and abstract mental image. But such findings need not totally refute Piaget. What may develop at 18 or 24 months may be the ability to *manipulate* these images in his head, or some greater generality of the images, so that they are less situation-specific. We are left, then, with a picture of an infant who is indeed busily *constructing* schemes, concepts, and memories but who seems to start out at a far higher level of skill in this process than Piaget had believed (Karmiloff-Smith, 1993).

> Rovee-Collier's findings have surprised a lot of developmental psychologists. Do you find them surprising? Why or why not?

Cognitive Development in the Preschool Period

Much the same picture emerges from the current studies of thinking in the preschool-age child. This is an area of great theoretical and research ferment at the moment, much of it stimulated originally by two of Piaget's observations about children of this age: that their thinking is egocentric and that they are captured by appearances. From these two starting points has come a rich and intriguing body of evidence suggesting that preschoolers are a great deal less egocentric than Piaget thought but that they must struggle with the problem of distinguishing between appearance and reality. Many of us have been immensely surprised by the evidence that one of the products of that struggle is the development by age 4 or 5 of a remarkably sophisticated "theory of mind." By that age, amazingly enough, a child seems to realize that other people's actions are governed by what they think and believe, not by "facts" or "reality."

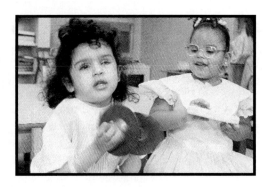

The 3-year-old on the right is able to adapt her speech and her play to the needs of her blind friend, which is one sign that preschoolers are less egocentric than Piaget thought.

Perspective Taking

Research on the child's ability to take others' perspectives shows that children as young as 2 and 3 have at least *some* ability to understand that other people see or experience things differently than they do. For example, children this age will adapt their speech or their play to the demands of their companion. They play differently with older or younger playmates and talk differently to a younger or a handicapped child (Brownell, 1990; Guralnick & Paul-Brown, 1984).

But such understanding is clearly not perfect at this young age. John Flavell has proposed two levels of such perspective-taking ability. At level 1 the child knows *that* some other person experiences something differently. At level 2 the child develops a whole series of complex rules for figuring out precisely *what* the other person sees or experiences (Flavell, Green, & Flavell, 1990). Two- and 3-year-olds have level 1 knowledge but not level 2. We begin to see some level 2 knowledge in 4- and 5-year-olds.

Appearance and Reality

This shift seems to be part of a much broader change in the child's understanding of appearance and reality. Flavell has studied this in a variety of ways, such as by showing objects under colored lights to change the apparent color or putting masks on animals to make them look like another animal. He finds that 2- and 3-year-olds consistently judge things by their appearance. By age 5 the child begins to be able to separate the appearance from the underlying reality and knows that some object isn't "really" red, even though it looks red under a red-colored light, or that a cat with a dog mask is still "really" a cat (Flavell, Green, & Flavell, 1989; Flavell et al., 1987).

In the most famous Flavell procedure, the experimenter shows the child a sponge that has been painted to look like a rock. Three-year-olds faced with this odd object will say either that the object looks like a sponge and is a sponge or that it looks like a rock and is a rock. But 4- and 5-year-olds can distinguish the two; they realize that it looks like a rock but *is* a sponge (Flavell, 1986). Thus, the older child now understands that the same object can be represented differently, depending on one's point of view.

Using the same type of materials, investigators have also asked if a child can grasp the principle of a *false belief.* After the child has felt the sponge/rock and has answered questions about what it looks like and what it "really" is, you can ask something like this: "John [a playmate of the subject's] hasn't touched this, he hasn't squeezed it. If John just sees it over here like this, what will he think it is? Will he think it's a rock or will he think that it's a sponge?" (Gopnik & Astington, 1988, p. 35). By and large, 3-year-olds think that John will believe it is a sponge, while 4- and 5-year-olds realize that because John hasn't felt the sponge, he will have a false belief that it is a rock. Thus, the child of 4 or 5 understands that someone else can believe something that isn't true *and will act on that belief.*

Theories of Mind

Evidence like this has led a number of theorists (e.g., Astington & Gopnik, 1991; Gopnik & Wellman, 1994; Harris, 1989) to propose that the 4- or 5-year-old has developed a new and quite sophisticated **theory of mind.** The child this age has begun to understand that you cannot predict what other people will do solely from observing the

Cultures and Contexts
Understanding of Appearance and Reality in Other Cultures

A number of studies from widely differing parts of the globe, and in widely different cultures, suggest that this shift at about age 4 in children's understanding of appearance and reality and of false belief may well be a universal developmental pattern.

Jeremy Avis and Paul Harris (1991) adapted the traditional false belief testing procedure for use with a pygmy tribe, the Baka, who live in Cameroon. The Baka are a hunter-gatherer people who live together in camps. Each child was tested in his or her own hut, using materials with which she was completely familiar. She watched one adult, named Mopfana (a member of the tribe), put some mango kernels into a bowl. Mopfana then left the hut and a second adult (also a tribe member) told the child they were going to play a game with Mopfana: They were going to hide the kernels in a cooking pot. Then he asked the child what Mopfana was going to do when he came back. Would he look for the kernels in the bowl or in the pot? And he asked the child whether Mopfana's heart would feel good or bad before he lifted the lid of the bowl and after he lifted the lid. Younger children—2-, 3-, and early 4-year-olds—were much more likely to say that Mopfana would look for the seeds in the pan or to say that he would be sad before he looked in the bowl, while older 4- and 5-year-olds were nearly always right on all three questions.

Similarly, when Flavell used his sponge/rock task with children in mainland China, he found that Chinese 3-year-olds were just as confused about this task as are American or British 3-year-olds, whereas 5-year-old Chinese children had no difficulty with the problem (Flavell et al., 1983).

Using a somewhat different kind of problem, but one that still touches on the difference between appearance and reality, Paul Harris and his colleagues (1989) have asked children in several cultures how characters in a story *really* feel and what emotion *appears* on their faces. For example:

Diana is playing a game with her friend. At the end of the game Diana wins and her friend loses. Diana tries to hide how she feels because otherwise her friend won't play any more. (Harris, 1989, p. 134)

Four-year-old children in Britain and the United States, faced with such stories, have no trouble saying how the character will really feel, but they have more trouble saying how the character would look. By 5 or 6, however, the child grasps the possible difference. Harris and his colleagues have found that the same age shift occurs in Japan (Gardner et al., 1988), and Joshi and MacLean (1994) found a similar shift in India, despite the fact that both the Japanese and Indian cultures put far more emphasis on the disguising of emotions than is true in British or American culture.

In these very different cultures, then, something similar seems to be occurring between ages 3 and 5. In these years, all children seem to understand something general about the difference between appearance and reality and seem to develop a type of theory of mind.

situation itself; the other person's desires and beliefs also enter into the equation. So the child develops various theories about other people's ideas, beliefs, and desires, and about how they will affect others' behaviors.

Such a theory of mind does not spring forth full-blown at age 4. Three-year-old children already understand some aspects of the links between people's thinking or feeling and their behavior. For example, they know that a person who wants something will try to get it. They also know that a person may still want something even if she can't have it (Lillard & Flavell, 1992). But they do not yet understand the basic principle that each person's actions are based on his own *representation* of reality and that a person's representation may differ from what is "really" there. People act on the basis of what they believe or feel, even if what they believe is incorrect or what they feel is unexpected or apparently inconsistent in a given situation. Thus, a person who feels sad even though she has succeeded at something will act on that sadness, not on the visible success. It is this new aspect of the theory of mind that seems to be absent in the 3-year-old but that clearly emerges at about 4 or 5.

The theories of mind of the 3- and 4-year-old differ in other ways as well. The 3-year-old seems to assume that everyone knows and experiences the world in the same way he does—a classic form of egocentrism. The 4-year-old seems to understand that there are many worlds and that other people not only know (or experience) different things, but may "know" or believe something that is untrue and can change their beliefs. He also understands that he himself may have experienced things differently at different times. He can remember that he used to think something different—that he used to think that the sponge was a rock but no longer believes that—which is one hint of the development of the ability to be *aware* of what one knows and thinks.

Consider your own theory of mind. What assumptions do you make about the way other people's behavior is affected by their beliefs, feelings, or ideas? You operate on the basis of such a theory all the time, but can you articulate it?

Still, there is much that the 4- or 5-year-old doesn't yet grasp about other people's thinking. The child of this age understands that other people think but does not yet understand that those same other people think about *him*. In the famous infinite regress, the 4-year-old understands "I know that you know." But he does not yet fully understand that this process is reciprocal, namely, that "You know that I know." Such an understanding of the reciprocal nature of thought seems to develop between ages 5 and 7 for most children (Perner & Wimmer, 1985; Sullivan, Zaitchik, & Tager-Flusberg, 1994)—a particularly important development, because it would seem to be a necessary element for the creation of genuinely reciprocal friendships, which we begin to see in the elementary school years.

Metacognition and Metamemory. Such an increased awareness of the ways in which thinking operates is also apparent in other areas. For example, between 3 and 5, children figure out that in order to tell if a rock painted like a sponge is really a sponge or a rock, a person would need to touch or hold it. Just looking at it doesn't give you enough information (Flavell, 1993; O'Neill, Astington, & Flavell, 1992). In a similar vein, 4-year-olds (but not 3-year-olds) understand that to remember or forget something, one must have known it at a previous time (Lyon & Flavell, 1994). These developments are important because they seem to be the first signs of what psychologists now call **metamemory** and **metacognition**—knowing about the process of memory and the process of thinking. By about age 4 or 5, children seem to have some beginning grasp of these processes, but they still have a long way to go.

John Flavell's most recent research (Flavell, Green, & Flavell, 1995) suggests that by age 4, a child understands that there is some kind of process called thinking that people do and that is distinct from knowing or talking. They also understand in some preliminary way that people can think about imaginary objects or events as well as real ones. But despite these major advances, 4- and 5-year-olds do not yet understand that thinking is a process or that it occurs continuously (Wellman & Hickling, 1994). In particular, they don't realize that *other people* are thinking all the time. They don't assume that another person is thinking all the time, and when asked, they are bad at guessing what the other person might be thinking about, even when the clues are quite clear—such as when the other person is reading or listening to something. All these skills are much more highly developed in 7- and 8-year-olds, who seem to have figured out that their own and other people's thinking goes on constantly and follows certain rules.

All this new work on the child's theory of mind not only has opened up a fascinating new area of research, but has clearly demonstrated that the preschool child is vastly less egocentric than Piaget supposed. By age 4, and in more limited ways at earlier ages, the child has a remarkably sophisticated ability to understand other points of view and can predict other people's behavior on the basis of deductions about their beliefs. I don't know about you, but I think this is an amazing—and surprising—achievement.

Understanding and Regulating Emotions

Another ability that expands greatly in the preschool years is the child's ability to understand emotions—a process that is clearly linked to the emerging theory of mind. You already know that by 10 to 12 months, babies can tell the difference between positive or negative facial expressions on others' faces, because at that age they already show *social referencing*. By age 4, children's emotional vocabulary has expanded enough that they can recognize facial expressions and situations that convey the emotions happy, sad, mad, loving, and scared. More than that, though, preschoolers begin to understand the links between other people's emotions and their circumstances. For example, a child this age understands another person will feel sad if she fails or happy if she succeeds. The preschool child also begins to figure out that particular emotions occur in situations involving specific relationships between desire and reality. Sadness, for example, normally occurs when someone fails to acquire some desired object or loses something desired (Harris, 1989).

During these same years, the child also learns to regulate or modulate her *own* expression of emotion (Dunn, 1994). Part of this process is the development of *impulse control*—the growing ability to inhibit a response, to wait rather than to weep, to protest verbally rather than to hit. When an infant is upset, it is the parents who help to regulate that emotion, by cuddling or soothing. Over the preschool years, this regulation process is gradually taken over more and more by the child. Two-year-olds are only minimally able to modulate their feelings in this way, but by 5 or 6, most children have made great strides in controlling the intensity of their expression of strong feelings.

A second aspect to this regulation of emotion—one that is clearly linked to the cognitive processes I'm talking about in this chapter—is the need for the child to learn the social rules of specific emotional expressions. When and where is it permissible to express various feelings? What form may that expression take? When should you smile? When should you *not* frown or smile, regardless of the feeling you may be experiencing? For example, as early as age 3 children begin to learn that there are times when they ought to smile—even when they do not feel completely happy. Thus begins the "social smile," a facial expression that is quite distinct from the natural, delighted smile. Similarly, over the

Preschoolers develop their first individual friendships at about the same age that they become more skilled at reading other people's emotions. Might these two things be causally linked? What kind of research could you do to find out?

years of childhood, children learn to use abbreviated or constricted forms of other emotions, such as anger or disgust (Izard & Malatesta, 1987), and they learn to conceal their feelings in a variety of situations. Such concealment appears to rest on the child's emerging theory of mind. For example, for a child to conceal some emotion in order not to hurt someone else's feelings requires that she have some sense of what will cause the other person's feelings to be hurt. Equally, the preschool child learns to use her own emotional expression to get things she wants, crying, smiling as needed. And this control of emotions also rests on her understanding of the links between her behavior and others' understanding of her behavior, an understanding that develops rapidly between ages 3 and 4.

Other Aspects of Preschool Thought: Conservation and Classification

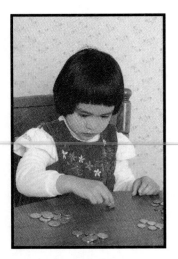

Three-year-old Stacie, busily sorting coins, shows that by this age, children are readily able to put similar things together.

Other work on this same age period also points to the inescapable conclusion that Piaget badly underestimated the cognitive abilities of the preschool child. For example, studies of classification show that 3- and 4-year-olds are able to classify objects into groups quite readily if you simplify the task or if you make it clear that you want them to use some kind of superordinate category for classifying. For example, Sandra Waxman and Rochel Gelman (1986) told 3- and 4-year-olds that a puppet really liked pictures of food (or animals, or furniture). The children were then given 12 pictures and asked to put the ones the puppet would like in one bin and the ones the puppet would not like in another bin. When they were given the category label in this way, these young children could quite easily classify the pictures into food and nonfood categories, or furniture and nonfurniture categories.

Even at 18 months babies may be capable of some classification. In one study, Alison Gopnik and Andrew Meltzoff (1992) gave toddlers this age sets of objects to play with, such as four different finger rings and four different rocks. The objects were laid out in front of the child in a random array, without any specific instructions except encouragement to the child to handle the objects. Fully half of these young children physically separated the two types of objects into distinct piles or groups.

All in all, this research shows that the basic understanding that things go together in groups is present by at least age 2 (and perhaps earlier). But whether the child can display this understanding will depend on the way you set up the task. Piaget happened to pick a relatively difficult version of the task for his own studies, so he ended up underestimating the child's understanding.

In contrast, studies of conservation have generally confirmed Piaget's basic observations. Although younger children can demonstrate some understanding of conservation if the task is made very simple (Gelman, 1972; Wellman, 1982), most children cannot consistently solve conservation problems until age 5 or 6 or later.

The relatively late development of the child's understanding of conservation makes sense if we think of conservation tasks as a particularly sophisticated form of question about appearance and reality; the amount of juice appears to change, even though in reality it remains the same. In addition, to grasp the basic principle of conservation the child also has to understand rules about what kinds of manipulations will change quantities (such as adding makes something more). But the understanding of the distinction between appearance and reality seems to be a precursor or requirement for conservation tasks.

Overview of the Preschool Child's Thinking

How can we add up the bits and pieces of information about the preschool child's thinking? At the least, we can say that preschool children are capable of forms of logic that Piaget thought impossible at this stage. In particular, by age 4, and certainly by age 5, they not only can take others' perspectives, but can understand, at least in a preliminary way, that other people's behavior rests on inner beliefs and feelings.

One possibility is that Piaget simply got the age wrong and that the transition he saw at 6 or 7 really happens at around age 4 or 5. Certainly the various understandings that children seem to come to at about that age—about false belief, about appearance and reality, about other people's physical perspective, and about the meanings of emotional expressions—are remarkably stagelike.

Another possibility is that while preschoolers can do some seemingly sophisticated things, their understanding remains specific rather than general. It is still tied heavily to specific situations or can be displayed only with a good deal of support. Studies of both conservation and children's logic show that sophisticated performances can be *elicited* in 2-, 3-, and 4-year-old children, but preschoolers do not typically show such skills spontaneously. For the preschool child to demonstrate these relatively advanced forms of thinking, you have to make the task quite simple, eliminate distractions, or give special clues. The fact that children this age can solve these problems at all is striking, but it is still true that preschool children think differently from older children. The very fact that they can perform certain tasks *only* when the tasks are made very simple or undistracting is evidence for such a difference.

More broadly, preschoolers do not seem to experience the world or think about it with as general a set of rules or principles as we see in older children and thus they do not easily generalize something they have learned in one context to a similar but not identical situation. It is precisely such a switch to general rules that Piaget thought characterized the thinking of the school-age child. So let's see if he was right.

Cognitive Development in the School-Age Child

As was the case for the two age periods we've already explored, research on thinking among school-age children divides fairly neatly into two groups: early studies that tested one or another of Piaget's observations directly and newer research that introduces new themes. Let me give you an example of each.

Direct Tests of Piaget's Ideas

Unlike researchers who have studied the first two of Piaget's stages, those who have followed up on Piaget's descriptions of the concrete operational period have generally found that Piaget was right about the ages at which children first show various skills or understandings. Studies of conservation, for example, consistently show that children grasp conservation of amount or mass by about age 6 and conservation of weight at about 7 or 8. And studies of classification skills show that only at about age 7 or 8 does the child grasp the principle of *class inclusion*—described in the *Research Report* box on page 190.

Preschool children understand that dogs are *also* animals, but they do not yet fully understand the nature of the relationship.

A good illustration of these changes and of the early research on this age period is a longitudinal study of concrete operations tasks by Carol Tomlinson-Keasey and her colleagues (Tomlinson-Keasey et al., 1979). They followed a group of 38 children from kindergarten through third grade, testing them with several traditional concrete-operations tasks each year, including *class inclusion, hierarchical classification,* and three kinds of conservation, *mass, weight,* and *volume.* You can see in Figure 7.3 that children got better at all these tasks over the three-year-period, with a particularly rapid improvement between the end of kindergarten and the start of first grade (about the age when Piaget thought that concrete operations really began). However, it is also obvious in the figure that the several tasks were not equally easy, even though all of them appear to require similar levels of concrete operational thought.

Tomlinson-Keasey also found that a child's skill on these tasks, relative to the other children, stayed approximately the same throughout the three years of testing. A 6-year-old who had developed conservation of mass early continued to be ahead of other children later on; a late-developing child went through the same sequence about two years later.

Studies like Tomlinson-Keasey's pointed to the conclusion that these more complex forms of thinking do indeed develop during the elementary school years but that the whole process is less clearly stagelike than Piaget proposed.

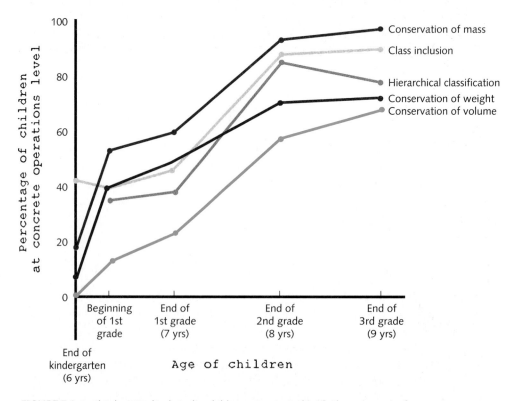

FIGURE 7.3 In this longitudinal study, children were tested with the same set of concrete operations tasks five different times, beginning in kindergarten and ending in the third grade. (*Source:* Tomlinson-Keasey et al., 1979, adapted from Table 2, p. 1158.)

New Themes: Memory and Strategy Development

Some researchers, rather than simply repeating Piaget's tasks, have tried to devise other ways to test the proposition that school-age children approach tasks in ways that are more general, based on broader principles, than do younger children. In particular, researchers have focused on the child's intentional and conscious use of *strategies* in solving problems or for remembering things. Work on memory and memory strategies is a particularly good example.

Rehearsal Strategies. Suppose you're about to go out the door to run some errands. You need to stop at the cleaners, buy some stamps, copy your IRS forms, and buy milk, bread, orange juice, carrots, lettuce, spaghetti, and spaghetti sauce at the grocery store. How do you remember all those things? You could use any one of a variety of strategies, some of which I have listed (with examples) in Table 7.2. You could rehearse the list, you could organize the route in your mind, you could remember your menu for dinner when you get to the grocery store.

Do children do these things when they try to remember? One classic, early study (Keeney, Cannizzo, & Flavell, 1967) indicated that school-age children do but that younger children do not. Keeney showed children a row of seven cards with pictures on them and told them to try to remember all the pictures in the same order they were laid

How do you remember lists of things to buy, or a set of errands you have to run? Do you write them down? What other strategies do you use?

Table 7.2
Some Common Strategies Involved in Remembering

Rehearsal	Perhaps the most common strategy, which involves either mental or vocal repetition, or repetition of movement (as in learning to dance). May occur in children as young as 2 years under some conditions.
Clustering	Grouping ideas or objects or words into clusters to help you remember them, such as "all animals," "all the ingredients in the lasagna recipe," or "the chess pieces involved in the move called castling." This is one strategy that clearly benefits from experience with a particular subject or activity, since possible categories are learned or are discovered in the process of exploring or manipulating a set of material. Primitive clustering occurs in 2-year-olds.
Elaboration	Finding shared meaning or a common referent for two or more things that need to be remembered. The helpful mnemonic for recalling the names of the lines on the musical staff ("Every Good Boy Does Fine") is a kind of elaboration, as is associating the name of a person you have just met with some object or other word. This form of memory aid is not used spontaneously by all individuals and is not used skillfully until fairly late in development, if then.
Systematic searching	When you try to remember something, you can "scan" the memory for the whole domain in which it might be found. Three- and 4-year-old children can begin to do this to search for actual objects in the real world but are not good at doing this in memory. So search strategies may be first learned in the external world and then applied to inner searches.

Source: Flavell, 1985.

out. A space helmet, then placed over the child's head, kept the child from seeing the cards but allowed the experimenter to see if the child seemed to be rehearsing the list by muttering under his breath. Children under 5 almost never showed any rehearsal, while 8- to 10-year-old children usually did. Interestingly, when 5-year-olds were *taught* to rehearse, they were able to do so and their memory scores improved. But when these same 5-year-olds were then given a new problem without being reminded to rehearse, they stopped rehearsing. That is, they could use the strategy if they were reminded, but they did not produce it spontaneously—a pattern described as a *production deficiency*.

Studies of children's use of the strategy of *clustering* show a similar age pattern. Studies of clustering often involve having children or adults learn lists of words that have potential categories built into them. For example, I might ask you to remember a list of words that includes a mixture of names for furniture, animals, and foods. I let you learn the list any way you wish, but when you name off the items later, I can check for the kind of organization you used by seeing whether you name the same-category words together.

School-age children do show this kind of internal organization when they recall things, while preschoolers do not. And within the school years, older children use this strategy more and more efficiently, using a few large categories rather than many smaller ones (Bjorklund & Muir, 1988) and discovering and using more methods for their clustering. For example, if you ask children and adults to list all the furniture in their house, 10-year-olds typically cluster the items by category, such as beds, tables, and chairs. By age 12 or 14, though, many teenagers discover the even more efficient spatial clustering strategy and name the furniture in each room in turn (Plumert, 1994).

However, preschool children do show some kinds of memory strategies if the task is quite simple, such as the game of hide-and-seek (DeLoache, 1989). In one of Judy DeLoache's studies, the child watches the experimenter hide an attractive toy in some obvious place (e.g., behind a couch) and is then told that when a buzzer goes off, she can go and find the toy. While playing with other toys during the four-minute delay interval, 2-year-olds often talked about the toy's hiding place, or pointed to or looked at the hiding place—all of which seem clearly to be early forms of mnemonic strategies.

These results and others like them tell us that no magic shift occurs at age 5, 6, or 7 from nonstrategic to strategic behavior. Primitive strategies are used by children as young as 2, perhaps younger. But there is clearly a shift toward greater and greater strategy use over the elementary school years. This shift has several characteristics.

First, in the use of any given strategy, children appear to move from a period in which they don't use it at all, or use it only under highly simplified conditions, to a period in which they use it if reminded or taught but not spontaneously, to one in which they use it spontaneously. Second, older children use strategies more and more skillfully and flexibly. For example, when learning a list of words, 8-year-olds are more likely to practice the words one at a time ("cat, cat, cat"), while still older children practice them in groups ("desk, lawn, sky, shirt, cat"). When the 8-year-olds are tested again a year later, they show signs of a shift toward the more efficient strategy (Guttentag, Ornstein, & Siemens, 1987).

Finally, elementary school children, unlike preschoolers, understand something of the process of strategy use and can describe the strategies they are using (Alexander & Schwanenflugel, 1994). Taking all this together, it looks as if Piaget was at least partially right about the existence of a significant change in children's thinking at around ages 5 to

The Real World

Memory and the Child as Witness

In England, a 7-year-old was able to provide the police with details of her experience after a sexual assault and was later able to identify her attacker in a lineup (Davies, 1993). In several famous cases in the United States, children as young as 3 years old have testified in court about physical or sexual abuse by nursery school teachers, testimony that has sometimes (but not always) led to convictions. Testimony by children has become more frequent as courts have relaxed their rules about child witnesses (Penrod, 1993), but such testimony continues to raise a storm of controversy, centering on two main issues: (1) Can young children accurately remember faces or events and report on their experiences, even after a period of time has passed? (2) Are children more suggestible than adults about what they might have seen or experienced? Will they report what they have been told to say, what may have been suggested to them, or what they actually saw or felt?

A few answers have begun to emerge from a growing body of research addressing these questions, although in many areas we are a long way from definitive answers. Among other things, there is still a good deal of controversy about whether stress improves or worsens children's memory for events—a highly relevant issue, given the fact that most of the events children would be asked to testify about in a court are likely to have been highly stressful. Nonetheless, a few things seem fairly clear.

1. Recall of specific events or of the faces of people seen at a previous time does improve with age, but even preschoolers can recall action-related events with considerable accuracy. When experimenters have staged various crises or happenings and later asked children about them or asked children to identify someone involved in a witnessed event, preschoolers and school-age children can describe what happened and can pick out a photo of the "culprit" almost as well as adults can. They report less detail than adults do, but they rarely report something that didn't actually occur (Baker-Ward et al., 1993; Ceci & Bruck, 1993; Davies, 1993). In one real-life study, Steward (1993) asked preschool children to describe their experiences on a recent visit to a medical clinic—visits that had been videotaped. The children reported only a quarter of the actual occasions when they had been touched on some part of their body by a medical person, but virtually all the reports they did give (94 percent) were accurate.

2. Over longer periods of time, such as a year or two, however, children's accuracy in recall may decline more than an adult's does. In one study, Debra Poole (Poole & White, 1993) found that 6-, 8-, and 10-year-olds were all less accurate than adults in a report of a staged event that had occurred two years earlier. More troublesome from a legal perspective was the finding that the children were more likely than the adults in this study to report false actions or to attribute an action to the wrong person two years later.

3. Younger children, particularly preschoolers, are also more suggestible than older children or adults. This has often been studied by showing a film or telling a story to children and adults. The researchers then ask questions about what the subject saw and inject some misleading question into the set—a question that assumes something that didn't really happen (e.g., "he was carrying a pipe wrench when he came into the room, wasn't he?"). Some days or weeks later, the subjects are again asked to describe what happened in the film or story. In this way you can check to see whether the inaccurate or misleading suggestion has been absorbed into the story. Young children are more affected than are older children or adults by such misleading suggestions. Of particular importance is the finding that it is possible to mislead young children enough in this way so that they will report inaccurately about specific physical events they have experienced, such as having been kissed while being bathed, having been spanked, or having been hurt by a shot when they visited a doctor a year or more earlier (Bruck et al., 1995; Ceci & Bruck, 1993). This is much more true of preschoolers than of school-age children, although no one is quite sure what mechanism is involved in this age difference.

Thus, it *is* possible for an interviewer—psychologist, social worker, attorney, whoever—to nudge a child's testimony in one direction or another. When the misinformation comes from parents, children are particularly likely to incorporate the parents' version into their own free recall. Even questioning a child about some event that did not occur sometimes leads children to generate false descriptions, including descriptions of bodily touches (Poole & Warren, 1995). Adult witnesses are *also* susceptible to suggestions of various kinds. So the difference here is one of degree and not of kind. From the legal point of view, this does not mean that children should not testify; it speaks only to the weight one might give their recollections and the care that should be used in framing questions.

7. The shift is more gradual than he proposed, but it does involve qualitative as well as quantitative changes. Older children are approaching problems differently than younger children, using a different repertoire of skills.

Expertise

However—and this is a big however—all these apparent developmental changes may well turn out to be as much a function of expertise as of age. Piaget obviously thought that children apply broad forms of logic to all their experiences in any given stage. If that's true, then the amount of specific experience a child has had with some set of material shouldn't make a lot of difference. A child who understands hierarchical classification but who has never seen pictures of different types of dinosaurs still ought to be able to create classifications of dinosaurs about as well as a child who had played a lot with dinosaur models. A child who understands the principle of transitivity (that if A is greater than B, and B is greater than C, then A is greater than C) ought to be able to demonstrate this ability with sets of strange figures as well as she could with a set of toys familiar to her. But in fact that seems not to be the case.

We now have a great deal of research showing that specific knowledge makes a huge difference. Children and adults who know a lot about some subject or some set of materials (dinosaurs, baseball cards, mathematics, or whatever) not only categorize information in that topic area in more complex and hierarchical ways, but also are better at remembering new information on that topic and better at applying more advanced forms of logic to material in that area. Expertise not only fosters greater speed in performing some well-practiced task, but also changes the way we think about that material and the way we go about solving problems in that domain. Furthermore, such expertise seems to generalize very little to other tasks.

Much of the most interesting work on expertise has been done by Michelene Chi and her various colleagues (Bedard & Chi, 1992; Chi & Ceci, 1987; Chi, Hutchinson, & Robin, 1989). In her now classic early study (1978), she showed that expert chess players can remember the placement of chess pieces on a board much more quickly and accurately than can novice chess players, *even when the expert chess players are children and the novices are adults.* To paraphrase Flavell (1985), expertise makes any of us look very smart, very cognitively advanced; lack of expertise makes us look very dumb.

These school-age chess players, unless they are rank novices, would remember a series of chess moves or the arrangement of pieces on a chessboard far better than I could, since they have expertise and I do not.

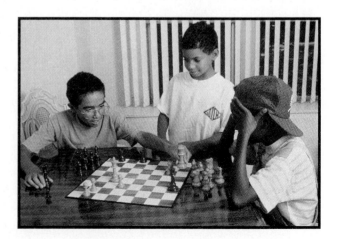

Since young children are novices at almost everything, while older children are more expert at many things, perhaps the apparent age difference in the use of cognitive strategies, including memory strategies, is just the effect of more specific knowledge, more experience, and *not* the result of any basic qualitative change in the child's cognitive structures.

Overview of the Schoolchild's Thinking

When we look at what we know about the thinking of children between 6 and 12, we find a sort of paradox. On the one hand, Piaget seems to have been more accurate in his descriptions of this period than any other. He did not underestimate the schoolchild's abilities as he had the abilities of infants and preschoolers. Nor did he overestimate them, as he did the skills of the teenager—a point I'll come to in a moment. What we see in this age period is the emergence, or perhaps the more consistent use, of more complex sorts of analysis and strategy. Children this age, much more than younger children, also know what they know and can reflect on the ways they use to learn or remember things.

This all sounds very like Piaget's description of this period. Yet it looks very much as if these cognitive skills do not arise at all from the mechanism Piaget suggested, which was some kind of general *equilibration*—a broad reorganization of schemes—at about age 6. The developmental process now appears to be far more gradual and is affected heavily by the amount of experience the child has had in a particular domain. At the same time, it *is* true that the 8-year-old approaches new tasks differently. He is more likely to attempt a more complex strategy, and if that strategy fails, he is more likely to try another one. So although the process may be gradual, there still appears to be genuine qualitative change.

Cognitive Development in Adolescence

Many of the same paradoxes emerge in the research on adolescent thinking. Early research, following Piaget's ideas, did indeed indicate that, as Edith Neimark put it,

> *An enormous amount of evidence from an assortment of tasks shows that adolescents and adults are capable of feats of reasoning not attained under normal circumstances by [younger] children, and that these abilities develop fairly rapidly during the ages of about 11 to 15. (1982, p. 493)*

Furthermore, many of the qualities of adolescent thought Piaget identified do seem to emerge during this period. Adolescents, much more than school-age children, operate with possibilities in addition to reality, and they are more likely to use deductive logic. As Flavell puts it (1985, p. 98), the thinking of the school-age child "hugs the ground of . . . empirical reality," while the teenager is more likely to soar into the realm of speculation and possibility. An 8-year-old thinks that "knowing" something is a simple matter of finding out the facts; a teenager is more likely to see knowledge as relative, as less certain (Bartsch, 1993).

Some additional illustrations would probably make the change clearer. In an early cross-sectional study, Susan Martorano (1977) tested 20 girls at each of four grades (sixth, eighth, tenth, and twelfth) on 10 different tasks that require one or more of what Piaget called formal operations skills. Indeed, many of the tasks she used were those Piaget himself had devised. Results from two of these tasks are given in Figure 7.4. The pendulum problem is the same one I described earlier; the "balance" problem requires a youngster to

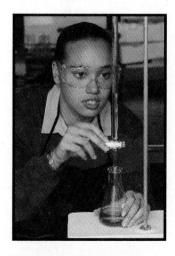

One aspect of formal operations is the use of deductive logic, which is normally required first in high school, especially in math and science classes, like this chemistry class.

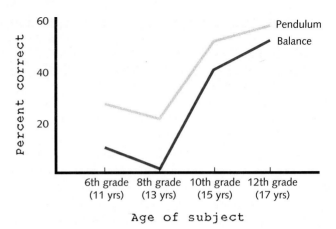

FIGURE 7.4 These are the results from 2 of the 10 different formal operational tasks used in Martorano's cross-sectional study. (*Source:* Martorano, 1977, p. 670. Copyright by the American Psychological Association.)

predict whether or not two varying weights, hung at varying distances on either side of a scale, will balance. To solve this problem using formal operations, the teenager must consider both weight and distance simultaneously. You can see in the figure that older students generally did better, with the biggest improvement in scores between eighth and tenth grades (between ages 13 and 15).

In a more practical vein, Catherine Lewis (1981) has shown that these new cognitive abilities alter the ways teenagers go about making decisions. Older teenagers are more focused on the future, on possibilities and options, when they consider decisions. Lewis asked eighth-, tenth-, and twelfth-grade students to respond to a set of dilemmas, each of which involved a person facing a difficult decision, such as whether or not to have an operation to remove a facial disfigurement or how to decide which doctor to trust when the doctors give differing advice. Forty-two percent of the twelfth graders but only 11 percent of the eighth graders mentioned future possibilities in their answers to these dilemmas.

In answer to the cosmetic surgery dilemma, for example, a twelfth grader said:

> *Well, you have to look into the different things . . . that might be more important later on in your life. You should think about, will it have any effect on your future and with, maybe, the people you meet. . . . (p. 541)*

An eighth grader, in response to the same dilemma, said:

> *The different things I would think about in getting the operation is like if the girls turn you down on a date, or the money, or the kids teasing you at school. . . . (p. 542)*

The eighth grader, as is characteristic of her age group, is focused on the here and now, on concrete things. The teenager is considering things that *might* happen in the future.

But note that even among the twelfth graders in Lewis's study nearly three-fifths did not show this type of future orientation. And take another look at Figure 7.4; only about 50 to 60 percent of twelfth graders solved the two formal operations problems. In Martorano's study, in fact, only 2 of the 20 twelfth-grade subjects used formal operations logic on all 10 problems.

These findings reflect a common pattern in research on adolescent thinking: By no means all teenagers (or adults) use these more abstract forms of logic and thought. Keating (1980) estimates that only about 50 to 60 percent of 18- to 20-year-olds in Western countries seem to use formal operations at all, let alone consistently. In non-Western countries the rates are even lower.

What was the last major decision you had to make? Think for a minute about how you went about it. What factors did you consider? Did you think about future consequences or only about the here and now?

Why Doesn't Every Teenager Use Formal Logic?

Why? There are several possibilities. One is that the usual methods of measuring formal operations are simply extremely difficult or unclear. When the instructions are made clearer or the subjects are given hints or rules, they can demonstrate some aspects of formal operations (Danner & Day, 1977)—just as preschoolers can display some "concrete operations" skills when tasks are made simpler or clearer.

A related possibility is that expertise is once again the crucial element. That is, most of us have some formal operational ability, but we can only apply it to topics or tasks with which we are familiar. For example, I use formal operations reasoning about psychology because it is an area I know well. But I am a lot less skillful at applying the same kind of reasoning to fixing my car—about which I know next to nothing. Willis Overton and his colleagues (1987) have found considerable support for this possibility in their research. They found that as many as 90 percent of adolescents could solve quite complex logic problems if the problems were stated using familiar content, while only half could solve the identical logical problem when it was stated in abstract language.

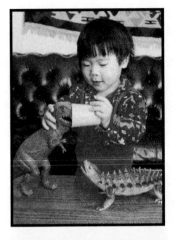

Still a third possibility is that most of our everyday experiences and tasks do not require formal operations. Inductive reasoning or other simpler forms of logic are quite sufficient most of the time. So we get into a cognitive rut, applying our most usual mode of thinking to new problems as well. We can kick our thinking up a notch under some circumstances, especially if someone reminds us that it would be useful to do so, but we simply don't rehearse formal operations very much.

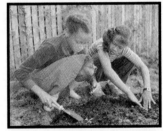

The fact that formal operations thinking is found more often among young people or adults in Western cultures may be interpreted in the same way. Because of their high level of technology and the complexity of life-styles, industrialized cultures demand formal operational thought much more. By this argument, all nonretarded teenagers and adults are thought to have the *capacity* for formal logic, but only those of us whose lives demand its development will actually acquire it.

Notice that all these explanations undermine the very notion of a universal "stage" of thinking in adolescence. Yes, more abstract forms of thinking may develop in adolescence, but these more complex forms are neither universal nor broadly used by individual teenagers or adults. Whether one develops or uses these forms of logic depends heavily on experience, expertise, and environmental demand.

Preliminary Conclusions and Questions

I have been raising a variety of questions as I have gone along, so you already know that many puzzles about cognitive development remain to be solved. To set the stage for a discussion of the third approach, information processing, let me pause for a quick review.

The child comes a long way in only about 15 years. As Robert Siegler puts it,

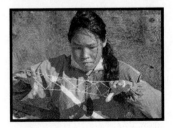

> *Among the most remarkable characteristics of human beings is how much our thinking changes with age. When we compare the thinking of an infant, a toddler, an elementary school student, and an adolescent, the magnitude of the change is immediately apparent. (1994, p. 1)*

In broad outline, Piaget's observations about this sequence have been frequently confirmed. Children do clearly change not only in what they know but in the way they approach problems.

Everything we know about children's cognitive development tells us that this toddler, these school-age children, and this teenager are using different types of thinking, different forms of logic or strategies. But we are still a long way from having a good explanation of how or why the change occurs.

But it now seems quite unlikely that this developmental progression involves coherent, general stages of the kind Piaget envisioned. Children's performance is much more variable than that. The same child may use quite sophisticated strategies for one kind of problem and very primitive strategies on another (Siegler, 1994). The expert child chess player, who can demonstrate quite extraordinary feats of memory and conceptual sophistication playing chess has no better memory for strings of numbers than does another child of the same age. In the current language used by cognitive theorists, children's thinking is quite *domain specific* (Hirschfeld & Gelman, 1994).

Nor do new cognitive skills emerge full-blown. Rather, they are preceded by more rudimentary or partial versions of the same skills at earlier ages. For example, virtually all the achievements of the concrete operational period are present in at least rudimentary or fragmentary form in the preschool years. This observation undermines the basic notion of a stage as Piaget proposed it.

But even if we are now able to reject Piaget's highly "domain-general" theory, we are still left with a wide range of possibilities. Development might be *totally* situation (domain) specific, or it might have at least some generality, with some basic skills or understandings changing with age and being applied across several different domains or tasks. We see some sign of just such a semigeneral, almost stagelike shift in children's theory of mind at about age 4. Indeed, the very use of the word *theory* in this label implies that the child has some kind of coherent model that gets applied to a variety of situations (Gopnik & Wellman, 1994). On the other side of the coin, the research on expertise makes thinking look highly domain specific.

A second major puzzle is just how to explain the broad sweep of changes that we do observe. Are these really qualitative changes involving the emergence of genuinely new skills? If so, then what is pushing those changes? Alternatively, perhaps children simply become more and more efficient at using the same basic set of cognitive processes.

The third theoretical approach to the study of intelligence, the information-processing approach, has offered new ways to think about and study both of these disputes.

Information Processing in Children

Theorists who study cognitive power ask *how well* a child does intellectual tasks compared to others; those who study structure ask *what type* of logic the child uses in solving problems, and how those structures change with age. The **information-processing** theorists ask what the child is *doing* intellectually when faced with a task, what intellectual *processes* she brings to bear, and how those processes might change with age. The information-processing approach is not really a theory of cognitive development; it is an approach to studying thinking and remembering—a set of questions and some methods of analysis.

This third approach has a whole series of theoretical fathers and grandfathers. The direct line of inheritance is from studies of adult intelligence, particularly computer simulations of adult intelligence. In fact, the basic metaphor underlying the entire information-processing approach has been that of the human mind as computer. Like a computer, we can think of the "hardware" of cognition (the physiology of the brain, the nerves, and connective tissues) and the "software" of cognition (the program that uses the basic hardware). To understand thinking in general, we need to understand the processing capacity of the hardware and just what programs have to be "run" to perform any given task. What inputs (facts or data) are needed? What coding, decoding, remembering, or analyzing are required? To understand cognitive *development,* we need to discover whether there are any changes with age in the basic processing capacity of the system and/or in the nature of the programs used. Do children develop new types of processing (new programs)? Or do they simply learn to use basic programs on new material?

In studies of children's thinking, we can see at least two branches to the information-processing family tree. On one side is a group of researchers and theorists with a somewhat Piagetian flavor who have given up the notion of stages but are still committed to the notion of qualitatively changing sequences of development (e.g., Siegler, 1981). On the other side are researchers interested in intellectual power who have been trying to identify a set of basic information-processing capacities or strategies that may underlie differences in IQ. What is different about the way "brighter" people go about solving a problem? These two approaches to the study of information processing are connected, but for the moment let me talk about them separately.

Developmental Approaches to Information Processing

Changes in Processing Capacity. One obvious place to look for an explanation of developmental changes in cognitive skills is in the hardware itself. Any computer has physical limits to the number of different operations it can perform at one time, or in a given space of time. As the brain and nervous system develop in the early years of life, with synapses formed and then pruned to remove the redundant ones, perhaps the capacity, the speed, or the efficiency of the system increases.

One type of evidence that is often mentioned to support the possibility of an age change in processing capacity is the finding that young children remember fewer items in lists of numbers, letters, or words than older children do. You can see the results of one typical study in Figure 7.5.

Such results are consistent with the hypothesis of an increase in basic processing capacity (including memory capacity) with age. An alternate explanation is that this pattern is the result of variations in experience/expertise. Younger children clearly have less experience with numbers, letters, and words. Perhaps their poorer performance on tests that measure memory span is simply another example of the fact that experts can do things better than novices. In fact, when the degree of experience is better matched, such as by having older children try to remember new letterlike figures, much of the age difference

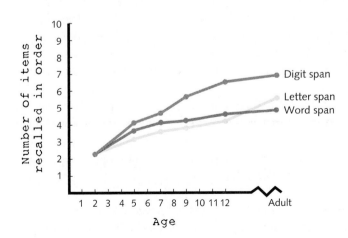

FIGURE 7.5 Psychologists have tried to measure basic memory capacity by asking subjects to listen to a list of numbers, letters, or words and then to repeat back the list in order. This figure shows the number of such items that children of various ages are able to remember and report accurately. (*Source:* Dempster, 1981, from Figures 1, 2, and 3, pp. 66, 67, 68.)

in memory span disappears. Competing arguments like this have made it difficult to resolve the question of whether a basic increase in capacity underlies cognitive development, although growing physiological evidence now supports such a change. Adele Diamond, for example (1991), has been able to link specific changes in the frontal lobes of the brain to the emergence of the object concept in the first year of life.

But whether a change in basic capacity occurs or not, psychologists agree that there is a steady increase in processing *efficiency* with age, a change that most developmentalists now see as the basis on which cognitive development occurs (Case, 1985; Halford et al., 1994; Kuhn, 1992).

Processing Efficiency.   The best evidence that cognitive processing becomes more efficient is that it gets steadily faster with age. Robert Kail (1991b; Kail & Hall, 1994) has found virtually the same exponential increase with age in processing speed for a wide variety of tasks, including such perceptual/motor tasks as tapping, simple response time to a stimulus (like pressing a button when you hear a buzzer), and cognitive tasks (like mental addition or subtests from the WISC). He has found virtually identical patterns of speed increases in studies in Korea as well as studies in the United States, which adds a useful bit of cross-cultural validity to the argument.

The most plausible explanation for this common pattern is that some fundamental change in the physical system itself occurs that allows greater and greater speed of both response and mental processing. The most likely candidate for such a basic change is the "pruning" of synapses—a process I talked about in Chapter 4. If pruning begins at about age 2 and then continues steadily throughout childhood, one effect could be to make the "wiring diagram" more efficient and thus faster.

Greater efficiency in processing is also gained as a result of the child's acquisition of new strategies for solving problems or recalling information. Of course the new strategies themselves may appear as a result of greater underlying capacity or efficiency. But once present, these more powerful strategies make the whole system more efficient, much as we see in the behavior of experts at some task, who can perform with remarkable speed and directness.

Rules for Problem Solving.   But how do these new strategies arise? Robert Siegler proposes that they emerge directly from experience—from repeated trial and error, from experimentation (1994). Some of Siegler's own early work on the development of *rules* illustrates how the system may operate (1976; 1978; 1981). Siegler's approach was a kind of cross between Piagetian theory and information processing. He argued that cognitive development consists in acquiring a set of basic rules, which are then applied to a broader and broader range of problems on the basis of experience. There are no stages, only sequences.

In one test of this approach, Siegler used a balance scale with a series of pegs on either side of the center, like the one in Figure 7.6. Discs can be placed on these pegs, and the child is asked to predict which way the balance will fall, depending on the location and number of discs. (You may recognize this as similar to the task Martorano used in her

FIGURE 7.6 This balance scale is similar to what Siegler used in his experiments. (*Source:* Siegler, 1981, p. 7.)

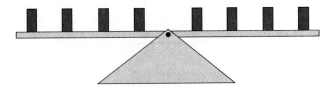

study of formal operations.) A complete solution requires the child to take into account both the number of discs on each size and the specific location of the discs.

Children do not develop such a complete solution immediately. Instead, Siegler predicted that four rules will develop, in order: Rule I is basically a "preoperational" rule, taking into account only one dimension, the number of weights. Children using this rule will predict that the side with more discs will go down, no matter which peg they are placed on. Rule II is a transitional rule. The child still judges on the basis of number, except when the same number of weights are on each side, and in that case she takes distance from the fulcrum into account. Rule III is basically a concrete operational rule, since the child tries to take both distance and weight into account simultaneously, except that when the information is conflicting (such as when the side with weights closer to the fulcrum has more weights), the child simply guesses. Rule IV is basically the formal operational rule—the one that Martorano counted as "correct" in her study (recall Figure 7.4). At this point the child/youth figures out the actual formula (distance × weight for each side).

Siegler has found that virtually all children perform on this and similar tasks as if they were following one or another of these rules and that the rules seem to develop in the given order. Very young children behave as if they don't have a rule (they guess or behave randomly so far as Siegler can determine). When a rule develops, Rule I always comes first. But progression from one rule to the next depends heavily on experience. If children are given practice with the balance scale so that they can make predictions and then check which way the balance actually falls, many show rapid shifts upward in the sequence of rules.

Thus, Siegler is attempting to describe a logical sequence children follow, not unlike the basic sequence of stages that Piaget describes, but Siegler shows that the specific step in this sequence that we see in a particular child depends not so much on age as on the child's specific experience with a given set of material. In Piaget's terminology, this is rather like saying that when accommodation of some scheme occurs, it always occurs in a particular sequence, but the rate with which the child moves through that sequence depends on experience. Further, the effect of the experience is to increase the child's skill in using more advanced rules/strategies, which in turn improves the underlying efficiency of the entire system.

Metacognition and Executive Processes. A third area in which information-processing researchers have been active is in studying how children come to know what they know. If I gave you a list of things to remember and then asked you later to tell me how you had gone about trying to remember it, you would have little difficulty explaining your mental process. You may even have consciously considered the various alternative strategies and then selected the best one. You could also tell me good ways to study, or which kinds of tasks will be hardest, and why. These are all examples of metamemory or metacognition—knowing about remembering or knowing about knowing. Such skills are a part of a larger category that information-processing theorists refer to as **executive processes:** planning what to do, considering alternative strategies—all similar to what an executive may do.

These skills are of particular interest because there is some suggestion that it may be precisely such metacognitive or executive skills that emerge (gradually) with age. Performance on a whole range of tasks will be better if the child can monitor her own performance or recognize when a particular strategy is called for and when it is not. I pointed out earlier that 4- and 5-year-old children do show some preliminary signs of

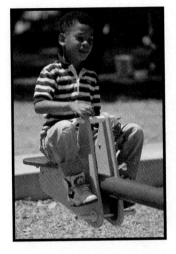

Experience with a teeter-totter may be one source of knowledge about how balance scales work.

Write down three good ways to study. In choosing one of these methods, does it matter what subject you are studying? How do you know all this? Do you think about it consciously when you are starting to study? The fact that you know these things and can think about them is evidence that you have metacognition—that you know what you know and how to think.

such monitoring, but it is rarely found earlier than that and it clearly improves fairly rapidly after school age. Such executive skills may well form the foundation of some of the age changes Piaget described.

A Summary of Developmental Changes in Information Processing. If I assemble all the bits and pieces of evidence about information-processing capacity and skills, I arrive at a set of tentative generalizations:

1. There may or may not be any increase in the basic processing capacity of the system (the hardware), but there is clearly an increase in the efficiency with which the hardware is used that results in steadily greater processing speed.

2. The sheer amount of specific knowledge the child has about any given task increases as the child experiments, explores, studies things in school. This leads to more and more "expert" approaches to remembering and solving problems, which in turn improves the efficiency of the processing system.

3. Genuinely new strategies are acquired, probably in some kind of order. In particular, the child seems to develop in middle childhood some "executive" or "metacognitive" abilities—she knows that she knows, and she can *plan* a strategy for the first time.

4. Existing strategies are applied to more and more different domains, and more and more flexibly. If a child learned to rehearse on one kind of memory problem, the older child is more likely to try it on a new memory task. The younger child (particularly younger than 5 or 6) is unlikely to generalize the strategy to the new task, although once again it is true that some transfer is seen in children as young as 2 when the conditions are carefully constructed (Crisafi & Brown, 1986).

5. With increasing age, a wider range of different strategies can be applied to the same problem, so that if the first doesn't work, a backup or alternative strategy can be used. If you can't find your misplaced keys by retracing your steps, you try a backup, such as looking in your other purse or the pocket of your jacket, or searching each room of the house in turn. Young children do not do this; school-age children and adolescents do.

Thus, some of the changes that Piaget observed and chronicled with such detail and richness seem to be the result simply of increased experience with tasks and problems (a quantitative change, if you will). But there also seems to be a qualitative change in the complexity, generalizability, and flexibility of strategies used by the child.

Individual Differences in Information Processing

While some researchers in the information-processing tradition have been asking about developmental changes or sequences, others have been trying to understand individual differences. IQ tests are intended to measure such underlying ability differences by giving people fairly complex cognitive tasks, each of which may require a whole series of more fundamental information-processing strategies. We might come closer to understanding individual differences in intelligence or intellectual performance if we shifted our attention to those more fundamental processes. Generally, the strategy has been to look at the relationship between IQ scores on standard tests and measures of specific information processing. This strategy has yielded a few preliminary connections.

Speed of Information Processing.   Since it is becoming clear that increases in speed or efficiency of processing are one of the underpinnings of age changes in cognitive skills, it makes sense to hypothesize that differences in speed may also underlie individual differences in IQ. A number of different investigators have found just such a link: Subjects with faster reaction times or speed of performance on a variety of simple tasks also have higher IQ scores on standard tests (Vernon, 1987). We even have a few studies in which speed of processing has been directly linked to central nervous system functioning and to IQ. For example, it is now possible to measure the speed of conduction of impulses along individual nerves, such as nerves in the arm. Philip Vernon (1993; Vernon & Mori, 1992) has found that such a measure correlates about .45 with IQ.

Most of this research has been done with adults, but a link between speed of reaction time and IQ has also been found in a few studies with children (Keating, List, & Merriman, 1985; Saccuzzo, Johnson, & Guertin, 1994). Furthermore, there are some pretty clear indications that such speed-of-processing differences may be built in at birth. The fact that measures of infant habituation and recognition memory are correlated so strongly with later IQ—a finding I talked about in Chapter 5—certainly points to such a possibility.

Other IQ-Processing Links.   Other researchers have explored the connections between IQ and information processing by comparing the information-processing strategies used by normal-IQ and retarded children. Two examples:

Judy DeLoache (DeLoache & Brown, 1987) has compared the searching strategies of groups of 2-year-olds who were either developing normally or showed delayed development. When the search task was very simple, such as searching for a toy hidden in a distinctive location in a room, the two groups did not differ in search strategies or skill. But when the experimenter surreptitiously moved the toy before the child was allowed to search, normally developing children were able to search in alternative, plausible places, such as in nearby locations; delayed children simply persisted in looking in the place where they had seen the toy hidden. They either could not change strategies or did not have alternative, more complex strategies in their repertoires.

Other research underlines this difference in the flexibility of strategy use. In several studies, Joseph Campione and Ann Brown (1984; Campione et al., 1985) have found that both retarded and normal-IQ children could learn to solve problems like items (a), (b), and (c) in Figure 7.7, but the retarded children could not transfer this learning to a more complex problem of the same general type, like item (d) in the figure, while normal-IQ children could. Both sets of studies suggest that flexibility of use of any given strategy may be another key dimension of individual differences in intelligence.

Putting the Three Approaches Together

I hope it is clear by now that the information-processing approach offers us some important bridges between the power and structure theories of intelligence in children. It now looks as if some basic, inborn strategies exist (such as noting differences or similarities) and as if these strategies change during the early years of life, with more complex strategies or rules emerging and old strategies used more flexibly. Plain old experience is a key part of the process of change. The more a child plays with blocks, the better she will be at organizing and classifying blocks; the more a person plays chess, the better he will be at seeing and remembering relationships among pieces on the board. So some of the changes that Piaget thought of as changes in underlying structure are instead specific task

FIGURE 7.7 For panels (a) through (c) the subject must figure out the "system" in each set and then describe what pattern should go in the empty box in the bottom right-hand corner. Panel (a) shows rotation; panel (b) shows addition of two elements; panel (c) shows subtraction. The figure in panel (d) is harder because the subject must apply *two* principles at once; in this case both addition and rotation rules. Retarded children could do problems like (a), (b), and (c) as well as normal-IQ children, but they did much more poorly on problems like (d). (*Source:* Campione et al., 1985, Figure 1, p. 302, Figure 4, p. 306.)

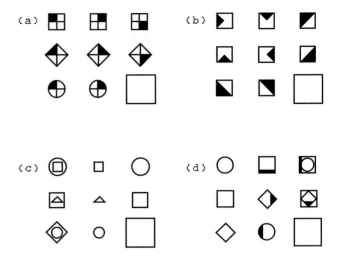

learning. But there seems to be some structural change as well, such as the emergence of new strategies, particularly metacognitive strategies.

Individual differences in what we normally think of as intelligence can then be conceived of as resulting both from inborn differences in the speed or efficiency of the basic processes (differences in the hardware perhaps) and from differences in expertise or experience. The child with a slower or less-efficient processing system is going to move through all the various steps and stages more slowly; he will *use* the experience he has less efficiently or effectively and may never develop as complete a range of strategies as does the initially quicker child. But when this less innately gifted child has sufficient expertise in some area, that specialized knowledge can compensate for the lower IQ.

This point is nicely illustrated in a study of expertise done in Germany (Schneider & Bjorklund, 1992). School-age children who were very knowledgeable about soccer (experts) had better recall of soccer-related lists than did nonexperts. But high-IQ novices did as well as low-IQ experts on these same tasks. So rich knowledge in some area can compensate somewhat for lower IQ, but it does not create equality. High-IQ experts are still going to be better than medium- or low-IQ experts in any given area.

The information-processing approach may also have some real practical applications. The studies of recognition memory in infancy, for example, may give us a way to identify retarded children very early in life or to sort out from among low-birth-weight infants those that seem at particular risk for later problems. By identifying the key differences between retarded and nonretarded children (or between brighter and less-bright children), we may also be able to identify specific kinds of training that would be useful for a retarded child or for a child with a learning disability.

I do not want to wax too rhapsodic about the information-processing approach. It is well to remember that we do not yet have any tests of information-processing ability that could realistically replace the careful use of IQ tests in schools and clinics, although a few psychologists believe that a clinically useful biological measure of IQ will be available within several decades (Matarazzo, 1992). Nor are the sequential theories of information-processing development far enough along yet to explain all the differences we see among infants, preschoolers, and older children in performance on various Piagetian tasks. In short, information processing is an important, integrative addition to our understanding of cognitive development, but it does not replace all the other approaches.

Summary

1   The study of cognitive "power" does not tell us what we need to know about the shared changes in the *way* children think about the world around them. Piaget's theory addressed this question.

2   Piaget assumed that the child was an active agent in his own development, constructing his own understandings and adapting to the environment by changing his basic schemes.

3   Schemes and their interrelationships are changed through the processes of assimilation, accommodation, and equilibration, beginning with primitive schemes at birth and progressing sequentially through several stages.

4   Piaget's first stage is the sensorimotor period, birth to 18 months, during which the baby understands the world in terms of her senses and motor actions.

5   In Piaget's preoperational period, from 18 months to 6 years, the child is able to use symbols to represent objects to himself internally. Piaget saw the child at this age as still egocentric and relatively unskilled.

6   In Piaget's third stage, concrete operations, from ages 6 to 12, the child acquires powerful new mental tools called operations, such as reversibility, addition, subtraction, multiplication, and serial ordering.

7   During the fourth Piagetian stage, formal operations, from age 12 onward, the young person is able to manipulate *ideas* as well as objects, to approach problems systematically, and to use deductive logic.

8   Post-Piagetian studies of infant cognition show infants to be far more cognitively skilled than Piaget thought. They can imitate from the earliest weeks and remember events, both of which appear to involve some kind of internal representation.

9   By about age 4, children become significantly less egocentric, can distinguish between appearance and reality in a variety of tasks, and develop a surprisingly sophisticated theory of how minds work. They understand that other people's actions are based on thoughts and beliefs, not on "reality."

10   By age 4 or 5, children also understand some of the links between specific situations and other people's likely emotions.

11   Studies of school-age children confirm many of Piaget's specific observations and indicate the importance of strategies in children's thinking at these ages. But it is clear that the development of the more complex forms of thought visible at these ages is gradual, not abrupt.

12   Children's cognitive skills are also highly dependent on specific knowledge and expertise.

13   In adolescence, more complex forms of logic and reasoning, similar to what Piaget described, become more prominent, but no more than half of young people display these advanced types of thinking.

14   Collectively, these findings make Piaget's strong stage concept untenable, but there is still disagreement about whether the observed changes nonetheless occur in clusters or groups and whether the changes are qualitative or quantitative.

15   Information-processing theorists ask not about structure, but about the basic processes that make up any cognitive activity, such as decoding, encoding, remembering, planning, or analyzing.

16   Information-processing specialists interested in development have asked what ways the basic processes change with age among children. There appear to be clear improvements with age in processing efficiency, perhaps resulting from synaptic pruning.

17 There also appear to be increases with age in the use of various strategies, including memory strategies, and executive processes.

18 Other information-processing specialists focus on individual differences in efficiency of basic processes. Higher-IQ individuals, for example, appear to process information more quickly and apply strategies or knowledge more broadly.

Key Terms

accommodation **(p. 183)**

assimilation **(p. 183)**

concrete operations **(p. 184)**

conservation **(p. 186)**

deductive logic **(p. 188)**

egocentrism **(p. 186)**

equilibration **(p. 183)**

executive processes **(p. 211)**

formal operations **(p. 184)**

inductive logic **(p. 188)**

information processing **(p. 208)**

metacognition **(p. 196)**

metamemory **(p. 196)**

operation **(p. 184)**

preoperational stage **(p. 184)**

scheme **(p. 182)**

sensorimotor stage **(p. 184)**

theory of mind **(p. 195)**

Suggested Readings

Flavell, J. H. (1992). Cognitive development: Past, present, and future. *Developmental Psychology, 28,* 998–1005.

This brief paper by one of the leading thinkers and researchers in the field of cognitive development gives you a quick tour of what Flavell thinks we now know, don't know, and are still arguing about. Flavell's 1985 book *Cognitive Development,* cited in the references, is also a wonderful source.

Goldstein, J. (Ed.). (1994). *Toys, play, and child development.* Cambridge, England: Cambridge University Press.

A collection of current papers on the role of play in children's development. Included is an interesting chapter on war toys and their effect.

Kuhn, D. (1992). Cognitive development. In M. H. Bornstein & M. E. Lamb (Eds.), *Developmental psychology: An advanced textbook* (3rd ed.). Hillsdale, NJ: Erlbaum.

A first-rate discussion of the strengths and limitations of both Piagetian and information-processing approaches.

Schneider, W., & Pressley, M. (1989). *Memory development between 2 and 20.* New York: Springer-Verlag.

An excellent discussion of research on memory in children.

Thomas, R. M. (1990). Basic concepts and applications of Piagetian cognitive development theory. In R. M. Thomas (Ed.), *The Encyclopedia of human development and education.* Oxford: Pergamon Press.

This is one of the very best short descriptions of Piaget's theory I have ever read. If you need another run at the basic ideas, expressed in someone else's language, this is a good place to look.

The Development of Language

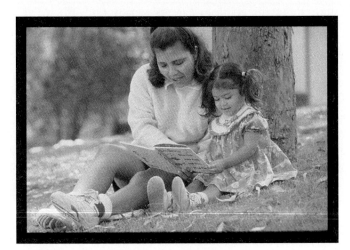

Afriend of mine listened one morning at breakfast while her 6-year-old and 3-year old daughters had the following conversation about the relative dangers of forgetting to feed the goldfish versus overfeeding the goldfish:

> 6-year-old: *It's worse to forget to feed them.*
>
> 3-year-old: *No, it's badder to feed them too much.*
>
> 6-year-old: *You don't say badder, you say worser.*
>
> 3-year-old: *But it's baddest to give them too much food.*
>
> 6-year-old: *No it's not. It's worsest to forget to feed them.*

Most of us are amused and charmed when we listen to children's language like this. It is so delightfully creative and unexpected, and yet completely clear. Linguists have also learned an enormous amount about children's language by studying "errors" like *baddest* or *worsest*—just as Piaget learned an enormous amount about the child's thinking by studying children's "wrong" answers. But one of the really remarkable things about language is that children make so few errors of this kind. Out of the enormously complex set of sounds they hear in the language of those around them, children somehow learn to speak their native tongue with fluency and accuracy within only a few years. At 6 or 8 months we hear a baby babbling a few sounds; by 18 months the child will probably be using 20 or 30 separate words; and by 3 years children construct long and complex sentences, like those of the 3-year-old in the conversation about the goldfish. Parents usually find this whole sequence fun to listen to, but most of us don't spend a lot of time worrying about just how a child manages all this.

For psychologists and linguists, though, the child's rapid and skillful acquisition of language has remained an enduring puzzle. Is some kind of language-learning faculty built into the organism? Is the child "taught" language in some direct way? Does the child "figure it out" on the basis of what he hears?

In attempting to answer such questions, the vast majority of linguists have looked at changes in both grammar (which the linguists call **syntax**) and word meaning (called **semantics**). Lately, some attempts have also been made to explain differences in the rate of language development from one child to the next and differences in individual children's style of language learning. But before I can explore any of these questions, I need to go back a step.

What Is Language Anyway?

What do we mean by *language?* What are we trying to explain? As most linguists use the term, it has several key features:

1. It is an "arbitrary system of *symbols*" (Brown, 1965, p. 246). Words (or gestures) *stand for* things. But the particular combination of sounds (or gestures) used to stand for some object, event, or relationship varies from one language to another, so the symbols are arbitrary.

2. It is *rule-governed.* Every language has certain rules for stringing together individual symbols, or creating new words, such as the rules for creating superlatives (like *nice, nicer, nicest*), past tenses, or the order of words in sentences.

3. Within those rules, language is *creative.* Speakers of a language combine symbols in new ways to create new meanings. When you talk, you are not restricted to some repertoire of sentences you have heard and learned; you create sentences according to your need at the moment.

Thus, language is not just a collection of sounds. Very young babies make several different sounds, but we do not consider that they are using language, since they do not appear to use those sounds to *refer* to things or events (that is, they do not use the sounds as symbols), and they do not combine individual sounds into different orders to create varying meaning. So far as we know, for example, the meaning does not change if a 6-month-old says "kikiki bababa" versus "bababa kikiki."

Some other animals, most notably primates like chimps and possibly other mammals like dolphins, can also learn to use sound or gestural systems in the symbolic way that we define as language. Chimps, for example, can learn to use sign language or point to se-

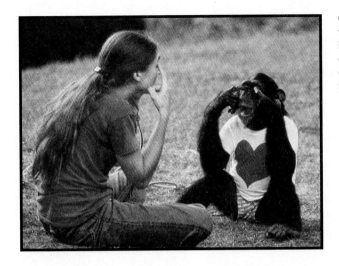

Chimps like Nim Chimpsky can fairly easily learn signs for individual objects or actions and can understand and follow quite complex instructions. Here he signs "I see."

quences of symbols, even creating new combinations of such symbols. Like human children, chimps also understand a good deal more than they can express, and they can follow quite complex verbal requests. But in most cases it takes a good deal of effort to teach them to use expressive language in creative ways (Savage-Rumbaugh et al., 1993). In contrast, as Flavell puts it, "Draconian measures would be needed to *prevent* most children from learning to talk" (1985, p. 248). And as any parent can tell you, once they learn, it is virtually impossible to shut them up!

The developmental process in infants and young children, from prelanguage sounds and gestures to language, follows a remarkably common set of steps.

Before the First Word: The Prelinguistic Phase

Given the definition I've just offered, you may wonder why language researchers would be interested in the sounds or gestures of infants. The baby's early sounds are not yet language, so why not start by studying the first obvious words or the first meaningful gestures? But investigators have recently discovered that the sounds and gestures that infants make during the **prelinguistic phase** are intimately linked to the emergence of the first words. So let's go back to the beginning.

Early Perception of Language

Recall from Chapter 5 that babies are born with or very soon develop remarkably good ability to discriminate speech sounds. By 1 or 2 months they pay attention to and can tell the difference between many individual letter sounds; within a few more months they clearly can discriminate among syllables or words. They also have figured out that these speech sounds are matched by the speaker's mouth movements. Researchers have also found that babies in these early months are sensitive to the intonational and stress patterns of the speech they are listening to. You'll remember from Chapter 5, for example, that 8-month fetuses respond differently to familiar than to unfamiliar rhymes (DeCasper et al., 1994). This sensitivity to stress and pattern becomes even more evident in the early months of life. For example, Anne Fernald has found that 5-month-olds will smile more when they hear tapes of adults saying something in an approving tone than when they speak in a prohibiting tone, whether the words are in Italian, German, or

English (1993). Even more impressive is a study showing that by 9 months of age, babies listening to English prefer to listen to words that have the typical English stress pattern of stressing the first syllable (such as *falter, comet,* or *gentle*) rather than those that stress the second syllable (e.g., *comply* or *assign*) (Jusczyk, Cutler, & Redanz, 1993). Presumably, babies listening to other languages would come to prefer listening to whatever stress pattern was typical of that language. All this research shows that from very early—perhaps from birth—the baby is paying attention to crucial features of the language she hears, such as stress and intonation.

Early Sounds

This early perceptual skill is not matched right away by much skill in producing sounds. From birth to about 1 month of age, the most common sound an infant makes is a cry, although infants also make other fussing, gurgling, and satisfied sounds. This sound repertoire expands at about 1 or 2 months, when we begin to hear some laughing and **cooing** vowel sounds, like *uuuuuu.* Sounds like this are usually signals of pleasure in babies and may show quite a lot of variation in tone, running up and down in volume or pitch.

Consonant sounds appear only at about 6 or 7 months, frequently combined with vowel sounds to make a kind of syllable. Babies this age seem to play with these sounds, often repeating the same sound over and over (such as *babababababa* or *dahdahdah*). This new sound pattern is called **babbling,** and it makes up about half of babies' noncrying sounds from about 6 to 12 months of age (Mitchell & Kent, 1990).

Any parent can tell you that babbling is a delight to listen to. It also seems to be an important part of the preparation for spoken language. For one thing, we know that infants' babbling gradually acquires some of the intonational pattern of the language they are hearing—a process Elizabeth Bates refers to as "learning the tune before the words" (Bates, O'Connell, & Shore, 1987). At the very least, infants seem to develop two such "tunes" in their babbling. When they babble with a rising intonation at the end of a string of sounds, it seems to signal a desire for a response; a falling intonation requires no response.

A second important thing about babbling is that when babies first start babbling, they typically babble all kinds of sounds, including some that are not part of the language they are hearing. But at about 9 or 10 months, their sound repertoire gradually begins to drift toward the set of sounds they are listening to, with the nonheard sounds dropping out (Oller, 1981)—a pattern that clearly parallels the findings from the Werker and Tees study I described in Chapter 5 (recall Figure 5.6, page 140). Findings like these do not tell us that babbling is *necessary* for language development, but they certainly make it look as if babbling is part of a connected developmental process that begins at birth.

Early Gestures

Another part of that connected developmental process appears to be a kind of gestural language that develops at around 9 or 10 months. At this age we first see babies "demanding" or "asking" for things using gestures or combinations of gestures and sound. A 10-month-old baby who apparently wants you to hand her a favorite toy may stretch and reach for it, opening and closing her hand, making whining sounds or other heartrending noises. There is no mistaking the meaning. At about the same age, babies will enter into

Why do you suppose babies babble? Do you think it is just the vocal equivalent of rhythmic foot kicking, or can you think of some other purpose it might serve?

Research Report
Early Gestural "Language" in the Children of Deaf Parents

Children of deaf parents are a particularly interesting group to study if we want to understand language development. The children do not hear oral language, but they are exposed to *language*—sign language. Do these children show the same early steps in language development as do hearing children, only using gestural language?

The answer seems to be yes. Deaf children show a kind of "sign babbling" between about 7 and 11 months of age, much as hearing children babble sounds in these same months. Then at 8 or 9 months of age, deaf children begin using simple gestures, such as pointing, which is just about the same time that we see such gestures in hearing babies of hearing parents. At about 12 months of age, deaf babies seem to display their first *referential* signs—that is, signs in which a gesture appears to stand for some object or event, such as signaling that they want a drink by making a motion like a cup being brought to the mouth (Petitto, 1988).

Folven and Bonvillian (1991) have studied an equally interesting group—hearing children of deaf parents. These babies are exposed to sign language from their parents and to spoken language from their contacts with others in their world, including TV, teachers, other relatives, and playmates. In this small sample of nine babies, the first sign appeared at an average age of 8 months, the first referential sign at 12.6 months, and the first spoken word at 12.2 months. What is striking here is that the first referential signs and the first spoken words appear at such similar times and that the spoken words appear at such a completely normal time, despite the fact that these children of deaf parents hear comparatively little spoken language.

This marked similarity in the sequence and timing of the steps of early language in the deaf and the hearing child provides strong support for the argument that the baby is somehow primed to learn "language" in some form, be it spoken or gestural.

those gestural games much loved by parents, like "patty-cake," "soooo-big," or "wave bye-bye" (Bates et al., 1987).

Receptive Language

Interestingly, the infant's earliest ability to understand the meaning of individual words (which linguists call **receptive language**) also occurs at about 9 or 10 months. Larry Fenson and his colleagues (1994) asked hundreds of mothers about their babies' understanding of various words. The mothers of 10-month-olds identified an average of about 30 words their infants understood; by 13 months, that number was up to nearly 100 words. Since infants of 9 to 13 months typically speak few, if any, individual words, findings like these make it clear that receptive language comes before **expressive language.** Children understand before they can speak.

Adding up these bits of information, we can see that a whole series of changes seems to come together at 9 or 10 months: the beginning of meaningful gestures, the "drift" of babbling toward the heard language sounds, imitative gestural games, and the first comprehension of individual words. It is as if the child now understands something about the process of communication and is intending to communicate to the adult.

The First Words

Somewhere in the midst of all the babbling, the first words appear, typically at about 12 or 13 months (Fenson et al., 1994). The baby's first word is an event that parents eagerly await, but it's fairly easy to miss. A *word,* as linguists usually define it, is any sound or set

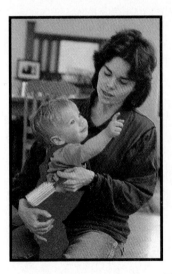

What do you think this young fellow is "saying" with his pointing gesture? Before they speak their first words, babies successfully use gestures and body language in consistent ways to communicate meaning.

Table 8.1
Brenda's Vocabulary at 14 and 19 Months

14 Months	19 Months[a]		
aw u (I want, I don't want)	baby	nice	boat
nau (no)	bear	orange	bone
d di (daddy, baby)	bed	pencil	checkers
d yu (down, doll)	big	write	corder
nene (liquid food)	blue	paper	cut
e (yes)	Brenda	pen	I do
ada (another, other)	cookie	see	met
	daddy	shoe	Pogo
	eat	sick	Ralph
	at	swim	you too
	(hor)sie	tape	climb
	mama	walk	jump
	mommy	wowow	

[a] Brenda did not actually pronounce all these words the way an adult would. I have given the adult version since that is easier to read.

Source: R. Scollon, *Conversations with a one-year-old.* Honolulu: The University Press of Hawaii, 1976, pp. 47, 57–58.

of sounds that is used consistently to refer to some thing, action, or quality. But it can be *any* sound. It doesn't have to be a sound that matches words the adults are using. Brenda, a little girl studied by Ronald Scollon (1976), used the sound *nene* as one of her first words. It seemed to mean primarily liquid food, since she used it for milk, juice, and bottle. But she also used it to refer to mother and sleep. (You can see some of Brenda's other early words in the left-hand column of Table 8.1.)

Often, a child's earliest words are used only in one or two specific situations, and in the presence of many cues. The child may say "doggie" or "bow-wow" only to such promptings as "How does the doggie go?" or "What's that?" Some linguists describe this period as one in which the child "learns what words do" (Nelson, 1985). The child learns a few words that communicate in particular interactional situations but has not yet understood that words are *symbolic*—that they refer to objects or events. In this early period children typically learn words very slowly, after many repetitions. It is quite common for children to take 6 months to acquire a vocabulary of 30 words.

The Naming Explosion

Somewhere between 16 and 24 months this pattern shifts, and most children begin to add new words rapidly, as if they had figured out that "things have names." According to mothers' reports, the average 16-month old has a speaking vocabulary of about 50 words; by 24 months this has multiplied more than sixfold, to about 320 (Fenson et al., 1994). If you look again at Table 8.1, you'll see that young Brenda had made this shift into linguistic high gear between 14 and 19 months. In this new phase, children seem to learn new words with very few repetitions, and they generalize these new words to many more situations.

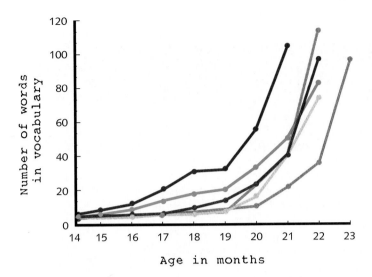

FIGURE 8.1 Each of the lines in this figure represents the vocabulary growth of one of the children studied by Goldfield and Reznick in their longitudinal study. (*Source:* Goldfield & Reznick, 1990, Figure 3, p. 177.)

It is helpful to speak in terms of the "average" child, because that gives you a sense of the normal pattern. But averages collected from cross-sectional studies like Fenson's conceal the fact that for the majority of children, vocabulary gains in the second year of life are not gradual; instead, vocabulary "spurts," beginning about the time that the child has acquired 50 words. You can see this pattern in Figure 8.1, which shows the vocabulary growth curves of six children studied longitudinally by Goldfield and Reznick (1990)—a pattern found by other researchers as well (e.g. Bloom, 1993).

Not all children show precisely this pattern. In Goldfield and Reznick's study, for example, 13 children showed a vocabulary spurt; 11 other children in the study followed varying growth patterns, including several who showed no spurt at all but only gradual acquisition of vocabulary. But a rapid increase over a period of a few months is the most common pattern.

During this early period of rapid vocabulary growth, most observers agree that most new words are names for things or people, like *ball, car, milk, doggie, he,* or *that.* Verblike words tend to develop later, perhaps because they label *relationships* between objects rather than just a single object (Gleitman & Gleitman, 1992). For example, more than half the first 50 words of the eight children Katherine Nelson studied were nounlike words, while only 13 percent were action words (1973). And in Fenson's large cross-sectional study (1994), 63 percent of the words mothers said their children knew by age 2 were nouns, while only 8.5 percent were verbs.

Recently, Lois Bloom and others have raised some doubts about this well-accepted conclusion that early vocabularies are mostly nouns (Bloom, Tinker, & Margulis, 1993). In Bloom's own longitudinal study of 14 children, for example, only about one-third of the early words were nouns. Results like these mean we need to go back and look again. But for now the bulk of the evidence—including studies of children learning other languages, as you can see in the *Cultures and Contexts* box on page 224—supports the conclusion that the early words are most likely to be names of one sort or another.

Later Word Learning

During the preschool years, children continue to add words at the astonishing speed of about one new word every two hours (Pinker, 1994). By age 2½, the average vocabulary

Cultures and Contexts
Early Words by Children in Many Cultures

Cross-cultural studies of children's early language support the generalization that in their earliest word learning, children learn words for people or things before they learn words for actions or other parts of speech. Here are some (translated) samples from the very early vocabularies of one child from each of four cultures, all studied by Dedre Gentner (1982). It is impressive how very similar these early vocabularies are. Of course there are some variations, but all these children had names for Mommy and Daddy, for some other relative, for other live creatures, for food. All but the Chinese child had words for toys or clothes. All four had also learned more naming words than any other type, with very similar proportions. They don't know the *same* words, but the pattern is remarkably similar.

	German boy	English girl	Turkish girl	Chinese girl
Some of the words for people or things	Mommy	Mommy	Mama	Momma
	Papa	Daddy	Daddy	Papa
	Gaga	babar	Aba	grandmother
	baby	baby	baby	horse
	dog	dog	food	chicken
	bird	dolly	apple	uncooked rice
	cat	kitty	banana	cooked rice
	milk	juice	bread	noodles
	ball	book	ball	flower
	nose	eye	pencil	wall clock
	moon	moon	towel	lamp
Some of the nonnaming words	cry	run	cry	go
	come	all gone	come	come
	eat	more	put on	pick up
	sleep	bye-bye	went pooh	not want
	want	want	want	afraid
	no	no	hello	thank you
Total percentage of naming words	67%	69%	57%	59%

is about 600 words; by age 5 or 6, the average vocabulary is roughly *15,000* words. Children can accomplish this feat because by age 3 or 4 they seem to pay attention to words in whole groups, such as words that name objects in a single class (e.g., types of dinosaurs or kinds of fruit) or words with similar meanings.

In middle childhood, children continue to add vocabulary at the rate of 5000 to 10,000 words per year. This estimate comes from a recent, careful study by Jeremy Anglin (1993), who tested the vocabulary knowledge of first-, third-, and fifth-grade children on a sample of words drawn at random from a large dictionary. Anglin's analysis is especially interesting because he broke down the total vocabulary into several different types of words. *Root words* are basic, uninflected words, such as *closet, flop, hermit,* and *pep. Inflected words* are those to which at least one of what linguists call "inflections" has been added, such as an *ed* to make a past tense or an *s* for plural. The third category, *derived words,* often has a root word as a base, to which some other piece has been added, result-

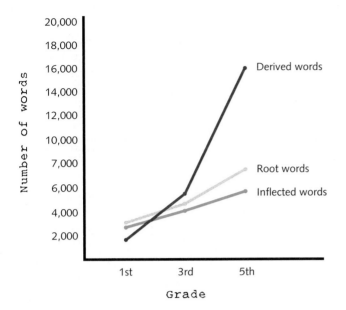

FIGURE 8.2 Anglin's study shows a very large overall increase in children's vocabularies during the school years, but the biggest increase is in "derived" words, which suggests that children of this age have understood some new aspects of grammar and word construction. (*Source:* Anglin, 1993, adapted from Figure 1, p. 65.)

ing in a change in the part of speech, such as happ*ily* or happi*ness*. You can see in Figure 8.2 that between the first and fifth grades, children increased their knowledge of all three types of words, but the biggest increase, occurring between third and fifth grades, was in derived words.

Anglin argues that what is happening is that at about third grade, the child shifts to a new level of understanding of the structure of language, figuring out relationships between whole categories of words, such as between adjectives and adverbs, (*happy* and *happily, sad* and *sadly*) or between adjectives and nouns (*happy* and *happiness*). Having understood these relationships, the child can now understand and create a whole class of new words, and his vocabulary thus increases rapidly.

As a personal aside, I found this result especially intriguing because it matched so closely my own experience of learning vocabulary during my recent year in Germany. Certainly I found many cognates—words that are the same or similar in English and German—and those I learned quickly. But other types of words I first learned laboriously, one at a time, requiring seemingly endless repetitions. In a second phase that lasted several months, this laborious process got quite a lot faster but was still not smooth. Finally, toward the end of my eight months, I began to understand and pay attention to such regularities as prefixes and word roots, and suddenly I could learn and remember a dozen words at a time—although even at the end I think I had roughly the vocabulary of a 4-year-old!

If you have learned another language, think about whether your experience matched mine. What about learning something other than language: Do you think that the acquisition of expertise on any kind of intellectual task follows similar steps?

Speaking in Sentences: The Development of Grammar

After the first word, the next big step is when the child begins to string words into sentences, initially using only two words together, then three, four, and more. The first two-word sentences usually appear between 18 and 24 months. This is not a random or independent event. Recent research, such as Fenson's large cross-sectional study, suggests that sentences only appear when a child has reached some threshold level of vocabulary size—somewhere around 100 to 200 words.

Just as the first spoken words are preceded by apparently meaningful gestures, the first two-word sentences have gestural precursors as well. Toddlers often combine a single word with a gesture to create a "two-word meaning" before they actually use two words together in their speech. Elizabeth Bates (Bates et al., 1987) suggests an example: The infant may point to Daddy's shoe and say "Daddy," as if to convey "Daddy's shoe." Or she may say "Cookie!" while simultaneously reaching out her hand and opening and closing her fingers, as if to say "Give cookie!" In both cases a sentencelike meaning is conveyed by the use of gesture and body language combined with a word. Linguists call these word-and-gesture combinations **holophrases,** and they are common between the ages of 12 and 18 months.

Once the actual speaking of two-word sentences begins, the child moves rapidly through a series of steps or stages, so that within a year or two, most children are able to create remarkably complex sentences—as witness the 3-year-old I quoted at the beginning of this chapter.

First Sentences: 18 to 27 Months

The first sentences, which Roger Brown, a famous observer of child language, called Stage I grammar, have several distinguishing features: They are *short*—generally two or three words—and they are *simple.* Nouns, verbs, and adjectives are usually included, but virtually all the purely grammatical markers (which linguists call **inflections**) are missing. At the beginning, for example, children learning English do not normally use the *s* for plurals or put the *ed* ending on verbs to make the past tense, nor do they use the *'s* of the possessive or auxiliary verbs like *am* or *do.* Because only the really critical words are present in these early sentences, Brown (Brown, 1973; Brown & Bellugi, 1964) describes this as **telegraphic speech.** The child's language sounds rather like what we say when we send a telegram. We keep in all the essential words—usually nouns, verbs, and modifiers—and leave out all the prepositions, auxiliary verbs, and the like.

Interestingly, linguists are no longer sure that precisely this form of telegraphic speech occurs in children learning all languages. Some research seems to show that what determines the words that children use in their early sentences is the amount of *stress* normally placed on such words when that particular language is spoken. In English (and in many other languages) nouns, verbs, and adjectives are stressed in speech while the inflections are not. But in languages like Turkish, in which inflections are more stressed, children seem to use inflections much earlier (Gleitman & Wanner, 1988). Findings like these certainly raise some interesting questions about the universality of some of the patterns Brown and others have described.

In contrast, there is no dispute about the assertion that even at this earliest stage children create sentences following rules. Not adult rules, to be sure, but rules nonetheless. They focus on certain types of words and put them together in particular orders. They also manage to convey a variety of different meanings with their simple sentences.

For example, young children frequently use a sentence made up of two nouns, such as *Mommy sock* or *sweater chair* (Bloom, 1973). We might conclude from this that a "two-noun" form is a basic grammatical characteristic of early child language. But that misses the complexity. For instance, the child in Bloom's study who said *Mommy sock* said it on two different occasions. The first time was when she picked up her mother's sock and the second was when the mother put the child's own sock on the child's foot. In the first case, *Mommy sock* seems to mean Mommy's sock (a possessive relationship). But in the second

Table 8.2
Some of the Different Meanings Children Express in Their Earliest Simple Sentences

Meaning	Examples
Agent-action	Sarah eat; Daddy jump
Action-object	Eat cookie; read book
Possessor-possessed object	Mommy sock; Timothy lunch
Action-location	Come here; play outside
Located object-location	Sweater chair; juice table
Attribute-modified object	Big book; red house
Nomination	That cookie; it dog
Recurrence	More juice; other book

Source: Maratsos, 1983.

instance the child seems to convey "Mommy is putting a sock on me," which is an *agent* (Mommy)–*object* (sock) relationship.

Table 8.2 lists some other different meanings that children convey with their earliest sentences. Not all children express all these relationships or meanings in their early word combinations, and there does not seem to be a fixed order in which these meanings or constructions are acquired, but all children appear to express at least several of these patterns in their earliest, simplest sentences (Maratsos, 1983).

Grammar Explosion: 27 to 36 Months

Just as there is a vocabulary explosion following an early, slow beginning, there is also a grammar explosion following these first simple sentences. Beginning some time in the third year, most children quickly add many of the inflections and function words, a period Roger Brown refers to as Stage II grammar.

This grammar explosion is strongly linked to vocabulary development. In his large cross-sectional study, Fenson finds a correlation of .84 between the complexity of a child's sentences and the size of her speaking vocabulary—an astonishingly high correlation for behavioral research (Fenson et al., 1994). That is, children whose grammar is more complex and advanced also have larger vocabularies. Just what such a link may tell us about how children learn language is still a matter of debate. Is a large vocabulary *necessary* for grammar development? Alternatively, perhaps having begun to understand the ways in which sentences can be constructed, a child also understands new words better and hence learns them more readily. Whatever the eventual explanation, Fenson's research gives us an important new piece of data to work with.

What sorts of changes occur during this grammar explosion? Within a few months, children use plurals, past tenses, auxiliary verbs such as *is* or *does*, prepositions, and the like. They also begin to create negative sentences and to ask questions with the auxiliary

Table 8.3
Examples of Daniel's Stage I and Stage II Sentences

Stage I (Simple) Sentences	Stage II (More Complex) Sentences
Age 21 Months	**Age 23 Months**
A bottle	A little boat
Here bottle	Doggies here
Hi Daddy	Give you the book
Horse doggie	It's a boy
Broke it	It's a robot
Kitty cat	Little box there
Poor Daddy	No book
That monkey	Oh cars
Want bottle	That flowers
	Where going?

Source: Reprinted by permission of the publisher. D. Ingram, Early patterns of grammatical development, in R. E. Stark (Ed.), *Language behavior in infancy and early childhood,* Tables 6 and 7, pp. 344–345. Copyright © 1981 by Elsevier Science Publishing Co., Inc.

verb in the correct order. You can get a feeling for the sound of the change from Table 8.3, which lists some of the sentences of a little boy named Daniel, recorded by David Ingram (1981). The left-hand column lists some of Daniel's sentences at about 21 months of age, when he was still using the simplest forms; the right-hand column lists some of his sentences only 2½ months later (age 23 to 24 months), when he had shifted into higher gear.

Adding Inflections. Daniel obviously did not add all the inflections at once. In this sample, he uses only a few, such as the *s* for plural, although the beginning of a negative construction is apparent in "no book" and the beginning of a question form shows in "where going?," even though he has not yet added the auxiliary verb to the question.

Within each language community, children seem to add inflections and more complex word orders in fairly predictable sequences. In a classic early study, Roger Brown (1973) found that the earliest inflection among children learning English is most often the *ing* added onto a verb, as in *I playing* or *doggie running.* Then come (in order) prepositions like *on* and *in,* the plural *s* on nouns, irregular past tenses (such as *broke* or *ran*), possessives, articles (*a* and *the* in English), the *s* that we add to third-person verbs such as *he wants,* regular past tenses like *played* and *wanted,* and the various forms of the auxiliary verb, as in *I am going.*

Questions and Negatives. We also hear predictable sequences in the child's developing use of questions and negatives. In each case, the child seems to go through periods when he creates types of sentences that he has not heard adults use but that are consistent with the particular set of rules he is using. For example, in the development of questions there is a point at which the child gets a *wh* word (*who, what, when, where, why*) at the front end of a sentence but doesn't yet have the auxiliary verb in the right place, for example, *Why it is resting now?* Similarly, in the development of negatives, there is a stage in which the *not* or *n't* or *no* is put in but the auxiliary verb is omitted, as in *I not crying, there no squirrels,* or *this not fits* (Bloom, 1991). Then children rather quickly figure out the correct forms and stop making these "mistakes."

Overregularization. Another intriguing phenomenon of this second phase of sentence construction is **overregularization** or overgeneralization. This is what the two little girls were doing in the conversation about the goldfish when they created new regularized forms of superlatives (*badder, baddest, worser,* and *worsest*). We can hear the same thing in children's creation of past tenses like *wented, blowed, sitted* or in plurals like *teeths* or *blockses* (Fenson et al., 1994; Kuczaj, 1977; 1978). Stan Kuczaj pointed out that young children initially learn a small number of irregular past tenses and use them correctly for a short time. But then children rather suddenly seem to discover the rule of adding *ed* and overgeneralize this rule to all verbs. Then they relearn the exceptions one at a time. Even among preschoolers this type of "error" is not hugely common (only about 2 to 3 percent of all past tenses in English according to one recent study [Marcus et al., 1992]). But these overregularizations stand out because they are so distinctive and because they illustrate yet again that children create forms that they have not heard but that are logical within their current grammar.

Complex Sentences: 30 to 48 Months

After children have figured out the inflections and basic sentence forms like negation and questions, they soon begin to create remarkably complex sentences, using conjunctions like *and* or *but* to combine two ideas or using embedded clauses. Here are some examples from de Villiers and de Villiers (1992):

> *I didn't catch it but Teddy did!*
>
> *I'm gonna sit on the one you're sitting on.*
>
> *Where did you say you put my doll?*
>
> *Those are punk rockers, aren't they?*

Past these early stages, children's language continues to develop in various ways. In particular, more complex and difficult sentence forms are added throughout elementary school, and recurrent overregularization errors are eliminated (Bowerman, 1985). For instance, passive forms, like *the food is eaten by the cat,* are not well understood even by 5- and 6-year-olds and are not used much in spontaneous speech until several years later. But these are refinements. The really giant strides occur between ages 1 and about 4, as the child moves from single words to complex questions, negatives, and commands.

The Development of Word Meaning

To understand language development, it is not enough to know how children learn to string words together to form sentences. We also have to understand how the words in those sentences come to have meaning. Linguists are still searching for good ways to describe (or explain) children's emerging word meaning. So far, several sets of questions have dominated the research.

Which Comes First, the Meaning or the Word?

The most fundamental question is whether the child learns a word to describe a category or class he has *already* created through his manipulations of the world around him or

Children learning English also learn the rules for "tag questions" quite late—those questions we put on the end of a sentence to make it a question, like "isn't it?" or "haven't you?" or "aren't they?" Can you figure out the rule that you use to decide what is the correct tag?

The Real World
Bilingual Children

What I've said so far about early language development describes what happens when a child learns a *single* language. But what about children who are exposed to two or more languages from the beginning? How confusing is this for a child? And how can parents ease the process? At least two important practical questions surround this issue of bilingualism:

- Should parents who speak different native languages try to expose their children to both, or will that only confuse the child and make any kind of language learning harder? What's the best way to do this?
- If a child arrives at school age without speaking the dominant language of schooling, what is the best way for the child to acquire that second language?

Learning Two Languages at the Same Time

Parents should have no fears about exposing their child to two or more languages from the very beginning. Such simultaneous exposure does seem to result in slightly slower early steps in word learning and sentence construction, and the child will initially "mix" words or grammar from the two languages in individual sentences (Genesee, 1993). But bilingual children catch up rapidly to their monolingual peers.

The experts agree that the best way to help a child to learn two languages fluently is to speak both languages to the child from the beginning, *especially* if the two languages come at the child from different sources. For example, if Mom's native language is English and Dad's is Italian, Mom should speak only English to the infant/toddler and Dad should speak only Italian. (The parents will of course speak to each other in whatever language they have in common.) If both parents speak both languages to the child or mix them up in their own speech, this is a much more difficult situation for the child and language learning will be delayed (McLaughlin, 1984). It will also work if one language is always spoken at home and the other is spoken in a day-care center, with playmates, or in some other outside situation.

Bilingual Education

For many children, the need to be bilingual does not begin in the home, but only at school age. In the United States today, there are 2.5 million school-age children for whom English is not the primary language of the home (Hakuta & Garcia, 1989). Many of those children arrive at school with little or no facility in English. Educators have had to grapple with the task of teaching children a second language at the same time that they are trying to teach them subject matter such as reading and mathematics. The problem for the schools has been to figure out the best way to do this. Should the child be immediately immersed in the new language? Should the child learn basic academic skills in his native language and only later learn English as a second language? Or will some combination of the two work?

The research findings are messy. Still, one thread does run through it all: Neither full immersion nor English-as-a-second-language programs are as effective as truly bilingual programs in which the child is given at least some of her basic instruction in subject matter in her native language in the first year or two of school but is also exposed to the second language in the same classroom (Padilla et al., 1991; Willig, 1985). After several years of such combined instruction, the child makes a rapid transition to full use of the second language for all instruction. Interestingly, in her analysis of this research, Ann Willig has found that the ideal arrangement is very much like what works best at home with toddlers: If some subjects are always taught in one language and other subjects in the other language, children learn the second language most easily. But if each sentence is translated, children do not learn the new language as quickly or as well.

Note, though, that even such ideal bilingual education programs will not be effective for children who come to school without good spoken language in their native tongue. Learning to read, in any language, requires that the child have a fairly extensive awareness of the structure of language—a point I will explore later in this chapter. Any child who lacks such awareness—because she has been exposed to relatively little language or was not read to or talked to much in infancy and preschool years—will have difficulty learning to read, whether the instruction is given in the native language or in English.

whether the existence of a word forces the child to create new cognitive categories. This may seem like a highly abstract argument, but it touches on the fundamental issue of the relationship between language and thought. Does the child learn to represent objects to himself *because* he now has language, or does language simply come along at about this point and make the representations easier?

Not surprisingly, the answer seems to be both (Clark, 1983; Cromer, 1991; Greenberg & Kuczaj, 1982). On the cognitive side of the argument are several pieces of evidence I described in Chapter 7, such as the fact that young babies are able to remember and imitate objects and actions over periods of time long before they have language to assist them.

Further evidence of cognitive primacy comes from the study of the child's use of various prepositions like *in, between,* or *in front of,* each of which seems to be used spontaneously in language only after the child has understood the concept (Johnston, 1985).

The naming explosion may also rest on new cognitive understandings, in particular the new ability to categorize things. In several studies, Alison Gopnik and Andrew Meltzoff (1987; 1992) have found that the naming explosion typically occurs just after, or at the same time as, children first show spontaneous categorization of mixed sets of objects. Having discovered "categories," the child may now rapidly learn the names for already existing categories.

But once the child understands in some primitive way that names refer to categories, learning a new name suggests the existence of a new category (Waxman & Hall, 1993); thus, the name affects the child's thinking.

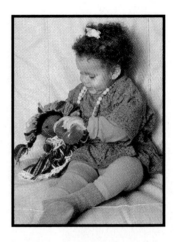

Does this 18-month-old know the word *doll* because she first had a concept of doll and later learned the word, or did she learn the word first and then create a category or concept to go with the word?

Extending the Class

What kinds of concepts does the child start with? Suppose your 2-year-old, on catching sight of the family tabby, says, "See kitty." No doubt you will be pleased that the child has the right word applied to the animal. But this sentence alone doesn't tell you much about the word meaning the child has developed. What does the word *kitty* mean to the child? Does he think it is a name only for that particular fuzzy beast? Or does he think it applies to all furry creatures, all things with four legs, things with pointed ears, or what?

One way to figure out the kind of class or category the child has created is to see what *other* creatures or things a child also calls a kitty. That is, how is the class *extended* in the child's language? If the child has created a kitty category that is based on furriness, then many dogs and perhaps sheep would also be called kitty. If having a tail is a crucial feature for the child, then some breeds of cat that have no tails might not be labeled as a kitty. Or perhaps the child used the word *kitty* only for the family cat, or only when petting the cat. This would imply a very narrow category indeed. The general question for researchers has been whether children tend to use words narrowly or broadly, overextending or underextending them.

Our current information tells us that underextension is most common at the earliest stages, particularly before the naming explosion (Harris, 1992), although even at this early point, overextension can also occur. Once the naming explosion starts, however, overextension seems to be more common. At that stage, we're more likely to hear the word *cat* applied to dogs or guinea pigs than we are to hear it used for just one animal or for a very small set of animals or objects (Clark, 1983). All children seem to show overextensions, but the particular classes the child creates are unique to each child. One child Eve Clark observed used the word *moon* for cake, round marks on windows, writing on

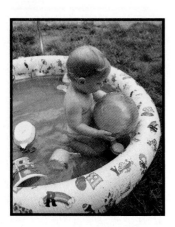

Chances are this toddler has a word for *ball,* and chances are also good that he uses the word *ball* to refer to a variety of other round things, which would be an example of overextension.

windows and in books, round shapes in books, tooling in leather book covers, round postmarks, and the letter *O.* Another used the word *ball* to refer not only to toy balls, but also to radishes and stone spheres at park entrances. Still another child used the word *ball* to refer to apples, grapes, eggs, squash, and a bell clapper (Clark, 1975).

These overextensions *may* tell us something about the way children think, such as that they have broad classes. But linguists like Eve Clark remind us that part of the child's problem is that he simply doesn't know very many words. A child who wants to call attention to a horse may not know the word *horse* and so may say "dog" instead. Overextensions may thus arise from the child's desire to communicate and may not tell us that the child fails to make the discriminations involved (Clark, 1987). As the child learns the separate labels that are applied to the different subtypes of "fuzzy four-legged creatures" the overextension disappears.

Parents may also contribute to a child's overextensions. Carolyn and Cynthia Mervis (1982) have found that mothers use labels that they think match the child's categories, rather than using the more precise labels. So they may call leopards and lions "kitty cats" or a toy fire engine a "car." Such a pattern undoubtedly aids communication between mother and child in the early stages of language development, but it also may contribute to what we hear as overextensions in the child's early language.

Constraints on Word Learning

Another of the fundamental questions about word meanings, the subject of hot debate among linguists in recent years, is just how a child figures out which part of some scene a word may refer to. The classic example: A child sees a brown dog running across the grass with a bone in its mouth. An adult points and says "doggie." From such an encounter the toddler is somehow supposed to figure out that *doggie* refers to the animal and not to running, bone, dog-plus-bone, brownness, ears, grass, or any other combination of elements in the whole scene.

Many linguists have proposed that a child could only conceivably cope with this monumentally complex task if he operated with some built-in biases or *constraints* (e.g., Golinkoff, Mervis, & Hirsh-Pasek, 1994; Markman, 1992; Waxman & Kosowski, 1990). For example, the child may have a built-in assumption that words refer to objects *or* events but not both, or an assumption that words refer to whole objects and not to their parts or attributes. Toddlers of 19 to 20 months, for example, already know that if you

If Dad says "goose" while he and his toddler are looking at this scene, how does the boy know that "goose" means the animal and not "white," "dirt," "honk honk," or some other feature? In fact, in this case, as in most instances, the child first *points* and then the father labels, which greatly simplifies the problem.

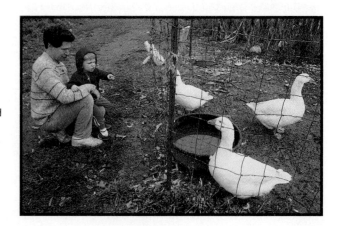

point at something and give a word, it is the label for that object (Baldwin, 1993) and not a name for some other feature of the scene.

Another possible built-in constraint is the *principle of contrast,* which is the assumption that every word has a different meaning, so if a new word is used, it must refer to some different object or a different aspect of an object (Clark, 1990). For example, in a widely quoted early study, Carey and Bartlett (1978) interrupted a play session with 2- and 3-year-old children by pointing to two trays and saying, "Bring me the chromium tray, not the red one, the chromium one." These children already knew the word *red* but did not know the word *chromium.* Nonetheless, most of the children were able to follow the instruction by bringing the nonred tray. Furthermore, a week later about half of the children remembered that the word *chromium* referred to some color and that the color was "not red." Thus, they learned the meaning by contrast.

Early proponents of constraints argued that the constraints are innate—built into the brain in some fashion. More recent proposals in this same vein place greater weight on the child's learning of the various principles over time. For example, Carolyn Mervis and Jacquelyn Bertrand (1994) have found that not all children between 16 and 20 months use the principle of contrast to learn the name of a new, unknown object. Furthermore, they found that those children who were using this principle had larger vocabularies and were more likely to be good at sorting objects into sets. Results like these tell us that constraints may be a highly useful way for children to learn words quickly but that they are probably a product of cognitive/linguistic development, not the basis for it.

A somewhat different argument against the notion of built-in constraints comes from Katherine Nelson (1988), who points out that the child rarely encounters a situation in which the adult points vaguely and gives some word. By far the most common scenario is that the parent follows the child's lead, labeling things the child is already playing with or pointing at (Harris, 1992). In fact, children whose parents do more of such responsive, specific labeling seem to learn language somewhat faster (Dunham, Dunham, & Curwin, 1993; Harris, 1992). To the extent that this is true, then, the child doesn't *need* a whole collection of constraints in order to figure out new words.

As these few examples illustrate, the study of the development of word meanings has been much more difficult to conceptualize than has been the development of grammar. Linguists are obviously searching for the rules that govern this process, so that we can understand how and why children use words the way they do. The study of constraints, whether they are ultimately conceived of as built in or as acquired, has moved us some distance forward, but there is still a long road to travel.

Using Language: Communication and Self-direction

In the past decade or so, linguists have also turned their attention to a third aspect of children's language, namely, the way children learn to *use* speech, either to communicate with others (an aspect of language often called **pragmatics**) or to regulate their own behavior. How early do children know what kind of language to use in specific situations? How early do they learn the "rules" of conversation, such as that you are supposed to take turns?

Language Pragmatics.   Children seem to learn the pragmatics of language at a remarkably early age. For example, children as young as 18 months show adultlike gaze patterns when they are talking with a parent: They look at the person who is talking, look

Do you recognize this pattern? Next time you are in a two-person conversation, monitor yourself and your partner and see if this isn't how it works.

away at the beginning of their own speaking turn, and then look at the listener again when they are signaling that they are about to stop talking (Rutter & Durkin, 1987).

Furthermore, a child as young as 2 years adapts the form of his language to the situation he is in or the person he is talking to—a point I made in the last chapter as well, when talking about children's egocentrism. He might say "gimme" to another toddler as he grabs the other child's glass but might say "more milk" to an adult. Among older children, language is even more clearly adapted to the listener: Four-year-olds use simpler language when they talk to 2-year-olds than when they talk to adults (Tomasello & Mannle, 1985); first graders explain things more fully to a stranger than to a friend (Sonnenschein, 1986) and are more polite to adults and strangers than to peers. Both of these trends are still clearer among fourth graders. Thus, from very early, probably from the beginning, the child's language is meant to *communicate,* and the child adapts the form of his language in order to achieve better communication.

Language and Self-control. Language seems to have another function for the child as well, namely, to help control or monitor her own behavior. Such "private speech," which may consist of fragmentary sentences, muttering, or instructions to the self, is detectable from the earliest use of words and sentences. For example, when 2- or 3-year-olds play by themselves, they give themselves instructions, stop themselves with words, or describe what they are doing: "No, not there," "I put that there," or "Put it" (Furrow, 1984). Piaget thought that this was *egocentric* speech, but the Russian psychologist Lev Vygotsky thought Piaget was quite wrong about this. Vygotsky insisted instead that the child is communicating with herself for the explicit purpose of guiding her own behavior. He believed that self-directing use of language is central to all cognitive development.

In young children such self-directing speech is audible; in older children it is audible when the child is facing a challenging task but has otherwise gone "underground." For example, you may recall from Chapter 7 that Flavell found that elementary school children muttered to themselves while they were trying to remember lists; among 9- or 10-year-olds this is much less common (Bivens & Berk, 1990). If we connect this set of findings with the work on information processing I talked about in the last chapter, it begins to sound as if the child uses language audibly to remind himself of some new or complex processing strategy; as the strategy becomes better rehearsed and more flexibly learned, overt language is no longer needed. Such an interpretation is bolstered by the observation

Can you think of times when you do this? Do you do it more for hard problems? How does whispering or speaking out loud help you?

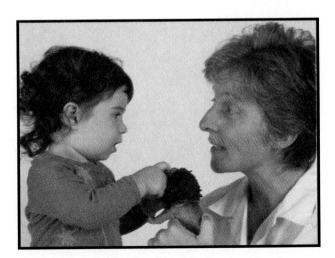

Twenty-month-old Clare already knows many of the social rules about how language is used, including rules about who is supposed to look at whom during a conversation.

that even adults will use audible language in problem solving when they are faced with especially difficult tasks.

Even this brief foray into the research on the child's use of language points out that a full understanding of language development is going to require understanding of both cognitive development and of the child's social skills and understanding. Lois Bloom, one of the foremost theorists and observers of children's language, argues that indeed "children learn language in the first place because they strive to . . . *share* what they and other persons are feeling and thinking" (Bloom, 1993, p. 245). From birth, the child has been able to communicate feelings and thoughts through facial expressions, somewhat later through gestures. But these are imperfect vehicles for communication; language is much more efficient. Such an argument reminds us once again that the child is not divided into tidy packages labeled "physical development," "social development," or "language development" but is instead a coherent, integrated system.

Explaining Language Development

If merely describing language development is hard—and it is—explaining it is still harder. Indeed, explaining how a child learns language has proven to be one of the most compelling, and one of the most difficult, challenges within developmental psychology. This may surprise you. I suspect that most of you just take for granted that a child learns to talk by listening to the language she hears. What is magical or complicated about that? Yet the more you think about it, the more amazing and mysterious it becomes. For one thing, as Steven Pinker (1987) points out, there is a veritable chasm between what the child hears as language input and the language the child must eventually speak. The input consists of some set of sentences spoken to the child, with intonation, stress, and timing. They are spoken in the presence of objects and events, and the words are given in a particular order. All that may be helpful, even essential. But what the child must acquire from such input is nothing less than a set of rules for *creating* sentences. How does the child accomplish this feat? Theories abound. Let me start on the nurture end of the theoretical continuum.

Imitation and Reinforcement

The earliest theories of language were based either on learning theory or on the commonsense idea that language was learned by imitation. Imitation obviously has to play some part, because the child learns the language she hears. Babbling drifts toward the sounds in the heard language; children imitate sentences they hear; they learn to speak with the accent of their parents. And those babies who show the most imitation of actions and gestures are also those who later learn language most quickly (Bates et al., 1982). So the tendency to imitate may be an important ingredient. Still, imitation alone can't explain all language acquisition because it cannot account for the creative quality of the child's language. In particular, children consistently create types of sentences and forms of words that they have never heard—words like *goed* or *beated* or *worser.*

Reinforcement theories such as Skinner's (1957) fare no better. Skinner argued that parents shape language through systematic reinforcements, gradually rewarding better and better approximations of adult speech. But in fact parents don't appear to do any-

Research Report
The Importance of Reading to the Child

One intriguing piece of evidence showing the importance of the child's environment in early language learning comes from a series of studies by G. J. Whitehurst and his colleagues. In their first study (Whitehurst et al., 1988), they trained some parents to read picture books to their toddlers and to interact with them in a special way during the reading, a pattern called *dialogic* reading. Specifically, they were trained to use questions that could not be answered just by pointing. So a mother reading *Winnie the Pooh* might say, "There's Eeyore. What's happening to him?" Or the parent might ask, pointing to some object shown in a book, "What's the name of that?" or ask a question about some character in a story, such as "Do you think the kitty will get into trouble?" Other parents were encouraged to read to the child but were given no special instructions. After a month, the children in the experimental group had shown a larger gain in vocabulary than had the children in the comparison group.

Whitehurst has now replicated this study in day-care centers for poor children in both Mexico and New York City (Valdez-Menchaca & Whitehurst, 1992; Whitehurst et al., 1994) and in a large number of Head Start classrooms (Whitehurst et al., 1995). In the Mexican study, one teacher in a day-care center was trained in dialogic reading. She then spent 10 minutes each day for six or seven weeks reading with each of ten 2-year-olds. A comparison group of children in the same day-care center spent an equivalent amount of time with the same teacher each day but was given arts and crafts instruction rather than reading. At the end of the intervention, the children who had been read to had higher vocabulary scores on a variety of standardized tests and used more complex grammar when talking in a special test conversation with another adult.

In Whitehurst's U.S. day-care and Head Start studies, children were read to in this special way either by their teacher or by both their mother and the teacher, while control group children experienced normal interactions with day-care workers or teachers. In both studies, the children who had participated in dialogic reading gained in vocabulary significantly more than did the control group children, and the effect appears to last.

Similarly, Catherine Crain-Thoreson and Philip Dale (1995) found that they could significantly increase language skills in language-delayed children by teaching either parents or teachers to read to them in this special way.

The fact that we now have evidence of the same types of effects in two different cultures, with two different languages, with both teachers and parents, with both poor and middle-class children, and with language-delayed children, strengthens the argument that richer, interactive language between adult and child is one important ingredient in fostering the child's language growth.

thing like this. Instead, parents are remarkably forgiving of all sorts of peculiar constructions and meaning (Brown & Hanlon, 1970; Hirsh-Pasek, Trieman, & Schneiderman, 1984). In addition, children learn many forms of language, such as plurals, with relatively few errors. In sum, it is plain that some process other than shaping must be involved.

Newer Environmental Theories: Talking to the Child

Still, it seems obvious that what is said to the child has to play *some* role in the process. At the simplest level, we know that children whose parents talk to them often, read to them regularly, and respond to the child's own verbalizations begin to talk a little sooner. So at least the *rate* of development is affected by the amount of input.

Motherese. The quality of the parents' language may also be important. In particular, we know that adults talk to children in a special kind of very simple language, originally called **motherese** by many linguists, now more scientifically described as **infant-directed speech.** This simple language is spoken in a higher-pitched voice and at a slower pace than is talk between adults. The sentences are short, with simple, concrete vocabulary, and they

Imagine yourself talking to an infant you are holding in your arms. Can your hear yourself using "motherese"?

are grammatically simple. When speaking to children, parents also repeat a lot, with minor variations. ("Where is the ball? Can you see the ball? Where is the ball? There is the ball!") They may also repeat the child's sentence but in a slightly longer, more grammatically correct form—a pattern referred to as an *expansion* or a *recasting.*

Parents don't talk this way to children in order to teach them language. They do so with the hope that they will communicate better by using simpler language. But infant-directed speech may nonetheless be very useful, even necessary, for the child's language acquisition. We know, for example, that some kind of higher-pitched, simplified, repetitious language to babies and children occurs in virtually all cultures and language communities, even among deaf parents using sign language to their infants (Masataka, 1992).

We also know that babies as young as a few days old can discriminate between motherese and adult-directed speech and that *they prefer to listen to motherese,* whether it is spoken by a female or a male voice (Cooper & Aslin, 1994; Pegg, Werker, & McLoed, 1992). This preference exists even when the motherese is being spoken in language other than the one normally spoken to the child. Janet Werker and her colleagues, for example (Werker, Pegg, & McLeod, 1994), have found that both English and Chinese infants prefer to listen to infant-directed speech, whether it is spoken in English or in Cantonese (one of the major languages of China). The quality of motherese that seems to be particularly attractive to babies is its higher pitch. Once the child's attention is drawn by this special tone, the very simplicity and repetitiveness of the adult's speech may help the child to pick out repeating grammatical forms.

Children's attention also seems to be drawn to recast sentences. For example, Farrar (1992) found that 2-year-old children were twice or three times as likely to imitate a correct grammatical form after they had heard their mother recast their own sentences than they were when that same correct grammatical form appeared naturally in the mother's conversation. Experimental studies confirm this effect of recastings. Children who are deliberately exposed to higher rates of specific types of recast sentences seem to learn the modeled grammatical forms more quickly than do those who heard no recastings (Nelson, 1977).

Sounds good, doesn't it? But this theory has some holes in it. For one thing, while children who hear more expansions or recastings may learn grammar sooner, in normal parent-toddler conversations, recasts are actually relatively rare, in some cases almost nonexistent. Yet children nevertheless acquire a complex grammar, which suggests that the kind of feedback provided by recastings is unlikely to be a major source of grammatical information for most children (Morgan, Bonamo, & Travis, 1995). And while motherese does seem to occur in the vast majority of cultures and contexts, it does not occur in *all.* For example, Pye (1986) could find no sign of motherese in one Mayan culture, and studies in the United States show it is greatly reduced among depressed mothers (Bettes, 1988). Children of these mothers nonetheless learn language. Thus, while infant-directed speech may be helpful, it cannot be *necessary* for language.

Innateness Theories

On the other side of the theoretical spectrum we have the innateness theorists, who argue that much of what the child needs for learning language is built into the organism. Early innateness theorists like Noam Chomsky (1965; 1975; 1986; 1988) were especially struck by two phenomena: the extreme complexity of the task the child must accomplish and the apparent similarities in the steps and stages of children's early language development across languages and among all children. Newer cross-language comparisons now make it clear that more variability exists than first appeared—a set of findings I've described in the *Cultures and Contexts* box on the facing page. Nonetheless, innateness theories are alive and well and increasingly accepted.

One particularly influential innateness theorist is Dan Slobin (1985a; 1985b), who assumes a basic language-making capacity in any child, made up of a set of fundamental *operating principles*. Just as the newborn infant seems to come programmed with "rules to look by," so, Slobin argues, infants and children are programmed with "rules to listen by."

You've already encountered a good deal of evidence consistent with this proposal in earlier chapters. We know that from earliest infancy, babies focus on individual sounds and on syllables in the stream of sounds they hear, that they pay attention to sound rhythm, and that they prefer speech of a particular pattern, namely motherese. Slobin also proposes that babies are preprogrammed to pay attention to the beginnings and endings of strings of sounds and to stressed sounds—a hypothesis supported by research (e.g., Morgan, 1994). Together, these operating principles would help to explain some of the features of children's early grammars. In English, for example, the stressed words in a sentence are normally the verb and the noun—precisely the words that English-speaking children use in their earliest sentences. In Turkish, on the other hand, prefixes are stressed, and Turkish-speaking children learn prefixes very early. Both these patterns make sense if we assume that what is built in is not "verbness" or "nounness" or "prefixness" but "pay attention to stressed sounds."

The fact that this model is consistent with the growing information about apparently built-in perceptual skills and processing biases is certainly a strong argument in its favor. But other compelling theoretical alternatives have also been proposed. In particular, some theorists argue persuasively that what is important is not the built-in biases, but the child's *construction* of language as part of the broader process of cognitive development. In this view, the child is a "little linguist," applying her emerging cognitive understanding to the problem of language, searching for regularities and patterns.

Constructivist Theories

Melissa Bowerman (1985) is one proponent of this view. She puts the proposition this way: "When language starts to come in, it does not introduce new meanings to the child. Rather, it is used to express only those meanings the child has already formulated independently of language" (1985, p. 372). In a similar vein, Lois Bloom suggests that "words a child hears from others will be learned if they connect with what the child is thinking and feeling" (1993, p. 247).

If this is true, then we should observe clear links between achievements in language development and the child's broader cognitive development. And, in fact, we do. For example, symbolic play (such as drinking from an empty cup) and imitation of sounds and gestures both appear at about the same time as the child's first words, suggesting some broad "symbolic" understanding that is reflected in a number of behaviors. In children whose language is significantly delayed, both symbolic play and imitation are normally delayed too (Bates et al., 1987; Ungerer & Sigman, 1984).

A second example occurs later: At about the point at which two-word sentences appear, we can also see children begin to combine several gestures into a sequence in their pretend play, such as pouring imaginary liquid, drinking, and then wiping the mouth. Those children who are the first to show this sequencing in their play are also the first to

Cultures and Contexts
Universals and Variations in Early Language

In the early years of research on children's language development, linguists and psychologists were strongly impressed by the apparent similarities across languages in children's early language. You've already seen some of the evidence that supports this impression in an earlier *Cultures and Contexts* box (p. 224), illustrating large similarities in early vocabularies. Studies in a wide variety of language communities, including Turkish, Serbo-Croatian, Hungarian, Hebrew, Japanese, a New Guinean language called Kaluli, German, and Italian, have revealed other important similarities in early language:

- The prelinguistic phase seems to be identical in all language communities. All babies coo, then babble; all babies understand language before they can speak it; babies in all cultures begin to use their first words at about 12 months.
- In all language communities studied so far, a one-word phase precedes the two-word phase, with the latter beginning at about 18 months.
- In all languages studied so far, prepositions describing locations are added in essentially the same order. Words for *in, on, under,* and *beside* are learned first. Then the child learns the words *front* and *back* (Slobin, 1985a).
- Children seem to pay more attention to the ends of words than to the beginnings, so they learn suffixes before they learn prefixes.

At the same time, cross-linguistic comparisons show that children's beginning sentences are not nearly so similar as the early innateness theorists had supposed. For example:

- The specific word order that a child uses in early sentences is not the same for all children in all languages. In some languages a noun/verb sequence is fairly common, in others a verb/noun sequence may be heard.
- Particular inflections are learned in highly varying orders from one language to another. Japanese children, for example, begin very early to use a special kind of marker, called a *pragmatic* marker, that tells something about the feeling or the context. For instance, in Japanese the word *yo* is used at the end of a sentence when the speaker is experiencing some resistance from the listener; the word *ne* is used when the speaker expects approval or agreement. Japanese children begin to use these markers very early, much earlier than other inflections appear in most languages.
- Most strikingly, there are languages in which there seems to be no simple two-word sentence stage in which the sentences contain no inflections. Children learning Turkish, for example, use essentially the full set of noun and verb inflections by age 2 and never go through a stage of using uninflected words. Their language is simple but it is rarely ungrammatical from the adult's point of view (Aksu-Koc & Slobin, 1985).

Obviously, any theory of language acquisition must account for both the common ground and the wide variations from one language to the next.

show two- or three-word sentences in their speech (Bates et al., 1987; Brownell, 1988; McCune, 1995; Shore, 1986).

These apparent linkages between language and cognition are impressive, but an interesting bit of counterevidence comes from recent studies of children with Williams syndrome, a genetic disorder linked to mental retardation. Williams syndrome children and adults, like those with Down syndrome, have general deficiencies in most aspects of cognitive functioning. But unlike Down syndrome children, Williams syndrome children develop excellent language skills—large vocabularies and complex grammar. Their language is delayed in the early years, just as is the language of Down syndrome children, but their eventual language skill—both comprehension and production—is close to normal (Mervis et al., 1995; Wang & Bellugi, 1993). In these children, then, there is no linkage between overall cognitive development and language development, a result that obviously poses problems for Bowerman's model.

My own view is that at this stage we should not choose between Slobin's and Bowerman's approaches. Both may be true. The child may begin with built-in operating principles that aim the child's attention at crucial features of the language input. The child then processes that information according to her initial (perhaps built-in) strategies or schemes. But then she modifies those strategies or rules as she receives new information, such as by arriving at some of the constraints about word meanings. The result is a series of rules for understanding and creating language. The strong similarities we see among children in their early language constructions come about both because all children share the same initial processing rules and because most children are exposed to very similar input from the people around them. But because the input is not identical, because languages differ, language development follows less and less common pathways as the child progresses.

As these brief descriptions of theory make clear, linguists and psychologists who have studied language have made progress. We know a lot more now about how *not* to explain language. But we have not yet cracked the code. The fact that children learn complex and varied use of their native tongue within a few years remains both miraculous and largely mysterious.

Individual Differences in Language Development

The sequences of development of language I have been describing are accurate on the average, but as I have mentioned a few times in passing, the speed with which children acquire language skill varies widely. There also seem to be important style differences.

Differences in Rate

Some children begin using individual words at 8 months, others not until 18 months; some do not use two-word sentences until 3 years or even later. You can see the range of normal variation in sentence construction very clearly in Figure 8.3, which shows the average sentence length (referred to by linguists as the **mean length of utterance,** or MLU) of 10 children, each studied longitudinally. Eve, Adam, and Sarah were studied by Roger Brown (1973); Jane, Martin, and Ben (all African-American children), by Ira Blake (1994); and Eric, Gia, Kathryn, and Peter, by Lois Bloom (1991). I have drawn a line at the MLU level that normally accompanies a switch from simple, uninflected two-word sentences to more complex forms. You can see that Eve was the earliest to make this transition, at about 21 months, while Adam and Sarah passed over this point about a year later. These variations are confirmed in Fenson's much larger cross-sectional study of more than 1000 toddlers whose language was described by their parents. In this group, the earliest age at which parents reported more complex than simple sentences was about 22 months, with an average of about 27 months. However, as many as a quarter of children had not reached this point by 30 months (Fenson et al., 1994).

I should point out that most children who talk late catch up later, and earliness or lateness of complex speech is *not* predictive of later IQ or later reading ability. The exception to this statement is a small group of late talkers who also have poor *receptive* language. This group appears to remain behind in language development and perhaps in cognitive development more generally (Bates, 1993).

How can we explain these variations in speed of early language development? The alternative possibilities should be familiar by now.

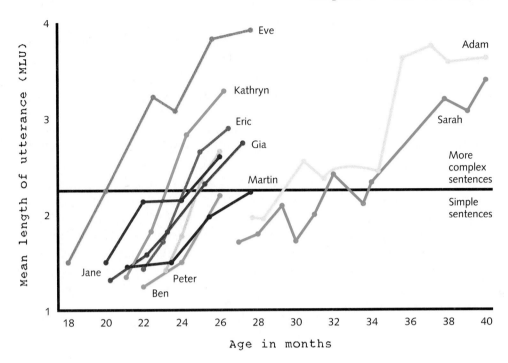

FIGURE 8.3 The 10 children whose language is charted here, studied by three different linguists, moved from simple one- and two-word sentences to more complex sentences at markedly different times. (*Sources:* Brown, 1973, Figure 1, p. 55; Bloom, 1991, Table 3.1, p. 92; Blake, 1994, Table 9.1, p. 169; and Figure 9.1, p. 171.)

Genetic Explanations. One possibility is that the rate of language development may be something you inherit—in the same way that intelligence or the rate of physical development may be partially influenced by heredity. Certainly if we assume that some language-processing patterns are built into the brain, it makes sense to think that some children may inherit a more efficient built-in system than others, just as some babies habituate faster to repeated stimuli.

Twin studies and adoption studies designed to test this possibility have yielded the typical mixture of findings. In twin studies, the common finding is that vocabulary size, but *not* grammatical complexity, is more similar in identical than in fraternal twins (Mather & Black, 1984). Adoption studies show that 2-year-olds' language skill can be predicted about equally well from the IQs or language skills of either the natural or the adoptive parents (Plomin & DeFries, 1985). And among adoptive families, those who talked the most and provided the most toys had children whose language was more advanced.

What this all looks like to me is that some aspects of language development are strongly related to the child's overall information-processing abilities, such as speed of learning new words and understanding other people's language. Since cognitive abilities have a significant genetic influence, so do these language abilities. But other aspects of language, such as pronunciation and possibly the rate of grammatical development, may be equally influenced by variations in the richness of the child's linguistic environment.

Environmental Explanations. I have already talked about some such influences. Parents who talk more, who read to the child more and elicit more language from the child, and who respond contingently to the child's language seem to have children who develop language more rapidly. The fact that this same set of relationships is found in families of *adoptive* children is impressive, since we can be fairly sure that what we are seeing here is not just genetic influence in disguise.

Overall, as with IQ, it seems obvious that both the particular genes the child inherits and the environment in which the child is growing up contribute to the rate of language development she will show. I should emphasize once again, though, that although children do differ widely in the timing of their language development, virtually all children progress adequately through the sequence of steps I have been describing. Nearly all children learn to communicate at least adequately; most do so with great skill, regardless of their early rate of progress. One moral for parents is that you should not panic if your child is still using fairly primitive sentences at 2½ or even 3—providing, of course, that the child appears to understand what is said to her. Instead of worrying, I would urge you to listen with pleasure to your child's emerging language—to the poetry of it, the wonderfully funny mistakes, the amazingly rapid changes. It is a fascinating process.

Differences in Style

A quite different kind of individual difference that has intrigued linguists far more than variations in rate is apparent differences in the style of children's early language. Katherine Nelson (1973) was the first to point our attention at such style differences. She noted that some toddlers use what she called an **expressive style.** For them, most early words are linked not to objects but to social relationships. They often learn pronouns (*you, me*) early and use many more of what Nelson calls "personal-social" words, such as *no, yes, want,* or *please.* Their early vocabulary may also include some multiword strings, like "Love you" or "Do it," or "Go away." This is in sharp contrast to the children who use what Nelson calls a **referential style,** whose early vocabulary is made up predominantly

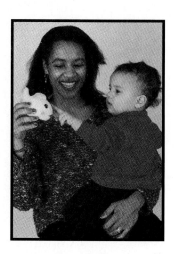

"Where is the fish's eye?" asks Mom. Seventeen-month-old Jesse obviously knows the answer. Moms who talk a lot to their babies and ask questions in this way have children who learn to talk sooner.

Table 8.4
Some Differences Between Expressive and Referential Children in Early Language

	Expressive	Referential
Early words	Low proportion of nouns and adjectives	High proportion of nouns and adjectives
Vocabulary growth	Slow, gradual; rarely any spurts	Rapid, with clear spurt at one-word stage
Articulation	Less-clear speech	Clearer speech
Early sentences	May have inflections at Stage I, because of high use of "rote strings" (formulas) inserted into sentences (e.g., "What do you want?")	Few rote strings at Stage I grammar; speech is clearly telegraphic at this stage, with no inflections

Sources: Thal & Bates, 1990; Shore, 1995.

of names for things or people. Later researchers have found further signs of such a difference in both grammar and articulation, as you can see in the summary in Table 8.4.

Elizabeth Bates and her colleagues (Bates, Bretherton, & Snyder, 1988; Thal & Bates, 1990) argue that the difference between these two styles may run fairly deep. Referential-style children are, in some sense, more cognitively oriented. They are drawn to objects, spend more of their time in solitary play with objects, and interact with other people more often around objects. They are much more likely to show a clear spurt in vocabulary development in the early stages, adding a whole lot of object names in a very short space of time, as if they—more than expressive children—had understood the basic principle that things have names. Such children are also advanced in their ability to understand complex adult language.

Expressive-style toddlers, on the other hand, are oriented more toward people, toward social interactions. Their early words and sentences include a lot of "strings" of words that are involved in common interactions with adults. Since many such strings include grammatical inflections, expressive children's early language often sounds more advanced than that of a referential child. But their vocabularies develop more slowly, with no obvious spurt.

Just how these differences come about is still being hotly debated. It could be that such children are simply matching the quality of the language they are hearing. For example, there are a few hints that firstborn children may be more likely to follow the referential pattern. Perhaps they receive much more intensive language input, with much more emphasis on learning names. Later-borns, who seem to be somewhat more likely to follow an expressive style, may encounter a different linguistic environment, with more emphasis on communication. The two styles might also reflect underlying temperamental variations, although the one study I know of that explores this possibility directly has not found such a link (Bates et al., 1988).

Whatever the source, the existence of such large differences in the form or style of early language raises serious questions about the assumption that the early stages of language development are the same for all children and about virtually all nativist theories of language development. If we assume that all children learn language based on the same built-in operating principles, then where do the style differences come from? Either there is more variability of process than innateness theories propose, or there must be substantial variations in the way parents talk to "referential" and "expressive" children—a possibility that is not well supported by the evidence. All in all, the literature on style differences in language learning, which seemed like an interesting sidelight when Nelson first described the phenomenon, has turned out to lead to a fascinating set of new questions.

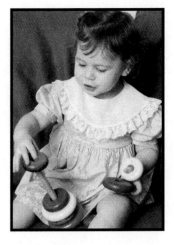

If you had to guess, which of the two styles of early language learning would you bet young Shifra shows?

There are some indications that girls are more likely to follow a referential pattern, while boys may be more often expressive. Can you think of any possible explanations of such a difference?

An Application of the Basic Knowledge: Learning to Read

In Chapter 5, I talked briefly about some of the *perceptual* aspects of learning to read. But of course reading involves language as well. Researchers have found that a child's knowledge of both the sound and the structure of language plays a very important role in early reading. Especially significant are two very specific bits of knowledge: (1) the child's ability to recognize individual letters, and (2) the child's awareness that spoken and written words are made up of individual sounds (Adams, 1990).

I already mentioned in Chapter 5 that very young babies pay attention to individual sounds, which linguists call *phonemes*. But the understanding that words are made up of strings of such sounds—an understanding referred to as *phonemic awareness*—seems to be a more advanced understanding, one that is essential to reading.

Suppose you say to a child, "Tell a word which starts the same as *tap*." To do this, the child has to be able to identify which sound in the string of sounds comes first in the word. He must also be able to recognize this same sound in other words. You can get at this same skill in other ways such as by asking children to recognize or produce rhyming words or by reading them two words that differ in only one sound, such as *sing* and *sink*, and asking if the two words are the same or different. We now have abundant evidence that children who are more skilled at such tasks at age 3, 4, or 5 later learn to read much more easily (Bryant et al., 1990; Hansen & Bowey, 1994; Whitehurst, 1995).

Letter recognition and phonemic awareness also interact with more basic cognitive skills. For instance, Tunmer and his colleagues (Tunmer, Herriman, & Nesdale, 1988) have found that the best predictor of reading skill at the end of first grade is the child's letter recognition at the beginning of the year. But among those children who began first grade with poor phonemic awareness or poor letter recognition, those with good concrete operational knowledge caught up much more quickly in reading than did those who lagged behind in these basic cognitive skills. Thus, good skills in either area—language awareness or logical abilities—can form the foundation for reading, but of the two, language awareness seems to be the more central.

Where does such early language awareness come from? How does it happen that some 5- and 6-year-olds have extensive understanding of the way words are put together, while others have little? The answer seems to be quite simple: exposure and expertise. For a child to learn about letters and sounds, he has to have had a great deal of exposure to language, both written and spoken. Such children are talked to a lot as infants, read to regularly, may have toy letters to play with, are told the sounds that go with each letter, or may be quite specifically taught the alphabet at an early age.

Nursery rhymes are also frequently a significant part of the early experience of good readers. In one study, researchers found that among a sample of children in England, those who knew more nursery rhymes at age 3½ later had greater phonemic awareness and learned to read more readily than did those who knew fewer rhymes (Maclean, Bryant, & Bradley, 1987). Because nursery rhyme knowledge was *not* predictive of the child's later mathematical ability in this study, it looks very much as if we are dealing here with a quite specific body of expertise.

Of all the types of early experience that may contribute to such expertise, the most crucial seems to be the experience of being read to, regularly and in a fashion that invites the child's attention and response—a point I already made in the *Research Report* earlier in the chapter (p. 236). Families that do not engage in such reading or do not encourage other prereading experiences have children who have far more difficulty learning to read once they begin school.

For those lacking such expertise at the start of school, the only solution is to try to build a parallel base of knowledge through many of the same kinds of experiences that more expert readers have had at home. This means that poor readers need a great deal of exposure to sound/letter combinations. But they also need to learn how to recognize patterns of letters in words. One need not—indeed must not—choose between those two hotly contesting educational systems, phonics and "whole word" training. Both are needed, along with instruction in syntax, so that the child will understand better what words *could* appear in certain places in sentences.

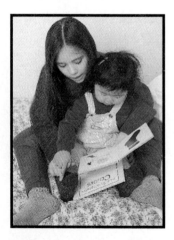

Children who are read to often have an easier time learning to read later. And it doesn't have to be the parent who does the reading: This 9-year-old is reading to her younger sister.

Marilyn Adams (1990), who has analyzed all the evidence, also makes a persuasive case that the poor reader must have maximum success in oral reading, preferably with texts that are full of the sort of rhyme and repetition that will help to foster phonemic awareness and learning of language regularities. Programs with this emphasis have been highly successful with poor readers, while more drill-like phonics programs have not (Hatcher, Hulme, & Ellis, 1994). In other words, poor readers seem to learn to read most easily through programs that to some degree mimic the naturally occurring home experiences of good readers: a great deal of reading, "play" with words, active questioning, and experimentation.

Summary

1   Language can be defined as an arbitrary system of symbols that permits us to say (in words or gestures), and to understand, an infinite variety of messages. It is rule governed and creative.

2   Many of the developments during the "prelinguistic" phase (before the first word) are significant precursors to language. The child discriminates language sounds, babbles sounds that more and more closely approximate the sounds he hears, and uses gestures in communicative ways.

3   At about 1 year of age the earliest words appear. Some of these early words are combined with gestures to convey whole sentences of meaning, a pattern called a holophrase.

4   Vocabulary grows slowly at first and then usually spurts in a "naming explosion." By 16 to 20 months, most children have a vocabulary of 50 or more words; by 30 months, the average vocabulary is 600 words. Children continue to add roughly one word every two hours through elementary school.

5   The first two-word sentences normally appear between 18 and 24 months and are short and grammatically simple, lacking the various grammatical inflections. The child can nonetheless convey many different meanings, such as location, possession, or agent–object relationships.

6   During a "grammar explosion," the child quickly adds the many grammatical inflections and learns to create questions and negative sentences.

7   By age 3 or 4, most children can construct remarkably complex sentences. Later skills are on the order of refinements, such as learning to understand and use passive sentences.

8   The development of word meanings (semantic development) follows a less-predictable course. Children appear to have many concepts or categories before they have words for them, but learning new words also creates new categories.

9   The earliest words are typically highly specific and context-bound in meaning; later, children typically "overextend" their usage.

10   Many (but not all) linguists have concluded that in determining word meanings, a child has built-in constraints or biases, such as the assumption that words refer to objects or actions but not both, or the principle of contrast. Others think that such constraints exist but are acquired rather than built in.

11   Children appear to have two uses for language: to communicate and to direct their own activity. Communication is the dominant use. As early as age 2 children adapt their language to the needs of the listener and begin to follow culturally specific customs of language usage.

12   Several theories have been offered to explain language development. Two early environmental explanations, based on imitation or reinforcement, have been largely set aside. More recently, emphasis has been placed both on the helpful quality of the simpler form of parent-to-child language called motherese or child-directed language and on the role of expansions and recastings of children's sentences.

13 Innateness theories are also common. They assume the child is born with a set of "operating principles" that focus the child on relevant aspects of language input. Others emphasize the child as a "little linguist" who constructs a language as he constructs all cognitive understandings.

14 Children differ in the rate of development of both vocabulary and grammar, differences explained by both heredity and environmental influences. Despite these variations in rate of early development, however, most children learn to speak skillfully by about age 5 or 6.

15 In the early years of language development, two styles of language can be distinguished, "referential" (focusing on objects and their description) and "expressive" (focusing on words and forms that describe or further social relationships).

16 Language research can also help us understand the development of reading skill. Metalinguistic awareness of grammar, semantics, and segmented sounds of language seems to be critical for reading.

Key Terms

babbling (**p. 220**)

cooing (**p. 220**)

expressive language (**p. 221**)

expressive style (**p. 242**)

holophrases (**p. 226**)

infant-directed speech (**p. 236**)

inflections (**p. 226**)

mean length of utterance (**p. 240**)

motherese (**p. 236**)

overregularization (**p. 229**)

pragmatics (**p. 233**)

prelinguistic phase (**p. 219**)

receptive language (**p. 221**)

referential style (**p. 242**)

semantics (**p. 218**)

syntax (**p. 218**)

telegraphic speech (**p. 226**)

Suggested Readings

Hakuta, K. (1986). *Mirror of language: The debate on bilingualism.* New York: Basic Books.

An elegant and readable discussion of many of the issues of bilingualism I've discussed in the *Real World* box on page 230.

Harris, M. (1992). *Language experience and early language development: From input to uptake.* Hove, England: Erlbaum.

Margaret Harris is a thoughtful researcher and theorist who argues in this book for the importance of the language input for the child's language development. She lays out the alternative theories nicely and presents a variety of evidence from her own research observations of mothers talking to their infants and toddlers.

Pinker, S. (1994). *The language instinct: How the mind creates language.* New York: Morrow.

This splendid book, written by one of the most articulate and easy-to-understand linguists, lays out the argument for a built-in language instinct.

Shore, C. M. (1995). *Individual differences in language development.* Thousand Oaks, CA: Sage.

A small book summarizing what we know about individual differences in rate and style of language development, and the alternative explanations of those differences.

de Villiers, P. A., & de Villiers, J. G. (1992). Language development. In M. H. Bornstein & M. E. Lamb (Eds.), *Developmental psychology: An advanced textbook* (3rd ed.) (pp. 337–418). Hillsdale, NJ: Erlbaum.

A remarkably thorough and clear review of this subject, much easier to read than many current discussions or descriptions of language development, and touching on many of the issues I have raised here. Strongly recommended as a next source.

Personality Development: Alternative Views

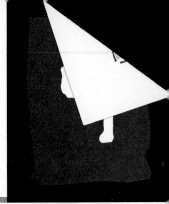

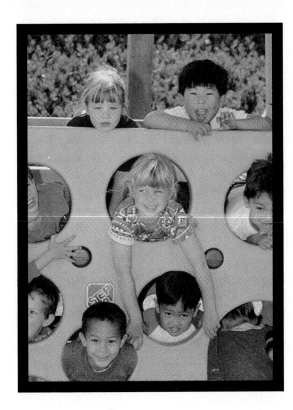

I magine yourself sitting in a day-care center, invisible to the eyes of the children but able to watch a group of 2-year-olds. Since you've just read all about cognitive and language development, your attention may be drawn at first to the ways the children play with toys or the way they talk to one another and to the teacher. But it won't take you long to notice that cognitive and language skills, however fascinating, are only part of the picture. The other part is the child's emerging *social* skills.

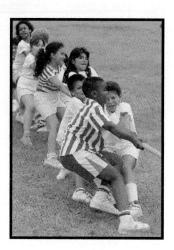

Each of these Texas second graders already has a distinct personality. Where do the differences come from?

You'll see conflict over toys ("Mine!"), often settled with physical aggression or tears, although signs of helpfulness or altruism are also likely to be visible. You'll see children playing and moving about pretty independently, but you will also see that they still turn to the teacher often for attention and reassurance, sometimes physically clinging to her. You'll see boys and girls playing together, but little sign of any real individual friendships.

If you watched the same group of children a few years later, many of these patterns would have changed. By age 5 or 6 we see some friendships formed, but almost entirely between children of the same gender. Clinging and obvious dependence on adults are less in evidence, and disputes are more likely to be dealt with by yelling and name calling than by grabbing or hitting.

These are all developmental changes, analogous to the changes in cognitive structure I talked about in Chapter 7. At the same time, you cannot watch children for very long without seeing the striking variations in children's approaches to these social tasks. The child who hung about on the edge of the group in nursery school is likely to show something similar in kindergarten; the child who clung more often to the teacher at age 2 or 3 is more likely to be the one who can hardly bear to let go of Mom on the first day of school. The gregarious toddler is probably the one who decides what game everyone will play at recess in first grade.

Psychologists normally use the word **personality** to describe these differences in the way children, and adults, go about relating to the people and objects in the world around them. Like the concept of intelligence, the concept of personality is designed to describe *enduring individual differences* in behavior.

Just as was true for cognition, we need to look at and try to understand both the common developmental patterns in children's social development and the individual differences in personality. Why do 5-year-olds normally show signs of individual friendships while 2-year-olds do not? What change makes that possible? Why are same-sex play groups much more obvious at school age than among preschoolers? And where do the personality differences come from? How does one child come to be shy and another gregarious? How does one child become a bully, another an accepted and popular friend? How does one child become securely attached, another insecurely attached, and what are the consequences of those variations over the long term?

I think the most helpful place to begin to try to answer this set of questions is to look at what we know about individual differences in personality and at the major theories that have been offered to explain personality development and variations. Then in the following two chapters, we can look more directly at the research on developmental changes in social behavior.

Defining Personality in Adults

Like the concept of intelligence, the concept of personality has been hard to define clearly. Most theorists and researchers have thought of personality in terms of variations on a set of basic traits or dimensions, such as shyness versus gregariousness or activity versus passivity. If we could identify the basic dimensions, we could then describe any individual's personality as a profile of those key traits. But coming to agreement on the nature of the key dimensions has been no simple task. Over the years, researchers and theorists

Table 9.1
The Big Five Personality Traits

Trait	Qualities of Individual High in That Trait
Extraversion	Active, assertive, energetic, enthusiastic, outgoing, talkative
Agreeableness	Affectionate, forgiving, generous, kind, sympathetic, trusting
Conscientiousness	Efficient, organized, planful, reliable, responsible, thorough
Neuroticism (also called emotional [in]stability)	Anxious, self-pitying, tense, touchy, unstable, worrying
Openness/intellect	Artistic, curious, imaginative, insightful, original, wide interests

Sources: McCrae & Costa, 1990; John et al., 1994, Table 1, p. 161.

have disagreed vehemently on how many such dimensions there might be, how they should be measured, or even whether there were any stable personality traits at all. But in the past decade, to the surprise of many psychologists, researchers in this disputatious field have reached consensus that adult personality can be adequately described as a set of variations along five major dimensions, often referred to as the **Big Five,** described in Table 9.1 (Digman, 1990; McCrae & John, 1992).

These same five dimensions have now been found in studies of adults in a variety of countries, including some non-Western cultures, which lends some cross-cultural validity for this list. At the very least, we know that this set of dimensions is not unique to American adults (Bond, Nakazato, & Shiraishi, 1975; Borkenau & Ostendorf, 1990). We also have good evidence that these five are stable traits; among adults, scores on these five dimensions have been shown to be stable over periods as long as a decade or two (Costa & McCrae, 1994). Finally, the usefulness of the Big Five as a description of personality has been validated by a variety of studies linking scores on these dimensions to behavior in a wide variety of real-life situations. For example, adults who are high in extraversion are more likely to be satisfied with their lives than are those low in extraversion. Similarly, those high in neuroticism have poorer health habits (they more often smoke, for example) and complain more about their health than do those low in neuroticism (Costa & McCrae, 1984). Thus, the Big Five, as measured either through self-reports or through reports by observers, appear to be both reliable and valid descriptions of personality.

How would you rate your own personality on each of the Big Five?

Defining Personality in Children

When we apply this new model to children's personality, things get more complicated. There are two tricky questions. First, do these same five dimensions accurately describe children's personality? Second, much of the study of individual differences in infant's and children's style and manner of interacting with the world has been couched in terms of temperament, not personality, so how do we connect these two bodies of research? I'll be coming back to this second question in a moment. But let me start with the first issue, whether the Big Five really describe children's personality.

The Big Five in Childhood

The answer seems to be yes. A small but growing body of research suggests that the same five factors that are a good description of adult personality also describe children's personality surprisingly well (Hartup & van Lieshout, 1995). For example, Cornelis van Lieshout and Gerbert Haselager, in a large study of children and adolescents in the Netherlands (1994), found that the five clearest dimensions characterizing their young subjects matched the Big Five very well, and this was as true among preschoolers as among adolescents, and among both boys and girls. In this sample, agreeableness and emotional (in)stability (equivalent to the neuroticism dimension) were the clearest dimensions, followed by conscientiousness, extraversion, and openness.

Similar results have come from a longitudinal study in the U.S. Oliver John and his colleagues (John et al., 1994) have studied a random sample of nearly 500 boys initially selected from among all fourth graders in the Pittsburgh public school system and followed up to age 13. Like the Dutch researchers, John has found strong evidence that the five-factor model captures the personality variations among these preteen boys. John's study is also helpful as a test of the five-factor model because he also has information on other aspects of the boys' behavior, such as their school success or their delinquent behavior. By comparing the personality profiles of boys who differ in some other way, he can check to see if the personality patterns differ in ways that make theoretical and conceptual sense. For example, Figure 9.1 contrasts the personality profiles of boys who reported delinquent activity versus boys who reported none. As John predicted, delinquent boys were markedly lower in both conscientiousness and agreeableness than nondelinquent boys. John also found that boys higher in conscientiousness do slightly better in school, just as you would expect.

A nice cross-cultural validation of the five-factor model comes from a study by Geldolph Kohnstamm and his colleagues (Havill et al., 1994; Kohnstamm et al., 1994), who asked parents in the U.S., the Netherlands, Belgium, and Surinam to describe their children, using whatever language they chose. He found that 70 to 80 percent

FIGURE 9.1 Twelve-year-olds who report more delinquent acts have quite different personality profiles from nondelinquent 12-year-olds—a set of results that helps to validate usefulness of the Big Five personality traits as a description of children's personality. (*Source:* John et al. 1994, Figure 1, p. 167.)

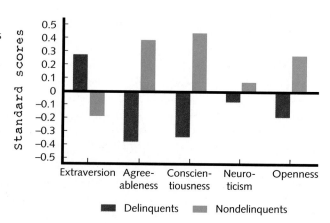

of the qualities mentioned by parents in every culture could be classified in one of the Big Five personality traits.

These early results are impressive and point to the usefulness of the five-factor model in describing children's personality. But it is still too soon to tell whether the Big Five will turn out to be the optimal way of describing children's personality. In particular, we may need more than five dimensions to describe children. For example, both John and his colleagues in their U.S. study and van Lieshout and Haselager in their Dutch study found two additional dimensions: irritability and activity level. Since both of these dimensions typically appear in descriptions of temperament, this brings us to the second hard question: What is the connection between all the Big Five research and studies of infant and child temperament?

Links to Temperament

I talked about temperament in Chapters 1 and 3, so the concept is not completely new. But what I am sure is not clear to you (and, honestly speaking, is not yet quite clear to most psychologists) is whether *temperament* is just another word for *personality*, or whether the two concepts are really different.

The clearest statement I can make, one that reflects most current thinking, is that **temperament** is the emotional *substrate* of personality—that set of core qualities or response patterns that are visible in infancy and reflected in such things as typical activity level, irritability or emotionality, soothability, fearfulness, and sociability (Hartup & van Lieshout, 1995, p. 658). According to this way of thinking, temperament is "the matrix from which later child and adult personality develops" (Ahadi & Rothbart, 1994, p. 190).

The distinction is a little like the difference between a genotype and a phenotype. The genotype sets the basic pattern, but the eventual outcome is the result of the basic pattern affected by specific experience. Thus, temperament may represent the basic pattern; what we measure as personality later in childhood or adulthood reflects the basic pattern affected by myriad life experiences.

If this model is correct, then variations in temperament ought to bear some (perhaps considerable) resemblance to the basic five personality dimensions we see in adulthood, although early temperament will probably not map directly onto the Big Five traits. Discovering whether this conceptualization actually matches the data has been made difficult by the fact that temperament researchers, unlike adult personality researchers, have not yet agreed on the best way to characterize the variations in early temperament. We don't have a nice, tidy list of "five basic temperament dimensions" to compare to the Big Five. Instead, we have many lists of temperamental variations.

Dimensions of Temperament.   You can get some feeling for the different views from Table 9.2, which lists the major dimensions of temperament proposed by three prominent temperament researchers. If you look carefully at these lists, you can see that there is a good deal of common ground, but no clear agreement—all of which has led to a good deal of confusion. However, the most recent writings of many of the key researchers offer some hope of consensus (Ahadi & Rothbart, 1994; Kagan, 1994; Martin, Wisenbaker, & Huttunen, 1994). Many theorists are now emphasizing a number of key dimensions and are actively exploring the possible links between these key dimensions of temperament and the Big Five. These often mentioned temperament dimensions are the following:

Table 9.2
Dimensions of Temperament Suggested by Various Theorists

Thomas and Chess[a]	Buss and Plomin	Rothbart
Activity level *Rhythmicity* *Approach/withdrawal* *Adaptability to new experience* *Threshold of responsiveness* *Intensity of reaction* *Quality of Mood* (+ or –) *Distractibility* *Persistence*	*Activity level:* variations in tempo, in vigor, and in endurance *Emotionality:* variations in the tendency to become distressed or upset easily or intensely (either with fear or anger) *Sociability:* variations in the tendency to seek and be gratified by rewards from social interaction; high level of responsivity toward others	*Extraversion/positive emotionality:* underlying tendency to approach rather than withdraw, with positive emotional tone *Negative affect/anxiety:* underlying tendency to respond with fear or withdrawal to novel experiences; sensitivity to threat *Effortful control:* variations in ability to regulate attention, self-soothing, behavioral inhibition, or the like

[a]Recall from Chapter 3 that Thomas and Chess describe three clusters based on these nine dimensions: the easy child, the difficult child, and the slow-to-warm-up child.

Sources: Thomas & Chess, 1977; Buss, 1989; Rothbart, Ahadi, & Hershey, 1994; Ahadi & Rothbart, 1994; Rothbart, Posner, & Hershey, 1995.

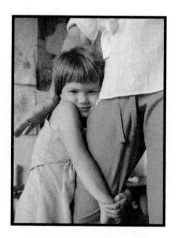

This child, clinging to her mom's leg, would probably be rated as relatively high in "behavioral inhibition," one of the commonly observed dimensions of temperament in infants and children.

- *Activity level.* A tendency to move often and vigorously, rather than to remain passive or immobile. High activity is most often hypothesized as a precursor to extraversion (Martin et al., 1994), although some high activity in infancy can also be part of strong negative emotion, which may link to later neuroticism.

- *Approach/positive emotionality.* A tendency to move toward rather than away from people, new things, objects, usually accompanied by positive emotion. This is similar to what Buss and Plomin call sociability and seems to be another obvious precursor to extraversion at later ages. It may also be a precursor to what is later measured as friendliness.

- *Inhibition.* The flip side of approach is a tendency to respond with fear or withdrawal to new people, new situations, new objects. This dimension has been intensely studied by Jerome Kagan and his colleagues (e.g., Kagan, 1994; Kagan, Reznick, & Snidman, 1990), who see this as the precursor to what is called "shyness" in everyday language. In the five-factor model, this would be reflected in very low scores on extraversion.

- *Negative emotionality.* A tendency to respond with anger, fussing, loudness, or irritability; a low threshold of frustration. An obvious precursor to what is later called neuroticism. This appears to be what Thomas and Chess are tapping with their concept of the "difficult" child, and what Buss and Plomin call emotionality.

- *Effortful control/task persistence.* An ability to stay focused, to manage attention and effort. This looks like a precursor to conscientiousness.

This is obviously not a final list; temperament researchers are still working their way toward common ground. But this set of traits or qualities is probably fairly close to the list temperament researchers will eventually agree on. At the very least, we know that babies and young children do differ on these dimensions, and we have at least some reasonable hypotheses about how these early variations may link to later stable personality characteristics. That's saying a lot.

But that still leaves us with several huge questions to answer: Where do these differences come from? And how are they transformed into adult personality? It is also important not to ignore the common developmental patterns. Are there phases or stages all children appear to go through in forming an adult personality?

Questions like these obviously take us into the realm of theory. So buckle up, folks; we're going on a fast trip through the theoretical landscape.

None of the basic dimensions of temperament listed here is an obvious precursor to either agreeableness or openness/intellect. Can you think of qualities of infants or young children that might be linked in some causal way to these two later facets of personality?

The Major Explanations of Personality Development

Three of the four major theoretical orientations I talked about in Chapter 1 are evident in theories of social and personality development: (1) *Biological explanations* focus on possible genetic, hormonal, or neurological bases for individual differences in temperament and personality; (2) *learning explanations* also focus on individual differences but explain them as products of each child's reinforcement history; (3) *psychoanalytically oriented explanations* offer a description of both developmental change and the origins of individual differences in personality. Let me lay out each of these alternative models as a set of propositions.

Genetic and Physiological Bases of Temperament and Personality

The biological argument runs like this:

Proposition 1: Each individual is born with genetically determined characteristic patterns of responding to the environment and to other people. Virtually every researcher who studies temperament shares the assumption that temperamental qualities are *inborn,* carried in the genes. The idea here is not so very different from the notion of "inborn biases" or "constraints" I have been talking about in earlier chapters, except that here we are talking about *individual* rather than shared behavioral dispositions.

Clear, strong evidence supports such an assertion (Rose, 1995), both in studies of adult personality (discussed in the *Research Report* on page 255) and in studies of children's temperament. Studies of twins in many countries show that identical twins are quite a lot more alike in their temperament or personality than are fraternal twins (Rose, 1995). One fairly typical set of results comes from a study by Robert Plomin, Robert Emde, and their many collaborators (Emde et al., 1992; Plomin et al., 1993). They have

Table 9.3
Similarity of Identical and Fraternal Twin Toddlers

Temperament Scale	14-Month Correlations		20-Month Correlations	
	Identical	Fraternal	Identical	Fraternal
Rated by Parents				
Emotionality	.35*	−.02	.51*	−.05
Activity	.50*	−.25	.59*	−.24
Sociability	.35*	.03	.51*	.11
Observed				
Behavioral inhibition	.57*	.26*	.45*	.17

*Indicates that the correlation is statistically significant.

Source: Plomin et al., 1993, from Table 2, p. 1364.

studied 100 pairs of identical and 100 pairs of fraternal twins at both 14 and 20 months. At each age, the toddlers' temperament was rated by their mothers using a modified version of the Buss and Plomin categories. In addition, each child's level of behavioral inhibition was measured at each age by observing how she reacted to a strange adult and strange toys in a special laboratory playroom. Did the child approach the novel toys quickly and eagerly, or did she hang back or seem fearful? Did she approach the strange adult, or did she remain close to Mom? You can see in Table 9.3 that the correlations between temperament scores of identical twins were consistently higher than those for fraternal twins, indicating a substantial genetic effect.

Proposition 2: These genetic differences operate via variations in fundamental physiological processes. Many (but not all) temperament theorists take the argument a step further and trace the basic differences in behavior to variations in underlying physiological patterns (Gunnar, 1994; Nelson, 1994; Rothbart, Derryberry, & Posner, 1994). For example, Jerome Kagan has suggested that differences in behavioral inhibition are based on differing thresholds for arousal in those parts of the brain, the amygdala and the hypothalamus, that control responses to uncertainty (1994; Kagan et al., 1990; Kagan, Snidman, & Arcus, 1993). Arousal of these parts of the brain leads to increases in muscle tension and heart rate. Shy or inhibited children are thought to have a *low* threshold for such a reaction. That is, they more readily become tense and alert in the presence of uncertainty, perhaps even interpreting a wider range of situations as uncertain. What we inherit, then, is not "shyness" or some equivalent, but a tendency for the brain to react in particular ways.

In support of this argument, Kagan reports correlations in the range of .60 between a measure of behavioral inhibition in children ages 2 to 5 and a series of physiological

Research Report

The Inheritance of Personality Patterns: Evidence from Adults

In the past decade, a number of methodologically careful new studies of adult twins have repeatedly demonstrated that identical twins are more like one another than are fraternal twins both on measures of the Big Five personality traits and on measures of temperament using Buss and Plomin's categories (Loehlin, 1992).

For example, a group of researchers including Nancy Pedersen and Robert Plomin (Bergeman et al., 1993; Pedersen et al., 1988) has taken advantage of the existence of an amazingly extensive and up-to-date twin registry in Sweden that includes 25,000 pairs of twins born between 1886 and 1958. From this set, they were able to identify 99 pairs of identical twins and 229 pairs of fraternal twins reared apart and could then compare these with similar groups of twins reared together. On each of the Big Five personality dimensions, identical twins were more similar than were fraternal twins. The degree of similarity was less for identical twins reared apart, but these pairs were nonetheless significantly more alike than were fraternal twins reared apart.

A smaller but much more famous study in the United States is the Minnesota Twin Study (Bouchard, 1984; Lykken et al., 1992; Tellegen et al., 1988)—a study that has been the subject of a great many articles in the popular press. These researchers have been particularly interested in identical twins reared apart, frequently arranging for them to meet one another for the first time. On standard personality tests they find the now familiar pattern: Identical twins are simply much more like one another than are fraternal twins, even when the identical twins did not grow up together. This was true on such measures as positive and negative emotionality (which may be similar to Buss and Plomin's dimension of emotionality), but also on less-obvious measures, such as a sense of "social potency" or a sense of well-being. Even a measure of "traditionalism"—an affinity for traditional values and a strong allegiance to established authority—shows slightly higher correlations among identical than among fraternal twins.

What has intrigued the popular press much more, though, are the less-precise but far more striking descriptions of the similarities in clothing preferences, interests, posture and body language, speed and tempo of talking, favorite jokes, and hobbies in pairs of identical twins reared apart:

One male pair who had never previously met arrived in England sporting identical beards, haircuts, wire-rimmed glasses and shirts. . . . One pair had practically the same items in their toilet cases, including the same brand of cologne and a Swedish brand of toothpaste. . . . [one pair] had the same fears and phobias. Both were afraid of water and had adopted the same coping strategy: backing into the ocean up to their knees. (Holden, 1987, p. 18)

It is difficult to imagine what sort of genetic process could account for similar preferences in hairstyles or for a particular brand of toothpaste. But we can't merely dismiss the results because they are hard to explain. At the very least, these findings certainly point to strong genetic components in many of the elements of personal style and emotional responsiveness that temperament researchers are trying to identify and track in children.

measures, such as muscle tension, heart rate, dilation of the pupil of the eye, and the chemical composition of both urine and saliva, all of which strongly suggests that temperament is based on physiological responses and is not simply a set of learned habits (1994; Kagan et al., 1990).

Proposition 3: Temperamental dispositions persist through childhood and into adulthood. No theorist in this tradition proposes that initial temperamental dispositions remain unchanged by experience—a point I'll come back to in a moment. But if temperamental patterns create a kind of "bias" in the system toward particular behaviors, we ought to see a fair amount of stability of temperament over time. Such stability ought to show itself in

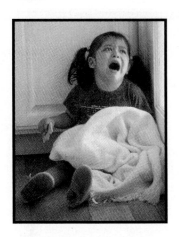

This preschooler may just be having a bad day. But if this is a typical reaction, one sign of a "difficult" temperament, she will be at higher risk for a variety of problems at later ages.

the form of at least modest correlations between measures of a given temperamental dimension from one age to another.

Although the research evidence is somewhat mixed, we have growing evidence of consistency in temperamental ratings over rather long periods of infancy and childhood. For example, Australian researchers studying a group of 450 children found that mothers' reports of children's irritability, cooperation/manageability, inflexibility, rhythmicity, persistency, and tendency to approach (rather than avoid) contact were all quite consistent from infancy through age 8 (Pedlow et al., 1993). Similarly, in an American longitudinal study covering the years from age 1 to age 12, Diana Guerin and Allen Gottfried (1994a; 1994b) found strong consistency in parent reports of their children's overall "difficultness" as well as approach versus withdrawal, positive versus negative mood, and activity level.

Kagan has also found considerable consistency over the same age range in his measure of inhibition, which is based on direct observation of the child's behavior rather than on the mother's ratings of the child's temperament. He reports that half of babies in his longitudinal study who had shown high levels of crying and motor activity in response to a novel situation when they were 4 months old were still classified as highly inhibited at age 8, while three-fourths of those rated as uninhibited at 4 months remained in that category eight years later (Kagan et al., 1993).

Thus, babies who readily and positively approach the world around them continue to be more positive as young teenagers, while cranky, temperamentally difficult babies continue to show many of the same temperamental qualities 10 years later, and strongly behaviorally inhibited babies are quite likely to continue to show such "shyness" at later ages.

Proposition 4: Temperamental characteristics interact with the child's environment in ways that may either strengthen or modify the basic temperamental patterns. Clearly, however, temperament does not inevitably determine personality. The child's experiences play a crucial role as well.

A number of temperament/environment interactions tend to strengthen the built-in qualities. For one thing, each of us—including young children—*chooses* our experiences. Highly sociable children seek out contact with others; children low on the activity dimension are more likely to choose sedentary activities like puzzles or board games than baseball. Similarly, temperament may affect the way in which a child *interprets* a given experience—a factor that helps to account for the fact that two children in the same family may experience the family pattern of interaction quite differently.

Imagine, for example, a family that moves often, such as a military family. If one child in this family has a strong built-in pattern of behavioral inhibition, the myriad changes and new experiences will trigger fear responses over and over. This child comes to anticipate each new move with dread and is likely to interpret his family life as highly stressful. A second child in the same family, with a more strongly approach-oriented temperament, finds the many moves stimulating and energizing, and is likely to think of his childhood in a much more positive light.

A third environmental factor that often reinforces built-in temperamental patterns is the tendency of parents (and others in the child's world) to respond differently to children with varying temperaments. The sociable child, who may smile often, is likely to elicit more smiles, more positive interactions with parents, simply because she has reinforced their behavior by her positive temperament. Buss and Plomin (1984) have proposed the general argument that children in the middle range on temperament dimensions typically

Research Report

Temperament and Behavior Problems

One of the consistent findings in the research on temperament is that children with difficult temperaments are much more likely to show various kinds of emotional disturbance or *behavior problems* than are children with less-extreme temperaments. Included in the category of behavior problems (which I'll be talking about in more detail in Chapter 15, when I discuss abnormal development) are such patterns as overaggressiveness, depression, anxiety, and hyperactivity.

The typical finding is that children who are rated as having aspects of difficult temperament are perhaps twice as likely to show one or another of these behavior problems as are children with less-difficult temperaments (Bates, 1989; Bates, Maslin, & Frankel, 1985; Chess & Thomas, 1984). So babies with more difficult temperaments are more likely to become preschoolers who show some behavior problem, and preschoolers whose temperament is rated as difficult or who are "lacking in control" are more likely to have behavior problems at age 10 or 15 or even as adults (Caspi et al., 1995).

Such findings may sound like a simple restatement of consistency of temperament. Perhaps hyperactivity, aggressiveness, or other behavior problems in 5-year-olds or 7-year-olds are simply further manifestations of a basically difficult temperament. But it is not so easy. The majority of children who are rated as showing "difficult" temperament in infancy or the preschool years do *not* develop behavior problems at later ages. They are more *likely* to exhibit such problems, but the relationship is not at all inevitable.

As usual, a complex interactive process is involved. The key seems to be whether the infant's or child's "difficultness" is acceptable to the parents or can be managed by the family in some effective way. For example, Fish, Stifter, and Belsky (1991) have studied changes and continuities in crying patterns in a small sample of infants. They found that those babies who had cried a great deal as newborns but cried much less at 5 months had mothers who were highly responsive and sensitive to the infants. Babies who cried a lot at both time points had much-less-responsive mothers. Thus, the responsive mother may have reshaped the baby's inborn temperamental behavior. Difficult temperament also seems to increase the risk of behavior problems when there are other stresses in the family system (such as divorce), or other deficits in the child, such as physical disability or retardation (Chess & Korn, 1980).

Thus, difficult temperament does not *cause* later behavior problems. Rather, it creates a *vulnerability* in the child. Such children seem to be less able to deal with major life stresses. But in a supportive, accepting, low-stress environment, many such children move through childhood without displaying any significant behavior problems.

The lesson for parents is not always an easy one. If you are under severe stress, that is precisely the moment when it is hard to provide a maximally supportive, accepting environment for any child, let alone a temperamentally difficult child. But it may still help to keep in mind that a child with a difficult temperament is going to need more attention, more help, more support than will a temperamentally less volatile child under any kind of stress, such as when the family moves, when the child changes schools or babysitters, or if the family pet dies.

adapt *to* their environment, while those whose temperament is extreme—like extremely difficult children—force their environment to adapt to them. Parents of difficult children, for example, adapt to the children's negativity by punishing them more and providing them with less support and stimulation than do parents of more adaptable children (Luster, Boger, & Hannan, 1993; Rutter, 1978). This pattern may well contribute to the higher rates of significant emotional problems in such children, a set of results I have explored in the *Research Report* above.

But Buss and Plomin's proposal, while accurate, doesn't convey the additional complexities of the process. First of all, sensitive and responsive parents can moderate the more extreme forms of infant or child temperament. A particularly nice example comes from the work of Megan Gunnar and her colleagues (1994), who have studied a group of highly inhibited toddlers who differed in the security of their attachment to their mothers. In a series of studies (Colton et al., 1992; Nachmias, 1993), they found that *inse-*curely attached inhibited toddlers showed the usual physiological responses to challenging or novel situations. But *securely* attached temperamentally inhibited toddlers showed no such indications of physiological arousal in the face of novelty or challenge. Thus, the secure attachment appears to have modified a basic physiological/temperamental response. Over time, this may shift the child's personality pattern away from extreme inhibition or shyness.

Thus, while many forces within the environment tend to reinforce the child's basic temperament and thus create stability and consistency of temperament/personality over time, environmental forces can also push a child toward new patterns or aid a child in controlling extreme forms of basic physiological reactions.

Critique of Biological Theories

This approach to the origins of personality has two great strengths. First, it is strongly supported by a large body of empirical research. There is simply no refuting the fact that built-in genetic and physiological patterns underlie what we think of as both temperament and personality. This approach thus provides a powerful counterweight to what had been an almost completely environmental model of personality development.

Paradoxically, the second strength I see is that this is not a *purely* biological approach; it is an interactionist approach, very much in keeping with much of the current theorizing about development. The child is born with certain behavioral tendencies, but the eventual outcome depends on the transactions between a child's initial characteristics and the responses of the environment.

On the other side of the ledger I see a number of problems, not the least of which is the continuing disagreement about just what the basic dimensions of temperament really are—a disagreement clear in Table 9.2. Because researchers have used such varying definitions and varying measures, it is often difficult to add up the results of different investigations.

A second problem, at least from my perspective, is that current biologically oriented temperament theories are not fundamentally *developmental* theories. They allow for change through the mechanism of interaction with the environment. But they do not tell us whether we might expect systematic age differences in children's responses to new situations or to people; they do not tell us whether the child's emerging cognitive skills have anything to do with changes in the child's temperamental patterns. They do not, in a word, tell us how the *shared* developmental patterns may interact with the inborn individual differences.

Neither of these concerns constitutes a refutation of any of the basic tenets of this theoretical approach. We can simply no longer ignore the importance of genetic differences and basic biology in shaping individual differences in temperament or personality.

Learning Explanations of Personality and Temperament

The emphasis shifts rather dramatically when we look at social learning approaches. Instead of looking at what the child brings to the equation, learning theorists have looked primarily at the reinforcement patterns in the environment as the primary cause of differences in children's patterns of behavior. Of course theorists in this tradition do not reject biology. Albert Bandura, arguably the most influential theorist in this group, grants that biological factors such as hormones or inherited propensities (such as temperament, presumably) also affect behavior. But he and others of this persuasion look to the environment as the major source of influence.

These are not new ideas for you. You have already read about the basic concepts in Chapter 1 and encountered a version of such a theory in Skinner's explanation of language acquisition. The question here is how to apply this theory specifically to such temperamental characteristics as activity level or gregariousness, or such social behaviors—often thought of as part of personality—as aggressiveness or dependency.

The "learning" camp includes several distinct schools of thought. Some, often called radical behaviorists, argue that only the basic principles of classical and operant conditioning are needed to account for variations in behavior, including personality. Others, like Bandura, emphasize not only observational learning but also important cognitive elements. Both groups would agree with the first two propositions I've listed next; the remaining propositions emerge primarily from Bandura's work.

Proposition 1: Behavior is "strengthened" by reinforcement. If this rule applies to all behavior, then it should apply to attachment, shyness, sharing, or competitiveness. Children who are reinforced for clinging to their parents, for example, should show more clinging than do children who are not reinforced for it. Similarly, a nursery school teacher who pays attention to children only when they get rowdy or aggressive should find that the children get steadily more rowdy and aggressive over the course of weeks or months.

Proposition 2: Behavior that is reinforced on a "partial schedule" should be even stronger and more resistant to extinction than behavior that is consistently reinforced. I talked briefly about this phenomenon in Chapter 1, so you have some idea of what is involved. Parents are nearly always inconsistent in their rewards to their children, so most children are on partial schedules of some kind, whether the parent intends that or not. That is, they are sometimes reinforced for a particular behavior, but not every time. Because behavior that is rewarded in this way is highly persistent—highly *resistant to extinction,* in the language of learning theory—partial reinforcement patterns are a major factor in the establishment of those distinctive and stable patterns of behavior defined as personality.

Can you think of other real-life examples of partial reinforcement in action? What about things you do to please your partner, for which you get a smile only some of the time?

An immense collection of studies supports these first two propositions. For example, in several studies, experimenters systematically rewarded some children for hitting an inflated rubber clown on the nose. When the researchers later watched the children in a play situation, they found that the children who had been rewarded showed more hitting, scratching, and kicking than did children who hadn't been rewarded for punching the clown (Walters & Brown, 1963). Partial reinforcement in the form of inconsistent behavior from parents also has the expected effect. For example, Sears, Maccoby, and Levin (1977) found that parents who permit fairly high levels of aggression in their children but occasionally react by punishing it quite severely have children who are more aggressive than are children whose parents neither permit nor punish aggression.

Gerald Patterson's research on families with aggressive or noncompliant children, which I described in Chapter 1, also illustrates the significance of these basic principles. If you go back and look at Figure 1.2 (p. 11), you'll see that the heart of Patterson's model is a link between "poor parental discipline" and resultant conduct problems in the child. He is arguing here that both normal personality patterns and deviant forms of social behavior have their roots in daily social exchanges with family members. For example,

The Real World

Applying Learning Principles at Home

It is a lot harder than you may think to apply basic learning principles consistently and correctly with children at home or in schools. Virtually all parents do try to reinforce some behaviors in their children by praising them or by giving them attention or treats. And most of us do our best to discourage unpleasant behavior through punishment. But it is easy to misapply the principles or to create unintended consequences because we have not fully understood all the mechanisms involved.

For example, suppose you have a favorite armchair in your living room that is being systematically ruined by the dirt and pressure of little feet climbing up the back of the chair. You want the children to *stop* climbing up the chair. So you scold them. After a while you may even stoop to nagging. If you are really conscientious and knowledgeable, you may carefully try to time your scolding so that it operates as a negative reinforcer, by stopping your scolding when they stop climbing. But nothing works. They keep on leaving those muddy footprints on your favorite chair. Why? It could be because the children *enjoy* climbing up the chair. So the climbing is intrinsically reinforcing to the children, and that effect is clearly stronger than your negative reinforcement or punishment. One way to deal with this might be to provide something *else* for them to climb on.

Another example: Suppose your 3-year-old son repeatedly demands your attention while you are fixing dinner (a common state of affairs, as any parent of a 3-year-old can tell you). Because you don't want to reinforce this behavior, you ignore him the first six or eight times he says "Mommy" or tugs at your clothes. But after the ninth or tenth repetition, with his voice getting louder and whinier each time, you can't stand it any longer and finally say something like "All right! What do you want?" Since you have ignored most of his demands, you might well be convinced that you have not been reinforcing his demanding behavior. But what you have actually done is to create a partial reinforcement schedule; you have rewarded only every tenth demand or whine. And we know that this pattern of reinforcement helps to create behavior that is *very* hard to extinguish. So your son may continue to be demanding and whining for a very long time, even if you succeed in ignoring it completely.

If such situations are familiar to you, it may pay to keep careful records for a while, keeping track of each incident and your response, and then see if you can figure out which principles are really at work and how you might change the pattern.

imagine a child playing in his very messy room. The mother comes into the room and tells the child to clean up his room. The child whines or yells at her that he doesn't want to do it, or won't do it. The mother gives in, leaves the room, and the child stops whining or shouting.

Patterson analyzes this exchange as a pair of negatively reinforced events. When the mother gives in to the child's defiance, her own behavior (giving in) is negatively reinforced by the ending of the child's whining or yelling. This makes it more likely that she will give in the next time. She has *learned* to back down in order to get the child to shut up. At the same time, the child has been negatively reinforced for yelling or whining, since the unpleasant event for him (being told to clean his room) stopped as soon as he whined. So he has learned to whine or yell. Imagine such exchanges occurring over and over, and you begin to understand how a family can create a *system* in which an imperious, demanding, noncompliant child rules the roost (Snyder et al., 1994).

As I pointed out in Chapter 1, Patterson's thinking has moved beyond the simple propositions I have outlined here. Like the current temperament theorists, he emphasizes that what happens in a given family, for a particular child, is a joint product of the child's own temperament or response tendencies, the parents' discipline skills, the parents' personalities, and the social context of the parents' lives. But Patterson is still assuming that basic learning principles can both describe and explain the ways in which the child's behavior pattern (his "personality") is formed or changed. And he and others have shown that it is possible to *change* the child's typical behavior by helping families learn new and more effective reinforcement and management strategies, and in this way to reduce the likelihood of later delinquency (Tremblay et al., 1995; Wierson & Forehand, 1994).

Proposition 3: Children learn new behaviors largely through modeling. Bandura has argued that the full range of social behaviors, from competitiveness to nurturance, is learned not just by direct reinforcement, but also by watching others perform those actions. Thus, the child who sees her parents taking a casserole next door to the woman who has just been widowed will learn generosity and thoughtful behavior. The child who sees her parents arguing or hitting each other when they are angry will most likely learn violent ways of solving problems.

Children learn from TV too and from their peers, their teachers, and their brothers and sisters. A boy growing up in an environment where he observes playmates and older boys hanging around street corners, shoplifting, or stealing hubcaps is going to learn all those behaviors. His continuous exposure to such antisocial models makes it that much harder for his parents to reinforce more constructive behavior.

These many effects of observational learning have been demonstrated experimentally in literally hundreds of studies (Bandura, 1973; 1977). One interesting—and very practical—sidelight to the process of modeling has been the repeated finding that modeling works better than preaching. So displaying the desired behavior yourself—such as generosity, fairness, or diligent work—works better than simply telling kids that it is good to be generous or fair or hardworking.

For example, in one early study, Joan Grusec and her co-workers (Grusec, Saas-Kortsaak, & Simutis, 1978) had elementary school children play a miniature bowling game, ostensibly to test the game. The children first observed an adult "test" the game and saw the adult win 20 marbles. Next to the bowling game was a poster that said "Help poor children. Marbles buy gifts." Under the poster was a bowl with some marbles in it. Half the time the adult model donated half his newly won marbles to this bowl; the other half of the time he did not. In addition, the model either "preached" about donating marbles or said nothing. To some of the children he preached in specific terms, saying that the child should donate half his marbles when he played the game, since it would be good to make poor children happy by doing that. To other children, he preached in more general terms, saying that the child should donate half his marbles because it is a good thing to make other people happy by helping them any way one can. The adult model then left the room and the child had an opportunity to play the bowling game and to decide whether to donate any marbles. You can see in Figure 9.2 how many children in each group (out of a maximum of 16) donated marbles. Clearly, modeling worked better than preaching. And when a conflict exists between what the model says and what the model does—such as when parents smoke but tell their kids that they should not smoke—children generally follow the behavior and not the verbal message. So the old adage "Do what I say and not what I do" doesn't seem to work.

However, learning from modeling is not an entirely automatic process. Bandura points out that what a child (or adult) learns from watching someone else will depend on four things: what she pays attention to, what she is able to remember (both *cognitive* processes), what she is physically able to copy, and what she is motivated to imitate. Because attentional abilities, memory, and other cognitive processes change with age

Suppose you were trying to learn a new sport, such as tennis or soccer, by observing an expert. Can you see how these four principles would affect what you were able to learn from the model?

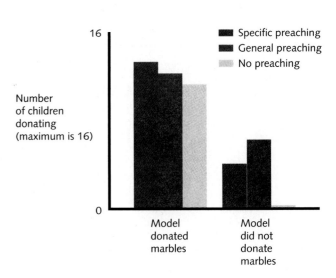

FIGURE 9.2 These results from Grusec's modeling study illustrate the general finding that modeling is more powerful than preaching in changing children's behavior. (*Source:* Grusec, Saas-Kortsaak, & Simutis, 1978, from Table 1, p. 922.)

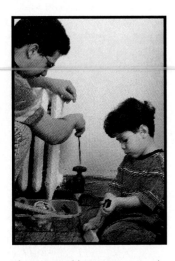

Three-year-old Marvin is not only learning something about how to use a screwdriver from observing his dad, but also is learning his father's attitudes about work and perhaps the beginnings of self-efficacy.

through infancy and childhood, what a baby or child can or will learn from any given modeled event will also change through development (Grusec, 1992).

Proposition 4: Children learn not only overt behavior but also ideas, expectations, internal standards, and self-concepts from reinforcement and modeling. The child learns standards for his own behavior and expectancies about what he can and cannot do (which Bandura calls *self-efficacy*) from specific reinforcements and from modeling. In this way, the child *internalizes* what he has learned. Once those standards and those expectancies or beliefs are established, they affect the child's behavior in consistent and enduring ways and form the core of what may be called personality.

Critique of Learning Models

Several implications of this overall theoretical approach are worth emphasizing. First of all, learning theorists can handle either consistency or inconsistency in children's behavior. If a child is friendly and smiling both at home and at school, this could be explained by saying that the child was being reinforced for that behavior in both settings rather than by assuming that the child has a "gregarious temperament." Or if the child is helpful at school but defiant at home, we need only invoke the principle that different reinforcement contingencies are at work in the two settings. To be sure, because individuals tend to choose settings that support or reward their accustomed behavior and because a person's behavior tends to *elicit* similar responses (reinforcements) from others in many settings, there is a bias toward consistency. But learning theorists have less trouble accounting for normal "situational variability" in behavior than do other theorists.

A related implication is that learning theorists are supremely optimistic about the possibility of change. Children's behavior can change if the reinforcement system (or their beliefs about themselves) changes, so "problem behavior" can be modified.

The great strength of this view of personality and social behavior is that it gives an accurate picture of the way in which many specific behaviors are learned. It is perfectly clear that children do learn through modeling; and it is equally clear that children (and adults) will continue to perform behaviors that "pay off" for them.

The addition of the cognitive elements to Bandura's theory adds further strength, since it offers a beginning integration of learning models and cognitive-developmental approaches. If we were to apply Piaget's language to Bandura's theory, we could talk about the acquisition of a "self-scheme"—a concept of one's own capacities, qualities, standards, and experiences. New experiences are then assimilated to that scheme. You will recall from Chapter 7 that one of the characteristics of the process of assimilation as Piaget proposed it is that new experiences or information are modified as they are taken in. In the same way, Bandura is saying that once the child's self-concept is established, it affects what behaviors she chooses to perform, how she reacts to new experiences, whether she persists or gives up on some new task, and the like. If a child believes he is unpopular, for example, then he will not be surprised if others do not choose to sit by him in the lunchroom; if someone does sit next to him, he's likely to explain it to himself in such a way that he retains his central belief, such as "there must have been no place else to sit." In this way the underlying scheme isn't modified (accommodated) very much.

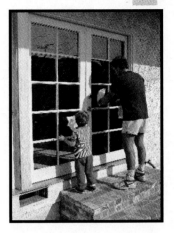

This toddler is happily helping his dad wash windows (yet another example of modeling). But there is no guarantee that he will be equally helpful to his mother—a kind of inconsistency that learning theorists can handle more easily than temperament theorists can.

Just as biological temperament theorists argue that inborn temperament serves as a central mediating process, shaping the child's choices and behavior, so in social learning theory, the self-concept or self-scheme acts as a central mediator, leading to stable differences in behavior of the kind we typically call personality. It *can* be modified (accommodated) if the child accumulates enough experience or evidence that doesn't fit with the existing scheme—in learning theory language, if the reinforcement contingencies change in some dramatic way. If the "unpopular" child noticed that classmates regularly chose to sit next to him at lunch even when there were other seats available, he might eventually change his self-scheme, coming to think of himself as "somewhat popular." But since the child (like the adult) will choose activities or situations that fit his self-concept, such as sitting in the corner where no one is likely to see him, he will be partially protected from such "nonconfirming" experiences.

To be sure, Bandura and Piaget would not agree on how this self-concept or self-scheme develops. Piaget emphasizes internal processes while Bandura emphasizes reinforcement and modeling as causal factors. But they agree on the impact that such a scheme will have once it has developed.

Think for a minute about the ways you choose activities that are consistent with your self-image or self-scheme. What would it take for you to change some of the key portions of your self-scheme?

At the same time, these learning theories have significant weaknesses, particularly the more radical versions. First, from the perspective of many psychologists, these theories still place too much emphasis on what happens *to* the child and not enough on what the child is doing with the information he has. Bandura's theory is much less vulnerable to this charge, but most learning theories of personality are highly mechanistic and focused on external events. Second, like biological temperament theories, these are not really *developmental* theories. They can say how a child might acquire a particular behavior pattern or belief, but they do not take into account the underlying developmental changes that are occurring. Do 3-year-olds and 10-year-olds develop a sense of self-efficacy in the same way? Do they learn the same amount or in the same way from modeling? Given Bandura's emphasis on the cognitive aspects of the modeling process, a genuinely developmental social learning theory could be proposed, although no such theory now exists. Still, despite these limitations, all the theories in this group offer useful descriptions of one source of influence on the child's developing pattern of behavior.

Psychoanalytic Models of Personality Development

Like many temperament theorists, and like social learning theorists of Bandura's stripe, psychoanalytic theorists believe that the interaction between the child's inborn characteristics and the environment plays a central role in shaping differences in personality. But unlike temperament or learning theories, psychoanalytic theories are clearly *developmental* as well, describing systematic changes in children's sense of self, in their needs or drives, and in their relationships with others.

In Chapter 1, I described a number of the key propositions of this approach. Here let me simply summarize Freud's and Erikson's views:

Proposition 1: Behavior is governed by unconscious as well as conscious motives and processes. Freud emphasized three sets of instinctual drives: the sexual drive (libido); life-preserving drives, including avoidance of hunger and pain; and aggressive drives. Erikson emphasizes a more cognitive process, the drive for identity.

Proposition 2: Personality structure develops over time, as a result of the interaction between the child's inborn drives/needs and the responses of the key people in the child's world. Because the child is often prevented from achieving instant gratification of his various drives, he is forced to develop new skills—planning, talking, delaying, and other cognitive techniques that allow gratification of the basic needs in more indirect ways. Thus, the ego is created, and it remains the planning, organizing, thinking part of the personality. The superego, in turn, develops because the parents try to restrain certain kinds of gratification; the child eventually incorporates these parental standards into his own personality.

Proposition 3: Development of personality is fundamentally stagelike, with each stage centered on a particular task or a particular form of basic need. I'll describe both Freud's and Erikson's stages in some detail in a moment. For now the key point is only that there *are* stages in these theories.

Proposition 4: The specific personality a child develops depends on the degree of success the child has in traversing these various stages. In each stage, the child requires a particular kind of supportive environment for successfully resolving that dilemma or for meeting that need. A child lacking the needed environment will have a very different personality than one whose environment was partially or wholly adequate. However, while each stage is important, all the psychoanalytic theorists strongly emphasize the crucial significance of the very earliest stages and focus especially on the adequacy of the relationship between the baby and the central caregiver, usually the mother. This is not quite like saying that infancy is a sensitive period for personality development; rather, Freud and later psychoanalytic theorists argue that the earliest relationship establishes a pattern and sets the child on a particular pathway through the remainder of the stages.

Some Differences Between Freud and Erikson

All four of these general propositions are contained in both Freud's and Erikson's theories, but both the details and the emphases differ in important respects. In Freud's theory, for example, cognitive skills develop only because the child needs them to obtain gratification; they have no independent life. In Erikson's theory (and in many other variations of psychoanalytic theory), cognitive skills are part of a set of ego functions that are presumed to develop independently, rather than being entirely in the service of basic gratification.

Basic physical maturation is also more central to Freud's theory than to Erikson's. In Freud's theory, the stages shift from one to the next in part because of maturation of the nervous system. In each stage, the child is attempting to gratify basic physical ("sexual") needs through stimulation of a particular part of the body—that part of the body that is most sensitive at that time. As neurological development proceeds, maximum body sensitivity shifts from the mouth to the anus to the genitals, and this maturational change is part of what drives the stage changes. Erikson grants such physical changes but places greater emphasis on shifts in the demands of the social environment. Each stage centers on a specific social conflict, resulting in a psychosocial crisis. For example, stage 4 (industry versus inferiority) begins at about age 6 because that is when the child goes off to school; in a culture in which schooling was delayed, the timing of the developmental task might be delayed as well.

Because of such theoretical differences, Erikson and Freud have described the stages of development differently. Because both sets of stages have become part of the vocabulary of developmental psychology, you need to be conversant with both, so let me describe each.

Freud's Psychosexual Stages

Freud proposed five **psychosexual stages,** which I've summarized in Table 9.4.

The Oral Stage: Birth to 1 Year. The mouth, tongue, and lips are the first center of pleasure for the baby, and his earliest attachment is to the one who provides pleasure in the mouth, usually his mother. For normal development the infant requires some optimum amount of oral stimulation—not too much and not too little. If the optimum amount of stimulation is unavailable, then some libidinal energy may remain attached to (*fixated* on, in Freud's terms) the oral mode of gratification. Such an individual, so Freud thought, will continue to have a strong preference for oral pleasures in later life, as you can see in the right-hand column in Table 9.4.

The Anal Stage: 1 to 3 Years. As the trunk matures, the baby becomes more and more sensitive in the anal region. At about the same time, her parents begin to place great emphasis on toilet training and show pleasure when she manages to perform in the right place at the right time. These two forces together help to shift the major center of physical/sexual energy from the oral to the anal erogenous zone.

The key to the child's successful completion of this stage (according to Freud) is whether the parents allow the child sufficient anal exploration and pleasure. If toilet training becomes a major battleground, then some fixation of energy at this stage may occur—with the possible adult consequences of excessive orderliness, stinginess, or the opposite.

The Phallic Stage: 3 to 5 Years. At about 3 or 4 years of age the genitals increase in sensitivity, ushering in a new stage. One sign of this new sensitivity is that children of both sexes quite naturally begin to masturbate at about this age.

In Freud's view, the most important event that occurs during the phallic stage is the so-called **Oedipus conflict.** He described the sequence of events more fully (and more believably!) for boys, so let me trace that pattern for you.

The theory suggests that first the boy somehow becomes "intuitively aware of his mother as a sex object" (Rappoport, 1972, p. 74). Precisely how this occurs is not completely spelled out, but the important point is that the boy at about age 4 begins to have a sort of sexual attachment to his mother and to regard his father as a sexual rival. His father sleeps with his mother, holds her, and kisses her, and generally has access to her body

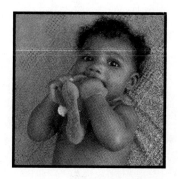

Freud thought that babies put things into their mouths because that is where they have the most pleasurable sensations. If babies don't get enough oral stimulation, he argued, they may become fixated at the oral stage.

Table 9.4
Freud's Stages of Psychosexual Development

Stage	Age	Erogenous Zones	Major Developmental Task (potential source of conflict)	Some Adult Personality Traits of Children Who Have Been "Fixated" at This Stage, According to Freud
Oral	0–1	Mouth, lips, tongue	Weaning	Oral behavior, such as smoking and over-eating; passivity and gullibility
Anal	2–3	Anus	Toilet training	Orderliness, parsi-moniousness, obsti-nacy, or the opposite
Phallic	4–5	Genitals	Oedipus complex; identification with parent of same sex	Vanity, recklessness, and the opposite
Latency	6–12	No specific area; sexual energy quiescent	Development of ego defense mechanisms	None; fixation does not normally occur
Genital	13–18 and adulthood	Genitals	Mature sexual intimacy	Adults who have successfully integrat-ed earlier stages should emerge with a sincere interest in others and mature sexuality

in a way that the boy does not. The boy also sees his father as a powerful and threatening figure who has the ultimate power—the power to castrate. The boy is caught between desire for his mother and fear of his father's power.

Most of these feelings and the resultant conflict are unconscious. The boy does not have overt sexual feelings or behavior toward his mother. But unconscious or not, the result of this conflict is anxiety. How can the little boy handle this anxiety? In Freud's view, the boy responds with a defensive process called **identification:** The boy "incorporates" his image of his father and attempts to match his own behavior to that image. By trying to make himself as like his father as possible, the boy not only reduces the chance of an attack from the father, but also takes on some of the father's power. Furthermore, it is this "inner father," with his values and moral judgments, who serves as the core of the child's superego.

A parallel process is supposed to occur in girls. The girl sees her mother as a rival for her father's sexual attentions and has some fear of her mother (though less than is true for

Can you think of any kind of study that would tell us whether Freud was right or not about the Oedipus conflict?

the boy, since the girl may assume she has already been castrated). In this case too, identification with the mother is thought to be the "solution" to the girl's anxiety.

The Latency Stage: 5 to 12 Years. Freud thought that after the phallic stage came a sort of resting period before the next major change in the child's sexual development. The child has presumably arrived at some preliminary resolution of the Oedipus conflict and now goes through a kind of calm after the storm. One of the obvious characteristics of this stage is that the identification with the same-sex parent that defined the end of the phallic stage is now extended to others of the same sex. So it is during these years that children's peer interactions are almost exclusively with members of the same sex and that children often have "crushes" on same-sex teachers or other adults.

The Genital Stage: 12 to 18 and Older. The further changes in hormones and the genital organs that take place during puberty reawaken the sexual energy of the child. During this period a more mature form of sexual attachment occurs. From the beginning of this period, the child's sexual objects are people of the opposite sex. Freud placed some emphasis on the fact that not everyone works through this period to a point of mature heterosexual love. Some have not had a satisfactory oral period and thus do not have a foundation of basic love relationships. Some have not resolved the Oedipus conflict with a complete or satisfactory identification with the same-sex parent, a failure that may affect their ability to cope with rearoused sexual energies in adolescence.

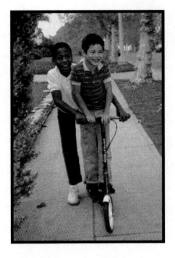

In elementary school, boys play with boys, girls play with girls. How would Freud explain this?

Optimum development at each stage, according to Freud, requires an environment that will satisfy the unique needs of each period. The baby needs sufficient oral and anal stimulation; the 4-year-old boy needs a father present with whom to identify and a mother who is not too seductive. An inadequate early environment will leave a residue of unresolved problems and unmet needs, which are then carried forward to subsequent stages.

This emphasis on the formative role of early experience, particularly early family experience, is a hallmark of psychoanalytic theories. In this view, the first five or six years of life are a kind of sensitive period for the creation of the individual personality.

Does the idea that one carries unresolved issues forward into adulthood make sense to you? Can you think of any examples from your own experience?

Erikson's Psychosocial Stages

Erikson shares most of Freud's basic assumptions, but there are some crucial differences between the two theories. First, Erikson deemphasizes the centrality of sexual drive and instead focuses on a step-wise emergence of a sense of identity. Second, although he agrees with Freud that the early years are highly important, he argues that identity is not fully formed at the end of adolescence but continues to move through further developmental stages in adult life. You can see in Table 9.5 that he proposes eight stages, three of which are reached only in adulthood.

In Erikson's view, maturation plays relatively little role in the sequence of stages. Far more important are common cultural demands for children of a particular age, such as the demand that the child become toilet trained at about 2, that the child learn school skills at age 6 or 7, or that the young adult form an intimate partnership. Each stage, then, centers on a particular dilemma, a particular social task. Thus, he calls his stages **psycho*social* stages** rather than psycho*sexual* stages. Let me give you a bit more detail on the five stages that Erikson described in childhood.

Basic Trust Versus Basic Mistrust: Birth to 1 Year. The first task (or "dilemma," as Erikson sometimes says) occurs during the first year of life, when the child must develop

Table 9.5
The Eight Stages of Development Proposed by Erikson

Approximate Age	Ego Quality to Be Developed	Some Tasks and Activities of the Stage
0–1	Basic trust versus basic mistrust	Trust in mother or central caregiver and in one's own ability to make things happen; a key element in an early secure attachment
2–3	Autonomy versus shame, doubt	Walking, grasping, and other physical skills lead to free choice; toilet training occurs; child learns control but may develop shame if not handled properly
4–5	Initiative versus guilt	Organize activities around some goal; become more assertive and aggressive. Oedipus-like conflict with parent of same sex may lead to guilt
6–12	Industry versus inferiority	Absorb all the basic cultural skills and norms, including school skills and tool use
13–18	Identity versus role confusion	Adapt sense of self to physical changes of puberty, make occupational choice, achieve adultlike sexual identity, and search for new values
19–25	Intimacy versus isolation	Form one or more intimate relationships that go beyond adolescent love; marry and form family groups
26–40	Generativity versus stagnation	Bear and rear children, focus on occupational achievement or creativity, and train the next generation
41+	Ego integrity versus despair	Integrate earlier stages and come to terms with basic identity; accept self

a sense of basic trust in the predictability of the world and in his ability to affect the events around him. Erikson believes that the behavior of the major caregiver (usually the mother) is critical to the child's successful or unsuccessful resolution of this crisis. Children who emerge from the first year with a firm sense of trust are those whose parents are loving and respond predictably and reliably to the child. A child who has developed a sense of trust will go on to other relationships, carrying this sense with him. But those infants whose early care has been erratic or harsh may develop *mis*trust, and they too carry this sense with them into later relationships.

Erikson never said, by the way, that the ideal position on any one of the dilemmas is at one extreme pole. In the case of the first stage, for example, there is some risk in being too trusting. The child also needs to develop some healthy mistrust, such as learning to discriminate between dangerous and safe situations.

Autonomy Versus Shame and Doubt: 2 to 3 Years. Erikson sees the child's greater mobility during the toddler years as forming the basis for the sense of independence or autonomy. But if the child's efforts at independence are not carefully guided by the parents and she experiences repeated failures or ridicule, then the results of all the new opportunities for exploration may be shame and doubt instead of a basic sense of self-control and self-worth. Once again the ideal is not for the child to have *no* shame or doubt; some doubt is needed for the child to understand which behaviors are acceptable and which are not, which are safe and which are dangerous. But the ideal does lie toward the autonomy end of the continuum.

Initiative Versus Guilt: 4 to 5 Years. This phase, roughly equivalent to Freud's phallic stage, is again ushered in by new skills or abilities in the child. The 4-year-old is able to plan a bit, to take the initiative in reaching particular goals. The child tries out these new cognitive skills, attempts to conquer the world around him. He may try to go out into the street on his own; he may take a toy apart, then find he can't put it back together and throw it—parts and all—at his mother. It is a time of vigor of action and of behaviors that parents may see as aggressive.

The risk is that the child may go too far in his forcefulness or that the parents may restrict and punish too much—either of which can produce guilt. Some guilt is needed, since without it there would be no conscience, no self-control. The ideal interaction between parent and child is certainly not total indulgence. But too much guilt can inhibit the child's creativity and free interactions with others.

Industry (Competence) Versus Inferiority: 6 to 12 Years. The beginning of schooling is a major force in ushering in this stage. The child is now faced with the need to win approval through specific competence—through learning to read, do sums, and practice other school skills. The task of this period is thus simply to develop the repertoire of abilities society demands of the child. If the child cannot develop the expected skills, he will develop instead a basic sense of inferiority. Yet some failure is necessary so that the child can develop some humility; as always, balance is at issue. Ideally, the child must have sufficient success to encourage a sense of competence but should not place so much

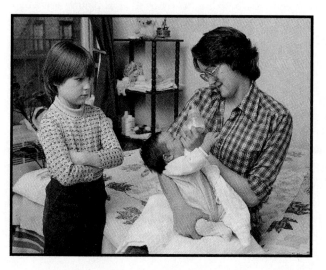

If looks could kill! This child is clearly jealous of the new baby and may well be harboring all sorts of angry and aggressive thoughts. A younger child would probably act out those thoughts and feelings directly. But a child of this age, probably in the period Erikson calls *initiative versus guilt,* feels guilty about these feelings and inhibits the angry actions.

emphasis on competence that failure is unacceptable or that she becomes a kind of "workaholic."

Identity Versus Role Confusion: 13 to 18 Years. The task occurring during puberty is a major one in which the adolescent reexamines his identity and the roles he must occupy. Erikson suggests that two "identities" are involved—a "sexual identity" and an "occupational identity." What should emerge for the adolescent from this period is a reintegrated sense of self, of what one wants to do and be, and of one's appropriate sexual role. The risk is that of confusion, arising from the profusion of roles opening to the child at this age.

Other Psychoanalytic Views: Bowlby's Model of Attachment

Before looking at some of the evidence supporting (or refuting) the psychoanalytic view, I want to reemphasize that Erikson is not the only influential modern theorist whose thinking has been strongly affected by Freud or psychoanalysis. Among those interested particularly in very early child development, John Bowlby's theory of the development of attachment has had a major impact (1969; 1973; 1980). He offers an interesting blend of psychoanalytic and biological approaches. Like Freud, Bowlby assumes that the root of human personality lies in the earliest childhood relationships. Significant failure or trauma in those relationships will permanently shape the child's development. Bowlby focused his attention on the child's first attachment to the mother because it is usually the earliest and is arguably the most central.

To describe how that attachment comes about, Bowlby introduced several concepts from *ethological theory*, which brings evolutionary concepts to bear on the study of behavior. Human evolution, Bowlby suggested, has resulted in the child being born with a repertoire of built-in, instinctive behaviors that elicit caregiving from others—behaviors like crying, smiling, or making eye contact. Similarly, the mother (or other adult) is equipped with various instinctive behaviors toward the infant, such as responding to a baby's cry or speaking to the baby in a higher-pitched voice. Together these instinctive patterns bring mother and infant together in an intricate chain of stimulus and response that causes the child to form a specific attachment to that one adult—a process I'll be talking about in some detail in Chapter 11.

Although Bowlby's theory is not a full-fledged stage theory of development in the manner of Freud or Erikson, it is nonetheless based on many of the underlying psychoanalytic assumptions. It has also stimulated and profoundly influenced the large body of current research on attachment.

Evidence and Applications

Empirical explorations of Freud's or Erikson's theories are relatively rare, largely because both theories are so general that specific tests are very difficult. For example, to test Freud's notion of fixation we would need much more information about how to determine if a given child is fixated at some stage. What is a sign that a child is fixated at the oral or the anal stage? Should we expect some automatic connection between how early a child is weaned and such ostensibly oral adult behavior as smoking or overeating? When researchers have searched for such direct linkages they have not found them. However, this does not rule out the possibility of a process akin to fixation, albeit perhaps at a subtler level.

Despite these difficulties, researchers have managed to devise tests of some of the basic propositions. Let me mention two bodies of work of this type, studies of the Oedipal period and studies of the security of attachment.

The Oedipal Period. A 4-year-old boy, after his mother told him that she loved him, said, "And I love you too, and that's why I can't ever marry someone else" (Watson & Getz, 1990a, p. 29). In their studies of Oedipal behavior, Malcolm Watson and Kenneth Getz (1990a; 1990b) have indeed found that children of about 4 or 5 are likely to make comments like this. More precisely, they have found that 4-year-olds, more than any other age group, show more affectionate behavior toward the opposite-sex parent and more aggressive or antagonistic behavior toward the same-sex parent. You can see the second half of this result in Figure 9.3. Whether Freud's explanation of this phenomenon is the correct one remains to be seen, but these results are certainly consistent with his theory.

Security of Attachment. A second research area that has its roots in psychoanalytic theory is the current work on the security or insecurity of children's early attachments. Both Erikson and Freud argue that the quality of the child's first relationship with the central caregiver will shape her relationships with other children and with other adults at later ages. And of course Bowlby's theory is designed specifically to examine that earliest relationship. I'll be talking a great deal more about early attachments in Chapter 11, but let me give you at least a taste of the research in this area, since it provides a good deal of support for the basic psychoanalytic hypothesis that the quality of the child's earliest relationship affects the whole course of the child's later development. This is particularly clear in the work of Alan Sroufe and his colleagues (Sroufe, Carlson, & Schulman, 1993). In a number of studies, they have first rated children on the security of their attachments to their mothers at about age 1. Later, at preschool, school age, or early adolescence, the same children are observed at school or at special summer camps where they must deal with new relationships or strange adults. The consistent finding from studies like this is that securely attached infants are later more capable, more friendly, more open to new relationships, more skillful with peers. Thus, the relationship formed during the earliest

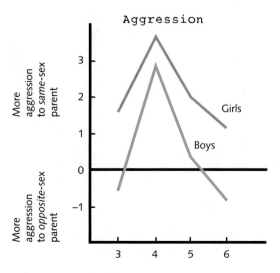

FIGURE 9.3 The data in this figure are based on the detailed reports of parents on the affectionate and aggressive behavior of their child toward them. Scores above 0 mean that the child was more aggressive toward the same-sex parent than toward the opposite-sex parent, while scores below 0 mean the reverse. (*Source:* Watson & Getz, 1990b, Table 3, p. 499.)

The Real World

The Effects of Divorce: One Test of Psychoanalytic Theory

Roughly 40 percent of children born in the United States in 1980 will experience their parents' divorce by the time they are 16 (Cherlin, 1992). What is the effect on the child of such an experience? I'll talk much more broadly about the effects of divorce in Chapter 13; for now, let me focus on just one issue, because it is a kind of test of psychoanalytic theory. If Freud is correct, the negative impact of divorce should be greatest if the divorce occurred before or during the Oedipal period (ages 3 to 5 approximately), since the successful resolution of the Oedipus conflict and the resulting identification process require the presence of both parents. Further, if the children live with their mother after a divorce, then the detrimental effect should be much greater for boys than for girls. A girl still has her mother to identify with, so at least her sex-role identification is appropriate. But the boy, lacking a father, may never go through the identification process properly and may end up with a very confused sex-role orientation and perhaps a weaker superego.

The results of studies of children in divorced families give partial support to the second, but not the first, of these hypotheses. Virtually all children show some negative effects of divorce, but the most common finding is that boys experience more problems (Hetherington, 1989; Kline et al., 1989). They are more likely than are girls to show behavior problems or have increased difficulty in school after a divorce. Among teenagers, there are a few hints that girls whose mothers have remarried may show higher rates of problems (Lee et al., 1994), although this point is not yet fully clear. What is clear is that preschool-age children do *not* have more profound or more lasting negative effects than do children of other ages, which calls some of Freud's hypotheses about the Oedipus conflict into question.

stage of psychosocial development seems to create a prototype for later relationships, as Bowlby and Erikson proposed. Recall, too, Megan Gunnar's finding that I described earlier: Temperamentally inhibited toddlers who have formed a secure attachment to their mothers show little or no physiological sign of fearfulness in a novel setting. Thus, the quality of the child's early attachment can at least partially override the basic temperamental tendencies in forming the child's personality.

Critique of Psychoanalytic Theories

Psychoanalytic theories like Freud's or Erikson's have several great attractions. Most centrally, they focus our attention on the importance of the emotional quality of the child's relationship with the caregivers. Furthermore, both these theories suggest that the child's needs or "tasks" change with age, so that the parents must constantly adapt to the changing child. One of the implications of this is that we should not think of "good parenting" as if it were a global quality. Some of us may be very good at meeting the needs of an infant but quite awful at dealing with teenagers' identity struggles; others of us may have the opposite pattern. The child's eventual personality, and her overall "health," thus depends on the interaction or transaction that develops in the particular family. This is an extremely attractive element of these theories because more and more of the research within developmental psychology is moving us toward just such a transactional conception of the process.

Psychoanalytic theory has also given us a number of helpful concepts, such as defense mechanisms and identification, that have been so widely adopted that they have become a part of everyday language as well as theory. These strengths have led to a resurgence of influence of both Erikson's theory and the several second-order or third-order psychoanalytic approaches such as Bowlby's.

The great weakness of all the psychoanalytic approaches is the fuzziness of many of the concepts. Identification may be an intriguing theoretical notion, but how are we to measure it? How do we detect the presence of specific defense mechanisms? Without more precise operational definitions, it is impossible to disconfirm the theory. Those areas in which the general concepts of psychoanalytic theory have been fruitfully applied to our understanding of development have nearly always been areas in which other theorists or researchers have offered more precise definitions or clearer methods for measuring some Freudian or Eriksonian construct, such as Bowlby's concept of security of attachment. Psychoanalytic theory may thus sometimes offer a provocative framework for our thinking, but it is not a precise theory of development.

A Tentative Synthesis

I have given you three different views of the origins of those unique, individual patterns of behavior we call personality. Each view can be at least partially supported with research evidence; each has clear strengths. Do we need to choose among them, or can we combine them in any sensible way? Some argue that theories as different as these cannot ever be combined because they make such different assumptions about the child's role in the whole process (Overton & Reese, 1973). I agree in part. I do not think we can simply add up the different sources of influence and say that personality is merely the sum of inborn temperament, reinforcement patterns, interactions with parents, and some kind of self-scheme.

But more complex combinations may still be fruitful. I have suggested one in Figure 9.4. In this model I am suggesting that the child's inborn temperament is a beginning point—an initial, highly significant bias in the system. Arrow number 1 shows a *direct* relationship between that inborn temperament and the eventual personality we see in the child and later in the adult.

Arrow number 2 indicates a second direct effect, between the pattern of the child's environment and his eventual personality and social behavior. Whether the parents respond reliably and contingently to the infant will affect his trust or the security of his attachment, which will show up in a range of behaviors later; whether the parents reinforce aggressive or friendly behavior will influence the child's future as well.

But most of what happens is much more complicated than that. The way the child is treated is influenced by her temperament (arrow 3), and both the basic temperament and the family environment affect the child's self-scheme—her expectations for others and herself, her beliefs about her own abilities (arrows 4 and 5). This self-scheme, or self-concept, in turn, helps to shape the behavior we see, the "personality" of the child.

This system does not exist in a vacuum. In keeping with the ecological approach of Bronfenbrenner and others, arrow 7 suggests that the parents' ability to maintain a loving and supportive relationship with their child is influenced by the parents' own outside experiences—whether they like their jobs, whether they have enough emotional support to help them weather their own crises.

For example, Mavis Hetherington (1989) reports that children with difficult temperaments show more problem behavior in response to their parents' divorce, but only if the mother is also depressed and has inadequate social support. In this study, those difficult children whose divorcing mothers were not depressed did not show heightened levels

In recent years the concept of "vulnerable" and "invulnerable" children has become prominent in developmental research. How might vulnerability be conceptualized or explained by theorists of each of the several persuasions described in this chapter?

A model of personality development

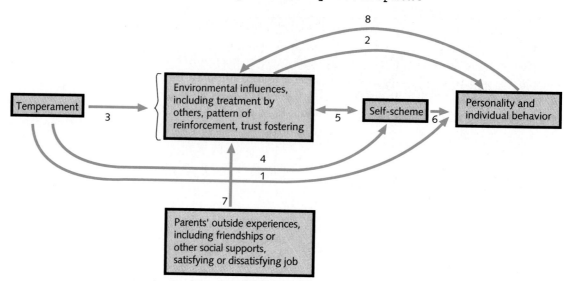

FIGURE 9.4 Here is my own proposal for a complex, interactive model describing the formation of individual personality. The effects of inborn temperament and environmental influences do not merely add. Each affects the other, helping to create the child's unique self-scheme, which in turn affects the child's experiences. This all occurs within the context of the family, which is itself influenced by the parents' own life experiences. What we think of as personality is a complex product of all these forces.

of problems. Thus, the child's temperament clearly seems to have an impact, but the effect of temperament can be and is modified by the parents' pattern of response.

Another illustration of the intricacy of the whole system comes from a study by Susan Crockenberg (1981), who studied a group of 46 mothers and infants over the first year of life. She measured each child's irritability (an aspect of temperament) when the baby was 5 to 10 days old and assessed the security of the child's attachment to the mother when the child was 12 months old. We might expect that irritable babies would be more likely to be insecurely attached, merely because they are more difficult to care for. In fact, Crockenberg found a small effect of this kind (see Table 9.6). But Crockenberg didn't stop there. She also measured the level of the mother's social support—the degree to which she had family and friends who were sufficiently helpful to assist her in dealing with the strains of a new child or other life changes she might be experiencing. The results of the study show that insecure attachment in the child was most likely when the mother had *both* an irritable infant *and* low levels of support. If the baby was irritable but the mother had good support, the child's attachment nearly always developed securely. Only when two difficult conditions occurred together did a poor outcome result for the child.

In a later study, Crockenberg (1987) found that a higher level of anger and noncompliant behavior (perhaps reflections of what is called "neuroticism" in the Big Five formula) was common in toddlers who had been irritable as infants *and* whose mothers were angry and punitive toward them. Furthermore, such angry and punitive behavior in the mother was more likely if the mother had experienced rejection in her own childhood and if she experienced little support from her partner. We are dealing here with a *system* of effects.

Table 9.6
Influence of Child's Temperament and Mother's Social Support on the Child's Secure or Insecure Attachment

Child's Irritability	Mother's Support	Number of Children with Secure Attachment	Number of Children with Insecure Attachment
High	Low	2	9
High	High	12	1
Low	Low	7	2
Low	High	13	2

Source: Crockenberg, 1981, Table 5, p. 862.

Finally, I have included arrow 8 in the diagram to underline the *transactional* elements of the system. Once the child's unique pattern of behaviors and attitudes (personality) is formed, this affects the environment she will encounter, the experiences she will choose, the responses of the people around her, which in turn affect her behavior (Scarr & McCartney, 1983; Sroufe et al., 1993).

No doubt even this fairly complex system underestimates the intricacy of the process of personality development in the child. Most of our research does not yet encompass all the pieces of the puzzle. But the very fact that developmental psychologists are turning toward such complex models seems to me to be a very good thing. Development *is* this complex, and we will not be able to describe it or explain it until we begin to examine and try to measure all these separate forces.

Summary

1 The word *personality* refers to the unique, individual, relatively enduring pattern of relating to others and responding to the world that is characteristic of each individual.

2 Researchers studying adult personality have agreed on a set of five dimensions (the Big Five) that capture most of the variation among individuals: extraversion, agreeableness, conscientiousness, neuroticism, and openness/intellect.

3 Recent research suggests that the same five dimensions may give us an accurate picture of variations in children's personality as well.

4 Researchers studying infants and young children have largely focused on the study of temperament, which is best thought of as the built-in patterns that form the emotional substrate of personality.

5   Sizable differences remain among temperament theorists on how best to characterize the basic dimensions of temperament among children, but reasonable agreement exists on the following: activity level, approach/positive emotionality, inhibition, negative emotionality, and effortful control/task persistence.

6   Explanations of personality variations center around three distinct theoretical approaches: biological/genetic theories, learning theories, and psychoanalytic theories.

7   Biological explanations of temperament/personality focus on genetic differences in patterns or styles of reacting to people and objects, an assertion well supported by research.

8   Evidence is also accumulating that specific differences in neurological and chemical responses underlie the observed variations in behavior.

9   Temperament is not totally determined by heredity or ongoing physiological processes, although the child's built-in temperament does shape the child's interactions with the world and affect others' responses to the child.

10 Traditional learning theorists emphasize the role of basic learning processes, such as reinforcement patterns, in shaping individual behaviors, including patterns of interaction with others.

11 Social learning theories such as Bandura's also emphasize the role of observational learning and the role of the child's learned expectancies, standards, and self-efficacy in creating more enduring patterns of response.

12 Psychoanalytic theorists emphasize the importance of unconscious motives and processes as well as the stagelike emergence of personality. In this approach, the relationship of the child with significant adults, particularly in early infancy, is seen as critical.

13 Freud's psychosexual stages are strongly affected by maturation. Particularly significant is the phallic stage, beginning at about age 4, when the Oedipus conflict is met and mastered through the process of identification.

14 Erikson's psychosocial stages are influenced both by social demands and by the child's physical and intellectual skills. Each of the major stages has a central task or "crisis," each relating to some aspect of the development of identity.

15 Bowlby's theory of attachment, with roots in psychoanalytic thought, is particularly influential today.

16 Psychoanalytic theory is difficult to test because of its imprecision, but in some areas it has been broadly confirmed, such as in studies of the impact of early attachments on later functioning.

17 Elements of all three views can be combined into an interactionist view of personality development. Temperament may serve as the base from which personality grows by affecting behavior directly and by affecting the way others respond to the child. Both the temperament and the specific pattern of response from the people in the child's environment affect the child's self-concept or self-scheme, which then helps to create stability in the child's unique pattern of behavior.

Key Terms

Big Five (personality dimensions) (**p. 249**)

identification (**p. 266**)

Oedipus conflict (**p. 265**)

personality (**p. 248**)

psychosexual stages (**p. 265**)

psychosocial stages (**p. 267**)

temperament (**p. 251**)

Suggested Readings

Bates, J. E. (1987). Temperament in infancy. In J. D. Osofsky (Ed.), *Handbook of infant development* (2nd ed.). New York: Wiley-Interscience.

A good basic source on this complex topic, although it does not include the current work on the links between temperament and the Big Five personality dimensions.

Erikson, E. H. (1980) *Identity and the life cycle.* New York: Norton (originally published 1959).

The middle section of this book, "Growth and Crises of the Healthy Personality," is the best description I have found of Erikson's model of the psychosocial stages of development.

Grusec, J. E. (1992). Social learning theory and developmental psychology: The legacies of Robert Sears and Albert Bandura. *Developmental Psychology, 28,* 776–786.

One of a series of papers to mark the centennial of the American Psychological Association, describing and celebrating the work of key theorists.

Kagan, J. (1994). *Galen's prophecy.* New York: Basic Books.

A detailed presentation, for the lay reader, of Kagan's ideas about the biological bases of temperament, particularly the aspect of temperament he calls behavioral inhibition.

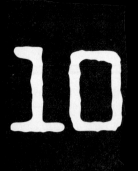

The Concept of Self in Children

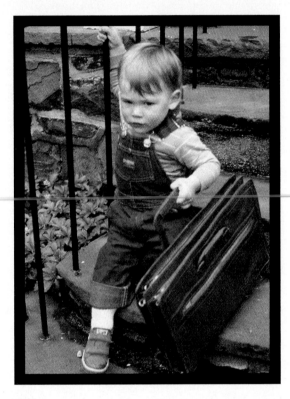

Try an experiment for me. Before you read any further, write down 20 answers to the question "Who am I?" Now look at your list and think about what you wrote. My own list includes items like these:

> *I am a logical, analytic person.*
> *I like closure and am uncomfortable with uncertainty.*
> *I am a stubborn, determined person who finishes what she starts.*
> *I am a person with many roles: wife, mother, stepmother, daughter, sister, friend, board member.*
> *I am lots taller than average and sometimes clumsy.*
> *I am not a traditionally feminine person.*

My list, as yours probably does, includes something about what I look like, something about the roles I occupy, and something about my qualities, attitudes, and beliefs about myself. These are all aspects of my **self-concept;** in Piagetian-style language, my *self-scheme.* For each of us, the self-concept serves as a sort of filter for experience, shaping our choices and affecting our responses to others. Our ideas about our own sex role form a powerful part of that self-concept. Because these beliefs and attitudes about ourselves are so central to our personality and hence to our behavior, it is important for us to try to understand how they develop. So in this chapter I want to explore the origins of both the common developmental pathways and the variations in such concepts from one child to the next.

The Concept of Self: Developmental Patterns

Our thinking about the child's emerging sense of self has been strongly influenced by both Freud and Piaget, each of whom assumed that the baby begins life with *no* sense of separateness. Freud emphasized what he called the *symbiotic* relationship between the mother and young infant in which the two are joined together as if they were one. He believed that the infant does not understand himself to be separate from the mother. Piaget emphasized that the infant's understanding of the basic concept of object permanence was a necessary precursor for the child's attaining *self*-permanence—a sense of himself as a stable, continuing entity. Both of these aspects of early self-development reappear in current descriptions of the emergence of the sense of self. Michael Lewis, for example (1990; 1991; Lewis & Brooks-Gunn, 1979), divides the process into two main steps or tasks.

The Subjective Self

Lewis argues that the child's first task is to figure out that he is separate from others and that this separate self endures over time and space. He calls this aspect of the self-concept the **subjective self.** We might fruitfully subdivide this stage still further, as Daniel Christie suggests (1995), beginning with the *fused self,* reflecting the initial symbiotic joining of infant and other, followed by the *existential self,* when the baby has understood that he is separate, that "I exist." Lewis places the germs of this existential understanding in the first two or three months of life. At that time, the baby grasps the basic distinction between self and everything else. In Lewis's view, the roots of this understanding lie in the myriad everyday interactions the baby has with the objects and people in his world. Over the early months, the baby learns that his behavior affects things or people around him. When he touches the mobile, it moves; when he cries, someone responds; when he smiles, his mother smiles back. By this process the baby begins to separate out self from everything else and a sense of *I* begins to emerge.

But it is not until the baby also grasps the concept of object permanence, at about 9 to 12 months, that we can say a subjective self has fully emerged. Just as he is figuring out that Mom or Dad continues to exist when they are out of sight, he is figuring out—at least in some preliminary way—that *he* exists separately and has some permanence.

The Objective Self

But it is not enough merely to understand yourself as an agent in the world or a person who has experiences. The second major step is for the toddler to come to understand that she is also an *object* in the world. Just as a ball has properties—roundness, the ability to roll, a certain feel in the hand—so the "self" also has qualities or properties, such as gender, size, a name, or qualities like shyness or boldness, coordination or clumsiness. It is this *self-awareness* that is the hallmark of the second phase of identity development. Lewis refers to this as the **objective self,** or sometimes the *categorical self,* because once the child achieves self-awareness, the process of defining the self involves placing oneself in a whole series of categories. Christie argues that here too we should distinguish two subperiods: the *concrete categorical self,* an early period in which the toddler or preschooler defines herself according to concrete, physical categories; and an *abstract, categorical self,* which emerges slowly over the years of childhood and adolescence, as the child gradually defines herself using more and more abstract categories, such as the ones I used to describe myself at the beginning of this chapter.

Studying Self-awareness. It has not been easy to determine just when a child has developed the initial self-awareness that defines the beginning of the categorical self. The most commonly used procedure involves a mirror. First the baby is placed in front of a mirror, just to see how she behaves. Most infants of about 9 to 12 months will look at their own images, make faces, or try to interact with the baby-in-the-mirror in some way. After allowing this free exploration for a time, the experimenter, while pretending to wipe the baby's face with a cloth, puts a spot of rouge on the baby's nose and then again lets the baby look in the mirror. The crucial test of self-recognition, and thus of awareness of the self, is whether the baby reaches for the spot on her *own* nose, rather than the nose on the face in the mirror.

The results from one of Lewis's studies using this procedure are shown in Figure 10.1. As you can see, none of the 9- to 12-month-old children in this study touched their noses, but by 21 months, three-quarters of the children showed that level of self-recognition. The figure also shows the rate at which children refer to themselves by name when they are shown a picture of themselves, which is another commonly used measure of self-awareness. You can see that this development occurs at almost exactly the same time as self-recognition in a mirror. Both are present by about the middle of the second year of life, a finding confirmed by other investigators (Bullock & Lütkenhaus, 1990).

We can see signs of this new self-awareness in a whole range of other behavior. It is only at this point in toddlerhood, for example, that toddlers begin to insist on doing things for themselves and show a newly proprietary attitude toward toys ("Mine!") or other treasured objects. Looked at this way, much of the legendary "terrible twos" can be understood as an outgrowth of self-awareness.

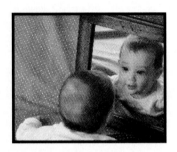

At 4 months, Lucy's pleasure at looking at herself in a mirror comes from the fact that this is an interesting moving object to inspect, not from any understanding that this is *herself* in the mirror.

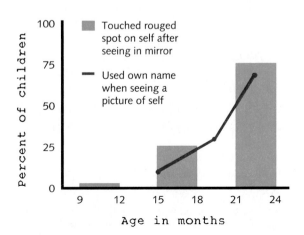

FIGURE 10.1 Mirror recognition and self-naming develop at almost exactly the same time. (*Source:* Lewis & Brooks, 1978, pp. 214–215.)

The Emergence of Emotional Expression. The developmental shifts in the child's understanding of self are also matched by parallel progressions in the baby's expression of emotions. You already know from Chapter 5 that babies are able to read others' emotions to at least some extent. They respond differently to their mothers' happy or sad expressions and by 10 months show social referencing. During the months of infancy, infants also develop a repertoire of their own emotional expressions.

At birth, infants have different facial expressions for interest, pain, and disgust, and an expression that conveys enjoyment develops very quickly. By the time the baby is 2 to 3 months old, adult observers can also distinguish expressions of anger and sadness, with expressions of fear appearing by 6 or 7 months (Izard & Harris, 1995). But it is only early in the second year of life, at about the same time that a child shows self-recognition in the mirror, that we see the emergence of such self-conscious emotional expressions as embarrassment, pride, or shame, all of which involve some aspect of self-evaluation (Lewis, Allesandri, & Sullivan, 1992; Lewis et al., 1989).

Early Self-definitions. Having achieved an initial self-awareness, the preschool child begins to define "who I am" by learning about her own qualities and her social roles. The 2-year-old not only knows her own name, but can probably tell you if she is a girl or a boy and whether she is big or little. By about age 5 to 7, a child can give you quite a full description of himself on a whole range of dimensions.

Beginning in the second year, children also seem to become aware of themselves as players in the social game. By age 2, the toddler has already learned a variety of social "scripts"—routines of play or interaction with others in her world. Over the preschool years, the toddler learns more about her own roles in these scripts. So she begins to think of herself as a "helper" in some situations or as "the boss" when she is telling some other child what to do. You have already seen one aspect of this in the emergence of roles in children's sociodramatic play—a pattern I talked about in Chapter 7. As part of the same process, the preschool child also gradually understands her place in the network of family roles. She has sisters, brothers, father, mother, and so on.

Can you think of some social scripts that a 2- or 3-year-old is likely to learn? What about bedtime rituals? What others?

These are major advances in the child's understanding. Yet this is still a *concrete* categorical self. For one thing, each facet of a preschool child's self-concept seems to be quite separate, rather like a list: "I'm good at running"; "I don't like to play with dolls"; "I'm a big girl." These separate aspects of the "self-scheme" or internal working model of the self have not yet coalesced into a *global* sense of self-worth (Harter, 1987; 1990; Harter & Pike, 1984). Children this age do not say things like "I am a terrible person," or "I really like myself." Their perceptions of themselves are more tied to specific settings and specific tasks.

The self-perceptions of a preschool-age child are also concrete in the sense that they are tied to visible characteristics, such as what he looks like, what or whom he plays with, where he lives, or what he is good or bad at doing, rather than more enduring, inner qualities, such as personality traits or basic abilities. This pattern obviously parallels what we see in cognitive development at the same ages, since it is in these same years that children's attention tends to be captured by the external appearance of objects rather than by their enduring properties.

Self-concept at School Age and Adolescence

Over the elementary school years this concrete self-concept gradually shifts toward a more comparative, more generalized self-definition—what Christie calls the *abstract categorical self*. A 6-year-old might describe herself as "smart" or "dumb"; a 10-year-old is more likely to say he is "smarter than most other kids" or "not as good at baseball as my friends" (Rosenberg, 1986; Ruble, 1987). At the same time, the child's self-concept becomes gradually less focused on external characteristics and more on stable, internal qualities. The school-age child also begins to see her own (and other people's) characteristics as relatively stable, and for the first time she develops a global sense of her own self-worth.

A number of these themes are illustrated nicely in an older study by Montemayor and Eisen of self-concepts in 9- to 18-year-olds (1977). Using the same "Who am I?" question I asked you to answer at the beginning of this chapter, these researchers found that the younger children in this study were still using mostly surface qualities to describe themselves, such as the description by this 9-year-old:

> My name is Bruce C. I have brown eyes. I have brown hair. I have brown eyebrows. I am nine years old. I LOVE! Sports. I have seven people in my family. I have great! eye site. I have lots! of friends. I live on 1923 Pinecrest Dr. I am going on 10 in September. I'm a boy. I have a uncle that is almost 7 feet tall. My school is Pinecrest. My teacher is Mrs. V. I play Hockey! I'm almost the smartest boy in the class. I LOVE! food. I love fresh air. I LOVE school. (pp. 317–318)

In contrast, look at the self-description of this 11-year-old girl in the sixth grade:

> My name is A. I'm a human being. I'm a girl. I'm a truthful person. I'm not very pretty. I do so-so in my studies. I'm a very good cellist. I'm a very good pianist. I'm a little bit tall for my age. I like several boys. I like several girls. I'm old-fashioned. I play tennis. I am a very good swimmer. I try to be helpful. I'm always ready to be friends with anybody. Mostly I'm good, but I lose my temper. I'm not well-liked by some girls and boys. I don't know if I'm liked by boys or not. (pp. 317–318)

This girl, like the other youngsters of this age in the Montemayor and Eisen study, not only describes her external qualities, but also emphasizes her beliefs, the quality of her relationships, and general personality traits. Thus, as the child moves through the concrete operations period, her self-definition becomes more complex, more comparative, less tied to external features, more focused on feelings, on ideas.

This trend toward greater abstraction in the self-definition continues during adolescence. Compare the answers of this 17-year-old to the "Who am I?" question with the ones you just read:

> I am a human being. I am a girl, I am an individual. I don't know who I am. I am a Pisces. I am a moody person. I am an indecisive person. I am an ambitious person. I am a very curious person. I am not an individual. I am a loner. I am an American (God help me). I am a Democrat. I am a liberal person. I am a radical. I am a conservative. I am a pseudoliberal. I am an atheist. I am not a classifiable person (i.e. I don't want to be). (p. 318)

Obviously, this girl's self-concept is even less tied to her physical characteristics or even her abilities than are those of the 11-year-old. She is describing abstract traits or ideology.

You can see the shift I'm describing graphically in Figure 10.2, which is based on the answers of all 262 subjects in the Montemayor and Eisen study. Each of the subjects' answers to the "Who am I?" question was placed in one or more specific categories, such as references to physical properties ("I am tall," "I have blue eyes") or references to ideology

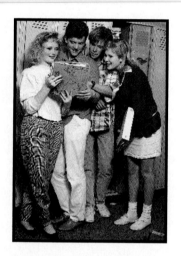

If you asked them to define themselves, these teenagers would surely give much more abstract and comparative answers than you would hear from a 6-year-old.

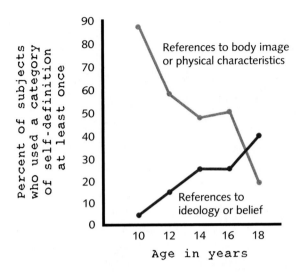

FIGURE 10.2 As they get older, children and adolescents define themselves less and less by what they look like and more and more by what they believe or feel. (*Source:* Montemayor & Eisen, 1977, Table 1, p. 316.)

("I am a Democrat," "I believe in God," etc.). As you can see, appearance was still a highly salient dimension in the preteen and early teen years but became less dominant in late adolescence, at a time when ideology and belief became more salient.

Self-judgments in School. The child's increasingly comparative self-assessments are particularly visible in school. Kindergarten and first-grade children pay relatively little attention to how well others do at a particular task; in fact, the great majority will confidently tell you that they are the smartest kid in their class. But by third grade or so, children begin to notice whether their classmates finish a test sooner than they did or whether someone else got a better grade or more corrections on his spelling paper.

Teachers' behavior shows a similar change: In the first few grades, teachers emphasize effort and work habits. Gradually they begin to use more comparative judgments. By junior high, teachers compare children not only to each other but also to fixed standards, other schools, or national norms (Stipek, 1992). These processes are sometimes subtle, but they can be powerful. Robert Rosenthal, in his famous "Pygmalion in the classroom" studies, has shown that a teacher's belief about a given student's ability and potential has a small but significant effect on her behavior toward that student and on the student's eventual achievement (Rosenthal, 1994)—a set of results that has now been replicated many times. Rosenthal's standard procedure is to tell teachers at the beginning of a school year that some of the children in the class are underachievers and just ready to "bloom" intellectually, although in fact the children labeled in this way are chosen randomly. At the end of the year, those students labeled as having more potential typically show more gains during the school year than do those who have not been labeled in this way. So the comparative judgments teachers make about individual children can have pervasive effects.

Similarly, parents' judgments and expectations also play a role. For example, you may recall from Chapter 6 that parents in the U.S. are more likely to attribute a daughter's good performance in math to hard work but a son's good math grades to ability. Children absorb these explanations and adjust their behavior accordingly.

The beliefs about their own abilities that students develop through this process are usually quite accurate. Students who consistently do well in comparison to others come to believe that they are academically competent. Further, and perhaps more important, they come to believe that they are in control of academic outcomes. Interestingly, this

There is clearly a chicken/egg problem here: Do children come to describe themselves more and more comparatively because that is a natural aspect of increasing cognitive complexity, or are they responding to the higher rate of comparisons made by teachers? How could you find out?

seems to be less true of girls than of boys, at least in American culture. On average, girls get better school grades than boys do, but they have lower perceptions of their own ability. When they do well, they are more likely to attribute it to hard work rather than to ability; when they do poorly, they see it as their own fault (Stipek & Gralinski, 1991).

Collectively, these experiences of comparative success and failure mean that by seventh or eighth grade, most students have very-well-established ideas about their own academic skills and their ability to control the events around themselves.

Identity in Adolescence

In adolescence, the basic process of creating the self-scheme takes on a new dimension, at least according to Erikson, who proposes that the central task of adolescence is that of establishing *identity versus role confusion.* Erikson argues that the child's early sense of identity comes partly unglued at puberty with the onset of both rapid body growth and sexual changes. He refers to this period as one in which the adolescent mind is in a kind of *moratorium* between childhood and adulthood. The old identity will no longer suffice; a new identity must be forged, one that must serve to place the young person among the myriad roles of adult life—occupational roles, sexual roles, religious roles. Confusion about all these role choices is inevitable. Erikson puts it this way:

> *In general it is primarily the inability to settle on an occupational identity which disturbs young people. To keep themselves together they temporarily overidentify, to the point of apparent complete loss of identity, with the heroes of cliques and crowds. . . . They become remarkably clannish, intolerant, and cruel in their exclusion of others who are "different," in skin color or cultural background . . . and often in entirely petty aspects of dress and gesture arbitrarily selected as the signs of an in-grouper or out-grouper. It is important to understand . . . such intolerance as the necessary defense against a sense of identity confusion, which is unavoidable at [this] time of life. (1980, pp. 97–98)*

The teenage clique or crowd thus forms a base of security from which the young person can move toward a unique solution of the identity process. Ultimately, each teenager must achieve an integrated view of himself, including his own pattern of beliefs, occupational goals, and relationships.

Nearly all the current work on the formation of adolescent identity has been based on James Marcia's descriptions of *identity statuses* (1966; 1980), which are rooted in Erikson's general conceptions of the adolescent identity process. Following one of Erikson's ideas, Marcia argues that the formation of an adolescent identity has two key parts: a *crisis* and a *commitment.* By a "crisis" Marcia means a period of decision making when old values and old choices are reexamined. This may occur as a sort of upheaval—the classic notion of a crisis—or it may occur gradually. The outcome of the reevaluation is a commitment to some specific role, some particular ideology.

If you put these two elements together, as in Figure 10.3, you can see that four different "identity statuses" are possible.

- **Identity achievement:** The person has been through a crisis and reached a commitment.

- **Moratorium:** A crisis is in progress, but no commitment has yet been made.

- **Foreclosure:** A commitment has been made without the person's having gone through a crisis. No reassessment of old positions has been made. Instead the

The implication in Marcia's formulation is that the foreclosure status is less developmentally mature—that one must go through a crisis in order to achieve a mature identity. Does this make sense to you?

Degree of crisis

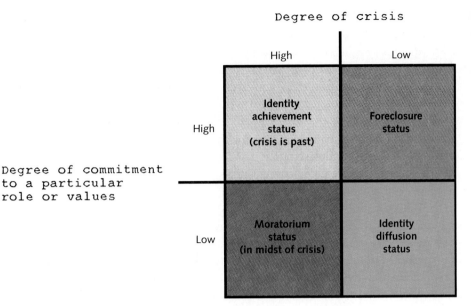

FIGURE 10.3 The four identity statuses proposed by Marcia, based on Erikson's theory. A fully achieved identity, according to this model, requires the young person to have examined his or her values or goals and to have reached a firm commitment. (*Source:* Marcia, 1980.)

young person has simply accepted a parentally or culturally defined commitment.

- **Identity diffusion:** The young person is not in the midst of a crisis (although there may have been one in the past) and no commitment has been made. Diffusion may represent either an early stage in the process (before a crisis) or a failure to reach a commitment after a crisis.

Whether every young person goes through some kind of identity crisis I cannot tell you, since there have been no longitudinal studies covering all the relevant years. Cross-sectional studies of the years of adolescence and early adulthood, however, suggest that the whole process of identity formation may occur later than Erikson thought, when it occurs at all. In one combined analysis of eight separate cross-sectional studies, Alan Waterman (1985) found that the identity achievement status occurred most often in college, not during the high school years. Among the subjects in these studies, a moratorium status was relatively uncommon except in the early years of college. So if most young people are going through an identity crisis, that crisis is fairly late and not lasting terribly long. What's more, about a third of the young people at every age were in the foreclosure status, which may indicate that many young people simply do not go through a crisis at all but follow well-defined grooves.

It is well to remember that all the subjects in the studies Waterman analyzed were in college or likely to attend college. It may be that young people who go to work immediately after high school will face the need to form at least an occupational identity earlier than is true for those who go to college. The college years involve a kind of postponement of full adult status, a period in which students are actively encouraged to question, doubt, and try out alternatives. Those who go directly into the working world do not have that luxury and thus must work out some kind of personal identity sooner, a possibility supported by at least some research (Munro & Adams, 1977).

It is also worth pointing out that the whole conception of an adolescent identity crisis has been strongly influenced by current cultural assumptions in Western societies. In such cultures today, full adult status is postponed for almost a decade after puberty, which leaves the adolescent in a kind of identity limbo—physically mature but not yet adult. In addition, young people in industrialized cultures do not normally or necessarily adopt the same roles or occupations as their parents. Indeed, they are encouraged to choose for themselves. In such a cultural system, adolescents are faced with what may be a bewildering array of options, a pattern that might well foster the sort of identity crisis Erikson described.

Initiation Rituals. In many less-industrialized countries, the problem of the change of identity and status at adolescence is handled with initiation rituals, most often at roughly the time of puberty. The content of such rituals varies enormously, but certain practices are especially common (Cohen, 1964).

One such practice, more common for boys than for girls, is the separation of the child from the family, referred to by anthropologists as *extrusion*. The child may spend the day with his family but sleep elsewhere, or may live in a separate dwelling with other boys or relatives. In traditional Hopi and Navaho cultures, for example, boys typically sleep apart from the family beginning at age 8 or 10. This practice obviously symbolizes the separation of the child from the birth family, marking a coming of age. But it also emphasizes that the child "belongs" not just to the family but to the larger group of kin or societal/tribal members.

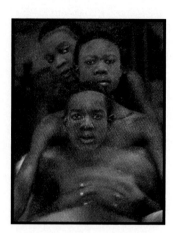

In the initiation rite of the Kota tribe of the Congo, boys' faces are painted blue to make them appear ghostlike, to symbolize the phantom of their now departed childhood.

A second pattern is a ritualized separation of boys and girls around the time of puberty, not only to strengthen incest taboos but also to signify the beginning of the time in life when males and females have quite different life patterns.

The initiation rituals themselves are typically fairly brief, often involving some kind of testing or trial, sometimes with physical mutilation of one sort or another (such as scarring or circumcision), to mark the individual as a member of that tribe or community. During the initiation, the adolescents are also indoctrinated by the elders into customary practices of their culture. They may learn special religious rituals or practices, such as the learning of Hebrew as preparation for the *bar mitzvah* or *bat mitzvah* in the Jewish tradition. They may learn the history and songs of their tribe or people. Often drama and pageantry are part of the entire process. Among the Hopi, for example, both boys and girls go through specific rituals in which they are taught the religious ceremonies of the kachina cult and are whipped. After these ceremonies, they may participate fully in the adult religious practices.

In Western industrialized cultures, a few pale remnants of such initiation practices remain, such as boot camp for those who enter the military or high school graduation ceremonies. But by and large, the shift to adult status is far more protracted and fuzzy, both characteristics that may well contribute to a greater sense of "identity crisis" among Western teens than is true in cultures in which the path to adulthood is more clearly signposted.

Ethnic Identity in Adolescence

Minority teenagers, especially those of color in a predominantly white culture, face another task in creating an identity in adolescence: They must also develop an ethnic or racial identity, including self-identification as a member of some specific group, commitment to that group and its values and attitudes, and some positive (or negative) attitudes about the group to which they belong.

Jean Phinney (1990; Phinney & Rosenthal, 1992) has proposed that in adolescence, the development of a complete ethnic identity moves through three rough stages. The first stage is an "unexamined ethnic identity," equivalent to what Marcia calls a foreclosed status. For some subgroups in U.S. society, such as African-Americans and Native

Americans, this unexamined identity typically includes the negative images and stereotypes common in the wider culture. Indeed, it may be especially at adolescence, with the advent of the cognitive ability to reflect and interpret, that the young person becomes keenly aware of the way in which his own group is perceived by the majority. As Spencer and Dornbusch (1990) put it, "The young African-American may learn as a child that black is beautiful but conclude as an adolescent that white is powerful" (p. 131). The same is doubtless true of other minority groups in the U.S.

Many youngsters in these and other minority groups initially prefer the dominant white culture or wish they had been born into the majority. An African-American journalist, Sylvester Monroe, who grew up in an urban housing project, clearly describes this initial negative feeling:

> *If you were black, you didn't quite measure up. . . . For a black kid there was a certain amount of self-doubt. It came at you indirectly. You didn't see any black people on television, you didn't see any black people doing certain things. . . . You don't think it out but you say, "Well, it must mean that white people are better than we are. Smarter, brighter—whatever." (Spencer & Dornbusch, 1990, pp. 131–132)*

Not all minority teenagers arrive at such negative views of their own group. Individual youngsters may have very positive ethnic images if that is the content of the identity conveyed by parents or others around the child. Phinney's point is, rather, that this initial ethnic identity is not arrived at independently but comes from outside sources.

The second stage is the "ethnic identity search," parallel to the crisis in Marcia's analysis of ego identity. This search is typically triggered by some experience that makes ethnicity salient—perhaps an example of blatant prejudice or merely the widening experience of high school. At this point the young person begins to compare her own ethnic group with others, to try to arrive at her *own* judgments.

This exploration stage is eventually followed by a resolution of the conflicts and contradictions—analogous to Marcia's status of identity achievement. This is often a difficult process. For example, some African-American adolescents who wish to try to compete in and succeed in the dominant culture may experience ostracism from their black friends, who accuse them of "acting white" and betraying their blackness. Latinos often report similar experiences. Some resolve this by keeping their own ethnic group at arm's length; others deal with it by creating essentially two identities, as expressed by one young Chicano interviewed by Phinney:

> *Being invited to someone's house, I have to change my ways of how I act at home, because of culture differences. I would have to follow what they do. . . . I am used to it now, switching off between the two. It is not difficult. (Phinney & Rosenthal, 1992, p. 160)*

Some resolve the dilemma by wholeheartedly choosing their own ethnic group's patterns and values, even when that choice may limit their access to the larger culture.

In both cross-sectional and longitudinal studies, Phinney has found that African-American teens and young adults do indeed move through these steps or stages toward a clear ethnic identity. Furthermore, there is evidence that among African-American, Asian-American, and Mexican-American teens and college students, those who have reached the second or third stage in this process—those who are searching for or who have reached a clear identity—have higher self-esteem and better psychological adjustment than do those who are still in the "unexamined" stage (Phinney, 1990). In contrast, among Caucasian students, ethnic identity has essentially no relationship to self-esteem or adjustment.

This stagelike model may be a decent beginning description of the process of ethnic identity formation. But let us not lose sight of the fact that the details and the content of the ethnic identity will differ markedly from one subgroup to another. Those groups that encounter more overt prejudice will have a different road to follow than will those who may be more easily assimilated; those whose own ethnic culture espouses values that are close to those of the dominant culture will have less difficulty resolving the contradictions than will those whose subculture is at greater variance with the majority. Whatever the specifics, young people of color and those from clearly defined ethnic groups have an important additional identity task in their adolescent years.

Self-esteem

So far, I have mostly talked about the self-concept as if there were no values attached to the categories by which we define ourselves. But the self-concept obviously contains an evaluative aspect as well. Note, for example, the differences in tone in the answers to the "Who am I?" question that I have already quoted. The 9-year-old makes a lot of positive statements about himself, while the two older subjects offer more mixed evaluations.

These evaluative judgments have several interesting features. First of all, over the years of elementary school and high school, children's evaluations of their own abilities become increasingly differentiated, with quite separate judgments about skills in academics or athletics, physical appearance, peer social acceptance, friendships, romantic appeal, and relationships with parents (Harter, 1990).

Paradoxically, however, it is at school age—around age 7—that children first develop a *global* self-evaluation. Seven- and 8-year-olds readily answer questions about how well they like themselves as people, how happy they are, or how well they like the way they are leading their lives. It is this global evaluation of one's own worth that is usually referred to as **self-esteem,** and this global evaluation is *not* merely the sum of all the separate assessments the child makes about his skills in different areas.

Instead, as Susan Harter's very interesting research on self-esteem tells us, a child's level of self-esteem is a product of two internal assessments or judgments (Harter, 1987; 1990). A child experiences some degree of discrepancy between what he would like to be (or thinks he *ought* to be) and what he thinks he is. When that discrepancy is low, the child's self-esteem is generally high. When the discrepancy is high—when the child sees himself as failing to live up to his own goals or values—self-esteem will be much lower.

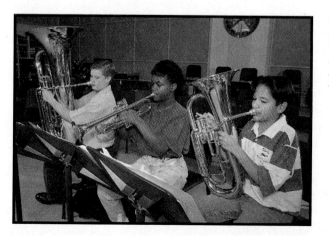

According to Harter's model, these teens' musical skill or the quality of their performance will only have an impact on their global self-esteem if musical skill is something they value.

The standards are not the same for every child. Some value academic skills highly, others value sports skills or having good friends. The key to self-esteem, Harter proposes, is the amount of discrepancy between what the child desires and what the child thinks he has achieved. Thus, a child who values sports prowess but who isn't big enough or coordinated enough to be good at sports will have lower self-esteem than will an equally small or uncoordinated child who does not value sports skill so highly. Similarly, being good at something, like singing, playing chess, or being able to talk to your mother, won't raise a child's self-esteem unless the child values that particular skill.

The second major influence on a child's self-esteem, according to Harter, is the overall sense of support the child feels from the important people around her, particularly parents and peers. Children who feel that other people generally like them the way they are have higher self-esteem scores than do children who report less overall support.

Both these factors are clear in the results of Harter's own research. She asked third, fourth, fifth, and sixth graders how important it was to them to do well in each of five domains and how well they thought they actually did in each. The total discrepancy between these sets of judgments comprised the discrepancy score. Remember that a high discrepancy score indicates that the child reported that he was *not* doing well in areas that mattered to him. The social support score was based on children's replies to a set of questions about whether they thought others (parents and peers) liked them as they were, treated them as a person, or felt that they were important. Figure 10.4 shows the results for the third and fourth graders; the findings for the fifth and sixth graders are virtually identical, and both sets of results strongly support Harter's hypothesis. Note that a low discrepancy score alone does not protect the child completely from low self-esteem if she lacks sufficient social support. And a loving and accepting family and peer group do not guarantee high self-esteem if the youngster does not feel she is living up to her own standards.

A particularly deadly combination occurs when the child perceives that the parents' support is *contingent* on good performance in some area—getting good grades, making the first-string football team, winning the audition to play the solo with the school orchestra, being popular with other kids. If the child does not measure up to the standard, he experiences both an increased discrepancy between ideal and achievement, and a loss of support from the parents.

Think about the following somewhat paradoxical proposition: If Harter's model is correct, then our self-esteem is most vulnerable in the area in which we may appear (and feel) the most competent. Does this fit with your experience?

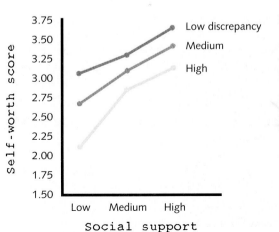

FIGURE 10.4 For these children in Harter's studies, self-esteem was about equally influenced by the amount of support the child saw herself as receiving from parents and peers and by the degree of discrepancy between the value the child places on various domains and the skill she sees herself having in each of those domains. (*Source:* Harter, 1987, Figure 9.2, p. 227.)

Consistency of Self-esteem Over Time

How stable are these self-judgments? Is a third grader with low self-esteem doomed to feel less than worthy for the rest of his life? A number of longitudinal studies of elementary-school-age children and teenagers show that global self-esteem is quite stable in the short term but somewhat less so over periods of several years. The correlation between two self-esteem scores obtained a few months apart is generally about .60. Over several years, this correlation drops to something more like .40 (Alsaker & Olweus, 1992), a level of consistency that has been found over periods as long as a decade, from early adolescence into early adulthood (Block & Robins, 1993). So it is true that a child with high self-esteem at age 8 or 9 is more likely to have high self-esteem at age 10 or 11. But it is also true that there is a good deal of variation around that stability.

Self-esteem seems to be particularly unstable in the years of early adolescence, especially at the time of the shift from elementary school to junior high school. Edward Seidman and his colleagues, for example (Seidman et al., 1994), studied a group of nearly 600 youngsters, including white, black, and Latino children, over the two years from sixth grade to junior high. Seidman found an significant drop in self-esteem over that period, a decline that occurred in every ethnic group included in this study. Such a decline in self-esteem, as well as a general instability in a child's sense of self-worth at this age, makes sense in Harter's terms, since these are years when the standards children set for themselves and the expectations of the school and parents are likely to change (Harter, 1990). In later adolescence, self-esteem appears to become more stable, although still not totally fixed.

Consequences of Variations in Self-esteem

When we look at the consequences of variations in self-esteem, the clearest research finding is that self-esteem is *strongly* negatively correlated with depression in both middle childhood and adolescence. That is, the lower the self-esteem score, the more depressed the child describes himself to be. The correlations in several of Harter's studies range from −.67 to −.80—numbers that are quite astonishingly high for research of this type (Harter, 1987; Renouf & Harter, 1990). Bear in mind, though, that this is still correlational evidence. These findings don't prove the existence of a causal connection between low self-esteem and depression. They only tell us that the two tend to go together. More persuasive is Harter's finding from her longitudinal studies that when the self-esteem score rises or falls, the depression score drops or rises accordingly.

Origins of Differences in Self-esteem

Where do differences in self-esteem come from? There are at least three sources. First, of course, a child's own direct experience with success or failure in various arenas plays an obvious role. If I take ballet lessons, it will not take me long to figure out whether I am any good at it or not. Comparative information is also involved here, of course. Just as the child learns a good deal about her academic ability by comparing herself to other students in school, so she gains information about other arenas through comparison with others' performances.

Second, the value a child attaches to some skill or quality is obviously affected fairly directly by peers' and parents' attitudes and values. For example, peer (and general cultural) standards for appearance establish benchmarks for all children and teens—which is one reason why the present Western cultural emphasis on extreme thinness in girls has led

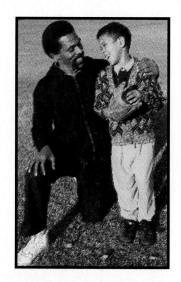

Playing catch with Dad is a classic father-son activity in American culture. One of the side effects is likely to be that the son comes to believe that skill in sports is highly valued by his dad.

to so many eating disorders. Similarly, the degree of emphasis parents place on the child performing well in some domain, whether it is school, athletics, or playing chess, is an important element in forming the child's aspirations in each area.

Finally, labels and judgments from others play a highly significant role. To a very considerable extent, we come to think of ourselves as others think of us (Cole, 1991). Children who are repeatedly told that they are "pretty," "smart," or "a good athlete" are likely to have higher self-esteem than are children who are told that they are "dumb," "clumsy," or a "late bloomer." A child who brings home a report card with Cs and Bs on it and hears the parents say, "That's fine, honey; we don't expect you to get all As" draws conclusions both about the parents' expectations and about their judgments of his abilities. From all these sources, the child fashions his ideas (his internal model) about what he should be and what he is.

The Self-concept: A Summing Up

Obviously, many questions remain to be answered. But I want to emphasize once again that a child's self-concept, including her level of self-esteem, appears to be a highly significant mediating concept. Once such a "theory" of the self is well established, once a global judgment of one's self-worth is established, we can see reverberations throughout the child's behavior. Among other things, she systematically chooses experiences and environments that are consistent with her beliefs about herself. The child who believes she can't play baseball behaves differently from the child who believes that she can. She is likely to denigrate the importance of sports or to avoid baseballs, bats, playing fields, and other children who play baseball. If forced to play, she may make self-deprecating remarks like "You know I can't play," or she may play self-defeating games, such as refusing to watch the ball when she swings at it or not running after the ball in right field because she knows she couldn't catch it even if she did get there on time. (If you think all this sounds autobiographical, you're right!)

A child who believes that she can't do long division will behave quite differently in the classroom from the child whose self-concept includes the idea "I am good at math" (or, even more potently, "I am better at math than other kids"). If she believes she is less competent, she may not try to work long division problems on the theory that if you don't try, you can't fail. Or she may try much harder, paying the price in anxiety about failure. At a later age, such a child is much less likely to take further math courses, thus reducing her occupational options.

These beliefs are pervasive, many develop early, and although they are somewhat responsive to changing circumstances, they act as self-fulfilling prophecies. We need to know a good deal more about the origins of the child's self-definitions if we are to understand how to modify the inaccurate elements.

Can you think of examples of how your own self-concept affects your choices and your behavior?

The Development of Gender and Sex-Role Concepts

A central aspect of the child's self-concept that I have not yet discussed is the gender concept and the accompanying concept of sex roles. How do children come to understand that they are a boy or a girl, and when and how do they learn to identify behaviors and attitudes considered appropriate for their gender in their particular culture? I have saved this set of questions for a separate discussion partly because this has been an area of hot debate and extensive research in the past several decades (so there is a lot to say) and partly because this set of questions has such central personal relevance for so many of us. Women's and men's roles are changing rapidly in most industrialized societies. But our stereotypes about men and women, and our own inner sense of what it means to be "male" or "female" have not always kept pace. If we are to understand ourselves (and perhaps rear our children with less confusion), we need to know more about the ways in which children learn about gender and sex roles.

The child has several related tasks. On the cognitive side, she must learn the nature of the gender category itself—that boyness or girlness is permanent, unchanged by such things as modifications in clothing or hair length. This understanding is usually called the **gender concept.** On the social side, she has to learn what behaviors go with being a boy or a girl. That is, she must learn the **sex role** (also often called the *gender role*) defined as appropriate for her gender in her particular culture.

All roles involve sets of expected behaviors, attitudes, rights, duties, and obligations. Teachers are supposed to behave in certain ways, as are employees, mothers, or baseball managers—all roles in our culture. Sex roles are somewhat broader than most other roles, but they are nonetheless roles, so we can think of a sex role as the set of expected behavior, attitudes, rights, duties, and obligations involved in filling the role of "girl," "woman," "boy," or "man."

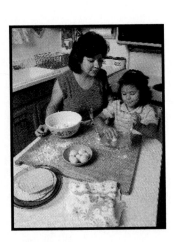

This mother is not only teaching her daughter how to cook, but also is transmitting information about sex roles and reinforcing traditional sex-typing.

A child's or adult's behavior is said to be **sex-typed** to the degree that it matches the sex-role expectations for his or her own gender. A girl may know quite well that she is a girl and be able to describe the cultural sex roles accurately but still behave in a tomboyish way. In this case we would say that her **sex-role behavior** is less sex-typed than is the behavior of a girl who adopts more traditional behavior patterns.

If we are going to understand the development of the child's concept of gender, we have to understand all these elements. How does the child come to know what gender she is? How and when does she develop ideas about sex roles? And how well and how early do children match their behavior to the sex roles or the stereotypes?

Developmental Patterns

The Development of the Gender Concept. How soon does a child figure out that she is a girl or he is a boy? It depends on what we mean by "figure out." There seem to be three steps. First comes **gender identity,** which is simply a child's ability to label his own sex correctly and to identify other people as men or women, boys or girls. By 9 to 12 months, babies already treat male and female faces as if they were different categories (Fagot & Leinbach, 1993). Within the next year, they begin to learn the verbal labels that go with these different categories. By age 2, if you show them a set of pictures of a same-sex child and several opposite-sex children and say "Which one is you?" most children can correctly pick out the same-sex picture (Thompson, 1975). By 2½ or 3, most children can correctly label and identify the sex of others as well (point out "which one is a girl" or "which one is a boy" in a set of pictures). Hair length and clothing seem to be especially important cues that children use for these early discriminations.

Accurate labeling, though, does not signify complete understanding. As is true with all the concepts I talked about in Chapter 7, which show increasing subtlety and complexity over the preschool and early school years, the gender concept undergoes further refinements. The second step is **gender stability,** the understanding that you stay the same gender throughout life. Researchers have measured this by asking children such questions as "When you were a little baby, were you a little girl or a little boy?" or "When you grow up will you be a mommy or a daddy?" Most children understand the stability aspect of gender by about age 4 (Slaby & Frey, 1975).

The final step is the development of true **gender constancy,** which is the recognition that someone stays the same gender even though he may appear to change by wearing different clothes or having different hair length. For example, girls don't change into boys by cutting their hair very short or by wearing boys' clothes. It may seem odd that a child who understands that he will stay the same gender throughout life (gender stability) can nonetheless be confused about the effect of changes in dress or appearance on gender. But numerous studies show this sequence, including studies of children growing up in other cultures, such as Kenya, Nepal, Belize, and Samoa (Munroe, Shimmin, & Munroe, 1984).

The underlying logic of this sequence may be a bit clearer if I draw a parallel between gender constancy and the concept of conservation I described in Chapter 7. Conservation of mass, number, or weight involves recognition that an object remains fundamentally the same even though it changes externally. Gender constancy is thus a kind of "conservation of gender" and is not typically understood until about 5 or 6, when the other conservations are first grasped.

The Development of Sex-Role Concepts and Stereotypes. Obviously, figuring out your gender and understanding that it stays constant is only part of the story. Learning what goes with, or ought to go with, being a boy or a girl is also a vital part of the child's task.

Researchers have studied this in two ways—by asking children what boys and girls (or men and women) like to do and what they are like (which is an inquiry about gender stereotypes) and by asking children if it is *okay* for boys to play with dolls or girls to climb trees or to do equivalent cross-sex things (an inquiry about roles).

In our society, adults have clear sex-role stereotypes. We think of men as being competent, skillful, assertive, aggressive, and able to get things done. Adults see women as warm and expressive, tactful, quiet, gentle, aware of others' feelings, and lacking in competence, independence, and logic (Williams & Best, 1990).

Studies of children show that such stereotyping occurs early. The 3-year-old daughter of a friend announced one day that mommies use the stove and daddies use the grill. Even 2-year-olds already associate certain tasks and possessions with men and women, such as vacuum cleaner and food with women and cars and tools with men. By age 3 or 4, children can assign occupations, toys, and activities to the stereotypic gender. By age 5, children begin to associate certain personality traits with males or females, and such knowledge is well developed by age 8 or 9 (Martin, 1993; Serbin, Powlishta, & Gulko, 1993). The most clearly stereotyped traits are weakness, gentleness, appreciativeness, and softheartedness for women, and aggression, strength, cruelty, and coarseness with males.

Studies of children's ideas about what men and women (or boys and girls) *ought* to be like add an interesting additional element. A study by William Damon (1977) illustrates the point particularly nicely. He told a story to children ages 4 through 9 about a little boy named George who likes to play with dolls. George's parents tell him that only little girls play with dolls; little boys shouldn't. They buy him some other toys, but still George prefers dolls. The children were then asked a batch of questions about this:

Why do people tell George not to play with dolls?

Are they right?

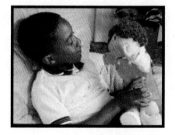

Does this little boy, like the mythical George in Damon's studies, have a right to play with dolls? Four-year-olds and 9-year-olds are likely to think that he does, but many 6-year-olds think it is simply wrong for boys to do girl things or for girls to do boy things.

Cultures and Contexts
Sex-Role Stereotypes Around the World

A child is shown a silhouette of a man, and one of a woman, and told a story: "One of these people is emotional. They cry when something good happens as well as when everything goes wrong. Which person is the emotional person?" Or, "One of these people is always pushing other people around and getting into fights. Which person gets into fights?" (Williams & Best, 1990).

In response to stories like these, third-grade children in the U.S. identify the male figure as aggressive 90 percent of the time and the female figure as emotional 79 percent of the time. Fourth graders give the stereotyped answer to both stories 100 percent of the time. Are these stereotypes unique to American culture, or does something similar exist in every culture? An amazing cross-cultural study by John Williams and Deborah Best (1990) gives us some answers.

They asked 5- and 8-year-old children in 24 countries these same questions, translated where necessary. Included were countries from every continent, with varying levels of industrialization.

Williams and Best had expected to find some common ground, but as they put it, "We were not prepared, however, for the high degree of pancultural generality that we found" (p. 303). In every country, the children had less-strong sex stereotypes than did adults in that same country, but in every country, the qualities associated with men were stronger and more active than those associated with women, and this was true of young children as well as adults.

Among the children, the characteristics most consistently ascribed to males were aggression, strength, and cruelty, and those most consistently ascribed to females were weakness, gentleness, and appreciativeness. These patterns become stronger with age in all countries, so 8-year-olds gave more stereotypic responses than 5-year-olds. And in virtually all countries, the male stereotype was clearer or more consistent than the female.

There were a few differences, naturally. Children in some countries seem to learn the sex stereotype very early, in others somewhat later. Five-year-olds in Pakistan and New Zealand, for example, already had very clear stereotypes, while those in Brazil and France showed little stereotyping at 5 but clearer stereotyping at 8—a pattern also found among African-Americans. Sex stereotypes in particular countries also contain unique content. German children, for instance, choose "adventurous," "confident," "jolly," and "steady" as female items, although these are more normally male items in other cultures. Pakistani children identify "emotional" with men; Japanese children associate independence and severity with neither sex. But these are variations on a common theme. In *all* 24 countries, 8-year-olds choose the male figure for stories about aggression, strength, cruelty, coarseness, and loudness, and they choose the female figure for stories about weakness. In 23 of 24 countries, 8-year-olds also choose the female story for gentleness, appreciativeness, and softheartedness. Thus, not only does every culture appear to have clear sex-role stereotypes, but the content of those stereotypes is remarkably similar across cultures.

Is there a rule that boys shouldn't play with dolls?

What should George do?

Does George have a right to play with dolls? (p. 242)

Four-year-olds in this study thought it was okay for George to play with dolls. There was no rule against it and he should do it if he wanted to. Six-year-olds, in contrast, thought it was *wrong* for George to play with dolls. By about age 9, children had differentiated between what boys and girls usually do, and what is "wrong." One boy said, for example, that breaking windows was wrong and bad, but that playing with dolls was not bad in the same way: "Breaking windows you're not supposed to do. And if you play with dolls, well you can, but boys usually don't."

What seems to be happening is that the 5- or 6-year-old, having figured out that she is permanently a girl or he is a boy, is searching for a *rule* about how boys and girls behave (Martin & Halverson, 1981). The child picks up information from watching adults, from watching TV, from listening to the labels that are attached to different activities (e.g., "boys don't cry"). Initially they treat these as absolute, moral rules. Later they understand that these are social conventions, at which point sex-role concepts become more flexible (Katz & Ksansnak, 1994). In fact, many kinds of prejudice—such as bias against obese children, against those who speak another language, or against those of other races—are at their peak in the early school years and then decline throughout the remaining years of childhood and adolescence (Doyle & Aboud, 1995; Powlishta et al., 1994).

One of the interesting sidelights in the research on stereotyping is that the male stereotype and sex-role concept seems to develop a bit earlier and to be stronger than the female stereotype or sex-role concept—and this is true in virtually all countries studied. More children agree on what men are or should be like than on what women are or should be. This might happen because children have direct experience with women in several significant roles (mother and teacher, for example), while their primary experience with men is in the role of father. Or it could mean that the female role in our society is more flexible than the male role. At any rate, it is clear that in Western societies, the qualities attributed to the male are more highly *valued* than are the female traits (Broverman et al., 1970). We see it as "good" to be independent, assertive, logical, and strong; it is less good to be warm, quiet, tactful, and gentle. Perhaps girls recognize early that the male role is seen more positively and aspire to some of the valued male qualities. That would lead to a female role being perceived more broadly. Whatever the reason, it is an interesting finding—one with considerable relevance for understanding adult male and female sex roles and stereotyping.

The Development of Sex-Role Behavior. The final element in the equation is the actual behavior children show with their own sex and with the opposite sex. The unexpected finding here is that children's *behavior* is sex-typed earlier than are their ideas about sex roles or stereotypes.

By 18 to 24 months, children begin to show some preference for sex-stereotyped toys, such as dolls for girls or trucks or building blocks for boys, which is some months before they can normally identify their own gender (O'Brien, 1992). By age 3, children begin to show a preference for same-sex playmates and are much more sociable with playmates of the same sex—at a time when they do not yet have a concept of gender stability (Maccoby, 1988; 1990; Maccoby & Jacklin, 1987). By school age, peer relationships are almost exclusively same-sex. You can see the early development of this preference in Figure 10.5, which shows the results of a study of preschool play groups. The researchers counted how often children played with same-sex or opposite-sex playmates (La Freniere, Strayer, & Gauthier, 1984). You can see that by age 3, about 60 percent of play groups were same-sex groupings and that the rate rose from there.

The other intriguing pattern is that children in early elementary school seem to begin to pay more attention to the behavior of same-sex adults or playmates than to that of the opposite sex and to play more with new toys that are labeled as appropriate for their own sex (Bradbard et al., 1986). All in all, then, we see many signs that children are both aware of and affected by gender from very early, perhaps by age 1, certainly by age 2. But

How many explanations can you think of for the fact that children begin to prefer to play with same-sex peers as early as age 3?

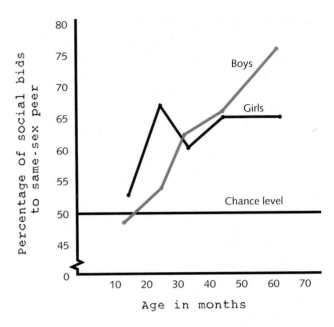

FIGURE 10.5 Same-sex playmate preference among preschoolers. (*Source:* La Freniere, Strayer, & Gauthier, 1984, Figure 1, p. 1961. Copyright by The Society for Research in Child Development, Inc.)

gender becomes a still more potent force in guiding behavior and attitudes at around age 5 or 6.

Explaining Sex-Role Development

Theorists from most of the major traditions have tried their hand at explaining this pattern of development. Freud relied on the concept of identification to explain the child's adoption of appropriate sex-role behavior, but his theory founders on the fact that children begin to show clearly sex-typed behavior long before age 4 or 5, when Freud thought identification occurred.

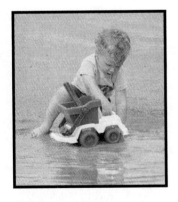

Social learning theorists would argue that little boys prefer to play with trucks because parents buy them more trucks and reinforce them directly for such play. Does this make sense to you?

Social Learning Theory. Social learning theorists, such as Bandura (1977) and Walter Mischel (1966; 1970), have naturally emphasized the role of both direct reinforcement and of modeling in shaping children's sex-role behavior and attitudes. This notion has been far better supported by research. Parents do seem to reinforce sex-typed activities in children as young as 18 months old, not only by buying different kinds of toys for boys and girls, but by responding more positively when their sons play with blocks or trucks or when their daughters play with dolls (Fagot & Hagan, 1991; Lytton & Romney, 1991). Such differential reinforcement is particularly clear with boys. New evidence also suggests that toddlers whose parents are more consistent in rewarding sex-typed toy choice or play behavior and whose mothers favor traditional family sex roles learn accurate gender labels earlier than do toddlers whose parents are less focused on the gender-appropriateness of the child's play (Fagot & Leinbach, 1989; Fagot, Leinbach, & O'Boyle, 1992)—findings clearly consistent with the predictions of social learning theory.

Interestingly, researchers have also accumulated a fair amount of evidence that differential treatment of sons and daughters is more common among fathers than mothers and that fathers are particularly likely to be concerned with the appropriate sex-role behavior of their sons (Siegal, 1987). Many fathers seem to be especially uncomfortable with "girlish" behavior in their sons and are much more likely to show disapproval of such behavior in their sons than they are to disapprove of "tomboyish" behavior in their daughters—

which may be one reason that the male stereotype develops earlier and is stronger than is the female stereotype.

Cross-cultural evidence also supports a social learning view. Anthropologist Beatrice Whiting (Whiting & Edwards, 1988), after examining patterns of gender socialization in 11 different cultures, concludes that "we are the company we keep." In most cultures, girls and boys keep different company, beginning quite early, with girls spending more time with women as well as in child-care responsibilities. To the extent that this is true, it would provide each sex with more same-sex than opposite-sex models and more opportunity for reinforcement of sex-appropriate behavior, such as nurturance directed at younger siblings.

Still, helpful as it is, a social learning explanation is probably insufficient. In particular, there is less differential reinforcement of boy-behavior versus girl-behavior than you'd expect, and probably not enough to account for the very early and robust discrimination children seem to make on the basis of gender. Even children whose parents seem to treat their young sons and daughters in highly similar ways nonetheless learn gender labels and show same-sex playmate choices.

Cognitive-Developmental Theories. A third alternative, based strongly on Piagetian theory, is Lawrence Kohlberg's suggestion that the crucial aspect of the process is the child's understanding of the gender concept (1966; Kohlberg & Ullian, 1974). Once the child realizes that he is a boy or she is a girl forever, he or she becomes highly motivated to learn to behave in the way that is expected or appropriate for that gender. Specifically, Kohlberg predicted that we should see systematic same-sex imitation only *after* the child has shown full gender constancy. Most studies designed to test this hypothesis have supported Kohlberg: Children do seem to become much more sensitive to same-sex models after they have understood gender constancy (Frey & Ruble, 1992). But Kohlberg's theory cannot easily handle the obvious fact that children show clear, differential sex-role behavior, such as toy preferences, long before they have achieved full understanding of the gender concept.

Gender Schema Theory. The most fruitful current explanation is usually called **gender schema theory** (Martin, 1991; Martin & Halverson, 1981), a model that has its roots in information-processing theories of cognitive development as well as in Kohlberg's theory. Just as the self-concept can be thought of as a "scheme" or "self-theory," so the child's understanding of gender can be seen in the same way. The gender schema begins to develop as soon as the child notices the differences between male and female, knows his own gender, and can label the two groups with some consistency—all of which happens by age 2 or 3. Perhaps because gender is clearly an either/or category, children seem to understand very early that this is a key distinction, so the category serves as a kind of magnet for new information (Maccoby, 1988). In Piaget's terms, once the child has established even a primitive gender scheme, a great many experiences are assimilated to it. Thus, as soon as this scheme begins to be formed, children begin to show preference for same-sex playmates or for gender-stereotyped activities (Martin & Little, 1990).

Preschoolers first learn some broad distinctions about what kinds of activities or behavior go with each gender, both by observing other children and through the reinforcements they receive from parents. They also learn a few gender "scripts"—whole sequences of events that normally go with a given gender, such as "fixing dinner" or "building with tools" (Levy & Fivush, 1993)—just as they learn other social scripts at about this age.

The Real World

Sex Stereotyping on TV and in Children's Books

In modern cultures, one obvious source for children to acquire information for their sex-role schemas is through the TV programs they watch. From early preschool age, children in the United States spend an average of two to four hours a day in the presence of a TV set that is running. (I put it that way because we don't know how much of the time children actually *watch* the moving image.) Before they begin school, children have already been exposed to thousands of hours of TV; by the time they are 18 the average child has spent more time in front of a TV set than in a classroom (Calvert & Huston, 1987). How are men and women portrayed in all those TV programs and commercials?

Highly stereotypically (Huston et al., 1990). The most current estimates suggest that in U.S. television programs, males outnumber females by 2 to 1 or 3 to 1 on virtually every kind of programming, including children's cartoons. The frequency of males and females is more equal in commercials, but the "voice-over" on commercials is nearly always male. In both commercials and regular programming, women are more often shown at home or in romantic situations; men more often appear in work settings, with cars, or playing sports. Men are shown solving problems and being more active, aggressive, and independent. Women are shown as sex objects, and more often as dependent, overly emotional, or less able to deal with difficult situations (Golombok & Fivush, 1994).

A continuous exposure to these stereotyped males and females does seem to have at least a small effect on a child's vision of men and women and their roles. In two longitudinal studies, Morgan (1982; 1987) has found that among elementary and high school students, those who watched a lot of TV at the beginning of the study reported more traditional sex-role stereotyping a year later. They were more likely, for example, to think that household chores should be done by women than by men. Even more persuasive is an experiment by Emily Davidson

(Davidson, Yasuna, & Tower, 1979), who deliberately exposed some 5- and 6-year-olds to highly sex-stereotyped cartoons. Those who had seen such cartoons, compared to control children who had seen neutral cartoons, later gave more stereotyped answers to questions about the qualities of men and women.

At a more subtle level, Aletha Huston and her colleagues, in several studies (Huston et al., 1984), have found that toy commercials aimed at boys and those aimed at girls are simply designed differently. Boys' commercials are fast, sharp, and loud—lots of quick cuts, loud music, activity. Girls' commercials are gradual, soft, and fuzzy. They have camera fades and dissolves rather than sharp cuts and use softer background music. Children as young as first grade notice these differences too. They can watch a commercial of some nonstereotyped toy and tell you whether the *style* of the commercial is suited to a boys' or girls' toy.

Children's books are also quite stereotyped. Fifty years ago, three or four times as many boys as girls appeared as central characters in such books. Today the ratio is more like 2 to 1, but boys are still more common protagonists in picture books and early reading books (Kortenhaus & Demarest, 1993). Even in books that have won the Caldecott Medal, given to the most distinguished picture book each year, male characters outnumber females by about 2 to 1 (Golombok & Fivush, 1994). When girls do appear as leading characters in such books, they are often depicted as adventurous, but it is still comparatively rare for girls to be central figures.

TV and books are clearly not the only sources of information children have about sex roles. We know that children growing up without TV nonetheless acquire sex-role stereotypes. Yet TV and books do have an impact on children's ideas about men and women, and they accentuate rather than minimize gender stereotypes.

Then between ages 4 and 6 the child learns a more subtle and complex set of associations for his or her *own* gender—what children of his own gender like and don't like, how they play, how they talk, what kinds of people they associate with. Only at about ages 8 to 10 does the child develop an equivalently complex view of the opposite gender (Martin, Wood, & Little, 1990).

The key difference between this theory and Kohlberg's is that for the initial gender schema to be formed, the child need not understand that gender is permanent. When gender constancy is understood at about 5 or 6, she develops a more elaborated rule or schema of "what people who are like me do" and treats this "rule" the same way she treats other rules—as absolutes. Later, the child's application of the "gender rule" becomes more flexible. She knows, for example, that most boys don't play with dolls but that they *can* do so if they like.

Many of us, committed to the philosophical goal of equality for women, have taken the rigidity of children's early sex stereotypes as evidence that we have made little progress toward equality ("Mommy, you can't be a psychology doctor, you have to be a psychology nurse"). But gender schema theorists emphasize that such rule learning is absolutely normal, and so is the rigid stereotyping that we see in children's ideas about sex roles between ages 5 and 8 or 9. Children are searching for order, for rules that help to make sense of their experiences. And a rule about "what men do" and "what women do" is a helpful schema for children. Like grammatical rules, children first apply this new rule too rigidly and then later learn the exceptions. But the rule-learning process seems to be a natural one.

Gender schema theory is surely not the last word. It too has limitations. For example, when researchers have measured preschool children's understanding of gender and then looked at how sex-typed their behavior is, they often find only very weak connections (Bussey & Bandura, 1992; Martin, 1993). So 3-year-olds who show the clearest preferences for same-sex playmates are not necessarily the same ones who have the most advanced cognitive understanding of gender. Ultimately, some combination of social learning theory and gender schema theory may be devised that will handle the data better.

Individual Differences In Sex-typing and Sex-Role Stereotypes

The developmental patterns I have been describing seem to hold for virtually all children. Nevertheless, as usual, we also see quite a lot of variation from child to child in the rigidity of the rule they develop or in the sex-typing of their behavior.

As a group, boys usually have stronger (more rigid and more traditional) sex-role stereotypes. Among both boys and girls, however, children whose mothers work outside the home have *less* stereotypic views (more flexible rules) (Powell & Steelman, 1982). Parallel evidence comes from one recent study of children who were cared for in early life by the father instead of the mother. These children too later had less-stereotyped views of sex roles (Williams, Radin, & Allegro, 1992). This makes perfectly good sense if the child's sex-role schema is formed primarily (or at least originally) by observing the parents' roles.

Cross-sex Children. Another interesting group is children with cross-sex preferences—girls who would rather be boys and boys who would rather be girls. Having been a tomboy myself, I find such children especially intriguing. How does a child come to prefer to be the other sex or to choose cross-sex playmates or toys?

One possibility is that such children are directly trained that way. They may have been specifically reinforced for aspects of the opposite sex's role. Some girls are given trucks and carpentry tools and taught football by their fathers (or mothers). They may come to wish to be boys. We know that tomboy behavior is more accepted and reinforced than is "girlish" behavior in a boy, so it makes sense from a social learning perspective that many more girls say they would like to be boys than the reverse.

If you had as one of your goals of child rearing to rear totally "nonsexist" children, how might you try to go about it, given what you have read about the emergence of the child's gender concept?

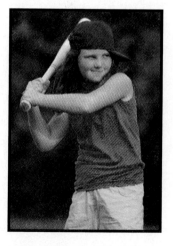

In our society, "tomboys" like this one are fairly common and largely accepted. But a boy this age who showed "girlish" behavior would experience much more pressure to change, perhaps especially from Dad.

How many explanations can you think of for the fact that there are more tomboys than there are "girlish" boys?

Social learning theory does not fare so well, though, in explaining the results of research by Carl Roberts and his colleagues (Roberts et al., 1987). They studied a group of boys who showed strong preference for female toys and playmates from their earliest years of life. When Roberts compared these boys to a group of boys with more typical masculine sex-role behaviors, he found little evidence that the more feminine boys had been specifically reinforced for these behaviors or that their fathers were providing models for such behavior. Rather, Roberts found that the feminine boys were more feminine in appearance from earliest babyhood, that they were more often ill or hospitalized early in life, and that they had relatively less contact with both their mothers and fathers on a daily basis, compared to the more masculine boys. This pattern of findings does not fit nicely with a simple social learning explanation.

Alternatively, there might be some biological differences. Roberts and his colleagues' finding that the more behaviorally feminine boys already looked more feminine from earliest infancy is at least consistent with such a possibility, as is their finding that in adulthood, three-quarters of the more feminine boys were homosexual or bisexual. Further evidence for some biological influence on cross-sex behavior comes from studies of girls who have experienced heightened levels of androgen prenatally. (Recall from Chapter 4 that androgen is largely a "male" hormone.) These "androgenized" girls, in comparison to their normal sisters, more often prefer to play with boys (Hines & Kaufman, 1994), show less interest in dolls or babies, and have fewer fantasies about being a mother (Meyer-Bahlburg, Ehrhardt, & Feldman, 1986). Some evidence also suggests that these androgenized girls are more interested in rough-and-tumble play, although here the findings are not consistent (Hines & Kaufman, 1994).

Findings like these suggest that actual sex-typing of behavior is at least partially affected by prenatal hormones. At the same time, it is also clear that a child's basic gender identity—the gender she thinks of herself as being—is strongly influenced by the label she is given and the treatment she receives from her parents. Children born with ambiguous genitalia, for example, will grow up to think of themselves as being whichever gender they were reared as, even if that gender does not match their genotype (Money, 1987).

Clearly, the gender a child *thinks* he is affects the gender *schema* he develops, and the environment is extremely potent in helping to shape that schema. But I think we must keep an open mind about the possible biological origins of some sex-role behaviors. The evidence is not all in yet.

Androgyny. A very different approach to the study of cross-sex sex-typing has emerged in the past decades in the study of **androgyny.** Until perhaps the early 1970s, psychologists had thought of "masculinity" and "femininity" as opposite ends of the same continuum. A person could be one or the other but couldn't be both. Following the lead of Sandra Bem (1974) and of Janet Spence and Robert Helmreich (1978), psychologists today conceive of masculinity and femininity as two separate dimensions. A person can be high or low on either or both. Thus, a person can be both compassionate and independent, both gentle and assertive.

This conceptualization creates four basic "types," as shown in Figure 10.6. The two traditional (strongly sex-typed) sex roles are the masculine and the feminine combinations. The two new "types" that become evident when we think about sex roles in this way are called *androgynous* and *undifferentiated*. Androgynous individuals think of themselves as having both masculine and feminine traits; undifferentiated individuals describe

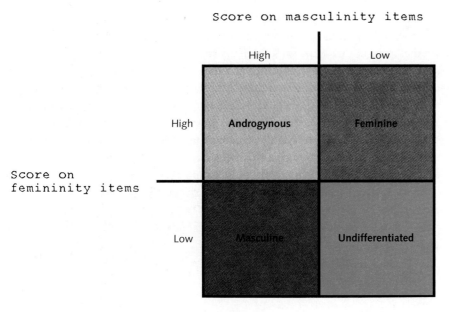

Score on masculinity items

FIGURE 10.6 Four sex-role types created when we think of masculinity and femininity as separate dimensions, rather than as two ends of the same dimension.

themselves as lacking both—a group that sounds a lot like those with a "diffuse" identity in Marcia's system.

This categorization system says nothing about the accuracy of the child's or the adult's rule or schema about sex roles. A teenage girl, for example, could have a clear notion of the norms for male or female behavior and still perceive *herself* as having some stereotypically masculine qualities. In some sense, then, when we study masculinity/femininity/androgyny, we are studying the intersection between the self-scheme and the gender scheme.

Perhaps because young children's ideas about sex roles are still quite rigid (or perhaps because we do not yet have good measures of androgyny for young children), we find little sign of androgyny among children younger than 9 or 10. But variations in androgyny, masculinity, and femininity clearly do exist among adolescents.

Several studies show that roughly 25 to 35 percent of high school students in the U.S. describe themselves as androgynous (Lamke, 1982a; Spence & Helmreich, 1978). More girls seem to show this pattern than do boys, and there are more girls in the "masculine" category than there are boys in the "feminine" group—just as there are more tomboys than the opposite. Furthermore, for *both* boys and girls in this culture, either a masculine or an androgynous sex-role self-concept is associated with higher self-esteem (Lamke, 1982a; 1982b), doubtless because both boys and girls value many of the qualities that are stereotypically masculine, such as independence and competence. Thus, a boy can achieve high self-esteem and success with his peers by adopting a traditionally masculine sex role. For girls, though, adoption of a traditionally feminine sex role without some balancing "male" characteristics seems to carry a risk of lower self-esteem, and even poorer relationships with peers (Massad, 1981).

Findings like these suggest the possibility that while the creation of rigid rules or schemas for sex roles is a normal—even essential—process in young children, a blurring of those rules may be an important process in adolescence (at least in Western cultures), particularly for girls, for whom a more androgynous self-concept is associated with positive outcomes.

I have been careful in the preceding few paragraphs to say, repeatedly, "in Western cultures." I have done so because it is not entirely obvious to me that androgyny or masculinity are the optimum patterns for adolescent self-esteem in every culture. Would we find this same link in a collectivist culture, in which cooperation and respectfulness are more highly valued than assertiveness and independence? The more general rule may be that higher self-esteem in teenagers (and in adults) is linked to a self-perception that matches the most valued traits in the culture in which one grows up. In the U.S., where assertiveness and independence are highly valued, adolescents who perceive themselves as having these qualities not only describe themselves as more masculine or androgynous, but also have higher self-esteem. In a collectivist culture, those teens who see themselves as having the more stereotypically feminine qualities of cooperativeness or respectfulness might have higher self-esteem. I know of no data that test this hypothesis, but it is yet another reminder that we have to be cautious about generalizing from U.S. or Western data to all cultures.

Summary

1   The child's emerging self-concept has several elements, including the awareness of a separate self and the understanding of self-permanence (which may be collectively called the subjective self) and awareness of oneself as an object in the world (the objective self).

2   The subjective self develops in the first year of life; we see real self-awareness and the emergence of the objective self in the second year.

3   In early childhood, the child begins to place herself in basic categories such as age, size, and gender. These early self-definitions are quite concrete, based primarily on physical attributes and things the child can do.

4   The self-concept becomes steadily more abstract in the elementary and high school years, coming to include not only actions but also likes and dislikes, beliefs, and more general personality characteristics. Beginning at about age 8 the child also has a global sense of self-worth (self-esteem).

5   At adolescence, there may also be a reevaluation of the self, a process Erikson talks of as the "identity crisis." In theory, adolescents move from a diffuse sense of future occupational or ideological identity, through a period of reevaluation (moratorium), to a commitment to a new self-definition. Whether this occurs to all adolescents or in all cultures is not so clear.

6   Self-concepts also include an evaluative dimension, usually called self-esteem. Self-esteem is shaped both by the degree of discrepancy between a child's goals and his accomplishments and by the degree of emotional support the child perceives from parents and peers. Children with high self-esteem show lower levels of depression.

7   Gender identity is part of the self-concept. Children generally acquire gender identity (labeling themselves and others correctly) by about age 2 or 3. They develop gender stability (knowing you stay the same gender throughout life) by about 4 and gender constancy (you don't change gender by changing appearance) by about 5 or 6.

8   Children in all cultures studied so far have knowledge of cultural sex-role stereotypes by age 7 or 8; these stereotypes are remarkably similar across cultures.

9   In early elementary school, children create maximally rigid rules about what boys and girls ought to do or are allowed to do. Older children are aware of the social conventions but do not treat them as incontrovertible rules.

10   Sex-typed behavior is visible from about 18 months of age; children this age begin to show sex-typed toy preferences; by 2½ or 3 they begin to choose same-sex playmates—*before* they have clearly understood gender stability.

11 Theorists of several different traditions have attempted to explain these patterns. Freud's theory, resting on the concept of identification, has little support.

12 Social learning theorists emphasize the role of reinforcement and modeling and argue that children are reinforced for imitating same-sex models. Parents do appear to treat boys and girls in systematically different ways, including punishing boys for girlish behavior, although differential reinforcement appears to be insufficient to account for the degree of early sex-typing.

13 Kohlberg proposed a cognitive-developmental model: Children begin to imitate same-sex models only after they have achieved gender constancy. Some evidence supports this, but the theory does not explain sex-typed behavior at age 2 or 3.

14 Gender schema theory offers a fourth alternative: Children begin to acquire a rule about what boys do and what girls do as soon as they figure out the difference, and this schema forms the basis of both stereotyping and sex-typed behavior.

15 More girls than boys show cross-sex preferences in toy choices and behavior. Both environmental and biological elements may play a part in such cross-sex choices.

16 Young people also differ in the extent to which they see themselves as having feminine and/or masculine qualities or traits. Those who describe themselves with both sets of qualities are called androgynous. Girls who describe themselves as androgynous or masculine have somewhat higher self-esteem—at least in U.S. culture.

Key Terms

androgyny (p. 300)

foreclosure (p. 284)

gender concept (p. 292)

gender constancy (p. 293)

gender identity (p. 292)

gender schema theory (p. 297)

gender stability (p. 292)

identity achievement (p. 284)

identity diffusion (p. 285)

moratorium (p. 284)

objective self (p. 280)

self-concept (p. 279)

self-esteem (p. 288)

sex role (p. 292)

sex-role behavior (p. 292)

sex-typing (p. 292)

subjective self (p. 279)

Suggested Readings

Golombok, S., & Fivush, R. (1994). *Gender development.* Cambridge, England: Cambridge University Press.

A basic, up-to-date description of all facets of gender development.

Harter, S. (1987). The determinants and mediational role of global self-worth in children. In N. Eisenberg (Ed.), *Contemporary topics in developmental psychology.* New York: Wiley-Interscience.

I think Harter's work is the best being done today on self-esteem. This paper is a very good introduction to her ideas.

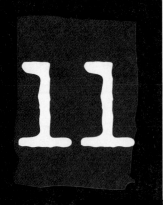

The Development of Social Relationships

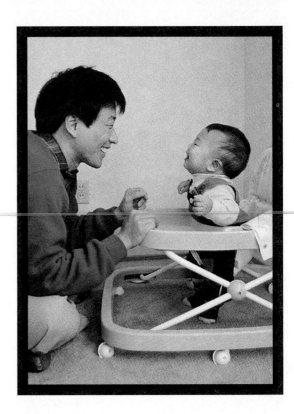

N ot long ago, as I had lunch in a restaurant with a friend, we were both happily distracted by the sight of an adorable baby at the next table. The baby, perhaps 4 or 5 months old, was sitting on her mom's lap, facing outward, and gazing with delight at an older woman sitting across from her—perhaps her grandmother. As the older woman talked to the baby in a high and lilting voice, smiled, and tickled the baby's tummy, the infant responded with one huge smile after another. My friend and I stopped talking as we watched and could hardly restrain ourselves from trying to join in the whole process. I had my "talking-with-baby voice" all warmed up and ready to go, and found myself smiling as if to try to entice an answering smile from the infant—although the baby didn't look our way at all.

But even as I was personally drawn into this small scene, the psychologist in me was also aware of many aspects of the interaction. The baby's social skills, her ability to entice, were on clear display, as were the skills of the older woman who was eliciting the baby's smiles. My guess was that this older woman was familiar to the baby and had played this interactive game many times before. Chances are good that had I tried to entice a smile or two, I would have had some success, but nothing like what we were watching. Just as dance partners need to learn each other's moves in order to dance smoothly, so babies and the adults who care for them adapt to one another's style and rhythms.

This brief scene focuses our attention on an aspect of development I have largely neglected so far, namely, the child's relationships with others—surely a central aspect of any child's (or adult's) life.

Willard Hartup, one of the most astute students of social development, suggests that each child needs experience in two rather different kinds of relationships: *vertical* and *horizontal* (1989). A vertical relationship involves an attachment to someone who has greater social power or knowledge, such as a parent, a teacher, or even an older sibling. Such relationships are complementary rather than reciprocal. The bond may be extremely powerful in both directions, but the actual behaviors the two partners show toward one another are not the same. For example, when a child bids for attention, the mother or father responds not with a matching bid for attention but with nurturance. Horizontal relationships, in contrast, are reciprocal and egalitarian. The individuals involved, such as same-age peers, have equal social power, and their behavior toward one another comes from the same repertoire.

Hartup's point is that these two kinds of relationships serve different functions for the child, and both are needed for the child to develop effective social skills. Vertical relationships are necessary to provide the child with protection and security. In these relationships the child creates his basic internal working models and learns fundamental social skills. But it is in horizontal relationships—in friendships and in peer groups—that the child practices his social behavior and acquires those social skills that can only be learned in a relationship between equals: cooperation, competition, and intimacy.

Let's begin by looking at the vertical relationships, particularly at the core relationship between child and parent.

Attachment Theory: Concepts and Terminology

The strongest theoretical influence in modern-day studies of infant-parent relationships is attachment theory, particularly the work of John Bowlby (1969; 1973; 1980; 1988a; 1988b), whose approach I described briefly in Chapter 9. You'll recall that his thinking has roots in psychoanalytic thought, particularly in the emphasis on the significance of the earliest relationship between mother and child. But he adds important evolutionary and ethological concepts. In his view, "The propensity to make strong emotional bonds to particular individuals [is] a basic component of human nature, already present in germinal form in the neonate" (1988a, p. 3). Such relationships have *survival* value, because they bring nurturance to the infant. They are built and maintained by an interlocking repertoire of instinctive behaviors that create and sustain proximity between parent and child or between other bonded pairs.

In Bowlby's writings and in the equally influential writings of Mary Ainsworth (1972; 1982; 1989; Ainsworth et al., 1978), the key concepts are those of an affectional bond, an attachment, and attachment behaviors.

Ainsworth defines an **affectional bond** as a "relatively long-enduring tie in which the partner is important as a unique individual and is interchangeable with none other. In an affectional bond, there is a desire to maintain closeness to the partner" (1989, p. 711). An **attachment** is a subvariety of emotional bond in which a person's sense of security is bound up in the relationship. When you are attached, you feel (or hope to feel) a special sense of security and comfort in the presence of the other, and you can use the other as a "safe base" from which to explore the rest of the world.

In these terms, the child's relationship with the parent is an attachment, but the parents' relationship with the child is not, since the parent presumably does not feel a greater sense of security in the presence of the infant or use the infant as a safe base. A relationship with one's adult partner or with a very close friend, however, is likely to be an attachment in the sense Ainsworth and Bowlby mean the term.

Since affectional bonds and attachments are internal states, we cannot see them directly. Instead, we deduce their existence by observing **attachment behaviors,** which are all those behaviors that allow a child or adult to achieve and retain proximity to someone else to whom he is attached. This could include smiling, making eye contact, calling out to the other person across a room, touching, clinging, crying.

It is important to make clear that there is no one-to-one correspondence between the number of different attachment behaviors a child (or adult) shows on any one occasion and the strength of the underlying attachment. Attachment behaviors are elicited primarily when the individual has need of care, support, or comfort. An infant is in such a needy state a good deal of the time, but an older child will be likely to show attachment behaviors only when he is frightened, tired, or otherwise under stress. It is the *pattern* of these behaviors, not the frequency, that tells us something about the strength or quality of the attachment or the affectional bond.

To understand the early relationship between the parent and the child, we need to look at both sides of the equation—at the development of the parents' bond to the child and of the child's attachment to the parent.

> Think about your own relationships. In Bowlby and Ainsworth's terms, which are attachments and which are affectional bonds?

> Pick one of your attachment relationships and make a list of all the attachment behaviors you show toward that person. Are any of these the same as the kind of attachment behaviors we see in an infant?

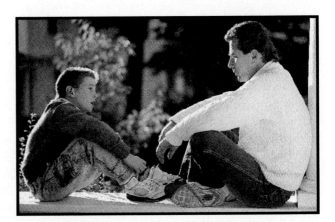

In this "vertical" social relationship, the son is attached to his dad, but in Ainsworth's terms, the father's relationship to his son is an "affectional bond" rather than an attachment.

The Parents' Bond to the Child

The Initial Bond

If you read the popular press at all, I am sure you have come across articles proclaiming that mothers (or fathers) must have immediate contact with their newborn infant if they are to become properly bonded with the baby. This belief has been based primarily on the work of two pediatricians, Marshall Klaus and John Kennell (1976). Two decades ago, they proposed the hypothesis that the first few hours after an infant's birth is a "critical period" for the mother's development of a bond to her infant. Mothers who are denied early contact, Klaus and Kennell thought, are likely to form weaker bonds and thus be at higher risk for a range of disorders of parenting.

Their proposal was one of many factors leading to significant changes in birth practices, including the now normal presence of fathers at delivery. I would certainly not want to turn back the clock on such changes. But it now looks as if Klaus and Kennel's hypothesis is essentially incorrect. Immediate contact does not appear to be either necessary or sufficient for the formation of a stable, long-term affectional bond between parent and child (Myers, 1987).

A few studies show some short-term beneficial effects of very early contact. In the first few days after delivery, mothers with such contact may show more tender fondling or more gazing at the baby than is true of mothers who first held their babies some hours after birth (e.g., de Chateau, 1980). But there is little indication of a lasting effect. Two or three months after delivery, mothers who have had immediate contact with their newborns do not smile at them more or hold them differently than do mothers who had delayed contact. Only among mothers who are otherwise at higher risk for problems with parenting—such as first-time mothers, mothers living in poverty, or very young mothers—are there a few signs that early contact may make a difference. Among such mothers, extended or early contact with the infant in the first days of life seems to help prevent later problems, such as abuse or neglect (O'Connor et al., 1980). But for the majority of mothers, neither early nor extended contact appears to be an essential ingredient in forming a strong affectional bond.

The Development of Synchrony

What *is* essential in the formation of that bond is the opportunity for the parent and infant to develop a mutual, interlocking pattern of attachment behaviors, a smooth "dance" of interaction. The baby signals his needs by crying or smiling; he responds to being held by quieting or snuggling; he looks at the parents when they look at him. The parents, in their turn, enter into this two-person dance with their own repertoire of caregiving behaviors. They pick the baby up when he cries, wait for and respond to his signals of hunger or other need, smile at him when he smiles, gaze into his eyes when he looks at them. Some researchers and theorists have described this as the development of *synchrony* (Isabella, Belsky, & von Eye, 1989).

One of the most intriguing things about this process is that we all seem to know how to do this particular dance, and we do it in very similar ways. In the presence of a young infant most adults will automatically display a distinctive pattern of interactive behaviors, including smiling, raised eyebrows, and very-wide-open eyes. And we all seem to use our voices in special ways with babies as well, as you'll remember from the discussion of motherese in Chapter 8. Parents all over the world use the characteristic high-pitched and lilting pattern of motherese; they also use similar intonation patterns. For example, in a

These two moms show almost identical expressions—the classic "mock surprise" expression characteristic of adults when interacting with a baby: raised eyebrows, open mouth, semismile.

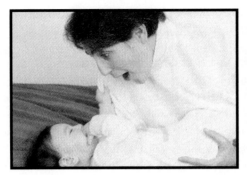 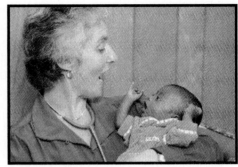

Watch yourself next time you interact with a baby. Does your facial expression match the "mock surprise" in the photos above? Does your intonation pattern follow the pattern in the Papousek study?

study of mother-infant interactions, Hanus and Mechthild Papousek (1991) found that Chinese, German, and United States mothers all tended to use a rising voice inflection when they wanted the baby to "take a turn" in the interaction and a falling intonation when they wanted to soothe the baby.

But while we can perform all these attachment *behaviors* with many infants, we do not form a bond with every baby we coo at in a restaurant or the grocery store. For an adult, the critical ingredient for the formation of a bond seems to be the opportunity to develop real synchrony—to practice the dance until the partners follow one another's lead smoothly and pleasurably. This takes time and many rehearsals, and some parents (and infants) become more skillful at it than others. In general, the smoother and more predictable the process becomes, the more satisfying it seems to be to the parents and the stronger their bond to the infant becomes.

This second step appears to be *far* more important than the initial contact at birth in establishing a strong parental bond to the child. But this second process too can fail. I've explored some of the possible reasons for such a failure in the *Real World* box on the facing page.

Father-Child Bonds

Most of the research I have talked about so far has involved studies of mothers. Still, many of the same principles seem to hold for fathers as well. The father's bond, like the mother's, seems more dependent on the development of mutuality or synchrony than on contact immediately after birth. Aiding the development of such mutuality is the fact that fathers seem to have the same repertoire of attachment behaviors as do mothers. In the early weeks of the baby's life, dads touch, talk to, and cuddle their babies in the same ways that mothers do (Parke & Tinsley, 1981).

Past these first weeks of life, however, we see signs of a kind of specialization of parents' behaviors with their infants and toddlers—at least among parents in the industrialized societies in which these observations have been done. Dads spend more time playing with the baby, with more physical roughhousing. Moms spend more time in routine caregiving, and they talk and smile more at the baby (Walker et al., 1992). This does not mean that fathers have a weaker affectional bond with the infant; it does mean that the attachment behaviors they show toward the infant are typically somewhat different from those mothers show.

We do not yet know whether such sex differences in parenting behaviors are reflections of culturally based role definitions or whether they might be instinctive, built-in

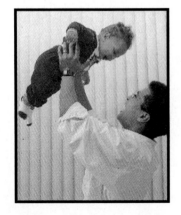

Ryan's dad, like most fathers, is far more likely to play with him by tossing him around than is his mom.

The Real World

Child Abuse and Other Consequences of Failure of Bonding

In any given year, roughly 1 million children in the United States suffer from neglect or from physical or sexual abuse (U.S. Bureau of the Census, 1994). Most such abuse is inflicted on older children; the average age of children in cases reported to child protective services is 7. But in many cases the origins of later abuse or neglect may lie in a failure of the parent to form a strong affectional bond to the baby in the first months of life. Such a failure can occur if either the baby or the parents lack the skills to enter into the "dance" of interaction fully. Of the two, the more serious problems seem to arise if it is the parent who lacks skills, but problems can also arise when the baby is handicapped or otherwise lacks the full repertoire of attachment behaviors (van IJzendoorn et al., 1992).

For example, blind babies smile less and do not show mutual gaze, and preterm infants are typically very unresponsive in the early weeks and months (Fraiberg, 1974; 1975). Most parents of handicapped or premature infants form a strong bond to the child despite the baby's problems, but the rate of abuse is higher among preterm than among term infants, and higher among families whose babies are sick a lot in the first few months (Belsky, 1993).

On the other side of the interaction, a parent might lack "attachment skill" because she or he did not form a secure attachment with her or his own parents, perhaps because of abuse (Crittenden, Partridge, & Claussen, 1991). The majority of parents who abuse their children were themselves abused as children—although it is important to emphasize that the reverse is not the case: The majority of adults who experienced abuse in childhood manage to break the cycle of violence and refrain from abusing their children (Zigler & Hall, 1989). Still, there appears to be a significant "intergenerational transmission" of such violence (Belsky, 1993). Those who are unable to break this cycle are typically those who lack other social

skills, who have no adequate social supports, or who are living under high levels of stress.

Another serious problem on the parents' side of the equation is depression, which not only disrupts the parents' nurturing behavior, but affects the child's response as well. Babies interacting with depressed mothers, or even with mothers who have been told to look depressed or "blank faced," smile less, show more sad and angry facial expressions, and are more disorganized and distressed (Field et al., 1990; Pickens & Field, 1993). Depressed mothers, for their part, are slower to respond to their infants' signals and are more negative—even hostile—to their infants (Rutter, 1990). All in all, these relationships appear to lack synchrony. That is, the mother and infant are not "dancing" well together. These deficiencies in the mother's behavior with the infant even persist after the mother is no longer depressed, and they generalize beyond the mother-infant dyad; babies with depressed mothers show similar distressed or nonsynchronous behaviors when they interact with a nondepressed adult (Field et al., 1988). Such children are also at higher risk for later behavior problems, including either heightened aggression or withdrawal (Cummings & Davies, 1994).

One common theme in all these findings is that a parent, regardless of depression or history of abuse, is more likely to abuse a child when her current life conditions are highly stressful. So abuse is more likely in families in which at least one parent is alcoholic (Famularo et al., 1986), in large families, in single-parent households, and in families living in poverty or in extremely crowded conditions (Garbarino & Sherman, 1980; Pianta, Egeland, & Erickson, 1989; Sack, Mason, & Higgins, 1985). Even these adverse conditions can be surmounted, though, if the parents have adequate emotional support, either from one another or from others outside the family.

differences. One crucial test would be to see if the parental behavioral roles are reversed in families in which the father is the primary caregiver. So far we have only pale imitations of this crucial test—studies in which the father had been a major caregiver for a few months of the child's early life. The three such studies I know of, done in Sweden, the United States, and Australia, have yielded totally contradictory results (Field, 1978; Lamb et al., 1982; Russell, 1982), which leaves the question still open.

The Baby's Attachment to the Parent

Like the parent's bond to the baby, the baby's attachment emerges gradually. Bowlby (1969) suggested three phases in the development of the infant's attachment, which I've sketched schematically in Figure 11.1.

Phase 1: Nonfocused Orienting and Signaling. Bowlby thought the baby begins life with a set of innate behavior patterns that orient him toward others and signal his needs. Mary Ainsworth describes these as "proximity-promoting" behaviors—they bring people closer. In the newborn's repertoire, these include crying, making eye contact, clinging, cuddling, and responding to caregiving efforts by being soothed. But at first, as Ainsworth says, "These attachment behaviors are simply emitted, rather than being directed toward any specific person" (1989, p. 710).

At this stage we see little evidence of an attachment. Nonetheless, the roots of attachment are to be found in this phase. The baby is building up expectancies, schemas, the ability to discriminate Mom and Dad from others.

Phase 2: Focus on One or More Figure(s). By 3 months of age, the baby begins to aim her attachment behaviors somewhat more narrowly. She may smile more at the people who regularly take care of her and may not smile readily at a stranger. Yet despite the change, Bowlby and Ainsworth have argued that the infant does not yet have a full-blown attachment. The child still favors a number of people with her "proximity-promoting" behaviors, and no one person has yet become the "safe base." Children in this phase show no special anxiety at being separated from their parent and no fear of strangers.

Phase 3: Secure Base Behavior. Bowlby thought that the baby forms a genuine attachment only at about 6 months of age. At the same time, the dominant mode of the baby's attachment behavior changes. Because the 6- to 7-month-old begins to be able to move about the world more freely by creeping and crawling, she can move *toward* the caregiver as well as entice the caregiver to come to her. Her attachment behaviors therefore shift from mostly "come here" signals (proximity promoting) to what Ainsworth calls "proximity seeking," which we might think of as "go there" behaviors. We also see a child of this age using the "most important person" as a safe base from which to explore the world around her—one of the key signs that an attachment exists.

I should note that not all infants have a *single* attachment figure, even at this early point. Some may show strong attachment to both parents or to a parent and another caregiver, such as a baby-sitter or a grandparent. But even these babies, when under stress, usually show a preference for one of their favored persons over the others.

FIGURE 11.1 This schematic may help you see how the various threads of development of attachment are woven together.

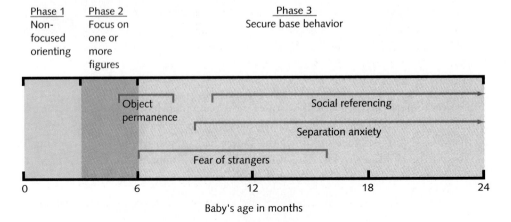

Cultures and Contexts

Attachment in a Very Different Cultural System

Is the sequence of phases Bowlby and Ainsworth describe universal? Do all babies go through this same sequence, no matter what kind of family or culture they live in? Maybe yes, maybe no. Ainsworth herself observed the same basic three phases in forming a clear attachment among children in Uganda, although they showed a more intense fear of strangers than is usually found in American samples. But among the Ganda, as in American and other Western families, the mother is the primary caregiver. What would we find in a culture in which the child's early care is much more communal?

Edward Tronick and his colleagues (Tronick, Morelli, & Ivey, 1992) have studied just such a culture, a pygmy group called the Efe, who forage in the forests of Zaire. They live in small groups of perhaps 20 individuals in camps, each consisting of several extended families, often brothers and their wives.

Infants in these communities are cared for communally in the early months and years of life. They are carried and held by all the adult women and interact regularly with many different adults. If they have needs, they are tended by whichever adult or older child is nearby; they may even be nursed by women other than the mother, although they normally sleep with the mother.

Tronick and his colleagues report two things of particular interest about early attachment in this group. First, Efe infants seem to use virtually any adult or older child in their world as a safe base, which suggests that they may have no single central attachment. But at the same time, beginning at about 6 months, the Efe infants seem to insist on being with their mother more and to prefer her over other women, although other women continue to help care for the child.

Thus, even in an extremely communal rearing arrangement, we can still see some sign of a central attachment, albeit perhaps less dominant. At the same time, it is clear, as Inge Bretherton says, that "attachment behavior is never purely instinctive, but is heavily overlain with cultural prescriptions" (1992b, p. 150).

Shortly after the child has developed a clear attachment, several related behaviors also appear. One of these is social referencing, which I talked about in Chapter 5. The 10-month-old begins to check out Mom's or Dad's expression before deciding whether to venture forth into some novel situation. At about the same age, babies also typically show both fear of strangers and separation protest.

Fear of Strangers and Separation Protest. Both these forms of distress are rare before 5 or 6 months, rise in frequency until about 12 to 16 months, and then decline. The research findings are not altogether consistent, but it looks as though fear of strangers normally appears first, while separation anxiety starts a bit later but continues to be visible for a longer period, a pattern I've marked in Figure 11.1.

Such an increase in fear and anxiety has been observed in children from a number of different cultures and in both home-reared and day-care-reared children in the United States, all of which makes it look as if some basic cognitive or other age-related developmental timetables underlie this pattern (Kagan, Kearsley, & Zelazo, 1978). But while the general timing of these two phenomena may be common to virtually all children, the intensity of the fearful reaction is not. Children differ widely in how much fear they show toward strangers or toward novel situations. Some of this difference may reflect basic temperamental variations, such as the pattern of behavioral inhibition Kagan describes and that I described in Chapter 9 (Kagan, 1994). Heightened fearfulness might also be a response to recent upheaval or stress in the child's life, such as a recent move or a parent changing jobs. It is also clear that the stranger's behavior makes a considerable difference. When a substitute caregiver is responsive and warm but does not approach too closely, babies show less fear than when the stranger pays little attention to the child or touches the child too soon (Gunnar et al., 1992; Mangelsdorf, 1992). Whatever the origin of such variations in fearfulness, the pattern does eventually disappear in most toddlers, typically by the middle of the second year. And even while it is going on, parents can take advantage of the existence of social referencing to try to reduce the child's fear: Your child is more likely to accept a stranger if he sees you talking and smiling to the stranger first.

Attachments in the Preschool and Elementary School Years

By age 2 or 3, most attachment behaviors have become less visible. Children this age are cognitively advanced enough to understand Mom if she explains why she is going away and that she will be back, so their anxiety at separation wanes. They can even use a photograph of their mother as a "safe base" for exploration in a strange situation (Passman & Longeway, 1982), which reflects another cognitive advance. Of course attachment behaviors have not completely disappeared. Two-year-olds still want to sit on Mom's or Dad's lap and are still likely to seek some closeness when Mom returns from some absence. But in nonfearful or nonstressful situations the child is able to wander further and further from her safe base without apparent distress.

An even broader change occurs at about age 4, when the quality of the child's attachment seems to change. Bowlby describes this new stage or level as a *goal-corrected partnership*. Just as the first attachment probably requires that the baby understand that his mother will continue to exist when she isn't there, so now the preschooler grasps that the *relationship* continues to exist even when the partners are apart.

Once this understanding has been achieved, visible attachment behaviors go underground even more. Among elementary school children, it is only in stressful situations that we see overt attachment behaviors. And because fewer experiences are new and potentially stressful to the 7- or 8-year-old than to the preschooler, we see much less obvious safe base behavior and less open affection from child to parent in this age group (Maccoby, 1984).

Parent-Child Relationships at Adolescence

In adolescence, the scene shifts somewhat, because teenagers have two, apparently contradictory, tasks in their relationships with their parents: to establish autonomy from the parents and to maintain their sense of relatedness with their parents. We can see both processes at work when we look at teen-parent relationships. The push for autonomy shows itself in increases in conflict between parent and adolescent; the maintenance of connection is seen in the continued strong attachment of child to parent.

Increases in Conflict.   The rise in conflict has been documented by a number of researchers (e.g., Flannery et al., 1993; Flannery, Montemayor, & Eberly, 1994; Steinberg, 1988). In the great majority of families, it seems to consist of an increase in mild bickering or conflicts over everyday issues like chores or autonomy (Laursen, 1995). Or as Hill and Holmbeck put it, the conflict is over "hair, garbage, dishes, and galoshes" (1986, p. 158). Teenagers and their parents also interrupt each other more often and become more impatient with one another.

This increase in discord is widely found, but we need to be careful not to assume that it signifies a major disruption of the quality of the parent-child relationships. Laurence

Can you think of anything other than the generally lower level of novelty or stress that might account for the elementary school child's rather sharp drop in overt affection displayed toward parents?

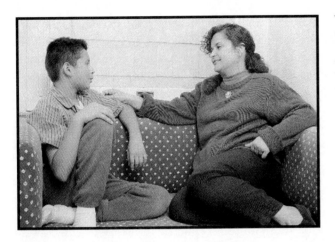

While it is true that conflict rises in many families when children reach puberty, it is a myth that parents and teenagers are constantly in conflict.

Steinberg, one of the key researchers in this area, estimates that only 5 to 10 percent of the families studied in the United States experience a substantial or pervasive deterioration in the quality of parent-child relationship in these years of early adolescence—a fact that flies in the face of the usual assumption that adolescence is a time of inevitable *sturm und drang* (storm and stress) (Steinberg, 1990).

But if the rise in conflict doesn't signal the relationship is falling apart, what does it mean? Steinberg and others have suggested that the temporary discord, far from being a negative event, may instead be developmentally healthy and necessary—a part of the process of individuation and separation. Among primates, we see the same kind of increase in conflict, especially between adult males and the newly adolescent males. The young males begin to make competitive gestures and may be driven off into a brief period of independent life before returning to the troop. Among humans, we have accumulating evidence that the increase in family conflict is linked with the hormonal changes of puberty, rather than age, which would lend further support to the argument that this is a normal and even necessary process.

For example, in a short-term longitudinal study, Steinberg (1988) followed a group of teenagers over a one-year period, assessing their stage of puberty and the quality of their relationship with their parents at the beginning and end of the year. He found that as the early pubertal stages began, family closeness declined, parent-child conflict rose, and autonomy in the child went up. Other researchers (Inoff-Germain et al., 1988) have taken this a step further by measuring actual hormone levels and showing links between the rise of the various hormones of puberty and the rise in aloofness toward or conflict with parents. Among girls, conflict seems to rise after menarche (Holmbeck & Hill, 1991).

The pattern of causes is obviously complex. Hormonal changes may be causally linked to increases in assertiveness, perhaps especially among boys. But parents' reactions to pubertal changes may also be highly important parts of the mix. Visible pubertal changes, including menarche, change parents' expectations for the child, and increase their concern about guiding and controlling the adolescent to help her avoid the shoals of too much independence.

In fact, adolescence may actually be more stressful to *parents* than to the young people themselves (Gecas & Seff, 1990). Almost two-thirds of parents perceive their children's adolescence as the most difficult stage of parenting, because of both loss of control over the adolescent and fear for the adolescent's safety resulting from increased independence.

In the midst of the increased conflict, and perhaps partially as a result of it, the overall level of the teenager's autonomy within the family increases steadily throughout the adolescent years. Parents give the youngster more and more room to make independent choices and to participate in family decision making. Steinberg argues that this "distancing" is an essential part of the adolescent development process.

Attachment to Parents.   Paradoxically, in the midst of this distancing and of the temporarily heightened family conflict, teenagers' underlying emotional attachment to their parents remains strong. Results from a recent study by Mary Levitt and her colleagues (1993) illustrate the point.

Levitt interviewed African-American, Hispanic-American, and Anglo children ages 7, 10, and 14. Each child was shown a drawing with a set of concentric circles and was asked to place in the middle circle those "people who are the most close and important to you—people you love the most and who love you the most." In the next circle outward from the middle, children were asked to place the names of "people who are not quite as close but who are still important—people you really love or like, but not quite as much as the people in the first circle." A third circle contained names of somewhat more distant members of this personal "convoy." For each person listed, the interviewer then asked about the kind of support that person provided.

Levitt found that for all three ethnic groups, at all three ages, parents and other close family members were by far the most likely to be placed in the inner circle. Even among 14-year-olds, friends were not often placed in this position. So the parents remain central. At the same time, it is clear from Levitt's results that peers become increasingly important as providers of support, as you can see in Figure 11.2. This figure shows the total amount of support the children and adolescents described from each source. Friends clearly provided more support among the 14-year-olds than among the younger children, a pattern that is clear for all three ethnic groups.

A recent large study in the Netherlands (van Wel, 1994) suggests that the teenager's bond with his parents may weaken somewhat in the middle of adolescence (ages 15 and 16) and then recover. But virtually all the current researchers who have explored this question find that, in general, a teenager's sense of well-being or happiness is more

---

You might find it interesting to complete such a "personal convoy" map for your own relationships. Are your parents in the center circle? Friends? Partner?

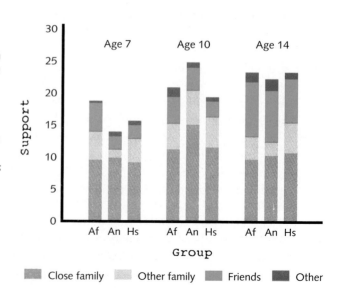

FIGURE 11.2 African-American (Af), Anglo-American (An), and Hispanic-American (Hs) children and teens were asked about the amount and type of support they received from various members of their "social convoy." Note that for teens, friends become more significant sources of support, but parents do not become substantially *less* important. (*Source:* Levitt, Guacci-Franco, & Levitt, 1993, Figure 2, p. 815.)

strongly correlated with the quality of his attachment to the parents than with the quality of his attachments to his peers (Greenberg, Siegel, & Leitch, 1983; Raja, McGee, & Stanton, 1992). Thus, even while the teenager is becoming more autonomous, the parents seem to continue to provide a highly important psychological safe base.

Attachments to Mothers and Fathers

I pointed out earlier that both fathers and mothers appear to form strong bonds with their infants, although their behavior with infants varies somewhat. But what about the child's half of this relationship? Are infants and children equally attached to their fathers and mothers?

In general, yes. From the ages of 7 to 8 months, when strong attachments are first seen, infants prefer *either* the father or the mother to a stranger. And when both the father and the mother are available, an infant will smile at or approach either or both, *except* when he is frightened or under stress. When that happens, especially between 8 and 24 months, the child typically turns to the mother rather than the father (Lamb, 1981).

As you might expect, the strength of the child's attachment to the father at this early age seems to be related to the amount of time the dad has spent with the child. In one early study, for example, Gail Ross (Ross et al., 1975) found she could predict a baby's attachment to the father by knowing how many diapers the dad changed in a typical week. The more diapers, the stronger the attachment! But greatly increased time with the father does not seem to be the only element, since Michael Lamb and his Swedish colleagues have found that infants whose father was the major caregiver for at least a month in the first year of the child's life were nonetheless more strongly attached to their mothers than their fathers (Lamb et al., 1983). For the father to be consistently *preferred* over the mother would probably require essentially full-time paternal care. As this option becomes more common in our society, it will be possible to study such father-child pairs to see if a preference for the father develops.

The fact that young Edwin's dad changes his diapers is probably not the crucial causal variable in Edwin's forming a strong attachment to his father, but diaper changing may signify a greater involvement by this father with his infant, and that greater involvement may be linked to the baby's stronger attachment.

Variations in the Quality of Infants' Attachments

Go to a day-care center sometime and watch the way the babies or toddlers greet their parents at the end of the day. Some are calmly pleased to see Mom or Dad, running to be hugged, showing a new toy, or smiling when picked up, showing no distress. Others may cry or cling strongly to the parent. All these babies have moved through the typical sequence from preattachment to attachment, but the *quality* of their attachments differs. In Bowlby's terminology, infants have different **internal working models** of their relationships with parents and key others. This concept introduces a distinctly cognitive flavor to the discussion, very like the concepts of the "self-scheme" or the "gender-schema" I talked about in the last two chapters. This internal working model of attachment relationships includes such elements as the child's confidence (or lack of it) that the attachment figure will be available or reliable, the child's expectation of rebuff or affection, and the child's sense of assurance that the other is really a safe base for exploration.

The internal model begins to be formed late in the child's first year of life and becomes more complex and firmer through the first 4 or 5 years. By age 5, most children have clear internal models of the mother (or other caregiver), a self-model, and a model of relationships. Once formed, such models shape and explain experiences and affect memory and attention. We notice and remember experiences that fit our model, and miss or forget experiences that don't match. More important, the model affects the child's behavior: The child tends to re-create, in each new relationship, the pattern with which he is familiar. Alan Sroufe gives a nice example that may make this point clearer:

> What is rejection to one child is benign to another. What is warmth to a second child is confusing or ambiguous to another. For example, a child approaches another and asks to play. Turned down, the child goes off and sulks in a corner. A second child receiving the same negative reaction skips on to another partner and successfully engages him in play. Their experiences of rejection are vastly different. Each receives confirmation of quite different inner working models. (1988, p. 23)

In a sense, these internal models are not unlike the social *scripts* that the preschooler develops in other areas (Bretherton, 1993). They contain expectations for sequences of behavior, rules for behavior with various individuals, and interpretations of others' actions.

Secure and Insecure Attachments

All the theorists in this tradition share the assumption that the first attachment relationship is the most influential ingredient in the creation of the child's working model. Variations in that first attachment relationship are now almost universally described using Mary Ainsworth's category system (Ainsworth et al., 1978). She distinguishes between **secure attachment** and two types of **insecure attachment,** which she has assessed using a procedure called the **Strange Situation.**

The Strange Situation consists of a series of episodes in a laboratory setting, typically used when the child is between 12 and 18 months of age. The child is first with the mother, then with the mother and a stranger, alone with the stranger, completely alone for a few minutes, reunited with the mother, left alone again, then reunited first with the stranger, and then with the mother. Ainsworth suggested that children's reactions to this situation could be classified into three types: *securely attached, insecure/avoidant,* and *insecure/ambivalent* (also sometimes called *resistant*). Mary Main (Main & Solomon, 1990) has suggested a fourth group, which she calls *insecure/disorganized/disoriented.* I have listed some of the characteristics of the different types in Table 11.1.

This category system and the theory that lies behind it have prompted an enormous amount of research and new theory, much of it fascinating and much of it with practical ramifications. So let me take some time to explore a few of the issues and implications.

Stability of Attachment Classification. One of the key questions is whether the quality of the child's attachment is stable over time. Does a child who is securely or insecurely attached to his mother at 12 months still show the same quality of attachment at 24 or 36 months, or at school age? This is a particularly important question for those researchers and therapists who are concerned about the possible permanence of effects of early abuse, neglect, or other sources of insecure attachment. Can children recover from such early treatment? Conversely, is a child who is securely attached at 1 year of age forever buffered from the effects of later difficult life circumstances?

The answer, perhaps not surprisingly, is that both consistency and inconsistency occur, depending on the circumstances. When the child's family environment or life circumstances are reasonably consistent, the security or insecurity of attachment does seem to remain consistent, even over many years. For example, Claire Hamilton has assessed current attachment security/insecurity in a small group of adolescents (Hamilton, 1995). Sixteen of the 18 adolescents who had been rated as insecurely attached at 12 months of

---

If internal working models tend to persist and to affect later relationships, is this the same as saying that the first few years of life are a critical period for the creation of patterns of relationships? How else could we conceptualize it?

Table 11.1
Categorization of Secure and Insecure Attachment in Ainsworth's Strange Situation

Securely attached	Child readily separates from the caregiver and easily becomes absorbed in exploration; when threatened or frightened, child actively seeks contact, is readily consoled, and does not avoid or resist contact if mother initiates it. When reunited with mother after absence, child greets her positively or is easily soothed if upset. Clearly prefers mother to stranger.
Insecurely attached: detached/avoidant	Child avoids contact with mother, especially at reunion after an absence. Does not resist mother's efforts to make contact, but does not seek much contact, and shows no preference of mother over the stranger.
Insecurely attached: resistant/ambivalent	Child shows little exploration and is wary of the stranger. Greatly upset when separated from mother but not reassured by mother's return or her efforts at comforting. Child both seeks and avoids contact at different times. May show anger toward mother at reunion and resists both comfort from and contact with stranger.
Insecurely attached: disorganized/disoriented	Dazed behavior, confusion, or apprehension. Child may show contradictory behavior patterns simultaneously, such as moving toward mother while keeping gaze averted.

Sources: Ainsworth et al., 1978; Main & Solomon, 1990; Carlson & Sroufe, 1995.

age were still rated as insecurely attached at age 17, while 7 of the 11 teens who had been classed as securely attached as infants were still rated as securely attached at 17. Similarly, in a shorter-term study in Germany (Wartner et al., 1994), 82 percent of a group of youngsters from stable, middle-class families were rated in the same category of attachment security at age 6 as they had been at age 1.

But when the child's circumstances change in some major way—such as when she starts going to day care or nursery school, grandma comes to live with the family, or the parents divorce or move—the security of the child's attachment may change as well, from either secure to insecure or the reverse. In poverty-level families, in which instability of circumstances is more common, changes in attachment security are also common.

The very fact that a child's security can change from one time to the next does not refute the notion of attachment as an internal working model. Bowlby suggested that for the first two or three years, the particular pattern of attachment a child shows is in some sense a property of each specific *relationship.* For example, studies of toddlers' attachments to mothers and fathers show that about 30 percent of the time the child is securely attached to one parent and insecurely attached to the other, with both possible combinations equally represented (Fox, Kimmerly, & Schafer, 1991). It is the quality of each relationship that determines the child's security with that specific adult. If that relationship changes markedly, the security of the baby's attachment to that individual may change too. But Bowlby argued that by age 4 or 5, the internal working model becomes more general, more a property of the *child,* more generalized across relationships, and thus

Cultures and Contexts

Secure and Insecure Attachments in Different Cultures

Studies in a variety of countries have pointed to the possibility that secure attachments may be more likely in certain cultures than in others. The most thorough analyses have come from a Dutch psychologist, Marinus van IJzendoorn, who has examined the results of 32 separate studies in eight different countries. You can see the percentage of babies classified in each category for each country in the table below (van IJzendoorn & Kroonenberg, 1988).

We need to be cautious about overinterpreting the information in this table, because in most cases there are only one or two studies from a given country, normally with quite small samples. The single study from China, for example, included only 36 babies. Still, the findings are thought-provoking.

The most striking thing about these data is their consistency. In each of the eight countries, a secure attachment is the most common pattern, found in more than half of all babies studied; in six of the eight, an avoidant pattern is the more common of the two forms of insecure attachment. Only in Israel and Japan is this pattern significantly reversed. How can we explain such differences?

One possibility is that the Strange Situation is simply not an appropriate measure of attachment security in all cultures. For example, because Japanese babies are rarely separated from their mothers in the first year of life, being left totally alone in the midst of the Strange Situation may be far more stressful for them, which might result in more intense, inconsolable crying and hence a classification of ambivalent attachment. The counterargument is that comparisons of toddlers' actual behavior in the Strange Situation suggest few cultural differences in such things as proximity seeking or avoidance of Mom, all of which gives us more confidence that the Strange Situation is tapping similar processes among children in many cultures (Sagi, van IJzendoorn, & Koren-Karie, 1991).

It is also possible that the *meaning* of a "secure" or "avoidant" pattern is different in different cultures, even if the percentages of each category are similar. German researchers, for example, have suggested that an insecure-avoidant classification in their culture may reflect not indifference by mothers, but explicit training toward greater independence in the baby (Grossmann et al., 1985).

On the other hand, research in Israel (Sagi, 1990) shows that the Strange Situation attachment classification predicts the baby's later social skills in much the same way as is found in United States samples, which suggests that the classification system is valid in both cultures.

At the moment the most plausible hypothesis is that the same factors in mother–infant interaction contribute to secure and insecure attachments in all cultures and that these patterns reflect similar internal models. But it will take more research like the Israeli work, in which the long-term outcomes of the various categories are studied, before we can be sure if this is correct.

Cross-Cultural Comparisons of Secure and Insecure Attachments

Percentage of Each Attachment Type

Country	Number of Studies	Secure	Avoidant	Ambivalent
West Germany	3	56.6	35.3	8.1
Great Britain	1	75.0	22.2	2.8
Netherlands	4	67.3	26.3	6.4
Sweden	1	74.5	21.6	3.9
Israel	2	64.4	6.8	28.8
Japan	2	67.7	5.2	25.0
China	1	50.0	25.0	25.0
United States	18	64.8	21.1	14.1
Overall Average		65.0	21.3	13.7

Source: Based on Table 1 of van IJzendoorn & Kroonenberg, 1988, pp. 150–151.

more resistant to change. At that point, the child tends to impose it upon new relationships, including relationships with teachers or peers.

Thus, a child may "recover" from an initially insecure attachment or lose a secure one. But consistency over time is more typical, both because children's relationships tend to be reasonably stable for the first few years and because once the internal model is clearly formed, it tends to perpetuate itself.

Origins of Secure and Insecure Attachments. Where do these differences come from? We know that insecurely attached infants are more likely to be found in poverty-level families, in families with a history of abuse, or in families in which the mother is diagnosed as seriously depressed (Cicchetti & Barnett, 1991; Spieker & Booth, 1988). But such a catalogue doesn't tell us what is actually happening between parents and children that may foster secure or insecure attachments. Studies of actual parent-child interactions suggest that for a secure attachment, the crucial ingredients seem to be both acceptance of the infant by the parents and *contingent responsiveness* from the parents toward the infant (Isabella, 1993; Pederson et al., 1990). Contingent responsiveness does not just mean that the parents love the baby or take care of the baby well, but rather that in their caregiving and other behavior toward the child they are sensitive to the child's own cues and respond appropriately. They smile when the baby smiles, talk to the baby when he vocalizes, pick him up when he cries, and so on.

Our certainty that this type of responsiveness is a key ingredient has been greatly strengthened by a recent study by Dymphna van den Boom, who has demonstrated the link experimentally. Van den Boom (1994) identified 100 lower-class Dutch mothers whose infants had all been rated as high in irritability shortly after birth. Half the mothers were then assigned randomly to participate in a set of three relatively brief training sessions aimed at helping them improve their responsiveness to their infant. The other mothers received no such help. When the babies were 12 months old, van den Boom observed the mothers interacting with their infants at home and observed the baby and mother in the standard Strange Situation. The effects were quite clear: The trained mothers had indeed become more responsive to their babies, and their babies were more likely to be securely attached, as you can see from the results in Table 11.2.

Table 11.2
The Effect of Mothers' Responsiveness Training on Infants' Attachment Security

	Attachment Classification	
	Number Secure	**Number Insecure**
Training	31	19
No training	11	39

Source: van den Boom, 1994, from Table 5, p. 1472.

A low level of responsiveness thus appears to be an ingredient in any type of insecure attachment. But each of the several subvarieties of insecure attachment has distinct antecedents. For example, a disorganized/disoriented pattern seems especially likely when the child has been abused and in families in which the parents had an unresolved trauma in their own childhoods, such as abuse or their own parents' early death (Cassidy & Berlin, 1994; Main & Hesse, 1990). An ambivalent pattern is more common when the mother is inconsistently or unreliably available to the child. Mothers may show such unavailability or periodic neglect for a variety of reasons, but a common ingredient is depression in the mother—a phenomenon I talked about briefly in the *Real World* box on page 309 (Teti et al., 1995). When the mother rejects the infant or regularly (rather than intermittently) withdraws from contact with the infant, the infant is more likely to show an avoidant pattern of attachment.

Long-Term Consequences of Secure and Insecure Attachment. Ainsworth's classification system has proven to be extremely helpful in predicting a remarkably wide range of other behaviors in children, both as toddlers and in later childhood. Dozens of studies show that children rated as securely attached to their mothers in infancy are later more sociable; more positive in their behavior toward others, including friends and siblings; less clinging and dependent on teachers; less aggressive and disruptive; more empathetic; and more emotionally mature in their approach to school and other nonhome settings (Carlson & Sroufe, 1995).

Most of this research has involved preschool or early elementary school children, so we cannot say with certainty that these early effects persist longer than age 6 or 7. But we do have at least one bit of evidence that the effects do last. Alan Sroufe and his colleagues, in a study I mentioned several times before (Chapters 1 and 9), have now followed 47 children from infancy up to ages 10 and 11 (Sroufe, Carlson, & Schulman, 1993; Urban et al., 1991). As preadolescents, the children were observed during a specially designed summer camp. The counselors rated each child on a range of characteristics, and observers noted how often children spent time together or with the counselors. Naturally, neither the counselors nor the observers knew what the children's initial attachment classification had been. The findings are clear: Those with histories of secure attachment were rated as more self-confident and as having more social competence. They complied more readily with counselor requests, expressed more positive emotions, and had a greater sense of their ability to accomplish things—what Bandura calls *self-efficacy* and Sroufe calls *agency*. They created more friendships, especially with other securely attached youngsters, and engaged in more complex activities when playing in groups. The majority of those with histories of insecure attachment showed some kind of deviant behavior pattern at age 11, such as isolation from peers, bizarre behavior, passivity, hyperactivity, or aggressiveness. Only a few of the originally securely attached children showed any of these patterns.

I should emphasize again that these 47 children are the only ones yet studied over this length of time, and it is risky to build too tall a theoretical edifice on such a small empirical foundation. But Sroufe's data fit very well with the results from studies of younger children as well as with newer studies that show links between adolescents' *current* attachment status (measured with interviews or questionnaires) and their emotional health or effective functioning. For example, teenagers who describe themselves as more securely attached to their parents have more intimate friendships and higher self-esteem (Black & McCartney, 1995; Lieberman, Doyle, & Markiewicz, 1995). Those with insecure attachments—particularly those with avoidant attachments—not only have less positive and supportive friendships, but also are more likely to become sexually active early and practice riskier sex (O'Beirne & Moore, 1995). Collectively, the findings point to potentially long-term consequences of attachment patterns or internal working models of relationships constructed in the first year of life. But fluidity and change also occur, and we need to know much more about the factors that tend to maintain, or alter, the earliest models.

Relationships with Peers

Because most theories of social and personality development have strongly emphasized the centrality of parent-child interactions, until recently most psychologists thought of relationships with peers as much less important. But that view is now changing as it becomes clear that peer relationships play a unique and significant role in a child's development.

Developmental Changes in Peer Relationships

Infants and Preschoolers. Children first begin to show some positive interest in other infants as early as 6 months of age. If you place two such babies on the floor facing each other, they will touch each other, pull each other's hair, reach for the other's clothing. By 10 months these behaviors are even more evident. Children this age apparently still prefer to play with objects but will play with each other if no toys are available. By 14 to 18 months, we begin to see two or more children playing together with toys—occasionally cooperating but more often simply playing side by side with different toys, a pattern often called *parallel play*. Babies are *interested* in one another. They gaze at other babies, smile, make noises at each other. But it isn't until around 18 months that we begin to see much coordinated play, such as when one toddler chases another or one imitates the other's action with some toy. At about this same age, babies also begin to show the first signs of playmate preferences, even some signs of individual friendships. For example, Carollee Howes (1983; 1987) noted that some children this young showed consistent preferences for one or more playmates over a full-year period in a day-care center. Still, these early peer interactions are quite primitive. Most of the time, toddlers ignore one another's bids for interaction, and when they play together it is mostly around common toys.

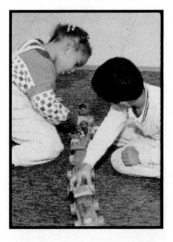

By age 3, most children play with one another in coordinated ways, rather than merely side by side.

By 3 or 4, children appear to prefer to play with peers rather than alone, and their play with one another is much more cooperative and coordinated. We see various forms of group pretend play, much of it already organized along gender lines. And friendships become clearer and somewhat more stable as well. Robert Hinde and his co-workers (1985) defined as friends any pair of children who spent at least a third of their playtime next to one another. By this criterion, only about 20 percent of a group of 3 ½-year-olds showed signs of a stable friendship; by age 4, half of these same children regularly played this often with one child. To be sure, these early friendships are based more on sheer proximity and shared play interests than is true of friendships among older children, but some kind of consistent preference is already visible at this early age.

School Age. Peers become even more important among school-age children. Indeed, among children of 7, 8, 9, and 10, playing with their pals (along with watching TV) takes up virtually all their time when they are not in school, eating, or sleeping (Timmer, Eccles, & O'Brien, 1985).

Shared play interests continue to form the major basis of these school-age peer relationships. Furthermore, kids this age *define* play groups in terms of common activities, rather than in terms of common attitudes or values. You can see this pattern in Figure

11.3, which shows the results of a study by Susan O'Brien & Karen Bierman (1988). They asked fifth- eighth-, and eleventh-grade subjects to tell them about the different groups of kids that hang around together at their school and then to say how they could tell that a particular bunch was "a group." For the fifth graders, the single best criterion of "a group" was that the children did things together. For eighth graders, shared attitudes and common appearance became much more important.

I'll be talking much more about the child's *understanding* of social relationships and processes in the next chapter, but let me just point out here that this "concreteness" in the elementary school child's view of peers is entirely consistent with what I've already told you about the character of the self-concept in children this same age, as well as with Piaget's ideas about the thinking of a concrete operational child.

Beyond the centrality of shared activities, the most striking thing about peer group interactions in the elementary school years is how sex-segregated they are, a pattern that appears to exist in every culture in the world (Cairns & Cairns, 1994; Harkness & Super, 1985) and that is frequently visible in children as young as 3 or 4. Boys play with boys, girls play with girls, each in their own areas and at their own kinds of games. There are some ritualized "boundary violations" between these separate territories, such as chasing games (e.g., "You can't catch me, nyah nyah," followed by chasing accompanied by screaming by the girls) (Thorne, 1986). But on the whole, girls and boys between the ages of 6 and 12 actively avoid interacting. Given a forced choice between playing with a child of the opposite gender or a child of a different race, researchers have found that elementary-school-age children will make the cross-race choice rather than the cross-gender choice (Maccoby & Jacklin, 1987).

Friendships in this age range are naturally also sex segregated. In one study, parents reported that about a quarter of the friendships of their 5- and 6-year-olds but *none* of the friendships of their 7- and 8-year-olds were cross-sex (Gottman, 1986).

School-age children spend more time with their friends than do preschoolers, and they gradually develop a larger collection of individual friendships. Second graders name about four friends each, while seventh graders name about seven (Reisman & Shorr, 1978). In these same years, friendships also become more stable—more likely to endure for a year or longer (Cairns & Cairns, 1994). At either age, children's behavior within friendships is quite different from what they display with strangers, although I suspect the differences are not always quite what you would predict: Children are more *polite* to strangers or nonfriends. They are more open and more supportive with chums, smiling, looking, laughing, and touching one another more than with nonfriends; they talk to one another more, and cooperate and help one another. Friends are also more critical toward one another than toward strangers, but when they have conflicts, they are more concerned about resolving their disagreements than is true among nonfriends. Thus, friendships are an arena in which children can learn how to manage conflicts (Newcomb & Bagwell, 1995).

There are also intriguing differences in the quality of relationship in boys' and girls' friendships in these years. Waldrop and Halverson (1975) refer to boys' relationships as *extensive* and to girls' relationships as *intensive*. Boys' friendship groups are larger and are more accepting of newcomers than are girls'. They play more outdoors and roam over a larger area in their play. Girlfriends are more likely to play in pairs or in smaller, more exclusive groups, and they spend more playtime indoors or near home or school (Benenson, 1994; Gottman, 1986).

How many different explanations can you think of for the fact that children begin to prefer to play with same-sex peers as early as age 3 or 4?

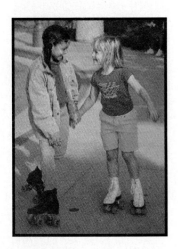

Even at this young age, girls like these form friendships that are less competitive and more compliant with one another than is true in friendships among boys the same age.

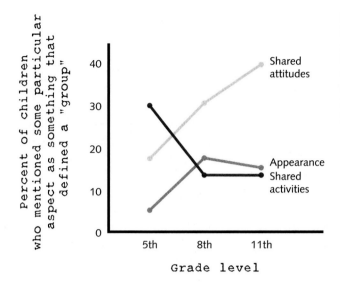

FIGURE 11.3 O'Brien and Bierman's results illustrate the change between elementary and high school in children's ideas about what defines a "group" of peers. (*Source:* O'Brien & Bierman, 1988, Table 1, p. 1363.)

At the level of actual interaction we also see sex differences. Boys' groups and boys' friendships appear to be focused more on competition and dominance than are girls' friendships. In fact, among school-age boys, we see *higher* levels of competition between pairs of friends than between strangers, which is the opposite of what we see among girls. Friendships between girls also include more agreement, more compliance, and more self-disclosure than is true for boys. For example, Leaper (1991) finds that "controlling" speech—a category that includes rejecting comments, ordering, manipulating or challenging, defiance or refutation, or resistance of the other's attempt to control—is twice as common among pairs of 7- and 8-year-old male friends as among pairs of female friends. Among the 4- and 5-year-olds in this study there were no sex differences in controlling speech.

None of this should obscure the fact that there are great similarities in the interactions of male and female friendship pairs in the years of middle childhood. As one example, collaborative and cooperative exchanges are the most common forms of communication in both boys' and girls' friendships. Nor should we necessarily conclude that boys' friendships are less important to them than are girls'. Nevertheless, it seems clear that there are differences in form and style that may well have enduring implications for the patterns of friendship over the full life span.

Adolescents.   Many of these patterns change at adolescence. Mixed-sex groups begin to appear, conformity to the peer group values and behaviors increases, and parents' influence on the child wanes (even while the attachment to the parents remains strong). Teenagers spend more than half their waking hours with other teenagers and less than 5 percent of their time with either parent. Their friendships are also increasingly intimate, in the sense that adolescent friends share more and more of their inner feelings and secrets and are more knowledgeable about each other's feelings. Loyalty and faithfulness become more valued characteristics of friendship. These friendships are also more likely to endure for a year or longer. In one longitudinal study, Robert and Beverly Cairns found that only about 20 percent of friendships among fourth graders lasted as long as a year, while about 40 percent of friendships formed by these same youngsters when they were tenth graders were long lasting (1994).

Do you think these same kinds of sex differences exist in adult friendships in our culture? Are adult men's friendships more competitive, women's friendships more intimate? Assuming this is true, what consequences do you think such a difference has for our society?

But beyond these changes in individual relationships, the *function* of the peer group changes in adolescence. In elementary school, peer groups are mostly the setting for mutual play and for all the learning about relationships and the natural world that is part of such play. But the teenager uses the peer group in another way. He is struggling to make a slow transition from the protected life of the family to the independent life of adulthood, and the peer group becomes the *vehicle* for that transition. As Erikson has pointed out, the clannishness and intense conformity to the group is a normal—even an essential—part of the process. Such conformity seems to peak at about age 13 or 14 (at about the same time that we see a drop in self-esteem, as you'll recall from Chapter 10) and then wanes as the teenager begins to arrive at a sense of identity that is more independent of the peer group.

However, while it is very clear that peers do indeed put pressure on each other to conform to peer group behavior standards, it is also true that peer group pressures are less potent and less negative than popular cultural stereotypes might lead you to believe (Berndt, 1992). For one thing, let us remember that adolescents *choose* their friends, their crowd. And they are likely to choose to associate with a group that shares their values, attitudes, and behaviors. If the discrepancy between their own ideas and those of their friends becomes too great, teens are more likely to move toward a more compatible group of friends than to be persuaded to shift toward the first group's values or behaviors. Furthermore, teenagers report that when explicit peer pressure is exerted, it is likely to be pressure toward positive activities, such as school involvement, and *away* from misconduct. Only in "druggie-tough" crowds does there seem to be explicit pressure toward misconduct or lawbreaking, and here the motive may be as much a desire to prove "I'm as tough as you are" as it is explicit pressure from peers (Berndt & Keefe, 1995; Brown, Dolcini, & Leventhal, 1995). Thus, while Erikson appears to be quite correct in saying that peers are a major force in shaping a child's identity development in adolescence, peer influence is neither monolithic nor uniformly negative.

Changes in Peer Group Structure in Adolescence. The structure of the peer group also changes over the years of adolescence. The classic, widely quoted early study is Dunphy's observation of the formation, dissolution, and interaction of teenage groups in a high school in Sydney, Australia, between 1958 and 1960 (Dunphy, 1963). He identified two important subvarieties of groups, using labels that until recently were widely adopted by other writers on adolescence. The first type, which Dunphy called **cliques,** is made up of four to six young people who appear to be strongly attached to one another.

In Dunphy's terms, what stage of teen group formation do you think this represents?

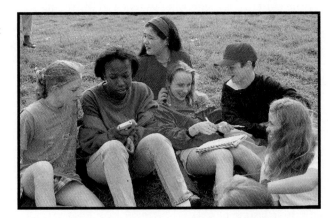

Research Report

Are African-American Adolescents More Susceptible to Peer Influence?

One assumption made by a great many adults, including many social scientists, is that African-American youth, more than any other group, are likely to be strongly peer-oriented and to be more vulnerable to peer pressure. One typical argument is that because black teenagers more often live in single-parent families, they are more likely to depend on peers for affiliation and support. Several recent studies call this assumption into question.

Peggy Giordano and her colleagues (Giordano, Cernkovich, & DeMaris, 1993) studied a group of 942 teenagers, chosen as a representative sample of all adolescents living in Toledo, Ohio. Half the group was black, the remainder was mostly non-Hispanic whites. These teens were asked a wide variety of questions about their friendships and their relationships with peers, such as:

"How important is it to you to do things your friends approve of?"

"How important is it to you to have a group of friends to hang around with?"

They were also asked about family intimacy (e.g., "I'm closer to my parents than a lot of kids my age are") and about parental supervision and control.

In this sample, African-American adolescents reported significantly *more* family intimacy, *more* parental supervision and control, *less* need for peer approval, and *less* peer pressure than did white teens.

Similarly, Vicki Mack (Mack et al., 1995), in a study of nearly 1000 teens in Detroit, found that the African-American youth described *lower* levels of compliance to friends and *higher* scores on measures of the importance of their relationship with their parents. These two studies certainly raise questions about widespread cultural assumptions.

Cliques have strong cohesiveness and high levels of intimate sharing. In the early years of adolescence, these cliques are almost entirely same-sex groups—a residual of the preadolescent pattern. Gradually, however, the cliques combine into larger sets Dunphy called **crowds,** made up of several cliques, some male and some female. Finally, the crowd breaks down again into heterosexual cliques and then into loose associations of couples. In Dunphy's study, the period of the fully developed crowd was roughly between ages 13 and 15—the very years when we see the greatest conformity to peer pressure.

Bradford Brown and others of the current generation of adolescence researchers have shifted the language somewhat. (1990; Brown, Mory, & Kinney, 1994; Youniss, McLellan, & Strouse, 1994). Brown uses the word *crowd* to refer to the "reputation-based" group with which a young person is identified, either by choice or by peer designation. In United States schools these groups have labels like *jocks, brains, nerds, dweebs, punks, druggies, radicals, normals, populars, outcasts, toughs, preppies,* or *loners.* Studies in American junior high and high schools make it clear that teenagers can readily identify and have quite stereotypic—even caricatured—descriptions of each of the major crowds in their school (e.g., "The partyers goof off a lot more than the jocks do, but they don't come to school stoned like the burnouts do"). Each of these descriptions serves as what Brown calls an "identity prototype" (Brown et al., 1994, p. 133): Labeling others and labeling oneself as belonging to one or more of these groups helps to create or reinforce the adolescent's own identity. Such labeling also help the adolescent identify potential friends or foes. Thus, membership in one crowd or another channels each adolescent toward particular activities and particular relationships.

Within any given school, these various crowds are organized into a fairly clear, widely understood pecking order. In U.S. schools, the groups labeled as some variant of "jocks," "populars," or "normals" are typically at the top of the heap, with "brains" somewhere in the middle and "druggies," "loners," and "nerds" at the bottom (Brown et al., 1994).

Through the years of junior high and high school, the social system of crowds becomes increasingly differentiated, with more and more distinct groups. For example, in one study in a Midwest school system (Kinney, 1993), there were only two major crowds in junior high, one small high-status group (called *trendies* in this school) and the great mass of lower-status students, called *dweebs*. In the early high school years, these same students identified five crowds, three with comparatively high social status and two low-status groups (*grits* and *punkers*.) By late high school, there were seven or eight identifiable crowds, but the groups appeared to be more fluid, less central to the social organization of the older students. Within (and sometimes across) these crowds, adolescents create smaller friendship groups Brown calls *cliques*—a usage that is very similar to Dunphy's meaning for the same term. These groups, as Dunphy observed, are almost entirely same-sex in early adolescence; by late adolescence they have become mixed in gender, often composed of groups of dating couples.

Whatever specific clique or crowd a teenager may identify with, theorists agree that the peer group performs the highly important function of helping the teenager make the shift from unisexual to heterosexual social relationships. The 13- or 14-year-old can begin to try out her new relationship skills in the wider group of the crowd or clique; only after some confidence is developed do we see the beginnings of dating and of more committed heterosexual pair relationships.

Heterosexual Relationships in Adolescence.   Of all the changes in social relationships in adolescence, perhaps the most profound is this shift from the total dominance of same-sex friendships to heterosexual relationships. There is a very large cultural element in all this, of course. Many cultures in the world still tightly control or prohibit heterosexual contact during puberty or before marriage; in others, few, if any, restrictions exist at all. Most Western cultures fall in between, with the current United States culture leaning strongly toward the no-restriction end of the continuum.

The heterosexual relationships we see in early and middle adolescence are clearly part of the preparation for assuming a full adult sexual identity. Physical sexuality is part of that role, but so are the skills of personal intimacy with the opposite sex, including flirting, communicating, and reading the form of social cues used by the other gender.

In Western societies, these skills are learned first in larger crowds or cliques and then in dating pairs (Zani, 1993). Studies of adolescents in the United States in the 1980s suggest that dating begins most typically at 15 or 16, as you can see from Table 11.3, which shows results from a representative sample of Detroit teenagers (Thornton, 1990).

You'll recall from Chapter 4 that there are some ethnic differences in such heterosexual behavior within American society. African-American teens begin dating and sexual experimentation earlier than do Anglos or Hispanics. Early dating and early sexual activity are also more common among the poor of every ethnic group and among those who experience relatively early puberty. Among girls, for example, those with early menarche are more likely to initiate sexual activity early than are same-age peers who have not yet reached menarche. Religious teachings and individual attitudes about the appropriate age for dating and sexual behavior also make a difference, as does family structure. Girls from divorced or remarried families, for example, report earlier dating and higher levels

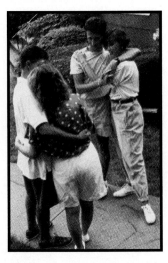

Dating and clear heterosexual (or homosexual) coupling comes fairly late in adolescence and represents the end point of the long sequence of changes in peer group structures.

Table 11.3
Age at First Date Among U.S. Adolescents (in percentages)

Age	Males	Females
13 or younger	21.2	8.6
14	17.9	16.2
15	21.2	33.6
16	29.5	29.3
17–18	7.2	10.0

Source: Thornton, 1990, Table 1, pp. 246–247.

of sexual experience than do girls from intact families, and those with strong religious identity report later dating and lower levels of sexuality (Bingham, Miller, & Adams, 1990; Miller & Moore, 1990). But for every group, these are years of experimentation with heterosexual relationships.

Prosocial Behavior and Aggression

This broad sketch of peer relationships from toddlerhood through adolescence makes clear the various roles that peers play in children's development over these years, and how central such relationships are. What it does not convey are all the changes in the actual content or quality of children's peer interactions. To fill in some of the gaps, let me say just a word or two about the two ends of the positive/negative continuum, namely, prosocial behavior and aggression.

Prosocial Behavior. This class of behavior is defined by psychologists as "intentional, voluntary behavior intended to benefit another" (Eisenberg, 1992, p. 3). In everyday language, this is essentially what we mean by **altruism,** and it changes with age, just as other aspects of peer behavior change.

We first see such **prosocial behaviors** in children of about 2 or 3—at about the same time that they begin to show real interest in play with other children. They will offer to help another child who is hurt, offer a toy, or try to comfort another person (Marcus, 1986; Zahn-Waxler & Radke-Yarrow, 1982). As I pointed out in Chapter 7, children this young have only a beginning understanding of the fact that others feel differently from themselves, but they obviously understand enough about the emotions of others to respond in supportive and sympathetic ways when they see other children or adults hurt or sad.

Past these early years, researchers have found a number of trends. Older children are more likely to share objects or money with others (such as donating marbles in the game I described in Chapter 9). School-age children and adolescents are also more likely than

The Real World

Homosexuality Among Adolescents

I have talked about the normal sequence of peer relationships in adolescence as moving gradually toward committed heterosexual partnerships. But of course heterosexual experience is not the only kind teenagers may have. In a recent study of nearly 35,000 youth in Minnesota public schools, Remafedi and his colleagues (1992) found that less than 1 percent of the adolescent boys and only 0.4 percent of the girls *defined* themselves as homosexual, but a much larger number said they were "unsure" of their sexual orientation, and 2 to 6 percent reported that they were attracted to others of the same sex. These figures are generally consistent with the newest and most comprehensive data on U.S. adults (Laumann et al., 1994): Two to 3 percent of adults say they think of themselves as homosexual or bisexual; roughly twice that many say they are attracted to those of the same sex.

Recent evidence has greatly strengthened the hypothesis that homosexuality has a biological basis (Gladue, 1994). For example, several new twin studies show that when one identical twin is homosexual, the probability that the other will also be homosexual is 50 to 60 percent, while this "concordance rate" is only about 20 percent for fraternal twins (Bailey & Pillard, 1991; Bailey et al., 1993; Whitam, Diamond, & Martin, 1993) and only about 11 percent among pairs of biologically unrelated boys adopted into the same families.

Studies of prenatal hormone effects also point to biological origins. For example, women whose mothers took the drug diethylstilbestrol (DES, a synthetic estrogen) during pregnancy are more likely to be homosexual as adults than are women who did not have such DES exposure (Meyer-Bahlburg et al., 1995).

Such biological evidence does not mean that there are no environmental causes of homosexuality. No behavior is entirely controlled by either nature or nurture, as I have said many times. At the very least, we know that 40 or 50 percent of identical twins do *not* share the same sexual orientation. Something beyond biology must be at work, although we do not yet know what environmental factors may be involved.

Whatever the cause, homosexual teenagers are a minority. These adolescents face high levels of prejudice and stereotyping. Many are physically attacked by their peers (Remafedi, Farrow, & Deisher, 1991). For these and other reasons, these young people are at high risk for a variety of problems. In Remafedi's study, for example, four fifths of homosexual teens interviewed in Minneapolis had deteriorating school performance, and more than a quarter dropped out of high school (Remafedi, 1987a). They must also cope with the decision about whether to "come out" about their homosexuality. Those who do come out are far more likely to tell peers than parents, although telling peers carries some risk: In his Minneapolis study, Remafedi found that 41 percent of homosexual male youths had lost a friend over the issue (Remafedi, 1987b). Some research suggests that as many as two thirds of homosexual youth have not told their parents (Rotheram-Borus, Rosario, & Koopman, 1991).

There is obviously much that we do not know about homosexual adolescents. But it is a reasonable hypothesis that the years of adolescence may be particularly stressful for this subgroup. Like ethnic-minority youth, homosexual teens have an additional task facing them in forming a clear identity.

are preschoolers to provide physical and verbal assistance to someone in need (Eisenberg, 1992). But not all prosocial behaviors show this pattern. Comforting another child, for example, appears to be more common among preschool and early-elementary-school children than at older ages (Eisenberg, 1988; 1990).

At any age, children vary a lot in the amount of altruistic behavior they show. For those of you interested in knowing more about how helpful or altruistic children come to be that way, I've explored some of the research in the *Real World* box on the facing page.

Aggression. If you have watched children together, you know that all is not sweetness and light in the land of the young. Children do support and share with their friends, and

The Real World
Rearing Helpful and Altruistic Children

If you wish to encourage your own children to be more generous or altruistic, here are some specific things you can do, based on the work of Eisenberg and others (1992):

1. *Create a loving and warm family climate.* This is especially effective if such warmth is combined with clear explanations.

2. *Explain why and give rules.* Clear rules about what *to* do as well as what *not* to do are important. Explaining the consequences of the child's action in terms of its effects on others is also good; for example: "If you hit Susan it will hurt her." Equally important is stating *positive* rules or guidelines; for example: "It's always good to be helpful to other people," or "We should share what we have with people who don't have so much."

3. *Provide prosocial attributions.* Attribute your child's helpful or altruistic action to the child's own internal character: "You're such a helpful child!" or "You certainly do a lot of nice things for other people." This strategy begins to be effective with children at about age 7 or 8, at about the same time that they are beginning to develop global notions of self-esteem. In this way you may be able to affect the child's self-scheme, which in turn may result in a generalized, internalized, pattern of altruistic behavior.

4. *Have children do helpful things.* Children can help cook, take care of pets, make toys to give away, teach younger siblings or tutor in school, and so forth. This can backfire if the coercion required to get the child to do the helpful thing is too strong: The child may now attribute his "good" behavior to the coercion ('Mother made me do it") rather than to some inner trait of his own ("I am a helpful/kind person"), and no future altruism is fostered.

5. *Model thoughtful and generous behavior.* Stating the rules clearly will do little good if your own behavior does not match what you say!

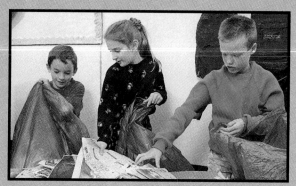

Having children do helpful things, as these third graders are doing by sorting recyclable material, is one way to increase altruistic behavior in kids.

they do show affectionate and helpful behaviors toward one another, but they also tease, fight, yell, criticize, and argue over objects and territory. Researchers who have studied this more negative side of children's interactions have looked mostly at **aggression,** which we can define as behavior with the apparent intent to injure some other person or object.

Every child shows at least some aggression, but the form and frequency of aggression change over the years of childhood. When 2- or 3-year-old children are upset or frustrated, they are more likely to throw things or hit each other. As their verbal skills improve, however, children shift away from such overt physical aggression toward greater use of verbal aggression, such as taunting or name calling. In the elementary school and adolescent years, physical aggression becomes still less common, and children learn the cultural rules about when and how much it is acceptable to display anger or aggression. In most cultures, this means that anger is more and more disguised, and aggression more and more controlled with increasing age (Underwood, Coie, & Herbsman, 1992).

One interesting exception to this general pattern is that in all-boy pairs or groups, at least in United States studies, physical aggression seems to remain both relatively high and constant over the years of childhood. Indeed, at every age, boys show more physical aggression and more assertiveness than do girls, both within friendship pairs and in general (Fabes, Knight, & Higgins, 1995). Table 11.4 gives some highly representative data from a very large, careful survey in Canada (Offord, Boyle, & Racine, 1991) in which both parents and teachers completed checklists describing each child's behavior—a study you may remember from Figure 1.4 in Chapter 1 (p. 25). In Table 11.4 I've listed only the information provided by teachers, but parent ratings yielded parallel findings. It is clear that boys are described as far more aggressive on nearly any measure of physical aggressiveness.

Results like these have been so clear and so consistent that most psychologists concluded that boys are simply "more aggressive" in every possible way. But that may turn out to be wrong. Instead, it begins to look as if girls simply express their aggressiveness in a different way, using what has come to be called *relational aggression* rather than physical aggression or nasty words. Physical aggression hurts others through physical damage or threat of such damage; relational aggression hurts others through damaging the other person's self-esteem or peer relationships, such as ostracism or threats of ostracism ("I won't invite you to my birthday party if you do that"), cruel gossiping, or facial expressions of disdain. Children experience such indirect aggression as genuinely hurtful, and they are likely to shun other kids who use this form of aggression a lot, just as they tend to reject peers who are physically aggressive (Casas & Mosher, 1995; Cowan & Underwood, 1995; Crick & Grotpeter, 1995). Girls are much more likely to use relational aggression than are boys, especially toward other girls, a difference that begins as early as the preschool years and becomes very marked by the fourth or fifth grade. For example, in one recent study of nearly 500 children third through sixth grades, Nicki Crick finds that

Table 11.4
Percentage of Boys and Girls Ages 4 to 11 Rated by Their Teachers as Displaying Each Type of Aggressive Behavior

Behavior	Boys	Girls
Mean to others	21.8	9.6
Physically attacks people	18.1	4.4
Gets in many fights	30.9	9.8
Destroys own things	10.7	2.1
Destroys others' things	10.6	4.4
Threatens to hurt people	13.1	4.0

Source: Offord, Boyle, & Racine, 1991, from Table 2.3, p. 39.

17.4 percent of the girls but only 2 percent of the boys were high in relational aggression—almost precisely the reverse of what we see for physical aggression (Crick & Grotpeter, 1995). Whether this difference in the form of aggression has some hormonal/biological basis or is trained at an early age, or both, we do not know. We do know that higher rates of physical aggression in males have been observed in every human society and in all varieties of primates. And we know that there is some link between rates of physical aggression and testosterone levels (Maccoby & Jacklin, 1974). But where the apparent propensity toward relational aggression comes from among girls is still a mystery.

Individual Differences in Peer Relationships

Collectively, children may move toward greater and greater ability to interact effectively with their peers, toward greater altruism and away from overt expression of aggression, toward greater intimacy in their relationships with peers. But there are clearly enormous differences in the degree to which children acquire such skills, and in their resulting popularity or lack of it. In recent years, the study of such individual differences in social skills and popularity has been one of the hottest topics in all developmental psychology. Researchers have struggled to understand why some children are rejected by their peers, while others are not.

Popularity and Rejection

Psychologists who study popularity in children have recently concluded that it is important to distinguish between several subgroups of unpopular children. The most frequently studied are those children who are overtly *rejected* by peers. If you ask children to list peers they would *not* like to play with or if you observe which children are avoided on the playground, you can get a measure of rejection of this type. A second type has come to be called *neglected*. Children in this category are reasonably well liked but lack individual friends and are rarely chosen as most preferred by their peers. Neglected children have been studied far less than have the rejected, but the preliminary evidence suggests that while neglect is much less stable over time than is rejection, neglected children are nonetheless more prone to depression and loneliness than are accepted children (Cillessen et al., 1992; Rubin et al., 1991). Where might such differences in popularity or peer acceptance come from?

Do you think it is a reasonable hypothesis that neglected children are likely to have been insecurely attached as infants? How could you test such a hypothesis?

Qualities of Rejected and Popular Children. Some of the characteristics that differentiate popular and unpopular children are things outside a child's control. In particular, attractive children and physically larger children are more likely to be popular—perhaps merely a continuation of the preference for attractive faces that Langlois detected in young infants and that I described in Chapter 5. The most crucial ingredient, though, is not how the child looks but how the child behaves.

Popular children behave in positive, supporting, nonpunitive, and nonaggressive ways toward most other children. They explain things, take their playmates' wishes into consideration, and take turns in conversation. Rejected children are aggressive, disruptive, and uncooperative. They interrupt their play partners more often and fail to take turns in a systematic way. To be sure, not all aggressive children are rejected. It is when they *also* lack compensating positive social skills that they are most likely to be overtly rejected by their peers (Coie & Cillessen, 1993; Newcomb, Bukowski, & Pattee, 1993).

If Christopher is this aggressive with his peers, and not just with his sister (as shown here), he is likely to be rejected by other children, a pattern with potential long-term consequences.

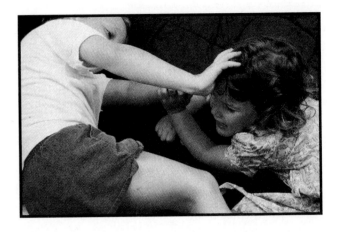

This conclusion emerges from a variety of types of research, including at least a few cross-cultural studies. For example, aggression and disruptive behavior are linked to rejection and unpopularity among Chinese children, just as they are among American children (Chen, Rubin, & Sun, 1992). Among the best sources of evidence are studies in which groups of previously unacquainted children are brought together to play for some number of hours over several weeks. At the end of these sessions, the children pick their favorite and least-favorite playmates from among the group. Since the researchers have observed the actual behavior of the children throughout the sessions, they can link the child's behavior with his or her later popularity. In these studies, children who are most consistently positive and supportive are those who end up being chosen as leaders or as friends. Those who consistently participate in conflicts are more often rejected.

Rejected children also seem to have quite different internal working models of relationships and of aggression from those of popular children. In a whole series of studies, Kenneth Dodge has shown that aggressive/rejected children are much more likely to see aggression as a useful way to solve problems. They are also much more likely to interpret someone else's behavior as hostile or attacking than is true for less-aggressive or more-popular children. Given an ambiguous event, such as being hit in the back with a ball while on the playground, aggressive or rejected children—especially boys—are much more likely to assume that the ball was thrown on purpose and to retaliate. In turn, such retaliation is likely to elicit hostility from others, further confirming the rejected boy's expectation that other people are hostile to him (Dodge et al., 1990; Quiggle et al., 1992).

This body of research can also be linked to Gerald Patterson's work, whose model I described in Chapter 1 (Figure 1.2, p. 11) and in Chapter 9. Patterson is persuaded that a child's excess aggressiveness can be traced originally to ineffective parental control. But once the child's aggressiveness is well established, the child displays this same behavior with peers, is rejected by those peers, and is then driven more and more toward the only set of peers who will accept him, usually other aggressive or delinquent youngsters. These antisocial kids are not friendless; but their friends are almost always other kids with similar antisocial patterns, and these friendships tend to be fairly transitory and focused on mutual coercion (Dishion, Andrews, & Crosby, 1995).

The seriousness of this set of connected problems is amply demonstrated in a growing body of research showing that rejection by one's peers in elementary school is one of the very few aspects of childhood functioning that consistently predicts behavior problems or emotional disturbances later in childhood, adolescence, and adulthood (Dishion, 1990; Eron, 1987; Farrington, 1991; Serbin et al., 1991).

For example, Melissa DeRosier (DeRosier, Kupersmidt, & Patterson, 1994) and her colleagues followed one group of more than 600 children over a four-year period in early elementary school. She finds that those children who were most chronically rejected by their peers showed higher rates of a whole variety of problems, including being absent from school, more depression or sadness, and more behavior problems.

Similarly, Janis Kupersmidt and John Coie (1990), in an even longer-term longitudinal study, from fifth grade through the end of high school, found that negative outcomes in high school—including poor school performance, regular truancy, dropping out of school, or juvenile court appearance—were considerably more common among rejected children than among the popular.

We might explain such a link between early unpopularity and later behavior problems in any of several ways. Early problems with peers might be merely the most visible reflection of a general maladjustment that later manifests itself as delinquency or emotional disturbance. It could also mean that a failure to develop friendships itself causes problems that later become more general. Or it could signify a seriously warped internal working model of relationships, or all of the above. Whatever the source of the problem, you will be glad to know that not all rejected children remain rejected or develop serious behavior problems or delinquency. The worst long-term prognosis is for those children who are rejected over a period of years; the best is for those who show some altruistic or prosocial behavior in addition to aggression (Tremblay, 1991).

Sex Differences

As a final word in this long and complex chapter, let me make a couple of additional brief points about a topic I have only touched on as we have gone along, namely, sex differences in social behavior. The most consistent difference is in the area of aggression/dominance/competitiveness. Boys show more of all these behaviors, beginning at an early age, just as the widespread gender stereotypes would suggest. But contrary to most expectations, we have little evidence that girls are consistently more nurturant or dependent on others, or more compliant to adults' wishes. Girls are also not more sociable; they do not, for example, have more friends than boys do.

But at a subtler level, we are beginning to understand that there are important differences in the *ways* boys and girls go about interacting with one another. I've already mentioned several of the bits of information that point us toward this conclusion, but let me pull them together for you:

- Pairs of boy friends are *more* competitive with each other than are pairs of strangers.

- Aggression between boys does not decline over the years of elementary school, while aggression between girls and between boys and girls does drop.

- Friendships between girls are much more intimate, with much more self-disclosure.

- Boy friends are more likely to gather in large groups than in paired chumships, and the boys are less likely to exchange confidences and more likely to engage in some mutual activity, such as sports.

We also have a variety of indications that the same differences in style of relationship are evident in adults. Eleanor Maccoby (1990) describes the girls'/women's pattern as an *enabling style.* Enabling includes such behaviors as supporting the partner, expressing agreement, making suggestions. All these behaviors tend to foster a greater equality and intimacy in the relationship and keep the interaction going. In contrast, boys and men are more likely to show what Maccoby calls a *constricting* or *restrictive* style. "A restrictive style is one that tends to derail the interaction—to inhibit the partner or cause the partner to withdraw, thus shortening the interaction or bringing it to an end" (p. 517). Contradicting, interrupting, boasting, or other forms of self-display are all aspects of this style. Campbell Leaper (1991) labels these two styles *cooperative* and *domineering,* which conveys much the same message.

These are subtle but profound differences and we still know little about how they arise in earliest childhood and whether equivalent differences occur across cultures. But if we are going to be able to make sense out of our own relationships, and out of the rapidly changing gender roles in modern society, we obviously need to know a great deal more about these apparently pervasive gender differences.

Summary

1   Both vertical relationships with adults and horizontal relationships with peers are of central significance in the child's social development. In particular, skills in forming and maintaining reciprocal relationships can only be learned with peers.

2   It is important to distinguish between an affectional bond (an enduring tie to a uniquely viewed partner) and an attachment, which involves the added element of security and a safe base.

3   An attachment is deduced from the existence of attachment behaviors.

4   For the parents to form a strong bond to the infant, what is most crucial is the learning and repetition of mutually reinforcing and interlocking attachment behaviors, and not immediate contact at birth.

5   Fathers as well as mothers form strong bonds to their infants, but fathers show more physically playful behaviors with their children than do mothers.

6   Initially, the infant shows attachment behaviors toward nearly anyone but no preferential attachment. By 5 to 6 months of age, most infants have formed at least one strong attachment, usually to the major caregiver.

7   Attachment behaviors become less visible during the preschool years except when the child is stressed. By age 4 or 5 the child understands the constancy of the relationship.

8   The basic attachment to the parents remains strong in adolescence, despite an increase in parent-child conflict, the greater independence of the teenager, and the increased role of the peer group.

9   Children differ in the security of their first attachments, and thus in the internal working model they develop. The secure infant uses the parent as a safe base for exploration and can be readily consoled by the parent.

10   The security of the initial attachment is reasonably stable and is fostered by contingent responsiveness and acceptance by the parent.

11   Securely attached children appear to be more socially skillful, more curious and persistent in approaching new tasks, and more mature.

12   Children's relationships with peers become increasingly significant for their social development past the age of about 2. In elementary school, peer interactions are focused mostly on common activities; in adolescence, peer groups also become the vehicle for the transition from dependence to independence.

13 Reputation-based groups, called "crowds" by current researchers, are an important part of adolescent social relationships, particularly in the early high school years. Smaller groups of friends, called "cliques," are also present and gradually shift from same-sex to mixed-sex to dating pairs.

14 On average in Western cultures, dating begins at about age 15, but there is wide variability.

15 By age 4 or 5 most children have formed individual friendships and show preferential positive behavior toward friends. Friendship becomes more common and more stable in the elementary school years, and more intimate in adolescence.

16 Prosocial behavior, such as helpfulness or generosity, is apparent as early as age 2 or 3 and generally increases throughout childhood.

17 Young children also show such negative social patterns as aggressiveness. Physical aggression peaks at 3 or 4 and is replaced more and more by verbal aggression among older children. Boys show more aggressiveness at every age.

18 Popularity among peers, in elementary school or later, is most consistently based on the amount of positive and supportive social behavior shown by a child toward peers.

19 Rejected children are typically those who show heightened levels of aggression toward peers and who lack social skills. Such children appear to have different internal working models than do nonrejected children. They are also at much higher risk for later behavior problems such as delinquency.

20 Boys and girls appear to have quite different styles of interacting with one another, with girls' pairs or groups showing a more "enabling" style.

Key Terms

affectional bond (**p. 306**)

aggression (**p. 329**)

altruism (**p. 327**)

attachment (**p. 306**)

attachment behavior (**p. 306**)

clique (**p. 324**)

crowd (**p. 324**)

insecure attachment (**p. 316**)

internal working model (**p. 315**)

prosocial behavior (**p. 327**)

secure attachment (**p. 316**)

Strange Situation (**p. 316**)

Suggested Readings

Bretherton, I. (1992a). The origins of attachment theory: John Bowlby and Mary Ainsworth. *Developmental Psychology, 28,* 759–775.

A clear, current, thoughtful review of both Bowlby's and Ainsworth's ideas, including new data from anthropology and other cross-cultural analyses.

Dunn, J. (1993). *Young children's close relationships.* Newbury Park, CA: Sage.

A wonderful small book, written in a clear and engaging style by one of the experts on children's social relationships.

Eisenberg, N. (1992). *The caring child*. Cambridge, MA: Harvard University Press.

A brief, clear, current summary of what we know about the development of prosocial and altruistic behavior.

Hartup, W. W. (1989). Social relationships and their developmental significance. *American Psychologist, 44,* 120–126.

Hartup has always been one of my favorite authors. His style is clear, his ideas interesting. Here he gives a brief review of some of the current work on social interactions.

Lickona, T. (1983). *Raising good children*. Toronto: Bantam Books.

One of the very best "how to" books for parents I have ever seen, with excellent, concrete advice as well as theory. His emphasis is on many of the issues I raised in the *Real World* box on rearing altruistic children.

Montemayor, R., Adams, R. G., & Gullotta, T. P. (Eds.). (1994). *Personal relationships during adolescence*. Thousand Oaks, CA: Sage.

A first-rate collection of papers, including an especially fascinating discussion of teen crowds by Bradford Brown.

Tannen, D. (1990) *You just don't understand*. New York: Morrow.

If you are at all interested in differences between women's and men's conversational and interactive styles, this book is a *must* read. I found it fascinating, and I learned a lot that has been a great help.

Thinking About Relationships: The Development of Social Cognition

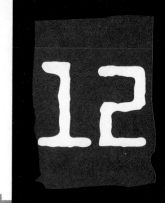

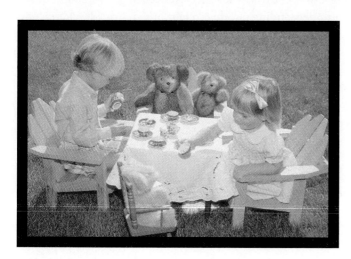

Think for a minute about the conversations you have with your friends. Haven't you said things like "I thought Jack was my friend, but now it turns out I can't really trust him," or "I've been trying to figure Jane out. Sometimes she's shy and sometimes she's the life of the party," or "Lots of people believe that I'm really the confident person I look like on the outside, but my friends know how insecure I really am"?

All these statements reflect some aspect of what psychologists have come to call **social cognition**—thinking about people, what they do and should do, how they feel. If you are anything like I am (and I assume you are), then you too spend a great deal of time and energy analyzing other people, trying to understand, trying to predict what your friends, partner, or co-workers will do. In fact, in our everyday life knowledge about people and relationships is probably more important than many of the more abstract kinds of knowledge or thinking I talked about in Chapters 6 and 7. Where does such social knowledge come from? How does children's thinking about people, about relationships, about right and wrong change over time?

These questions are not new in this book. I have touched on many facets of social cognition as I have gone along. The infant's emerging ability to recognize individuals and to use facial expressions and other body cues for social referencing is one kind of social cognition, as is the growing understanding of others' emotions and the development of a theory of others' minds in the preschool years. One could also argue that an "internal working model" of attachment is a kind of social cognition, as is the child's self-scheme. What I need to do now is to pull these various threads together and to describe some of the more general ideas about social cognition that have emerged in the past few years. In the process, I hope to build a few bridges between the earlier, separate discussions of thinking and social relationships.

Some General Principles and Issues

One way to think about social cognition is simply to conceive of it as the application of general cognitive processes or skills to a different topic, in this case people or relationships. In Chapter 7 I talked about all the ways in which children's thinking changes from infancy through adolescence. We might assume that at any given age a child applies these fundamental ways of thinking to his relationships as well as to objects. In this view, the child's understanding of self and others, of social relationships, reflects or is based on her overall level of cognitive development, such as her level of perspective-taking skills (Selman, 1980).

This approach has a powerful intuitive appeal. After all, as John Flavell points out (1985), it is the same head doing the thinking when a child works on a conservation problem and when she tries to understand people. Furthermore, as you will see very clearly as we go through the evidence, many of the same principles that seem to apply to general cognitive development hold here as well, such as the following:

- *Outer to inner characteristics.* Younger children pay attention to the surface of things, to what they look like; older children look for principles, for causes.

- *Observation to inference.* Young children base their conclusions initially only on what they can see or feel; later they make inferences about what ought to be or what might be.

- *Definite to qualified.* Young children's "rules" are very definite and fixed (such as sex-role rules); by adolescence, rules begin to be qualified.

- *Observer's view to general view.* Children also become less "egocentric" with time—less tied to their own individual view, more able to construct a model of some experience or some process that is true for everyone.

All these dimensions of change describe children's emerging social cognition, just as they describe the development of thinking about objects. But thinking about people and about relationships also has some special features that makes it different from thinking about physical objects.

One obvious difference is that people, unlike rocks or beakers of water, behave *intentionally*. In particular, people often attempt to conceal information about themselves, which makes the ability to "read" other people's cues one of the key social-cognitive skills. Further, unlike relationships with objects, relationships with people are mutual and reciprocal. Dolls, sets of blocks, or bicycles don't talk back, get angry, or respond in unexpected ways, but people do all these things. In learning about relationships, children must learn enough about other people's motives and feelings to predict such responses.

Children also have to learn special rules about particular forms of social interactions, such as rules about politeness, about when you can and cannot speak, or about power or dominance hierarchies—all forms of social *scripts* (Schank & Abelson, 1977), which is a concept I have mentioned several times before. Children presumably learn these scripts from their own experience, developing strong expectations about how people will behave, in what order, in which settings. Furthermore, these scripts probably change with age not just because children's cognitive skills change, but also because the rules (scripts) themselves change as children move from one social setting to another. One obvious example is the set of changes that occurs when children start school. The script associated with the role of "student" is quite different from the one connected with the role of "little kid." Classrooms are more tightly organized, expectations for obedience are higher, and there are more drills and routines to be learned than was probably true at home or even in nursery school. Similarly, the script changes when a 12-year-old moves into junior high school.

These illustrations make it clear, I hope, that the development of sophisticated social cognitive understanding is more than a simple process of applying basic cognitive processes and strategies to the arena of social interaction. The child must also come to understand the ways in which social relationships are *different* from interactions with the physical world and must learn special rules and strategies. Let's begin with the child's growing ability to read others' feelings.

Reading Others' Feelings

Think of sitting in a classroom while the professor hands back the midterm exams. The person on your right, after looking at her exam, raises her head and smiles widely. The person on your left stays hunched over his test and turns down his mouth as he shakes his head a bit. A third person near you breathes a huge sigh and sits in a more relaxed posture but does not smile. You easily deduce that the first person did well on the test and is happy; that the second person did less well than he expected or hoped and is distressed, perhaps even feeling guilty; and that the third person is relieved. How did you know that? What clues did you use? Presumably, you used three types of information: facial expression, other body language, and the context in which it all occurred. Because you knew that tests were being handed back, you were alert for both happy and sad reactions, and you interpreted the body language accordingly. The same body language in another setting might mean something a bit different.

Both cognitive skill and social information are obviously involved in this whole process. You need to be able to identify various body signals, including facial expressions; you need to understand various kinds of emotions and know that it is possible for people to feel several emotions at the same time; you need to understand the social context; and you need to have a theory of mind that helps you link the context and the feelings. In this

Think for a minute about how you tell when someone else is concealing some feeling. What clues do you use? How sure can you be of your interpretation?

Research Report

The Link Between a Child's Popularity and His Ability to Read Others' Intentions or Emotions

The study of children's social cognitions is not just a dry, obscure topic, interesting only for theoretical reasons. It turns out that whether a child is good or poor at reading cues from others has direct relevance to that child's success in social relationships. One good illustration comes from a series of studies by Kenneth Dodge and his colleagues: They have shown that unpopular children are significantly less skilled than are popular children at reading others' intentions.

In one study (Dodge, Murphy, & Buchsbaum, 1984), Dodge showed kindergarten, second-grade, and fourth-grade children videotapes, each of which showed an interaction in which one child destroyed the toy of a second child. These videos were carefully created so that the destroying child's intent was varied. In some vignettes, the intent was clearly hostile, in others it was accidental, in some it was ambiguous, and in others it was prosocial, such as knocking down the playmate's block tower in order to help clean up the room. Dodge found that in each age group, the popular children were better at detecting the actor's intent, with neglected and rejected children least accurate. In particular, neglected and rejected chil-

dren were more likely to see hostile intent when it was not present, a pattern that has been found in other studies, especially among rejected children (Dodge & Feldman, 1990; Graham & Hudley, 1994).

Of course this study does not tell us what is causing what. Does a child become unpopular because he sees hostility where it doesn't exist? Or does he see hostility in ambiguous situations because he has been rejected? Perhaps both, although we have at least some indications that such problems arise earlier in childhood as a result of harsh discipline from the parents (Strassberg et al., 1992; Weiss et al., 1992). Whatever the origin, it is clear that once such a "hostile attributional bias" has been established, it affects the child's later relationships. For example, when children are placed in new groups to interact with one another, those youngsters who begin such a process with a tendency to attribute hostile intent to others are more likely to be rejected later by their new playmates (Dodge & Feldman, 1990). And when highly aggressive children are given training specifically designed to reduce their hostile attributional bias, their level of aggression declines—an important real-life application (Hudley & Graham, 1993).

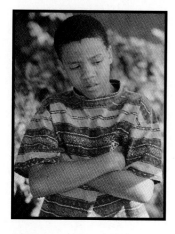

A preschool child would no doubt label this boy's emotion as "sad." A teenager would understand that the emotions might be much more complicated, such as sadness mixed with anger at himself, sadness and relief, or other forms of ambivalence.

case, you need the basic understanding that another person will be happy or sad, depending on how well he does on some task.

Research on children's understanding of others' emotions suggests that they acquire these various forms of knowledge gradually over the years from about age 1 to adolescence. You already know from Chapter 7 that by 10 to 12 months, babies can tell the difference between positive and negative expressions on others' faces, because at that age they already show *social referencing*. You also know that by age 3 or 4, children have some preliminary understanding of the links between other people's emotions and their situations, such as that someone would be sad if she failed.

All of this may make it sound as if 4- and 5-year-olds have already understood everything they need to know about others' emotions. In fact, a good deal of more sophisticated knowledge is still to come, such as understanding more complex or subtle emotions and grasping the fact that a person can have more than one emotion at the same time, even competing emotions. For example, 4-year-olds may be able to recognize the emotions of happiness, sadness, anger, love, and fear, but feelings like pride or shame are understood only in middle childhood (Harter & Whitesell, 1989). Similarly, by age 6, children understand that a person can switch rather rapidly from sadness to happiness if circumstances change, but it is only at about age 10 that children begin to understand that a person can feel opposite feelings (ambivalence) at the same moment

(Harter & Whitesell, 1989), and only in adolescence do they realize that a person can feel opposite feelings about the *same* object or event. "I was happy I was joining the new club but also a little worried because I didn't know anyone in it." "I was happy that I got a present but mad that it wasn't exactly what I wanted" (Harter & Whitesell, 1989, p. 86).

Emotions in Cross-cultural Perspective

One might reasonably ask—as one can about virtually all the developmental sequences I have given you in this book—whether children in every culture learn about emotions in this same way. In this case, we have a bit of evidence.

The Utka, an Inuit band in northern Canada, have two words for fear, distinguishing between fear of physical disaster and fear of being treated badly. In some African languages, there are no separate words for fear and sorrow. Samoans use the same word for love, sympathy, and liking, and Tahitians have no word at all that conveys the notion of guilt. These examples, drawn from the anthropological literature by James Russell (1989), remind us that we need to be very careful when we talk about the "normal" process of a child learning about emotional expression and emotional meaning. From our English-speaking, Western perspective, emotions like fear or anger seem like "basic" emotions that all infants would understand early and easily. But what would be the developmental sequence for a child growing up in a culture in which fear and sorrow are not distinguished?

At the same time, the work of Paul Ekman (1972; 1973; 1994) has given us evidence of a strong cross-cultural similarity in people's facial expressions when conveying certain of these same "basic" emotions, such as fear, happiness, sadness, anger, and disgust. (Figure 12.1 shows two such common expressions.) In all cultures studied so far, adults understand these facial expressions as having the same core meaning. One could argue that infants and toddlers are already quite good at discriminating and understanding these very basic, shared patterns. Even 2-year-olds can recognize and categorize happy and sad expressions. What the child must then learn are all the cultural overlays—the links between emotion and situation that hold in each culture, the specific meanings of emotional language (such as separate words for types of fear), the scripts that govern the appropriate expression of emotion in a given culture.

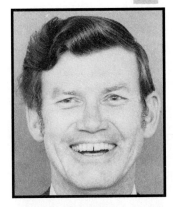

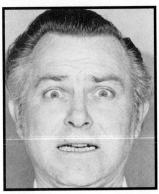

FIGURE 12.1 What emotion is being expressed in each of these photos? If you said happiness and fear, you agree with virtually all observers, in many countries, who have looked at these pictures. (Copyright © Paul Ekman.)

The Development of Empathy

Psychologists have also explored the development of the child's ability to read the emotions and cues of others by studying the development of **empathy.** Empathy involves two aspects, apprehending another person's emotional state or condition and then matching that emotional state oneself. An empathizing person experiences the same feeling that he imagines the other person to feel, or a highly similar feeling. *Sympathy* involves the same process of apprehending the other's emotional state, but it is accompanied not by a matching emotion but by a general feeling of sorrow or concern for the other (Eisenberg et al., 1989). Generally speaking, empathy seems to be the earlier response developmentally, and among older children and adults, sympathy often seems to grow out of an initial empathetic response.

The most thorough analysis of the development of empathy and sympathy has been offered by Martin Hoffman (1982; 1988), who describes four broad steps, which I've summarized in Table 12.1. The first stage, "global empathy," which is visible in infants,

Do you cry at weddings and funerals, even when you do not know the people involved really well? Is that a form of empathy?

Table 12.1
Stages in the Development of Empathy Proposed by Hoffman

Stage 1: **Global empathy**	Observed during the first year. If the infant is around someone expressing a strong emotion, he may match that emotion, such as beginning to cry when he hears another infant crying.
Stage 2: **Egocentric empathy**	Beginning at about 12 to 18 months, when the child has a fairly clear sense of his separate self, children respond to another's distress with some distress of their own but may attempt to "cure" the other person's problem by offering what they them-selves would find most comforting. They may, for example, show sadness when they see another child hurt and go to get their *own* mother to help.
Stage 3: **Empathy for another's feelings**	Beginning as young as 2 or 3 and continuing through elementary school, children note others' feelings, partially match those feel-ings, and respond to the other's distress in nonegocentric ways. Over these years, children distinguish a wider and wider (and more subtle) range of emotions.
Stage 4: **Empathy for another's life condition**	In late childhood or adolescence, some children develop a more generalized notion of others' feelings and respond not just to the immediate situation, but to the other individual's general situa-tion or plight. So a young person at this level may become more distressed over another person's sadness if he knows that that sadness is chronic or that the person's general situation is particu-larly tragic than if he sees it as a more momentary problem.

Sources: Hoffman, 1982, 1988.

seems to be a kind of automatic empathetic distress response, perhaps arising out of the earliest "fused self" I mentioned in Chapter 10. Hoffman says:

> *An 11-month-old girl, on seeing a child fall and cry, looked as if she was about to cry herself, and then put her thumb in her mouth and buried her head in her mother's lap, which is what she would do if she herself were hurt. (Hoffman, 1988, pp. 509–510)*

This changes as early as 12 or 18 months, as soon as the child has a clear understanding of the difference between self and other. The toddler still shows a matching emotion but un-derstands that the distress is the other person's and not her own. Nonetheless, her solu-tion to the other's distress is still likely to be egocentric, such as offering the distressed person a teddy bear.

Children's empathetic responses become more and more subtle over the preschool and elementary school years, as they become better readers of others' emotions. By mid-dle childhood, many children can even empathize with several different emotions at once, as when they see another child make a mistake and fall during a game. The observing

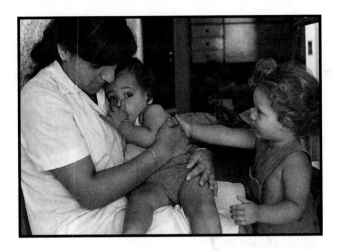

Children as young as 2 or 3 show this kind of empathetic response to other people's distress or delight.

child may see and empathize with both the hurt and the sense of shame or embarrassment and be aware that the victim may prefer *not* to be helped. In adolescence a still more abstract level emerges, when the child moves beyond the immediate situation and empathizes (or sympathizes) with another person's general plight.

Notice that both the developmental progressions I've been describing—in reading others' emotions and in empathizing with them—reflect several of the general principles I outlined earlier and parallel the changes Piaget described. In particular, we see a shift from observation to inference: With increasing age, the child's empathetic response is less and less guided by just the immediate, observed emotions seen in others, such as facial expressions or body language, and much more by the child's inferences or deductions about the other person's feelings. But this is not a swift change. For example, research in England by Paul Harris and his associates (Harris, Olthof, & Terwogt, 1981) shows that not until adolescence do young people become fully aware that other people may hide their emotions, or act differently from the way that they feel "inside."

As you might expect, not all children show equal amounts of such empathetic responses. We know little about where such differences may come from, but one clue is that children with histories of secure attachment show more empathy than do others (Kestenbaum, Farber, & Sroufe, 1989).

Describing Other People

We can see the same kind of shift from observation to inference in studies of children's descriptions of others, as well as a clear change in focus from outer to internal characteristics. There seem to be at least three steps. Up to perhaps ages 6 to 8, when children are asked to describe others, they focus almost exclusively on external features—what the person looks like, where he lives, what he does. This description by a 7-year-old boy, taken from a study in England by Livesley and Bromley (1973), is typical:

> *He is very tall. He has dark brown hair, he goes to our school. I don't think he has any brothers or sisters. He is in our class. Today he has a dark orange [sweater] and gray trousers and brown shoes. (p. 213)*

Before you read the rest of this section, write down a description of a friend or an acquaintance. Then as you read along, compare your descriptions to the ones children give.

When young children do use internal or evaluative terms to describe people, they are likely to use quite global terms, such as *nice* or *mean* or *good* or *bad*. Further, young children do not seem to see these qualities as lasting or general traits of the individual, applicable in all situations or over time (Rholes & Ruble, 1984). In other words, the young child has not yet developed a concept we might think of as "conservation of personality."

Then beginning at about age 7 or 8, at just about the same time that children seem to develop a global sense of self-esteem, a rather dramatic shift occurs in children's descriptions of others. The child begins to focus more on the inner traits or qualities of another person and to assume that those traits will be visible in many situations (Gnepp & Chilamkurti, 1988). Children this age still describe others' physical features, but now those descriptions are more by way of examples or elaborations of more general points about internal qualities. You can see the change when you compare the 7-year-old's description with this (widely quoted) description by a nearly 10-year-old:

> *He smells very much and is very nasty. He has no sense of humour and is very dull. He is always fighting and he is cruel. He does silly things and is very stupid. He has brown hair and cruel eyes. He is sulky and 11 years old and has lots of sisters. I think he is the most horrible boy in the class. He has a croaky voice and always chews his pencil and picks his teeth and I think he is disgusting. (Livesley & Bromley, 1973, p. 217)*

This description still includes many external, physical features but goes beyond such concrete, surface qualities to the level of personality traits, such as lack of humor or cruelty.

In adolescence, young people's descriptions begin to include more comparisons of one trait with another or one person with another, more recognition of inconsistencies and exceptions, more shadings of gray (Shantz, 1983), as in this description by a 15-year-old:

> *Andy is very modest. He is even shyer than I am when near strangers and yet is very talkative with people he knows and likes. He always seems good tempered and I have never seen him in a bad temper. He tends to degrade other people's achievements, and yet never praises his own. He does not seem to voice his opinions to anyone. He easily gets nervous. (Livesley & Bromley, 1973, p. 221)*

I can illustrate these changes less anecdotally with some findings from two studies by Carl Barenboim (1977; 1981). He asked children ranging in age from 6 to 16 to describe three people. Any descriptions that involved comparing a child's behaviors or physical features with another child, or with a norm, he called *behavioral comparisons* (such as "Billy runs a lot faster than Jason," or "She draws the best in our whole class"). Statements that involved some internal personality construct he called *psychological constructs* (such as "Sarah is so kind," or "He's a real stubborn idiot!"), while any that included qualifiers, explanations, exceptions, or mentions of changes in character he called *organizing relationships* (e.g., "He's only shy around people he doesn't know," or "Usually she's nice to me, but sometimes she can be quite mean"). Figure 12.2 shows the combined findings from the two studies. You can see that behavioral comparisons peaked at around age 8 or 9, psychological statements peaked at about age 14, and organizing relationships did not appear at all until age 10 and were still increasing at age 16.

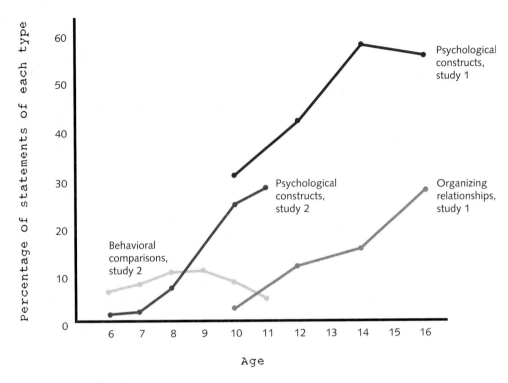

FIGURE 12.2 Barenboim's two studies of children's descriptions of others show clear shifts toward greater emphasis on psychological constructs. Study 1 involved children ages 10 to 16, study 2 involved children ages 6 through 11. (*Sources:* study 1: Barenboim, 1977, Table 1 p. 1471; study 2: Barenboim, 1981, Figure 1, p. 134.)

I am sure that many of you have noticed the strong resemblance between this series of changes and the development of children's self-descriptions that I outlined in Chapter 10 (Figure 10.2, p. 283). This parallel illustrates Flavell's basic point, that it is the same head doing the thinking about self and about others.

Thinking About Relationships

When we look at children's ideas about relationships, very much the same pattern holds, no matter what type of relationship we study—the relationship with parents, with other authority figures, with groups, or with friends. I'm going to focus on children's understanding of friendship because we can draw on a richer vein of research in this area than in any other.

In the last chapter I described the developmental changes in the actual relationships children have with their friends—what they do together, how enduring and intimate they are. Here I want to talk about how the child *understands* the nature of friendship itself.

Among preschool children, friendships seem to be understood mostly in terms of physical characteristics. If you ask a young child how people make friends, the answer is usually that they "play together" or spend time physically near each other (Damon, 1977; 1983; Selman, 1980). Friendship is understood to involve sharing toys or giving goods to one another.

Selman's research and extensive studies by Thomas Berndt (1983; 1986) show that in elementary school this early view of friendship gives way to one in which the key concept seems to be *reciprocal trust*. Friends are now people who help and trust one another. Since this is also the age at which children's understanding of others becomes less external, more psychological, we shouldn't be surprised that friends are now seen as special people, with particular desired qualities other than mere proximity. In particular, generosity and helpfulness become part of the definition of friendship for many children. Children this age also understand friendship to have a temporal dimension: Friends are people with whom one has a history of connection and interaction, rather than someone one has just met or played with once.

At adolescence Berndt finds a further change, as friends come to be seen as people who *understand* one another, who share their innermost thoughts or feelings. Friendships are also seen as more exclusive, more long term. Friends should comfort one another, be with one another, forgive one another. Friendships at this stage are often intense relationships, with many hours spent on the phone or talking in person, sharing every detail, every thought, every activity.

Damon suggests that still another change takes place for some young people in late adolescence or early adulthood, which is parallel to the shift to more qualified statements Barenboim found in his studies of children's descriptions of others. At this point young people understand that even very close friendships cannot fill every need and that friendships are not static: They change, grow, or dissolve, as each member of the pair changes. A really good friendship, then, is one that *adapts* to these changes. At this age, young people say things about friendship like "trust is the ability to let go as well as to hang on" (Selman, 1980, p. 141).

Let me again make these generalizations concrete with some actual research findings, this time from a cross-sectional study by Brian Bigelow and John La Gaipa (1975). They asked several hundred children in Canada to write an essay about how their expectations of best friends differed from their expectations of other acquaintances. The answers were scored along many dimensions, three of which I have shown in Figure 12.3. You can see that references to "demographic similarity" (e.g., "We live in the same neighborhood") were highest among fourth graders, while mentions of loyalty and commitment were highest among seventh graders. References to intimacy potential (e.g., "I can tell her things about myself I can't tell anyone else") did not appear at all until the seventh grade, and then increased further in eighth grade.

How would you define a friend or friendship? What do you expect from a friend that you do not expect from an acquaintance? What do you *give* to a friend that you would not give to an acquaintance? Think about it for a minute.

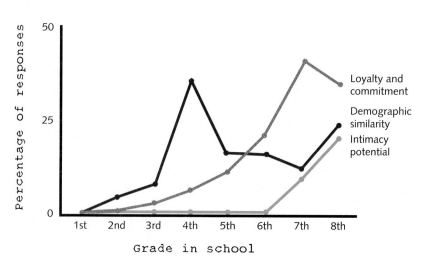

FIGURE 12.3 Some of the changes in children's ideas about friendship are clear from these findings from Bigelow and La Gaipa's study. (*Source:* Bigelow & La Gaipa, 1975, from Table 1, p. 858.)

Taking together all of what I have told you so far, it seems clear that the patterns of developmental change in children's understanding of themselves, of others, and of relationships are strikingly similar, shifting in all the ways I listed at the beginning of the chapter: from outer to inner characteristics, from observation to inference, from definite to qualified, from an egocentric to a general view.

Thinking About What People Ought to Do

A somewhat different facet of the child's emerging social understanding is her judgment or explanation of other people's actions. The aspect of this that has most intrigued developmental psychologists is the child's judgment of the "morality" of actions. How does a child decide what is good or bad, right or wrong in other people's behavior, and in his own behavior? You make these kinds of judgments often in your everyday life. Should you complain about the store clerk who seems to have given you back too little change? Should you turn in a classmate you see cheating on an exam? What do you think about someone who lies in a job interview? Does your judgment change if you know that the person desperately needs the job to support his handicapped child?

Kohlberg's Stages of Moral Development

Piaget was the first to offer a description of the development of moral reasoning (1932), but Lawrence Kohlberg's work has had the most powerful impact (e.g., Colby et al., 1983; Kohlberg, 1976; Kohlberg, 1981). Building on and revising Piaget's ideas, Kohlberg pioneered the practice of assessing moral reasoning by presenting a subject with a series of hypothetical dilemmas in story form, each of which highlighted a specific moral issue, such as the value of human life. One of the most famous is the dilemma of Heinz:

> In Europe, a woman was near death from a special kind of cancer. There was one drug that the doctors thought might save her. It was a form of radium that a druggist in the same town had recently discovered. The drug was expensive to make, but the druggist was charging ten times what the drug cost him to make. He paid $200 for the radium and charged $2000 for a small dose of the drug. The sick woman's husband, Heinz, went to everyone he knew to borrow the money, but he could only get together about $1000 which is half of what it cost. He told the druggist that his wife was dying, and asked him to sell it cheaper or let him pay later. But the druggist said, "No, I discovered the drug and I'm going to make money from it." So Heinz got desperate and broke into the man's store to steal the drug for his wife. (Kohlberg & Elfenbein, 1975, p. 621)

After hearing this story, the child or young person is asked a series of questions, such as whether Heinz should have stolen the drug. What if Heinz didn't love his wife? Would that change anything? What if the person dying was a stranger? Should Heinz steal the drug anyway?

On the basis of answers to dilemmas like this one, Kohlberg concluded that there were three main levels of moral reasoning, with two stages within each level, summarized briefly in Table 12.2.

At level I, **preconventional morality,** the child's judgments are based on sources of authority who are close by and physically superior to himself—usually the parents. Just as

Table 12.2
Kohlberg's Stages of Moral Development

Level I: Preconventional Morality

Stage 1:
Punishment and obedience orientation

The child decides what is wrong on the basis of what is punished. Obedience is valued for its own sake, but the child obeys because the adults have superior power.

Stage 2:
Individualism, instrumental purpose, and exchange

The child follows rules when it is in his immediate interest. What is good is what brings pleasant results.

Level II: Conventional Morality

Stage 3:
Mutual interpersonal expectations, relationships, and interpersonal conformity

Moral actions are those that live up to the expectations of the family or other significant group. "Being good" becomes important for its own sake.

Stage 4:
Social system and conscience (law and order)

Moral actions are those so defined by larger social groups or the society as a whole. One should fulfill duties one has agreed to and uphold laws except in extreme cases.

Level III: Principled or Postconventional Morality

Stage 5:
Social contract or utility and individual rights

Acting so as to achieve the "greatest good for the greatest number." The teenager or adult is aware that most values are relative and laws are changeable, although rules should be upheld in order to preserve the social order. Still, there are some basic nonrelative values, such as the importance of each person's life and liberty.

Stage 6:
Universal ethical principles

The adult develops and follows self-chosen ethical principles in determining what is right. These ethical principles are part of an articulated, integrated, carefully thought-out and consistently followed system of values and principles.

Sources: After Kohlberg, 1976, and Lickona, 1978.

his descriptions of others at this same stage are largely external, so the standards the child uses to judge rightness or wrongness are external rather than internal. In particular, it is the outcome or consequences of his actions that determine the rightness or wrongness of those actions.

In stage 1 of this level—the *punishment and obedience orientation*—the child relies on the physical consequences of some action to decide if it is right or wrong. If he is punished, the behavior was wrong; if he is not punished, it was right. He is obedient to adults because they are bigger and stronger.

In stage 2—*individualism, instrumental purpose, and exchange*—the child begins to do things that are rewarded and to avoid things that are punished. (For this reason the stage is sometimes called a position of "naive hedonism.") If it feels good or brings pleasant results, it is good. Some beginning of concern for other people is apparent during this phase, but only if that concern can be expressed as something that benefits the child as well. So he can enter into agreements like "If you help me, I'll help you."

As illustration, here are some responses to variations of the Heinz dilemma, drawn from studies of children and teenagers in a number of different cultures, all of which would be rated as stage 2:

> *"He should steal the food for his wife because if she dies he'll have to pay for the funeral, and that costs a lot" (Taiwan).*
>
> *He should steal the drug because "he should protect the life of his wife so he doesn't have to stay alone in life" (Puerto Rico).*
>
> *[Suppose it wasn't his wife who was starving but his best friend. Should he steal the food for his friend?] "Yes, because one day when he is hungry his friend would help" (Turkey). (All quotes from Snarey, 1985, p. 221)*

At the next major level, **conventional morality,** the young person shifts from judgments based on external consequences and personal gain to judgments based on rules or norms of a group to which the individual belongs, whether that group is the family, the peer group, a church, or the nation. What the chosen reference group defines as right or good *is* right or good in the child's view, and the child internalizes these norms to a considerable extent.

Stage 3 (the first stage of level II) is the stage of *mutual interpersonal expectations, relationships, and interpersonal conformity* (sometimes also called the *good boy/nice girl* stage). Children at this stage believe that good behavior is what pleases other people. They value trust, loyalty, respect, gratitude, and maintenance of mutual relationships. Andy, a boy Kohlberg interviewed who was at stage 3, said:

> *I try to do things for my parents, they've always done things for you. I try to do everything my mother says, I try to please her. Like she wants me to be a doctor and I want to, too, and she's helping me get up there. (Kohlberg, 1964, p. 401)*

Another mark of this third stage is that the child begins to make judgments based on intentions as well as on outward behavior. If someone "means well" or "didn't mean to do it," their wrongdoing is seen as less serious than if they did it "on purpose."

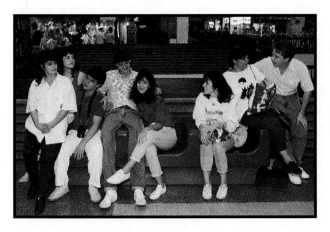

By this age, the majority of teenagers—like this group of Venezuelan adolescents—are using stage 3 moral reasoning: What is good is what family or peers define as good and right. Do you think that the level of moral reasoning a teenager shows has any connection to his or her conformity to peers at this same age?

Stage 4, the second stage of the conventional level, shows the child turning to larger social groups for her norms. Kohlberg labeled this the stage of *social system and conscience.* It is also sometimes called the *law-and-order orientation.* People reasoning at this stage focus on doing their duty, respecting authority, following rules and laws. The emphasis is less on what is pleasing to particular people (as in stage 3) and more on adhering to a complex set of regulations. The regulations themselves are not questioned.

The transition to level III, **principled morality** (also called *postconventional morality*), is marked by several changes, the most important of which is a shift in the source of authority. At level I, children see authority as totally outside themselves; at level II, the judgments or rules of external authority are internalized, but they are not questioned or analyzed; at level III, a new kind of personal authority emerges in which individual choices are made, with individual judgments based on self-chosen principles.

In stage 5 at this level—called the *social contract* orientation by Kohlberg—we see the beginning of such self-chosen principles. Rules, laws, and regulations are still seen as important because they ensure fairness. But people operating at this level also see times when the rules, laws, and regulations need to be ignored or changed. Our American system of government is based on moral reasoning of this kind, since we have provisions for changing laws and for allowing personal protests against a given law, such as during the civil rights protests of the 1960s, the Vietnam War protests of the 1960s and 1970s, or the protests against apartheid in the 1980s.

In his original writing about moral development, Kohlberg also included a sixth stage, the *universal ethical principles* orientation. People who reason in this way assume personal responsibility for their own actions on the basis of fundamental and universal principles, such as justice and basic respect for persons. Kohlberg later waffled a good bit on whether such a stage was the logical and necessary end point of the sequence and on whether people reasoning at such a level actually existed (Kohlberg, 1978; Kohlberg, 1984; Kohlberg, Levine, & Hewer, 1983). If they exist at all, it seems likely that such universal ethical principles guide the moral reasoning of only a few very unusual individuals—perhaps those who devote their lives to humanitarian causes, such as Mother Teresa or Gandhi.

In all of this, it is *very* important to understand that what defines the stage or level of a person's moral judgment is not the specific moral choice but the *form of reasoning* used to justify that choice. For example, either choice, that Heinz should steal the drug or that he should not, could be justified with logic at any given stage. I've already given you some examples of a stage 2 justification for Heinz's stealing the drug; here's a stage 5 justification of the same choice, drawn from a study in India:

> [*What if Heinz was stealing to save the life of his pet animal instead of his wife?*] *If Heinz saves an animal's life his action will be commendable. The right use of the drug is to administer it to the needy. There is some difference, of course—human life is more evolved and hence of greater importance in the scheme of nature—but an animal's life is not altogether bereft of importance. . . . (Snarey, 1985, p. 223, drawn originally from Vasudev, 1983, p. 7)*

If you compare this answer to the ones I quoted before, you can clearly see the difference in the form of reasoning used, even though the action being justified is precisely the same.

Imagine a society in which everyone handled moral issues at Kohlberg's stage 3. Now think about one in which everyone operated at stage 5. How would these two societies be likely to differ?

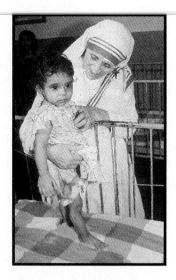

Kohlberg thought that there were at least a few people, perhaps like Mother Teresa, whose moral reasoning was based on universal ethical principles.

Kohlberg argued that this sequence of reasoning is both universal and hierarchically organized, just as Piaget thought his proposed stages of cognitive development were universal and hierarchical. That is, each stage follows and grows from the preceding one and has some internal consistency. Individuals should not move "down" the sequence, but only "upward" along the stages, if they move at all. Kohlberg did *not* suggest that all individuals eventually progress through all six stages, or even that each stage is tied to specific ages. But he insisted that the order is invariant and universal. Let me take a critical look at these claims.

Age and Moral Reasoning. Kohlberg's own findings, confirmed by many other researchers (e.g., Walker, de Vries, & Trevethan, 1987), show that preconventional reasoning (stages 1 and 2) is dominant in elementary school and that stage 2 reasoning is still evident among many early adolescents. Conventional reasoning (stages 3 and 4) emerges as important in middle adolescence and remains the most common form of moral reasoning in adulthood. Postconventional reasoning (stages 5 and 6) is relatively rare, even in adulthood. For example, in one study of men in their forties and fifties, only 13 percent were rated as using stage 5 moral reasoning (Gibson, 1990).

Let me give you two examples illustrating these overall age trends. The first, shown in Figure 12.4, comes from Kohlberg's own longitudinal study of 58 boys, first interviewed when they were 10 and now followed for more than 20 years (Colby et al., 1983). Table 12.3 shows cross-sectional data from a study by Lawrence Walker and his colleagues (Walker et al., 1987). They studied 10 boys and 10 girls at each of four ages and interviewed the parents of each child as well. Note that Walker scored each response on a nine-point scale rather than just scoring the five main stages. This system, which has become quite common, allows for the fact that many people's reasoning falls between two specific stages.

The results of these two studies are not identical, but they point to remarkably similar conclusions about the order of emergence of the various stages and about the approximate ages at which they predominate. In both studies, stage 2 reasoning dominates at age 10, and stage 3 reasoning is most common at about age 16.

Sequence of Stages. The evidence also seems fairly strong that the stages follow one another in the sequence Kohlberg proposed. There have been a number of long-term longitudinal studies of teenagers and young adults in the United States (Colby et al., 1983),

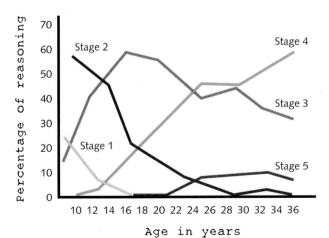

FIGURE 12.4 These findings are from Colby and Kohlberg's long-term longitudinal study of a group of boys who were asked about Kohlberg's moral dilemmas every few years from age 10 through early adulthood. Note that postconventional or principled reasoning was quite uncommon, even in adulthood. (*Source:* Colby et al., 1983, Figure 1, p. 46. Copyright © The Society for Research in Child Development.)

Table 12.3
Percentage of Children and Parents Who Show Moral Reasoning at Each of Kohlberg's Stages

| Age | Stage | | | | | | | | |
---	1	1–2	2	2–3	3	3–4	4	4–5	5
6 (first grade)	10	70	15	5	—	—	—	—	—
9 (fourth grade)	—	25	40	35	—	—	—	—	—
12 (seventh grade)	—	—	15	60	25	—	—	—	—
15 (tenth grade)	—	—	—	40	55	5	—	—	—
Parents	—	—	—	1	15	70	11	3	—

Source: Walker, de Vries, & Trevethan, 1987, Table 1, p. 849.

in Israel (Snarey, Reimer, & Kohlberg, 1985), and in Turkey (Nisan & Kohlberg, 1982). In each, the changes in subjects' reasoning nearly always occurred in the hypothesized order. Subjects did not skip stages, and only about 5 to 7 percent of the time was there any indication of regression (movement down the sequence rather than up). Similarly, when Walker retested the subjects in his study two years later, he found only 6 percent had moved down, mostly only half a stage, while 22 percent had moved up and none had skipped a stage (Walker, 1989). Such a rate of regression is about what you would expect to find, given the fact that the measurements of stage reasoning are not perfect. On the whole, I agree with James Rest (1983) that the evidence is "fairly compelling" that moral judgment changes over time in the sequence Kohlberg describes.

Universality. But is this sequence of stages only a phenomenon of Western culture? Or has Kohlberg uncovered a genuinely universal process? Thus far, variations of Kohlberg's dilemmas have been presented to children or adults in 27 different countries or subcultures, including both Western and non-Western, industrialized and nonindustrialized (Snarey, 1985).

John Snarey, who has reviewed and analyzed these many studies, notes several things in support of Kohlberg's position: (1) In studies of children, an increase in stage of reasoning with age is found consistently; (2) the few longitudinal studies report "strikingly similar findings" (1985, p. 215), with subjects moving upward in the stage sequence with few reversals; (3) cultures differ in the highest level of reasoning observed. In complex urban societies (both Western and non-Western), stage 5 is typically the highest stage observed, while in those cultures Snarey calls "folk" societies, stage 4 is typically the highest. Collectively, this evidence seems to provide quite strong support for the universality of Kohlberg's stage sequence.

Moral Development: A Critique. Kohlberg's theory about the development of moral reasoning has been one of the most provocative theories in all of developmental psychology. There have been more than 1000 studies exploring or testing aspects of the theory, and several competing theories have been proposed. The remarkable thing is how well the theory has stood the test of this barrage of research and commentary. There does appear to be a clear set of stages in the development of moral reasoning, and these stages seem to be universal.

Still, the theory has not emerged unscathed. Some psychologists are less impressed than Snarey with the data on universality (Shweder, Mahapatra, & Miller, 1987). Also troubling is the fact that so few teenagers or adults seem to reason at the postconventional level (stages 5 and 6). Shweder points out that the effective range of variation is really only from stage 2 to stage 4, which is not nearly so interesting or impressive as is the full range of stages.

But by far the most vocal critics have been those who have pointed out that Kohlberg is really not talking about all aspects of "moral reasoning." Instead, as Kohlberg himself acknowledged in his later writings (Kohlberg et al., 1983), he is talking about the development of reasoning about *justice and fairness*. But what about moral reasoning about doing good, or reasoning based on some other ethic than justice, such as an ethic resting on concern for others or for relationships? Let me take a quick look at two such alternative views.

Eisenberg's Model of Prosocial Reasoning

Most of the moral dilemmas Kohlberg posed for his subjects deal with wrongdoing—with stealing, punishment, disobeying laws. Few tell us anything about the kind of reasoning children use in justifying *prosocial behavior*. I mentioned in Chapter 11 that altruistic behavior is visible in children as young as 2 and 3; but how do children explain and justify such behavior?

Nancy Eisenberg and her colleagues (Eisenberg, 1986; Eisenberg et al., 1987) have explored such questions by proposing dilemmas to children in which self-interest is set against the possibility of helping another person. One story involves a child walking to a friend's birthday party. On the way, he comes upon another child who has fallen and hurt himself. If the party-bound child stops to help, he will probably miss the cake and ice cream. What should he do?

In response to dilemmas like this, preschool children most often use what Eisenberg calls *hedonistic* reasoning in which the child is concerned with self-oriented consequences rather than moral considerations. Children this age say things like "I'd help because she'd help me the next time," or "I wouldn't help because I'd miss the party." This approach gradually shifts to one Eisenberg calls *needs-oriented* reasoning, in which the child expresses concern directly for the other person's need, even if the other's need conflicts with the child's own wishes or desires. Children operating on this basis say things like "She'd feel better if I helped." At this stage, children do not express their choices in terms of general principles or indicate any reflectiveness about generalized values; they simply respond to the other's needs.

Still later, typically in adolescence, children say they will do good things because it is expected of them, a pattern highly similar to Kohlberg's stage 3 reasoning, and in late adolescence, some young people give evidence that they have developed clear, internalized values that guide their prosocial behavior: "I'd feel a responsibility to help because of my values," or "If everyone helped, society would be a lot better."

Figure 12.5 gives some sample data from Eisenberg's longitudinal study of a small group of American children that illustrate the shift from hedonistic to needs-oriented reasoning. By early adolescence, hedonistic reasoning has virtually disappeared (the lowest possible score on this scale is 4), while needs-oriented reasoning has become the dominant form. Eisenberg reports that similar patterns have been found among children in

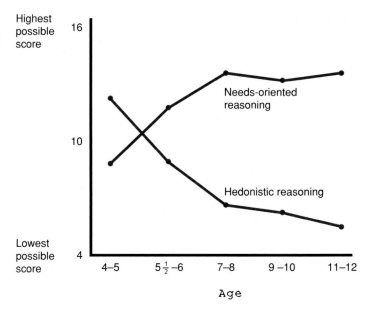

FIGURE 12.5 Every two years Eisenberg asked the same group of children what a person should do when confronted with each of a series of dilemmas about doing good, such as helping someone who is hurt. She then analyzed their form of reasoning, using a measure with a minimum score of 4 and a maximum of 16. (*Source:* Eisenberg et al., 1987, from Table 1, p. 715.)

West Germany, Poland, and Italy but that kibbutz-reared Israeli elementary school children show little needs-oriented reasoning (Eisenberg, 1986). Instead, this particular group of Israeli children is more likely to reason on the basis of the humanness of recipients and on internalized values and norms, a pattern consistent with the strong emphasis on egalitarianism and communal values in the kibbutzim. These findings point to perhaps a larger role of culture in children's prosocial reasoning than in reasoning about justice, although that is still a highly tentative conclusion.

There are obviously strong parallels between the sequences of changes in prosocial reasoning Eisenberg has described and Kohlberg's levels and stages of moral reasoning. Children seem to move from a self-centered orientation (what feels good to me is right) to a stance in which social approval guides reasoning about justice and about doing good. What is right is what other people define as right; one should do good things because others will approve of you if you do. Much later, some young people seem to develop internalized, individualized norms to guide both kinds of reasoning.

Despite these obvious parallels, though, researchers have typically found that children's reasoning about prosocial dilemmas such as Eisenberg's and their reasoning about Kohlberg's justice or fairness dilemmas are only moderately correlated. The sequences of steps may be similar, but as was true of so many of the developments I talked about in Chapter 7, children's reasoning in one arena doesn't necessarily generalize to a related area.

Eisenberg's research, as well as the work of others in the same vein, helps to broaden Kohlberg's original conception, without changing the fundamental arguments. In contrast, Carol Gilligan has questioned some of the basic tenets of Kohlberg's model.

Gilligan's Ethic of Caring

Carol Gilligan (1982; Gilligan & Wiggins, 1987) is fundamentally dissatisfied with Kohlberg's focus on justice and fairness as the defining features of moral reasoning. Gilligan argues that there are at least two distinct "moral orientations": justice and care. Each has its own central injunction: not to treat others unfairly (justice) and not to turn away from

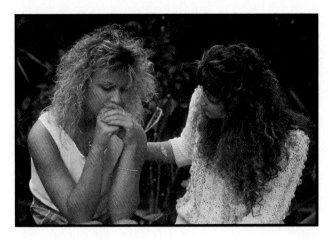

Gilligan argues that these young women are much more likely to be using an "ethic of caring" than an "ethic of justice" as a basis for their moral judgments, while the reverse is true among boys and men. Such a difference *may* exist among adults, but research on children and adolescents shows no such pattern.

someone in need (caring). Boys and girls learn both of these injunctions, but Gilligan has hypothesized that girls are more likely to operate from an orientation of caring or connection, while boys are more likely to operate from an orientation of justice or fairness. Because of these differences, she argues, they tend to perceive moral dilemmas quite differently.

Given the emerging evidence on sex differences in styles of interaction and in friendship patterns, which I talked about in the last chapter, Gilligan's hypothesis makes some sense. Perhaps girls, focused more on intimacy in their relationships, judge moral dilemmas by different criteria. But in fact, research on moral dilemmas has not shown that boys are more likely to use justice reasoning or that girls more often use care reasoning. Several studies of adults do show such a pattern (Lyons, 1983), but studies of children, adolescents, or college students generally have not (Jadack et al., 1995; Smetana, Killen, & Turiel, 1991; Walker et al., 1987).

For example, Lawrence Walker (Walker et al., 1987) scored children's answers to moral dilemmas using both Kohlberg's fairness scheme and Gilligan's criteria for a care orientation. He found no sex difference for either hypothetical dilemmas like the Heinz dilemma or the real-life dilemmas suggested by the children themselves. Only among adults did Walker find a difference, in the direction that Gilligan would expect.

Gilligan's arguments have often been quoted in the popular press as if they were already proven, when in fact the empirical base is really quite weak. Gilligan herself has done no systematic studies of children's (or adults') care reasoning. Yet despite these weaknesses, I am not ready to discard all her underlying points, primarily because the questions she is asking seem to me to fit so well with the newer research on sex differences in styles of relationship. The fact that we typically find no differences between boys and girls in their tendencies to use care versus justice orientations does not mean that there are no differences in the assumptions males and females bring to relationships or to moral judgments. This seems to me to be clearly an area in which we need to learn a great deal more.

Suppose Gilligan is right and adult women typically reason with an ethic of care while men reason with an ethic of justice. What do you think would be the implications of such a difference—for male/female relationships, for men and women as political leaders, or in other ways?

Social Cognition and Behavior

In Chapter 11, I talked about children's social behavior; in this chapter I have been talking about children's thinking about relationships. What is the connection between the two? Can we predict a child's behavior, such as his moral choices, his generous behavior, or the quality of his relationships, from knowing the stage or level of his social cognition? Yes and no. Knowing the form or level of a child's reasoning cannot tell us *precisely* what he will do in a real-life situation. But there are nevertheless some important links between thinking and behavior.

Empathetic Understanding, Prosocial Reasoning, and Behavior.   One possible link is the one between empathy and prosocial behavior. The findings are not completely consistent, but Eisenberg's research shows that more empathetic or other-oriented children are somewhat more likely to share or help others in real situations and less likely to show socially disruptive or highly aggressive behavior (Eisenberg & Mussen, 1989).

For example, George Bear and Gail Rys (1994) gave four of Eisenberg's dilemmas to a group of second- and third-grade students drawn from 17 different classrooms. The teacher in each classroom also rated each child's level of disruptive and aggressive behavior (collectively referred to as "acting out") as well as each child's positive social skills, including being friendly toward peers, having friends, being able to cope with failure, being comfortable as a leader, and so on. Bear and Rys found that children who used predominantly hedonistic reasoning were rated by their teachers as lower in social competence than were those who used mostly needs-oriented (empathetic) or higher levels of social reasoning. Teachers also described the hedonistic boys, but not the hedonistic girls, as more likely to act out, a pattern you can see in Figure 12.6. The hedonistic boys also had fewer friends and were more likely to be rejected by their peers. Bear and Rys argue that higher levels of prosocial moral reasoning help to curtail a child's acting-out behavior, keeping it at a socially acceptable level and thus preventing peer rejection.

Similarly, Eisenberg has found that certain types of prosocial reasoning are correlated with a child's altruistic behavior. For instance, in a group of 10-year-olds, she found that hedonistic reasoning was negatively correlated with a measure of the child's willingness to donate to UNICEF the nickels they earned for participating in the study (Eisenberg et al., 1987).

Friendship Understanding and Friendship Behavior.   Equivalent links appear in studies of reasoning about friendships. As a general rule, children with more mature reasoning about friendships are less likely to be aggressive with their peers and more likely to show sharing or other helpful behavior toward their friends in actual interactions.

In one study, Lawrence Kurdek and Donna Krile (1982) found that among children in the third through the eighth grades, those with higher scores on a measure of under-

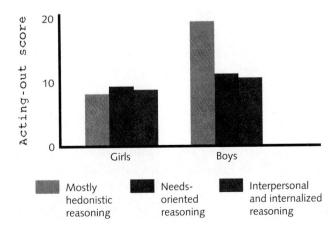

FIGURE 12.6 Bear and Rys find that among these second and third graders, boys with primarily hedonistic moral reasoning are more likely to act out in the classroom. (*Source:* Bear & Rys, 1994, Table 2, p. 636.)

standing of individuals and friendships were more likely to be involved in mutual friend-ships than were children with lower scores. Similarly, Selman (1980) compared children's scores on a measure of social reasoning with teachers' ratings of the children's social strengths and weaknesses. He found that children with more mature reasoning were more likely to be described by their teachers as showing higher levels of helpful or other proso-cial behaviors.

An intriguing exception to this pattern, however, is the finding I reported in the last chapter, that in friendships between boys, competition, not sharing or helpfulness, is of-ten the dominant pattern. Furthermore, Berndt finds that among boys, the level of com-petition or cooperation is unrelated to their level of social cognitive reasoning about either friendship or the justification for helpfulness (1983). Thus, while we usually find a correlation between the maturity of a child's social reasoning and his friend-making skills, more mature reasoning does not invariably increase the level of helpfulness or coopera-tion in actual friendship pairs among males. Once again, then, we have evidence that the "relationship rules" are different for boys than for girls, a pattern that I think is both fasci-nating and important.

Moral Judgment and Behavior. Kohlberg's theory has sometimes been criticized on the grounds that children's or adults' moral behavior does not always match their reason-ing. But Kohlberg never said that there should be a one-to-one correspondence between the two. Reasoning at stage 4 (conventional reasoning) does not mean that you will never cheat or always be kind to your mother. Still, the form of reasoning a young person typi-cally applies to moral problems should have at least *some* connection with real-life choices or behavior.

One such connection proposed by Kohlberg is that the higher the level of reasoning a young person shows, the stronger the link to behavior ought to become. Thus, young people reasoning at stage 4 or stage 5 should be more likely to follow their own rules or reasoning than should children reasoning at lower levels.

For example, Kohlberg and Candee (1984) studied students involved in the early "Free Speech" movement at Berkeley in the late 1960s (a precursor to the Vietnam War protests). They interviewed and tested the moral judgment levels of a group that had par-ticipated at a sit-in in the university administration building, plus a group randomly cho-sen from the campus population. Of those who thought it was morally right to sit in, nearly three-quarters reasoning at stages 4 or 5 actually did sit in, compared to only about

Do you think that a person's stage or level of moral reasoning has any impact on political behavior, such as whether a person votes or political party affiliations? Can you generate a hypothesis about such a link and figure out how you might test it?

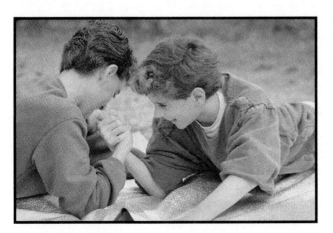

Why do you think it is that among boys, competition is such a strong feature of friendship interactions, no matter what level of reasoning the boys may otherwise have about relationships or morality?

a quarter of those reasoning at stage 3. Thus, the higher the stage of reasoning, the more consistent the behavior was with the reasoning.

In other research, Kohlberg and others approached the question simply by asking whether a link exists between stage of moral reasoning and the probability of making some "moral choice," such as not cheating. In one study, Kohlberg (1975) found that only 15 percent of students reasoning at the principled level (stage 5) cheated when they were given an opportunity, while 55 percent of conventional-level and 70 percent of pre-conventional students cheated.

A similar argument lies behind studies in which the moral reasoning of delinquents, or highly aggressive younger children, is compared to that of nondelinquent peers. The repeated finding is that delinquents (male or female) have lower levels of moral reasoning than do nondelinquents, even when the two groups are carefully matched for levels of education, social class, and IQ (Smetana, 1990). In one recent study, for example, Virginia Gregg and her colleagues (1994) found that only 20 percent of a group of incarcerated male and female delinquents were reasoning at stage 3 or higher, while 59 percent of a carefully matched comparison group of nondelinquents were reasoning at this level. Like younger children who act out more in school, delinquents are most likely to use highly hedonistic reasoning, scored at Kohlberg's stage 2 (Richards et al., 1992).

Yet despite this abundant evidence for a link between moral reasoning and behavior, no one has found the correspondence to be perfect. After all, in Kohlberg's studies, 15 percent of the principled moral reasoners did cheat, and a quarter of stage 4 and stage 5 reasoners who thought it morally right to participate in a sit-in did not do so. As Kohlberg says, "One can reason in terms of principles and not live up to those principles" (1975, p. 672).

What else besides level of reasoning might matter? We don't have all the answers to that question yet, but some influences are clear. First, simple habits are involved. Every day each of us faces small moral situations that we have learned to handle in a completely automatic way. Sometimes these automatic choices may be at a lower level of reasoning than we would use if we sat down and thought about it. For example, I may make the same donation to a particular charity every year without stopping to consider whether I could now afford more or whether that particular charity is really the place where my money could best be used.

Second, in any given situation, even though you might think it morally right to take some action, you may not see that action as morally *necessary* or obligatory. I might be able to make a good argument for the moral acceptability of a sit-in protest but still not see it as my *own* duty or responsibility to participate.

Third, the cost to the person of doing something helpful (or refraining from doing something morally "wrong," like cheating) may be an important factor. If helping someone else has little cost in time, money, or effort, then most children and adults will help, regardless of their overall level of social cognitive reasoning. But when there is some cost—as was the case for the children in Eisenberg's study who were asked if they wanted to donate some of the nickels they earned to help other children—we find a more consistent correlation between level of reasoning and behavior. This suggests the more general principle that moral reasoning becomes a factor in moral behavior only when something about the situation heightens the sense of moral conflict, such as when a cost is involved or when the individual feels personally responsible.

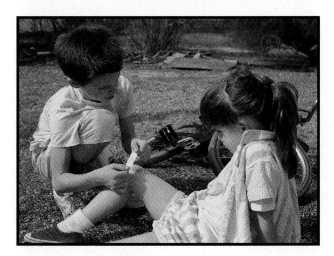

Most children and adults will readily show helpful actions like this if little personal cost is attached. But if the cost of helping goes up—as when you're in a hurry to get somewhere else—then those with higher levels of moral reasoning are more likely to help.

Finally, competing motives or ethics are often at work as well, such as the pressure of a peer group or motives for self-protection or self-reward. Gerson and Damon found this very clearly in a study in which they asked groups of four children to divide up 10 candy bars (1978). The candy was a reward for work the children had done on a project, and some of the group members had worked harder than others. When asked separately about how the candy bars ought to be divided, children usually argued for various kinds of fair arrangements, such as a model in which the child who worked the hardest should get the most. But when faced with the actual distribution of the candy bars, some children gave themselves the most; others went along with a group consensus and divided the candy equally. We might expect that in early adolescence, when the impact of the peer group is particularly strong, this group effect on moral actions might be especially strong too.

Thus, moral *behavior* results from a complex of influences, of which the level of moral reasoning is only one element. Our knowledge about these links is improving, but we badly need to know more, both about group pressure and about all the other factors that lead each of us to behave in ways that are less thoughtful, considerate, or fair than we "know how" to do. Kohlberg's own fascination with this set of questions, and with the question of how one raises a person's level of moral reasoning, led him and his colleagues to a series of bold attempts to apply the theory to schooling. I've explored some of this research in the *Real World* box on page 360.

Social Cognition and General Cognitive Development

Before I leave this subject, I need to explore one other set of linkages, namely, the potential connection between the sequences of development of social cognition, such as Kohlberg's stages of moral reasoning, and the broader sequences of cognitive development I described in Chapter 7. Earlier in this chapter I suggested several key dimensions that seem to characterize both sets of changes, such as a shift in focus from outer to inner characteristics. But I need to look at those possible connections more systematically.

The Real World

Application of Kohlberg's Theory to Education

A lot of what I have said about Kohlberg's theory may seem pretty abstract to you. In Kohlberg's own view, though, there were many potential practical implications for education. The question that interested him was whether children or young people can be taught higher stages of moral reasoning, and if so, whether such a change in moral reasoning would change their behavior in school.

We know from early research by Elliot Turiel (1966) that, at least under some conditions, exposing young people to moral arguments one step above their own level of reasoning can lead to an increase in their level of moral judgment. Young people who attend college also continue to show increases in moral stage scores, while those who quit school after high school typically show no further increase (Rest & Thoma, 1985). Because arguments about moral and philosophical issues in class and over coffee (or a few beers) in the wee small hours of the night are one of the hallmarks of the college experience for many young people, perhaps it is the discussion—the exposure to other people's ideas, other people's logic—that makes a difference.

If that's true, what would happen if high school students were given systematic opportunities to explore moral dilemmas? Would that change them too? Apparently it can.

One educational application has involved the creation of special discussion classes in which moral dilemmas similar to those Kohlberg devised are presented and argued. In the process, the teacher attempts to model higher levels of reasoning. Other programs are broader based, involving not just discussion but also cross-age teaching (to encourage nurturance and caring), empathy training, cooperation games, volunteer service work, and the like. The dozens of studies on the effectiveness of programs of this kind show that on average, the programs succeed in shifting young people's moral reasoning upward about a half a stage (Schaefli, Rest, & Thoma, 1985). The largest effects are generally found in programs focusing exclusively on discussions of moral dilemmas, but broader-based programs work too. Courses lasting longer than 3 or 4 weeks seem to work better than very short programs, and the effects are generally larger with older students—college students and even post-college-age adults. Among high school students, we see some impact, but it is not as large.

An even broader-based educational application, designed to change students' moral behavior as much as their moral reasoning, has been the development of the so-called *just community*. These experimental schools, typically set up as a "school within a school," operate as a kind of laboratory for moral education (Higgins, 1991; Kohlberg & Higgins, 1987).

Kohlberg insisted that the crucial feature of these just communities must be complete democracy: Each teacher and student has one vote, and community issues and problems have to be discussed in open forum. Rules are typically created and discussed at weekly community-wide meetings. In this way, students become *responsible* for the rules and for one another.

In experimental schools following this model, Kohlberg and his co-workers found that as students' level of Kohlbergian moral reasoning shifted upward, so did their reasoning about responsibility and caring. The link between moral reasoning and moral behavior was strengthened as well. For example, stealing and other petty crime virtually disappeared in one school after the students had repeatedly discussed the problem and arrived—painfully—at a solution that emphasized the fact that stealing damaged the whole community, and thus the whole community had to be responsible. For example, after one stealing episode the group agreed that if the stolen money had not been returned (anonymously) by a specified date, each community member would be assessed 15 cents to make up the victim's loss (Higgins, 1991).

This effect of just communities makes sense when you think about the factors that seem to affect moral behavior. In these schools, two elements were added that would tend to support more moral behavior: a sense of personal responsibility and a group norm of higher moral reasoning and caring.

Among teenagers, the emotional impact of the group pressure may be especially significant, in addition to whatever effect there may be from exposure to more mature arguments. If you find yourself in the minority in some argument about a moral issue, the "social disequilibrium" you feel may help to make you more open to other arguments and thus to change your view. Certainly in experimental schools like those studied by Kohlberg, this added emotional impact is no doubt part of the process (Haan, 1985).

Classes in moral education have not proven to be the "quick fix" that many educators hoped for. The gains in moral reasoning are not huge and may not be reflected in increases in moral behavior in the school unless there is an effort to alter the overall moral atmosphere of the entire school. But these programs do show that there are provocative and helpful applications of some of the abstract developmental theories.

We know that IQ is weakly linked to a child's level of social reasoning (Shantz, 1983). The correlations, which are in the range of +.20 to +.40, mean that children with higher IQs typically show slightly more advanced forms of social reasoning than do children of the same age with lower IQs.

Surprisingly, we know much less about any possible connections between overall cognitive *structure* and social-cognitive reasoning. The most concrete proposal was offered by Kohlberg, who hypothesized that the child first moves to a new level of logical thought, then applies this new kind of logic to relationships as well as objects, and only then applies this thinking to moral problems. More specifically, Kohlberg argued that at least some formal operations and at least some mutual perspective taking in relationships are necessary (but not sufficient) for the emergence of conventional moral reasoning. Full formal operations and still more abstract social understanding may be required for postconventional reasoning.

Why might it be important, either practically or theoretically, whether there is any link between children's approach to moral dilemmas and their level of Piagetian cognitive reasoning?

The research examining such a sequential development is scant, but it supports Kohlberg's hypothesis. Lawrence Walker (1980) found that among a group of fourth to seventh graders he had tested on all three dimensions (concrete and formal operations, social understanding, and moral reasoning), half to two-thirds were reasoning at the same level across the different domains, which makes the whole thing look unexpectedly stage-like. When a child was ahead in one progression, the sequence was always that the child developed logical thinking first, then more advanced social understanding, and then the parallel moral judgments.

This research seems to tell us that there is *some* coherence in a child's or young person's thinking or reasoning about quite different problems. Children who have not yet understood principles of conservation are not likely to understand that another person's behavior may not match his feelings. But once conservation is understood, the child begins to extend this principle to people and to relationships. Similarly, a young person still using concrete operations is unlikely to use postconventional moral reasoning. But the coherence is not automatic. The basic cognitive understanding makes advances in social and moral reasoning *possible* but does not guarantee them. Experience in relationships and with moral dilemmas is necessary too.

The moral of this (if you will excuse the pun) is that just because a young person or adult shows signs of formal operations does *not* necessarily mean that the teenager or young adult will show sensitive, empathetic, and forgiving attitudes toward friends or family. You may find it helpful to bear this in mind in your own relationships.

Summary

1   Many of the principles of developmental change that describe overall cognitive development also describe the changes in social cognition, including a shift in focus from outer to inner characteristics, from observation to inference, from definite to qualified judgment, and from a particular to a general view.

2   Social cognition differs from other aspects of cognition, however, in that the child must learn that people behave with intention, mask feelings, and operate by special socially defined scripts or rules.

3   Children learn to read many basic emotional expressions fairly early, but more complex emotions and emotional blends can be correctly "read" only later.

4   Empathy—being able to match or approximate the emotion of another—is seen in young infants but becomes less egocentric and more subtle through the preschool and elementary school years.

5   Children's descriptions of others shift from a focus on external features to a focus on personality traits and to a more qualified, comparative description at adolescence, paralleling the shifts in children's self-descriptions.

6   Children's thinking about their relationships, such as friendships, shows strongly parallel shifts, moving from definitions of friends as people who share physical space or activities to definitions emphasizing trust, and finally at adolescence to definitions emphasizing intimacy.

7   Children's reasoning about what people ought to do, usually called moral reasoning, has been most fully described by Kohlberg.

8   Kohlberg proposed six stages, divided into three levels. The child moves from preconventional morality, dominated by punishment and "what feels good"; to conventional morality, dominated by group norms or laws; to postconventional (principled) morality, dominated by social contracts and basic ethical principles.

9   Cross-sectional and longitudinal research shows that the stages occur in subjects from all countries studied, that the stages occur in the order listed, and that the modal level for young adults is conventional morality.

10   Alternative models of moral reasoning include Eisenberg's stages of prosocial reasoning (reasoning about why to do something good) and Gilligan's proposal about a parallel ethic of caring.

11   A child's level of social cognition is at least somewhat predictive of the type of social behavior she will show. Children with more hedonistic reasoning are more likely to act out in class and have lower general social competence; children with higher levels of reasoning about friendships have more and more intimate friendships; higher-level moral reasoning is associated with higher likelihood of "moral" behavior and a lower likelihood of delinquency.

12   Other factors that may influence moral behavior include group pressure, whether the individual sees the moral action as necessary or obligatory, the cost of some moral action, and the presence of other motivations, such as self-interest.

13   Social-cognitive development is somewhat related to broader sequences of cognitive development. In particular, conventional levels of moral reasoning seem to require (as a necessary but not sufficient condition) at least beginning formal operations, as well as fairly advanced reasoning about social relationships.

Key Terms

conventional morality (p. 349)

empathy (p. 341)

preconventional morality (p. 347)

principled morality (p. 350)

social cognition (p. 337)

Suggested Readings

Flavell, J. H. (1985). *Cognitive development* (2nd ed.). Englewood Cliffs, NJ: Prentice Hall.

I have recommended this excellent text before. In this case, you may want to look at the very good chapter on social cognition.

Hoffman, M. L. (1988). Moral development. In M. H. Bornstein & M. E. Lamb (Eds.), *Developmental psychology: An advanced textbook* (2nd ed.). Hillsdale, NJ: Erlbaum.

Not all psychologists are as persuaded as I am of the general validity of Kohlberg's stage theory. Hoffman is one of the articulate skeptics, so this paper would give you a look at an alternate view.

Kurtines, W. M., & Gewirtz, J. L. (Eds.). (1991). *Handbook of moral behavior and development.* Hillsdale, NJ: Erlbaum.

This is a massive three-volume work, prepared as a commemoration of the work of Lawrence Kohlberg. Volume 1 deals with theory, volume 2 with research, and volume 3 with application. If this area intrigues you, there is no more complete source.

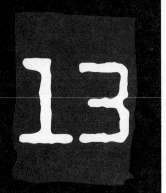

The Ecology of Development: The Child Within the Family System

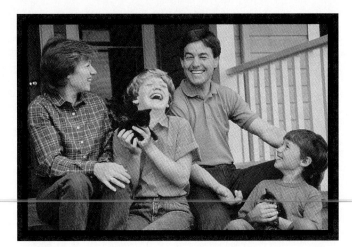

In the process of "downsizing," Sam McKenzie's company laid off several hundred workers. So six months ago Sam, age 35, lost his job as a machinist. Sam's wife, Edith, still has her job as a clerk in the local grocery store, but Sam's unemployment compensation is running out. Money is tight. Sam has tried hard to persuade himself that these things happen to people, but mostly he blames himself and his lack of education. He also thinks it is the man's job to support his family, so he finds it very difficult to have to rely so much on Edith's income. He also finds it very hard to take on pieces of the traditional wife's role, like getting the kids off to school or putting the meat loaf in the oven at 5:00 so that dinner will be ready when his wife comes home from work. Over the months, he has become increasingly gloomy and irritable. He drinks more, has trouble sleeping, and has been arguing more with Edith. The kids have also felt the change—not just in the things they can't buy now, but in the whole atmosphere at home. Sam snaps at them often and most of the time is much stricter with them—though sometimes he seems to pay no attention at all. The kids also notice that he hugs them a lot less. David, who is 13, has started yelling back much more frequently than he used to and has been spending more and more time with his school buddies. Nine-year-old Jennifer has reacted differently: She's become quite withdrawn and depressed, and no longer spends much time with her friends. Both the children have also had a lot more colds and other sicknesses than usual.

What the McKenzie family has experienced is fairly typical of families when the father loses his job or when a single mother loses her job (Crouter & McHale, 1993; McLoyd et al., 1994). It also illustrates two important points—points I made in a preliminary way in Chapter 1 but that may have gotten a bit lost in all the intervening chapters.

First, to understand the child's development we must go beyond the child himself and whatever intrinsic developmental patterns may exist; we must go beyond the dyad of child and mother, or child and father. We need to look at the whole ecology of development—at the pattern of interaction within the family and at the influences of the larger culture on that family. David and Jennifer McKenzie have been affected by Sam's job loss both directly and indirectly, and some of those effects may be very long-lasting. Glen Elder's studies of families in the Great Depression of the 1930s, for example (1974; 1981; 1984), show that some children whose families experienced major financial upheavals in the Depression continued to show the emotional scars well into adult life.

Second, the McKenzies' story illustrates a *system* of influences at work. Sam's job loss was not just an economic event. It affected Sam's attitudes, self-esteem, and behavior, and it reverberated through the entire family system, affecting every other person and every relationship.

In this chapter and the next I want to explore this larger psychological and ecological system in which the child's development occurs. I introduced some of the current thinking about such family and cultural influences in Chapter 1, but let me both refresh your memory and set the stage by delving a bit more deeply into the theoretical issues.

Theoretical Approaches

Thirty years ago, most child development texts and books of advice to parents emphasized the role of the parents in "molding" the child, as if the child were a blob of clay. The parents' task was thought to be to *socialize* the child, to shape the child's behavior so that it fit well into the expectations and rules of society. This clay-molding view has now given way to a far more complex model, most commonly called *systems theory.*

Systems Theory

Systems theorists such as Arnold Sameroff (1995) emphasize that any system—biological, economic, psychological—has certain properties. First and foremost, a system has "wholeness and order," which is another way of saying that the whole is greater than the sum of its parts. The whole consists of both parts and their *relationship* to one another. The usual analogy is that of a melody, which is far more than a set of individual notes. It is the relationship of those notes to each other that creates the melody.

A second key feature of a system is that it is *adaptive,* in precisely the same way that Piaget talks about the child's cognitive system being adaptive. When any part of the system changes, or some new element is added, the system will "assimilate" if it can but will "accommodate" if it must. So systems resist change as much as they can by absorbing new data or new parts into the existing structure, but if that doesn't work—as it often doesn't—then the system changes. For example, when a second child is born into a family, the parents may try to keep to their old routines as much as possible, but the presence of this new individual in the family system will inevitably force accommodations as well. And that will be particularly true if the new baby is temperamentally very different from the first child.

Combining these two features of systems, you can see that any change in any one part of a system will affect every other part. Furthermore, feedback loops occur. In the McKenzie family's experience, for example, Sam's distress led him to be more negative toward Edith, which made their relationship worse. Such a worsening of the marital relationship, along with Sam's own basic distress, led to changes in both parents' behavior toward the children, to which the kids reacted with changes of their own. Once set in motion, the changes in David's and Jennifer's behavior affected Sam and Edith. David became more defiant, to which Sam responded by becoming even more strict and demanding, which affected David's behavior in still more negative ways.

Although virtually all psychologists would now grant the general validity of such a systems approach, figuring out how to conceptualize the various parts of such systems has been no small task. Urie Bronfenbrenner, who originally coined the phrase "ecology of development," has offered one approach.

Bronfenbrenner's Ecological Approach

Bronfenbrenner (1979; 1989), whose work I talked about briefly in Chapter 1, proposes that we think of the ecological system in which the child develops as having a series of layers or concentric circles. The most central circle, which he calls *microsystems,* includes all those settings in which the child has direct personal experience, such as most crucially the family, but also the school, day-care center, or job setting where a teenager works.

The next layer, which Bronfenbrenner calls *exosystems,* includes a whole range of system elements that the child does not experience directly but that influence the child because they affect one of the microsystems, particularly the family. The parents' work and workplace are one such element, as is the parents' network of friends.

Finally, Bronfenbrenner describes a *macrosystem,* which includes the larger cultural or subcultural setting in which both the micro- and exosystems are embedded. The poverty or wealth of the family, the neighborhood in which the family lives, the ethnic identity of the family, and the larger culture in which the entire system exists are all parts of this macrosystem. The child's development is presumably some highly complex product of all these interacting layers.

I am sure it is obvious to you that trying to understand development in this way is *immensely* difficult. It is hard to keep all the elements of the system in mind at once, let alone to try to study all the relevant parts simultaneously. Perhaps frustrated by that difficulty or perhaps because of the long tradition of examining family and cultural effects in more linear ways, psychologists have continued to design research that explores only small pieces of the total system. Thus, much of what we know about family and cultural influences on children is piecemeal rather than systemic. But using Bronfrenbrenner's

We can also think of cultures as systems in this same sense. So when you change one aspect of a given culture, everything is affected. As an experiment, imagine that all violent TV, all highly aggressive games, and all handguns were banned. How might such a change reverberate through the entire cultural system?

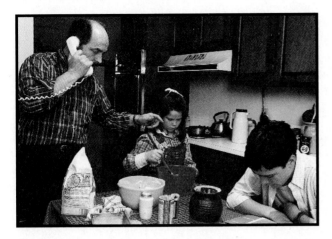

To understand any child's development, we must understand the "ecological niche" in which he is growing up: whether his parents are together or divorced; whether the family is poor or well-off; where he falls in the family sequence; whether his mother works or not; whether his parents find their jobs challenging or boring; whether he is a part of the dominant ethnic group in a culture or a part of a minority group; the quality of the school he attends; and so on and on.

model as a general framework, let us plunge in anyway. I want to begin in this chapter by looking more closely at that most studied and most obviously influential microsystem, the family. I'll also explore some of the exosystem influences on the family. Then in Chapter 14 I'll look at other microsystems affecting the child directly, as well as at the larger cultural influences.

Naturally, I have talked about family influences on the child many times already. You have seen how family interaction patterns affect the child's language or cognitive development, or the security of the child's attachment. But I have not talked about the family as a system, with all its complexities. To understand how that system works and how it might affect the child, we need first to have some way of describing the many possible patterns of interaction that can occur in families. Then we have to try to understand the ways in which other factors inside and outside of the family will affect those patterns—factors such as the parents' personalities, the family structure, and the parents' job experiences.

Dimensions of Family Interaction

Those researchers who have focused most directly on patterns of parent-child interaction have identified several major dimensions on which families differ that seem to be significant for the child. These include the emotional tone of the family, the responsiveness of the parent to the child, the manner in which control is exercised, and the quality and amount of communication.

The Emotional Tone of the Family

The first key element for the child seems to be the relative **warmth versus hostility** of the home. "Warmth" has been difficult to define and measure, but intuitively and theoretically it is clear that it is highly important for the child. A warm parent cares about the child, expresses affection, frequently or regularly puts the child's needs first, shows enthusiasm for the child's activities, and responds sensitively and empathetically to the child's feelings (Maccoby, 1980). On the other end of the continuum are parents who overtly reject their children—saying and expressing with their behavior that they do not love or want the child.

Such differences have profound effects. Psychologists have found that children in warm and loving families are more securely attached in the first two years of life; have

The Real World

The Long-Term Consequences of Hostility and Abuse

The other end of the warmth continuum is, of course, hostility, a pattern of parental behavior associated with a whole range of negative outcomes for children, especially when that hostility takes physical form as abuse. I talked a bit about abuse and some of its causes in a box in Chapter 11. Let me touch here on some of the consequences.

Physically abused children are far more likely than are nonabused children to become aggressive or delinquent later in childhood or to engage in violence as adults (including such behaviors as date rape or spousal abuse). They are more likely to be substance abusers in adolescence and adulthood; to attempt suicide; to have emotional problems, such as anxiety, depression, or more serious forms of emotional illness; and to have lower IQs and poorer school performance (Malinosky-Rummell & Hansen, 1993).

Sexually abused children also show a wide variety of disturbances, including fears, posttraumatic stress disor-

der, behavior problems, and poor self-esteem (Kendall-Tackett, Williams, & Finkelhor, 1993). Children who suffer either type of abuse do not typically show *all* these symptoms, but they are far more likely than are their nonabused peers to show some form of significant disturbance. The more lasting and severe the abuse, the greater the likelihood of problems of these types.

The picture is not totally bleak. Some abused children show no measurable symptoms, and when the abuse is stopped, many children show a decline in symptoms of distress, especially when the mother is supportive and protective toward the child. But let us not lose sight of the fact that long-term problems are common among children who experience this degree of hostility or hurt, nor of the fact that our society has not yet found good ways of reducing the incidence of such abuse.

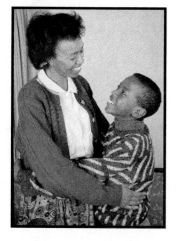

I am sure it is obvious to you that loving a child is a critical ingredient in the child's optimum development. But sometimes it helps to restate the obvious.

higher self-esteem; are more empathetic, more altruistic, more responsive to others' hurts or distress; and have higher IQs in preschool and elementary school (Maccoby, 1980; Simons, Robertson, & Downs, 1989). They are also less likely to show high levels of aggression or delinquent behavior in adolescence (Maughan, Pickles, & Quinton, 1995). Several studies show that among children and teens growing up in poor, tough neighborhoods, the lives of those who do *not* become delinquent are distinguished most by a single ingredient: They have experienced high levels of maternal love (Glueck & Glueck, 1972; McCord, McCord, & Zola, 1959).

I suspect that the role of warmth in fostering a secure attachment of the child to the parent is one of the key elements in this picture. You already know from Chapter 11 that securely attached children are more skillful with their peers, more exploratory, more sure of themselves. Warmth also makes children generally more responsive to guidance, so the parents' affection and warmth increase the potency of the things that parents say to their children and the efficiency of their discipline (MacDonald, 1992).

Responsiveness

A second key element is **responsiveness** by the parent to the child, a concept I've mentioned repeatedly in earlier chapters. Responsive parents are those who pick up on the child's signals appropriately and then react in sensitive ways to the child's needs. Parents who do more of this have youngsters who learn language somewhat more rapidly, show higher IQ and more speedy cognitive development, are more likely to be securely attached, are more compliant with adult requests, and are more socially competent (Bornstein, 1989b)

Methods of Control

It is the nature of children that they will often do things their parents do not want them to do, ask for things they cannot have, or refuse to obey their parents' requests or demands. From early days, parents are inevitably faced with the task of controlling the child's behavior, a process more popularly called *discipline*. Since I have not yet talked much about this aspect of parent-child interactions, I need to break the subject up into several elements.

One element of control is the *consistency of rules*—simply making it clear to the child what the rules are and what the consequences are of disobeying (or obeying) them, and then enforcing the rules consistently. Some parents are very clear and consistent; others waffle or are fuzzy about what they expect or will tolerate. Studies of families show that parents who are clear and consistent have children who are much less likely to be defiant or noncompliant—a pattern you'll remember from Gerald Patterson's research (recall Figure 1.2). But such clarity does not produce little robots. Children from families with consistent rules are also more competent, more sure of themselves, and less likely to become delinquent or show significant behavior problems.

One recent piece of research that nicely illustrates this pattern is Lawrence Kurdek and Mark Fine's study of 850 junior high school students (1994). They measured the level of control in the family by asking the young adolescents to say whether each of the following three questions was true or not true (on a seven-point scale) about their families:

Someone in my family makes sure that my homework is done.

Generally, someone in my family knows where I am and what I'm doing.

Someone in my family keeps a close eye on me.

Kurdek and Fine also had information about each child's self-esteem and sense of self-efficacy, which they combined into a measure of "psychological competence." You can see the relationship between these two pieces of information in Figure 13.1: Greater control was clearly linked with greater psychological competence.

A related element of parental control is the *level of expectations* the parents have for the child's behavior. Is the child expected to show relatively more mature behavior, or does the parent feel it is important not to expect too much too soon? Studies of such variations

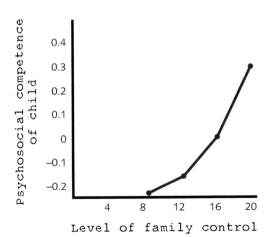

FIGURE 13.1 Junior-high-school students who report higher levels of parental control and supervision also describe themselves as having higher self-esteem and self-efficacy. (*Source:* Kurdek & Fine, 1994, from Figure 1, p. 1143.)

show that, within limits, higher expectations seem to be associated with better outcomes. Children whose parents make high demands on them, expecting them to help around the house or to show relatively mature behavior for their age, have higher self-esteem, show more generosity and altruism toward others, and have lower levels of aggression. Obviously, this can be carried much too far. It is unrealistic and counterproductive to expect a 2-year-old to set the table for dinner every day or to tie his own shoes. But when parents expect the child to be as independent and helpful as possible for his age, that does seem to foster a sense of competence in the child that carries over into other situations.

A third element of parental control is the degree of **restrictiveness** imposed. This is not the same thing as clear or consistent rule setting. A parent can be relatively low in restrictiveness and still have clear rules. For example, you might have a rule that your 10-year-old can stop off at another child's house after school without arranging it with you ahead of time, but he must call you to tell you where he is. That would be a clear rule, but with relatively low restrictiveness. On the other hand, a parent who insists on keeping a child within eyesight at all times or who puts a toddler in a playpen for most of the day rather than risk having the child pull the drawers open would be considered restrictive.

Restrictive parents also frequently use a distinctive form of language with their children, namely, *imperative* sentences, such as "Stop that" or "Come here" or "Do what I tell you." They are less likely to explain the rules to the children, but instead use their own power to control the child.

The other end of this continuum is usually listed as *permissive* parenting, which frequently also includes relatively few rules and few imperatives. Sometimes permissive parenting occurs because a parent feels helpless to control the child at all. In other cases permissiveness reflects a specific philosophy of child rearing that emphasizes the child's need for freedom and opportunity to explore.

You might think that children reared in permissive families have been specifically encouraged and reinforced for independence and decision making. Can you think of any reason why they would nonetheless show *less* independence and responsibility?

Neither high nor low restrictiveness is consistently linked to positive outcomes. Highly restrictive parents are likely to have quite obedient, unaggressive children. But such children are also likely to be somewhat timid and may have difficulty establishing close relationships with peers. Children with highly permissive parents—who may exert far too little control—are likely to show only moderate independence and to be relatively thoughtless of others. All in all, children seem to respond most positively to clear rules consistently enforced, to realistic demands and expectations, combined with only moderate restrictiveness.

Finally, to understand the process of control we have to understand the role of *punishment*. When a child does something you don't want (like writing on the wall, or hitting her brother, or staying out past a curfew) or fails to do something you do want (like cleaning his room), most parents respond with some kind of punishment, such as withholding privileges or treats, assigning extra chores, sending a child to his room, "grounding," verbal scolding, or spanking. The most controversial of these is spanking. Because of the importance of the question, I have explored the pros and cons of such physical punishment in the *Real World* box on the facing page. But I want to make a number of other points about punishment strategies in general.

First, as Gerald Patterson (1975) says, "Punishment 'works.' If you use it properly it will produce rapid changes in the behavior of other people" (p. 19). The operative word here, though, is *properly.* The most effective punishments—those that produce long-term

The Real World

To Spank or Not to Spank

Nine out of ten parents of preschoolers in the United States say that they spank their children at least occasionally; about half of parents of teenagers do so (Straus, 1991a; Straus & Donnelly, 1993). Most of these parents think of spanking as an effective way of discipline. But I think they are wrong, at least under most conditions and in most families.

Note please: I am not talking here about physical abuse, although certainly some parents do abuse their children by spanking excessively with a switch or a brush or other objects. I'm talking about the ordinary kind of spanking—two or three hard swats on the rear, or (more likely with older children) a quick slap—that most people think of as normal and helpful.

In the short term, spanking a child usually *does* get the child to stop the particular behavior you didn't like, and it seems to have a *temporary* effect of reducing the chance that the child will repeat the bad behavior. Since that's what you wanted, it may seem like a good strategy. But even in the short term there are some negative side effects. The child may have stopped misbehaving, but after a spanking he is likely to be crying, which may be almost as distressing as the original misbehavior. And crying is a behavior that spanking does not decrease: It is virtually impossible to get children to stop crying by spanking them! So you have exchanged one unpleasantness for another, and the second unpleasantness (crying) can't be dealt with by using the same form of punishment.

Another short-term side effect is that *you* are being reinforced for spanking whenever the child stops misbehaving after you spank her. Thus, you are being "trained" to use spanking the next time, and a cycle is being built up.

In the longer term, the effects are clearly negative. First, when you spank, the child observes you using physical force or violence as a method of solving problems or getting people to do what you want. You thus serve as a model for a behavior you do *not* want your child to use with others. Second, by repeatedly pairing your presence with the unpleasant or painful event of spanking, you are undermining your own positive value for your child. Over time, this means that you are less able to use *any* kind of reinforcement effectively. Eventually even your praise or affection will be less powerful in influencing your child's behavior. That is a very high price to pay.

Third, spanking frequently carries a strong underlying emotional message—anger, rejection, irritation, dislike of the child. Even very young children read this emotional message quite clearly (Rohner, Kean, & Cournoyer, 1991). Spanking thus helps to create a family climate of rejection instead of warmth, with all the attendant negative consequences.

Finally, we have research evidence that children who are spanked—just like children who are abused—at later ages show higher levels of aggression and less popularity with their peers, lower self-esteem, more emotional instability, and higher levels of delinquency and later criminality (Laub & Sampson, 1995; Rohner et al., 1991; Strassberg et al., 1994). And as adults, children who have been spanked are more likely to be depressed than are those who were never or rarely spanked (Straus, 1995). These effects are especially clear if the physical punishment is harsh and erratic, but the risks for these negative outcomes are higher even with fairly mild levels of physical punishment.

I am *not* saying that you should never punish a child. I *am* saying that *physical punishment,* such as spanking, is not a good way to go about it. However . . . there *may* be one exception to this general statement: Among families living in inner-city neighborhoods where there are high levels of crime and violence, it is especially crucial for parents to maintain tight monitoring and control over their child's activities. It is possible that in such conditions, mild forms of physical punishment may help such parents maintain the needed control. Still, the balance here is fairly delicate. When such physical punishment is not combined with warmth toward the child or when the physical punishment is regular and harsh, the effects are negative, even in these extremely dangerous environments (McCord, 1991).

Another important caveat is that strong verbal aggression by a parent toward a child is also linked to many poor outcomes in the child, including increased risk of delinquency and adult violence (Straus, 1991b). So resisting the impulse to hit the child and yelling at him instead is not a good tradeoff.

Despite these caveats, however, I think the bulk of the evidence is persuasive: Spanking and other forms of physical punishment have negative consequences for children.

Think about your own upbringing. What types of control strategies did your parents use? What kinds of punishment? How might you want to change these patterns in bringing up your own children?

changes in the child's behavior without unwanted or negative side effects—are those used early in some sequence of misbehavior, with the lowest level of emotion possible, and the mildest level of punishment possible. Taking a desired toy away when the child *first* uses it to hit the furniture (or a sibling) or consistently removing small privileges when a child misbehaves will "work," especially if the parent is also warm, clear about the rules, and consistent. It is far less effective to wait until the screams have reached a piercing level or until the fourth time a teenager has gone off without telling you where she's going and then weighing in with yelling, loud comments, and strong punishments.

Second, to a considerable degree, parents get back what they give out in the way of punishment. As I pointed out in Chapter 9, children learn by observation as well as by doing, so they learn the adults' ways of coping with stress and forms of punishment. Yelling at children to stop doing something, for example, may bring a *brief* change in their behavior (which thus reinforces the parent for yelling, by the way). But it also increases the chances that children will yell back on other occasions.

Communication Patterns

Two things about communication within the family seem to make a difference for the child: the amount and richness of language spoken *to* the child, and the amount of conversation and suggestions *from* the child that the parent encourages. Listening is important, as well as talking.

When I say "listening," I have in mind more than merely saying "uh-huh" periodically when the child talks. I also mean conveying to the child the sense that what he has to say is *worth* listening to, that he has ideas, that his ideas are important and should be considered in family decisions.

We have much less research on the quality of communication within families than on some of the other dimensions I have been describing, so we are a long way from understanding all the ramifications. In general, children from families with open communication are seen as more emotionally or socially mature (Baumrind, 1971; Bell & Bell, 1982).

Open communication may also be important for the functioning of the family as a unit. For example, in a study of a national sample of families with adolescents, Howard

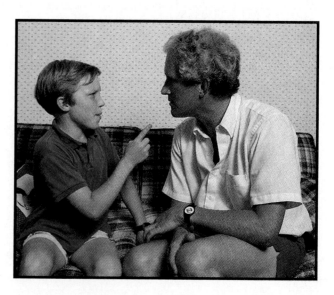

This dad seems to be willing to listen carefully to his son, even though the boy is angry and accusatory.

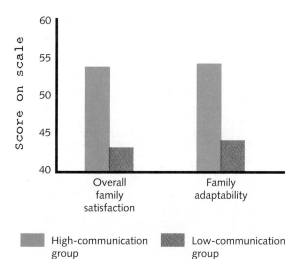

FIGURE 13.2 Good family communication was associated with both satisfaction and adaptability in this study of more than 400 adolescents and their parents. (*Source:* Barnes & Olson, 1985, Table 3, page 445.)

Barnes and David Olson (1985) measured communication by asking the parents and teenagers to agree or disagree with statements like "It is easy for me to express all my true feelings to my [mother/father/child]." As you can see in Figure 13.2, they found that those families in which parents and child reported good, open communication, compared to those with poorer communication, also described themselves as more adaptable to stress or change and more satisfied.

Patterns or Styles of Child Rearing

Each of these dimension of parental behavior has a demonstrable effect on the child, but if we are going to try to use a systems theory approach, it is not enough to look at each dimension independently. We also have to think about how they interact with one another to create *styles* or *patterns* of child rearing.

The most influential proposal about such styles has come from Diana Baumrind (1972), who has looked at combinations of four aspects of the dimensions I've just described: (1) warmth or nurturance; (2) level of expectations, which she describes in terms of "maturity demands"; (3) the clarity and consistency of rules; and (4) communication between parent and child. Baumrind saw three specific combinations of these characteristics:

- The **permissive parental style** is high in nurturance but low in maturity demands, control, and communication.

- The **authoritarian parental style** is high in control and maturity demands but low in nurturance and communication.

- The **authoritative parental style** is high in all four.

Eleanor Maccoby and John Martin (1983) have proposed a variation of Baumrind's category system, shown in Figure 13.3, that I find even more helpful. They emphasize two dimensions, the degree of demand or control, on the one hand, and the amount of acceptance/rejection or responsiveness on the other. The intersection of these two dimensions creates four types, three of which correspond fairly closely to Baumrind's authoritarian, authoritative, and permissive types. Maccoby and Martin's fourth type, the

FIGURE 13.3 Maccoby and Martin expanded on Baumrind's categories into this two-dimensional typology. (*Source:* Adapted from Maccoby & Martin, 1983, Figure 2, p. 39.)

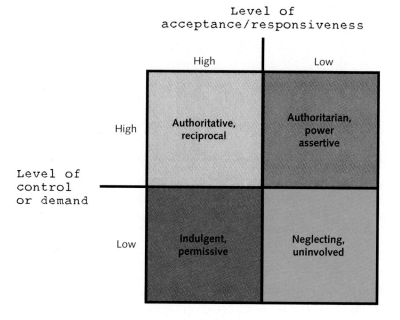

neglecting or uninvolved type, was not identified by Baumrind in her early work, although recent research makes it clear that this is an important group to study.

The Authoritarian Type. Children growing up in authoritarian families—with high levels of demand and control but relatively low levels of warmth or responsiveness—do less well in school, are typically less skilled with peers than are children from other types of families, and have lower self-esteem. Some of these children appear subdued; others may show high aggressiveness or other indications of being out of control. Which of these two outcomes occurs may depend in part on how skillfully the parents use the various disciplinary techniques. Patterson finds that the "out-of-control" child is most likely to come from a family in which the parents are authoritarian by inclination but lack the skills to enforce the limits or rules they set.

The Permissive Type. Children growing up with indulgent or permissive parents also show some negative outcomes. They do slightly less well in school in adolescence and are likely to be more aggressive—particularly if the parents are specifically permissive toward aggressiveness—and somewhat immature in their behavior with peers and in school. They are less likely to take responsibility and are less independent.

The Authoritative Type. The most consistently positive outcomes have been associated with the authoritative pattern, in which the parents are high in both control and warmth, setting clear limits but also responding to the child's individual needs. Children reared in such families typically show higher self-esteem, are more independent but at the same time more likely to comply with parental requests, and may show more altruistic behavior. They are self-confident and achievement oriented in school and get better grades. In late adolescence they are more likely to use postconventional moral reasoning (Boyes & Allen, 1993).

The Neglecting Type. The most consistently negative outcomes are associated with the fourth pattern, the neglecting or uninvolved type. You may remember from the discussion of secure and insecure attachments in Chapter 11 that one of the family characteristics often found in children rated insecurely attached is the "psychological unavailability" of the mother. The mother may be depressed or may be overwhelmed by other problems in her life and may simply not have made any deep emotional connection with the child. Whatever the reason, such children continue to show disturbances in their relationships with peers and with adults for many years. In less-extreme cases the effects are also detectable. At adolescence, for example, youngsters from neglecting families are more impulsive and antisocial and much less achievement oriented in school (Block, 1971; Pulkkinen, 1982).

A Research Example: The Work of Steinberg and Dornbusch

The best single piece of research demonstrating the effects of these several styles is a longitudinal study of more than 8000 high school students in California and Wisconsin, by Laurence Steinberg and Sanford Dornbusch and their colleagues (Dornbusch et al., 1987b; Lamborn et al., 1991; Steinberg, Elmen, & Mounts, 1989; Steinberg et al., 1992; Steinberg et al., 1994). They measured parenting styles by asking the teenagers themselves to complete a questionnaire about their relationship with their parents that focused on the dimensions of acceptance/involvement and strictness/supervision. For example, they were asked to indicate the extent to which each of the following statements was true or not true:

"I can count on my parents to help me out if I have some kind of problem."

"When he wants me to do something he explains why."

"My parents know exactly where I am most afternoons after school."

Steinberg and Dornbusch then looked at the relationship between these family styles and a variety of outcomes, finding that teenagers from authoritative families showed the optimum pattern on every measure they used. These teenagers had higher self-reliance, higher social competence, better grades, fewer indications of psychological distress, and lower levels of school misconduct, drug use, and delinquency. Teenagers from authoritarian families had the lowest scores on the several measures of social competence and self-reliance, but the young people with the highest rates of problem behavior and the poorest school achievement were those from neglectful families (Steinberg et al., 1994). Figure 13.4 gives two of these results, one showing variations in grade point average and the other, self-reported delinquent acts, including such things as carrying a weapon, theft, or getting into trouble with the police.

Steinberg and Dornbusch continued their contact with these teenagers over two years, which allowed them to look at possible links between the parents' style at the beginning of the study and the students' *later* behavior. In this longitudinal analysis, they found the same kinds of patterns: Those students who described their parents as most authoritative at the beginning of the study showed more *improvement* in academic competence and self-reliance and the smallest increases in psychological symptoms and delinquent behavior of any of the groups.

But the system is more complex than this makes it sound. For one thing, authoritative parents not only create a good family climate and thereby support and motivate their child optimally, but also behave differently *toward the school.* They are much more likely to be involved with the school, attending school functions or talking to teachers, and this involvement seems to play a crucial role in the process. When an otherwise authoritative parent is *not* also more involved with the school, the outcomes for the student are not so clearly positive. Similarly, a teenager whose parent is highly involved with the school but is not authoritative shows less optimal outcomes. It is the combination of authoritativeness and school involvement that is associated with the best results (Steinberg et al., 1992).

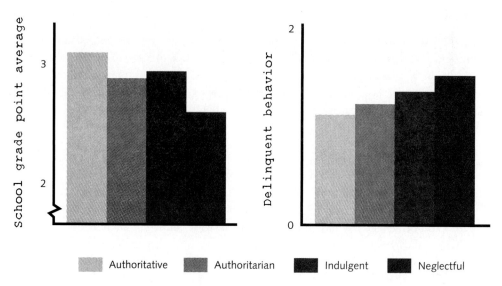

FIGURE 13.4 School grades and delinquency both vary as a function of parental style in Steinberg and Dornbusch's large sample of teenagers. Delinquent behavior in this case reflects the adolescent's own report of the frequency with which he or she carries a weapon, steals, or gets into trouble with the police. (*Source:* Steinberg et al., 1994, from Table 5, p.762.)

In another indication of the complexity, this research group has recently found that the young people in their study whose *friends* had more authoritative parents showed more optimum outcomes, regardless of the style of interaction in their own families. Even authoritatively reared teenagers had better grades and lower delinquency when they hung out with friends whose families were also authoritative than when they chose pals from families with other styles (Fletcher et al., 1995).

Ethnic Group Differences in Styles. Because the sample in the Steinberg and Dornbusch study is so large, it has also been possible for them to look separately at sub-groups of African-American, Hispanic-American, and Asian-American youth and their families (Steinberg et al., 1991). In the process, they have uncovered some very interesting patterns that point us both toward common processes and toward unique cultural variations.

Table 13.1 shows the percentages of families from each of the four ethnic groups involved in this study who can be described as authoritative, broken down further by social class and the intactness of the family. The authoritative pattern was most common among white families and least common among Asian-Americans, but in each ethnic group, authoritative parenting was more common among the middle class and (with one exception) more common among intact families than in single-parent or stepparent families.

More important, Steinberg and Dornbusch find that many of the relationships between authoritative parenting and positive outcomes occurred in all ethnic groups. In all four groups, teenagers from authoritative families had more self-reliance and less delinquency than did those from nonauthoritative families.

On the other hand, school performance is *not* linked to authoritative parenting in the same ways in all four groups: Good grades are linked to such a parenting style for whites and for Hispanic-Americans but only very weakly for Asian-Americans or African-Americans. In particular, Asian-Americans as a group do extremely well in school even though their parents are among the least authoritative.

Before you read any further, see if you can come up with any explanations of this apparent paradox. Why might Asian families be high in authoritarian style but still have children who do well in school? How many different hypotheses can you come up with?

Table 13.1
Ethnic Differences in Authoritative Parenting

| | Percentage of Authoritative Families | | | |
| | Working Class | | Middle Class | |
Ethnic Group	Intact[a]	Not Intact	Intact	Not Intact
White	17.2	11.5	25.0	17.6
Black	13.4	12.2	14.0	16.0
Hispanic	10.7	9.8	15.8	12.9
Asian	7.5	6.1	15.6	10.8

[a]*Intact* means the child is still living with both biological parents; *not intact* means either a single-parent family, stepfamily, or any family configuration other than one with both natural parents.

Source: Steinberg et al., 1991, from Table 1, p. 25.

How can we explain this paradox? One possibility is that the four styles of parenting simply don't capture the most crucial features of family interaction that affect academic performance. Steinberg and Dornbusch have pursued this possibility by examining a wide variety of other aspects of family and cultural systems (Steinberg, Dornbusch, & Brown, 1992). They conclude that an additional key element is the beliefs students and parents have about the importance of education for later success in life. All four ethnic groups they studied share a belief that doing well in school will lead to better chances later. But the groups disagree on the consequences of doing poorly in school. Asian students, more than any other group, believe that a good job is unlikely to follow a bad education, while both Hispanics and African-Americans are more optimistic (or more cavalier) about the risks associated with poor school performance. Perhaps as a result of their greater fear of failure, Asian students spend much more time on homework than do other groups.

Furthermore, Asian-American students (and whites) get very good peer support for academic achievement, while African-American teens get little peer support for such an activity, which undermines the beneficial effects of authoritative parenting in this subgroup. Indeed, interviews with the African-American students in the Steinberg and Dornbusch study suggest that academically oriented African-American youths find it very difficult to find a peer group that will support their academic goals. Those who nonetheless persist in their striving for achievement often resolve the issue by choosing peers primarily from other ethnic groups. Thus, the dilemma for African-American students, more than any other subgroup in American culture, seems to involve a choice between doing well in school and being popular.

Another possibility is that the four styles suggested by Maccoby and Martin are themselves ethnocentric and do not (perhaps cannot) capture the elements that make individual cultural patterns unique. For example, Ruth Chao (1994) notes that Chinese-American parents come out high on traditional measures of authoritarian parenting because they require obedience. But in Asian culture, strictness and a demand for obedience are perceived

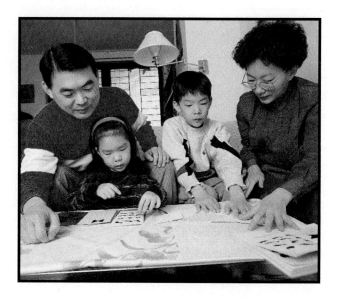

Asian parents very often score high on measures of authoritarian parental style. But their high level of strictness and control is embedded in a different set of cultural values and thus has a different meaning for the child, and a different effect on the child's behavior—yet another illustration of the fact that psychologists need to be careful in generalizing theories and results across cultures.

as aspects of concern and caring, not as signs of coldness. For the Chinese, says Chao, the key concept is that of *training,* which means teaching or educating and carries with it the element not only of control but also of high involvement and closeness to the child. Chinese parents control their children not to dominate—an aspect implicit in the authoritarian style as Baumrind described it—but to ensure that harmonious relations within the family and the culture will be maintained.

Chao devised a set of questions to tap "training" and asked these questions, as well as the usual questions used to measure authoritarian and authoritative styles, of Chinese and European-American mothers. As expected, she found that Chinese mothers were more likely to be rated as authoritarian on the traditional measure. But they were also higher on the measure of "training," agreeing more often with statements like "Parents must begin training the child as soon as he is ready," or "Mothers must train the child to work very hard and be disciplined," or "Mothers teach a child by pointing out good behavior in others." According to Chao, the traditional measures of the authoritarian style fail to capture these values and thus badly misrepresent the quality of the parent-child interaction within the Chinese family.

Adding Up What We Know About Parental Style

I think the accumulating evidence makes it clear that the concept of parental style has been and will continue to be highly useful descriptively and predictively. For one thing, it reminds us that it is the *pattern,* the *system,* that is critical, and not just the individual behaviors. And it seems clear that children are affected by the family "climate" or style. Although we do not have the sort of longitudinal data needed to be sure, I suspect that these effects persist well into adulthood.

However, we may not yet have zeroed in on the best ways to describe family styles. The four types Baumrind and Maccoby and Martin suggest are probably only a first approximation, and we need to find ways to bring cultural variations more fully into our descriptive systems.

In addition, we need to understand more fully the relationship between parental *styles* and parental *behavior*. Darling and Steinberg (1993) have recently argued that we should think of parenting style more as a kind of basic climate in the family, as a set of attitudes and values, rather than as a set of specific parenting behaviors. The basic attitudes and values are obviously reflected in the parent's behavior, but the family climate also affects the impact the parent has on the child. For example, both authoritative and authoritarian parents are more likely than are permissive or neglecting parents to be involved with the child's school, attending parents' nights, visiting the child's school advisor or teachers, and so on. But as I mentioned earlier, the beneficial effect of such high parental involvement on the teenager's school grades was greater among authoritative than among authoritarian parents (Steinberg et al., 1992). So even when the parenting *behavior* (high school involvement) was the same, the effect was different because the overall family climate was different. Authoritative parents, when they get involved, have more impact on their child's behavior because they have created a climate of greater acceptance and support of the child, so the child listens more and is more influenced.

Finally, we need to remember that a great many variables beyond parental style are involved in family dynamics. Each child brings her own temperament or other qualities to the mixture, parents bring their own personalities and habits, the relationship between siblings may have a powerful effect, and the structure of the family itself is clearly important.

Other Aspects of Family Dynamics

The Child's Characteristics

One of the first things to understand is that the influences in the parent-child system flow both ways. Children influence their parents as well as the other way around. I have already talked about one important influence of this type, namely, the child's temperament. Children with "difficult" temperaments seem to elicit more punishment (especially if the family is under some kind of stress) and may affect a parent's mood. More generally, such children may have much more difficulty adapting to any change in the family system, such as a family divorce.

The child's position in the family is also an important ingredient. Parents generally have higher expectations for maturity in their firstborn and may well be more responsive, more child-centered with the first child. Firstborns are also punished more, in part because parents may be less skilled in using noncoercive forms of control with their first child.

The child's age also makes a difference—a point that may seem obvious but that is well worth reemphasizing. As the child develops, very different demands are made on the parents. As any parent can tell you, caring for an infant is a quite different task from caring for a 2-year-old or a 12-year-old. The areas in which control will be needed change over time, the degree of push for independence changes, the child's intellectual and language abilities change. Parents quite naturally adapt to these changes, altering their own pattern—perhaps even their style—as the child grows older. At the same time, parents show some consistency in their behavior toward children of the same age. That is, parents behave similarly toward the second child when he is 2 as they had toward the first child when she was 2, even though they are now treating the older child as a 4-year-old (Boer,

Cultures and Contexts
China's One-Child Policy

A particularly fascinating cultural experiment regarding family size has been under way in China since 1979, when the government instituted an intense family-planning effort to reduce the normal family size to one child. This was done for economic and political reasons, since China has about 21 percent of the population of the world but only 7 percent of the arable land. The Chinese were facing the prospect of enormous food shortages with attendant social unrest if something was not done about their population explosion. What they did was adopt a one-child policy. At present, this policy is still rigorously followed in urban areas, although in rural areas families are generally allowed to have two children.

In the early years of the policy, the Chinese themselves had many fears that these only children would become family tyrants, spoiled by parents and grandparents. But recent studies do not confirm that fear. Toni Falbo (1992; Falbo & Poston, 1993), an American researcher who has been involved in a series of large survey studies of Chinese children, reports that she can find few differences between only and nononly children, either in school performance or in personality. Thus, by *Chinese* standards, the one-child policy has been a success. It has not led to a generation of "little emperors" as some had feared, although it is still early to know what effect this policy will have on the society as a whole in the decades to come, when the only children have become adults. A culture made up of only children is likely to differ in a whole variety of ways, many of them unanticipated, from one in which larger families prevail.

Godhart, & Treffers, 1992). Such a clearly rational set of changes in the parents' behavior as their children grow older has the effect of changing the family system over time.

Siblings

Such changes over time may be one contributor to a phenomenon that has been puzzling developmental psychologists more and more in recent years, namely, the fact that two children from the same family so often turn out quite differently. I think that until recently, most of us assumed that parental style was rather like the weather in a given location: If it's raining, it's raining equally hard on everyone in the same place. In just the same way, we assumed that if one child experienced an authoritative style, then such a style must characterize the *family;* all other children in the same household would experience the same style, and the children would therefore end up with similar skills, similar personalities, similar strengths and weaknesses. But both pieces of this assumption now look wrong. Children growing up in the same family turn out quite differently, and the family system, perhaps even the family style, can be quite different from one child to another.

Some of the best evidence comes from several studies by Judy Dunn (Dunn & McGuire, 1994) in both England and the United States. She has found that parents may express warmth and pride toward one child and scorn toward another, may be lenient toward one and strict with another. Here's an example from one of Dunn's observations, of 30-month-old Andy and his 14-month-old sister Susie.

> *Andy was a rather timid and sensitive child, cautious, unconfident, and compliant. . . .*
> *Susie was a striking contrast—assertive, determined, and a handful for her mother, who*
> *was nevertheless delighted by her boisterous daughter. In [one] observation of Andy and*
> *his sister, Susie persistently attempted to grab a forbidden object on a high kitchen*
> *counter, despite her mother's repeated prohibitions. Finally, she succeeded, and Andy*

Are you and your siblings alike in a lot of ways, or do you have quite different traits, skills, and attitudes? Can you trace any of those differences to variations in the way you were treated as children?

overheard his mother make a warm, affectionate comment on Susie's action: "Susie, you are a determined little devil!" Andy, sadly, commented to his mother, "I'm not a determined little devil!" His mother replied, laughing, "No! What are you? A poor old boy!" (1992, p. 6)

Not only are such episodes common in family interactions, but children are highly sensitive to such variations in treatment. Notice how Andy had monitored his mother's interaction with Susie and then compared himself to his sister. Children this age are already aware of the emotional quality of exchanges between themselves and their parents, as well as the exchanges between their siblings and parents. Dunn finds that those who receive less affection and warmth from their mothers are likely to be more depressed, worried, or anxious than are their siblings. And the more differently the parents treat siblings, the more rivalry and hostility brothers and sisters are likely to show toward one another (Brody et al., 1992).

Of course parents treat children differently for many reasons, *including* the child's age. Susie and Andy's mother may have been just as accepting of naughty behavior from Andy when he was a toddler. But Andy does not remember that. What he sees is the contrast between how he and Susie are treated now. Thus, even when parents are consistent in the way they respond to each child at a given age, at any moment they are *not* behaving consistently toward all children, and the children notice this and create internal models about the meaning of those differences in treatment.

Parents also respond to temperamental differences in their children, to gender differences, and to variations in the children's skills or talents, all of which creates a unique pattern of interaction for each child. It is becoming increasingly clear that such differences in treatment are an important ingredient in the child's emerging internal model of self and contribute greatly to variations in behavior between children growing up in the same families.

The Parents' Characteristics

The parents bring their own life histories, their own personalities, into the family dynamic as well. I could spend a whole chapter talking about the parents' half of this equation, but lacking such space, let me give only two brief illustrations.

First, when either parent is significantly depressed it has a profound effect on the entire family system. You already know from Chapter 11 that an insecure attachment is more likely when the mother is depressed. Depressed parents also perceive their children as more difficult and problematic, and are more critical of them, even when objective observers cannot identify any difference in the behavior of such children and the children of nondepressed mothers (Richters & Pellegrini, 1989; Webster-Stratton & Hammond, 1988). Thus, the parent's depression changes not only her behavior, but also her perception of the child's behavior, both of which alter the family system.

The parent's own internal working model of attachment also seems to have a very strong effect on the family system and thus on the child. Mary Main and her colleagues have devised an interview that allows them to classify the security or insecurity of an adult's attachment to his or her own parents (Main & Hesse, 1990; Main, Kaplan, & Cassidy, 1985). Using this interview, Main and others have now found that those adults who are themselves securely attached are much more likely to have a child who is also securely attached (Benoit & Parker, 1994; Ward & Carlson, 1995).

Can you think of other parental qualities, skills, or attributes that might affect the family system?

The history and personal qualities the parents bring with them to the family interactive system obviously help to shape the style of parenting they show with their children—whether authoritarian, authoritative, or some other. But they do more than that. They affect the parents' perceptions of the child as well as the parents' behavior, and thus affect the system in myriad subtle ways.

Family Structure

Another obvious aspect of the family system is the particular configuration of people who live together in a given family unit—an aspect usually called *family structure*. I suspect that many of us still harbor the illusion that the most common family structure is a father, a mother, and several children. And no doubt many of us still think that most children spend their childhood and adolescence with their biological mom and dad. But in the United States today, both assumptions are wrong.

Donald Hernandez, in his remarkable book *America's Children* (1993), estimates that only 40 to 45 percent of the children born in 1980—today's teenagers—will spend all their years up to age 18 living with both natural parents. Among African-Americans, Hernandez estimates, this figure is only 20 percent, while among American whites, it is about 55 percent. Interestingly, these numbers have not changed as much as you might expect through this century. In the 1920s, for example, 31 percent of whites and 57 percent of blacks spent at least some part of their childhood living with only one parent. But the *reasons* for the pattern have changed dramatically. In 1920, the most common reason for a child to be living with only one parent was that a parent had died; today the most common reasons are divorce or that the mother never married.

You can get some feeling for the variety of family structures in which children live today from Figure 13.5, which shows the percentages of five different structures in white, African-American, and Hispanic 13-year-olds in the U.S., based on a nationally representative sample of more than 21,000 children studied by Valerie Lee and her colleagues (Lee et al., 1994). But even this chart doesn't begin to convey the variety of family structures or the number of changes in family structure a child may experience over time. Divorced mothers, for example, may have had live-in relationships with one or more men before a remarriage, or they may have lived for a while with their own parents. And many children, especially children with never-married mothers, live in extended families with

If cultures are systems too, then this enormous increase in the number of children experiencing a single-parent family structure has to have some impact on the whole system. What might be the long-term effects of this change?

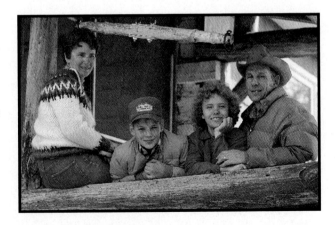

When we think of "the family," no doubt most of us think of a family with a father and mother and several children. But, in fact, in the United States it now is the exception rather than the rule for a child to spend his or her entire childhood and adolescence in such a family system.

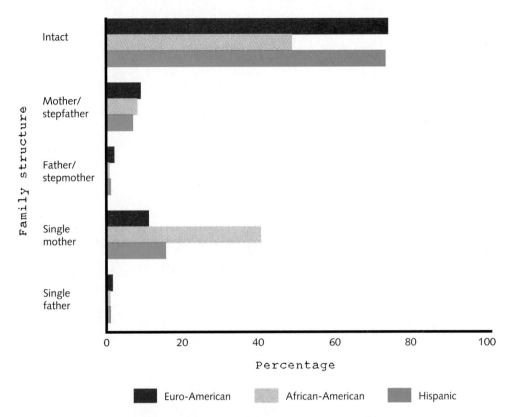

FIGURE 13.5 Variations in family structure among current-day 13-year-olds. (*Source:* Lee, Burkham, Zimiles, & Ladewski, 1994, from Table 2, p. 419.)

grandparents and other family members as well as a parent. All in all, the evidence makes it inescapably clear that the *majority* of children in the United States today experience at least two different family structures, often many more than that, in the course of their growing up. This is especially true of African-Americans, but it is increasingly true of other ethnic groups in our culture as well.

In other industrialized countries, single-parent families are less common, but they are on the rise everywhere. By the mid-1980s, the proportions ranged from less than 5 percent in Japan to about 15 percent in Australia, the United Kingdom, and Sweden, and to nearly 25 percent in the U.S. (Burns, 1992). Because cultures are complex, knowledge gleaned about the impact of family structure on children's development in one country may not hold elsewhere. But the issue is growing in importance in many parts of the world.

What do we know about the impact on children of being reared in such varied or varying family structures?

Single-Parent Families. One place to begin is to look at what happens to children reared with both natural parents versus those with only one natural parent. Sara McLanahan and Gary Sandefur, sociologists who have studied this question extensively, come to a sweeping, somewhat grim conclusion:

Children who grow up in a household with only one biological parent are worse off, on average, than children who grow up in a household with both of their biological parents,

Cultures and Contexts

The Benefits of Extended Families

Because single-parent families have become so common in the United States, researchers here tend to develop a kind of tunnel vision when it comes to studies of "family structure." For us, the question nearly always translates to a comparison of single-parent families with two-parent families. But in many parts of the world, the normative form of family life is not the nuclear or two-parent family, but an *extended* family, in which several generations live together in the same household. One recent study from the Sudan provides a kind of antidote to our typical cultural myopia.

Al Hassan Al Awad and Edmund Sonuga-Barke (1992) compared the incidence of childhood problems for children who lived in Western-style nuclear families (mother and father only) versus those who lived in traditional extended families, in which three generations lived in the same household. All these families lived in towns near Khartoum (the capital of Sudan), and the two groups were matched for social status and approximate income. The mothers were interviewed about their child's behavior and problems.

The findings are very clear: Children reared in extended households had fewer conduct problems, fewer sleep problems, and better self-care, and they were less likely to be overly dependent. The best single predictor of these good outcomes was the involvement of the child's grandmother in the child's care, and this was true within the group of nuclear families as well as in the comparison of nuclear and extended families.

How many different explanations for this result can you think of? Should we generalize this finding to Western cultures and conclude that extended families would be better for children in our society as well? How could you check out such a hypothesis?

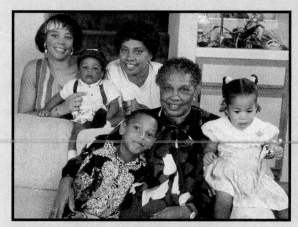

Extended families like this one have their own strengths, too often ignored. In the United States, such families are much more common among African-Americans and Hispanic-Americans than among European Americans.

regardless of the parents' race or educational background, regardless of whether the parents are married when the child is born, and regardless of whether the resident parent remarries. (1994, p. 1)

Such children are about twice as likely to drop out of high school, twice as likely to have a child before age 20, and less likely to have a steady job in their late teens or early twenties. This does *not* mean that single parenthood is the cause of all evil. Rather, as McLanahan and Sandefur point out, it is but one of many factors that increase the risk that a child will do poorly in school or become delinquent. Nor does living in an intact family buffer a child against all problems. Many young people whose parents are still together nonetheless drop out of school or experience other significant personal problems. But living with only one parent substantially increases the risks.

But why are the risks so much higher for this group? One obvious but nevertheless highly significant reason is that such families are simply much more likely to be poor. For

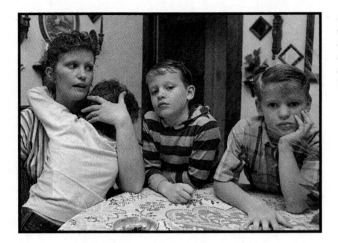

Many single parents manage to overcome the substantial obstacles and give their children the support and supervision they need. But on average, children of single parents have poorer life outcomes.

example, data from the U.S. indicate that after a divorce, a woman's income drops an average of 40 to 50 percent (Smock, 1993). Never-married mothers are also far more likely to be poor. Poverty, in turn, reduces the resources available to the child, increases the parent's stress, and makes it far less likely that the child will receive the financial or emotional support needed to finish high school or to go on to college.

Ethnicity, incidentally, is *not* a causal factor here. Yes, a larger percentage of African-American children grow up in single-parent families. But the same negative outcomes occur in white single-parent families, and the same positive outcomes are found in two-parent minority families. For example, the school dropout rate for a white child from a disrupted family is higher than for a Hispanic or African-American child reared in a two-parent family.

Stepparent Families. For a single parent, remarriage is not a quick fix for all these various problems. Adding a stepparent to the family system usually reduces the economic hardship, but it doesn't eliminate the other stresses associated with single-parent families. For example, Dornbusch, in the same large study I've been describing, finds that stepparent families show higher levels of authoritarian and lower levels of authoritative child-rearing

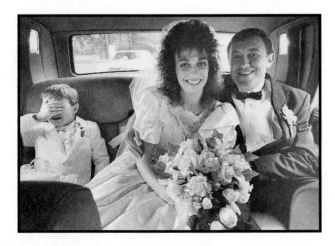

Five-year-old Keith is a whole lot less sure than his mother is that her second marriage is a joyous occasion!

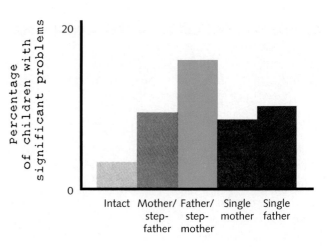

FIGURE 13.6 Children in stepparent families, especially father/stepmother, are more likely than are those in intact families to show behavior problems of one type or another. (*Source:* Lee et al., 1994, from Table 1, p. 417.)

styles (Dornbusch et al., 1987b), and the children have lower school grades and higher rates of delinquency than do children in intact families. Valerie Lee and her colleagues, in the study from which I drew the data in Figure 13.5, find something very similar, as you can see in Figure 13.6. In this large group of young adolescents, any family structure other than two biological parents was linked to higher levels of problems in the teenagers.

The literature on stepparent families also contains a curious finding, now replicated several times: In remarried families, the closer the new adult couple's own relationship is, the *more* problems the children display (Brand, Clingempeel, & Bowen-Woodward, 1988; Hetherington, 1989). This seems to be especially true in the years immediately following the remarriage, and in cases in which the mother and children lived alone for some years. What is striking about this finding is that in studies of nondivorced families, just the opposite is typically found. That is, the closer the parents' relationship, the better off the children are.

One can perhaps make sense of this finding within a systems perspective by assuming that after the original divorce, the children not only were given more independence, but also took on various family roles from which they were displaced when the new stepfather appeared on the scene. And the closer the relationship of the mother and stepfather, the more displaced the children feel. However we explain it, this finding illustrates how enormously complex the family system is. We simply cannot assume that something like high marital satisfaction is going to have precisely the same effect on every family. The effect will vary as a function of the family's history, the age of the children, the specific style of child rearing, and many other factors.

Can you think of any other explanation(s) for this odd finding?

Divorce

All of what I have just been saying about the impact of single parenthood and stepfamilies is obviously relevant to any discussion of the effects of divorce on children. But some special additional strains are associated with divorce, and some special questions are linked to this event.

The first several years after a divorce are a period of special strain. In these years, children typically become more defiant, more negative, more aggressive or depressed or angry. If they are of school age, their school performance often drops for at least a while

(Furstenberg & Cherlin, 1991; Hetherington & Clingempeel, 1992). Psychologists disagree about how long these more severe negative effects may persist for the child. Some investigators report lingering effects five and ten years later (Wallerstein, 1984, 1989). Others do not find such lasting effects (Hetherington, 1989), but all agree that in the short term, children are disturbed.

The same sort of disruption occurs in the parents' behavior. The adults may show wide mood swings, experience problems at work, or suffer from poor health. Their parenting style also changes, becoming much less authoritative, almost neglectful (Hetherington, 1989). In particular, they do much less well at monitoring their children's behavior and setting clear rules or limits, a pattern that typically persists for several years, even if the mother remarries (Hetherington & Clingempeel, 1992). In all of this, it is still unclear what the causal agent is, because so many changes happen at the same time when a couple divorces: the loss of one member of the family system; often a rise in conflict between the parents; increased economic hardship; and other stressful life changes. The disruption in the children's behavior, and in the adults' behavior, seems to result from some combination of these factors, although open conflict between the parents may well be the most critical (Amato, 1993).

Open parental conflict has negative effects on children whether the parents divorce or not. Children whose parents fight often, physically or verbally, show more distress, more anger, more aggression than do children whose parents fight less openly or less often (Davies & Cummings, 1994), even when the parents are still together. So we should be careful not to blame all the bad outcomes on divorce itself. But divorce has normally been preceded by a period of more parental conflict. And after a divorce, the former spouses often continue to argue or bicker, all of which increases the risk for the child.

These are not comforting findings. Still, divorcing parents can do some things to buffer their children from the more severe effects—strategies I've discussed in the *Real World* box on page 388.

Summing Up What We Know About Family Structure. So where does all this leave us in our effort to understand the impact of family structure? My own reading of this growing body of evidence is that single parenthood (or divorce) has negative effects for two principal reasons. First, it reduces the financial and emotional resources available to support the child. With only one parent, there is only one income and only one adult to respond to the child's emotional needs. Equally important, single parenthood or divorce increases the likelihood that the family climate or style will shift away from optimal patterns toward much less supportive ones. In particular, it reduces the likelihood of authoritative parenting.

The key thing to understand is that authoritative child rearing is linked to low levels of disturbed behaviors and higher levels of psychological adjustment in the child, *no matter what family structure the child grows up in.* And authoritarian or neglecting parenting is linked to poor outcomes, whether it is triggered by a divorce, the father's loss of a job, or any other stress (Goldberg, 1990). Ultimately, it is this *process* within the family that is significant for the child. The likelihood of a nonoptimal family process is greater in single-parent families, but this does not mean that the probability is 1.0. Many single parents are able to find the strength within themselves to maintain a supportive process with their children. After all, we know three-quarters of children reared in single-parent or step-families manage to finish high school, and roughly half of those high school graduates go on to at least some college (McLanahan & Sandefur, 1994). Similarly, the great majority

Given what you have just read, how would you answer someone who asks you whether it is worse for an unhappy couple to get divorced or to stay together even though they fight all the time? What kind of study might you do to try to answer this question better?

The Real World

Softening the Effects of Divorce

Given the rate of divorce in our culture, a significant percentage of you reading these words will go through a divorce when you have children still living at home. There is no way to eliminate all the short-term disruptive effects of such an event on your children, but here are some specific things you can do that are likely to soften or shorten the effects:

1. Try to keep the number of separate changes the child has to cope with to a minimum. If at all possible, keep the children in the same school, the same home, the same day-care setting, and so on.

2. If your children are teenagers, consider having each child live with the parent of the same gender. The data are not totally consistent, but it looks as if this may be a less stressful arrangement (Lee et al., 1994). Alternatively, consider an arrangement in which the children spend roughly equal time with each parent. Some research suggests that this arrangement provides marginally better psychological support for the child than one in which the child lives entirely with one parent (Buchanan, Maccoby, & Dornbusch, 1992).

3. If the children live with you full time, help your children stay in touch with the noncustodial parent. If you are the noncustodial parent, maintain as much contact as possible with your children, calling regularly, seeing them regularly, attending school functions, and so on. I should tell you that the evidence on this point is actually quite mixed; some studies show no special benefit to the child of continued regular contact with the noncustodial parent (Emery, 1988). The difficulty in interpreting these results is that contact with the noncustodial parent is often confounded with the quality of the relationship between the now divorced parents, which leads to the next point:

4. If you and your ex-spouse continue to have conflict, try very hard not to fight in front of the children. Conflict itself is not inevitably detrimental; it is the conflict that the child actually sees and hears that adds to the child's level of stress and disruption (Emery, 1988). If such conflict is low, then increased contact with the noncustodial parent is beneficial to the child.

5. Whatever else you do, do not use the child as a go-between or talk disparagingly about your ex-spouse to your child. Children who feel caught in the middle between the two parents are more likely to show various kinds of negative symptoms, such as depression or behavior problems (Buchanan, Maccoby, & Dornbusch, 1991).

6. Maintain your own network of support and use that network liberally. Stay in touch with friends, seek out others in the same situation, and join a support group. In whatever way you can, nurture yourself and your own needs (Hetherington & Camera, 1984).

In the midst of your own emotional upheaval from a divorce, these are not easy prescriptions to follow. But if you are able to do so, your children will suffer less.

of children reared by a single parent or in a stepfamily do not become delinquent or show significant behavior problems. Obviously, many single or divorced parents manage to surmount the extra problems. But we need to face up to the fact that such family systems are less stable and, on average, less supportive for children.

Some Exosystem Effects: Parents' Work and Social Support

Beyond family structure, the family process is affected by a wide range of experiences in the *parents'* lives—experiences that occur outside the family's interactions but that nonetheless affect those interactions. The two examples I want to talk about are the parents' jobs and their network of social support.

Parents' Jobs

The existing research on the effects of parents' work on children contains an odd quirk: Nearly all the research on mothers' employment compares mothers who work with those who do not, while nearly all the work on the impact of fathers' employment focuses on fathers who have *lost* their jobs. We have little research on mothers who lose their jobs or on stay-at-home fathers compared with employed fathers. Given our cultural history, I suppose this pattern of research makes sense, although it certainly leaves some significant gaps in our knowledge. Fortunately, a new body of work is beginning to emerge that asks a very different kind of question, namely: What is the impact of the *quality* of the parents' work experience on family life?

Mothers' Employment.   How is life different for children whose mothers work, compared with those whose mothers stay home? Do these two groups of children differ in any systematic way? These questions are obviously not entirely separable from all the issues about day care I'll be talking about in the next chapter, since it is precisely because the mother is working that most children are in alternate care. But the question is also relevant when we look at families with school-age children, where the impact of the mother's work is not so totally confounded with the effects of the child's alternative care.

Most of the research points to a generally positive effect of the mother's employment, at least in this culture at this time. Girls whose mothers work are more independent and admire their mothers more than do girls whose mothers do not work. And both boys and girls whose mothers work have more egalitarian sex-role concepts. The effects of the mother's employment on the children's academic performance are less clear. Many studies show no differences; some studies show that among boys, those whose mothers work full time do slightly less well in school (Hoffman, 1989). One recent large study (Muller, 1995), involving a nationally representative sample of 24,599 eighth graders, shows a very small negative effect of the mother's employment on adolescents' math grades and test scores—a difference that seems to flow from the fact that when mothers work, they are less involved with the child's school and are less likely to supervise the teenager's schoolwork during the after-school hours. Working mothers who find ways to provide such supervision and who remain involved with their child's school have kids who do as well as children of homemaker mothers.

These findings point to the fact that it is not the mother's job per se that produces the effects linked to maternal employment; instead, her employment alters the family system in various ways. For one thing, having a job may affect the mother's own view of herself by increasing her self-esteem or her morale and thereby changing the way she relates to the rest of the family. For example, a woman who begins working generally acquires more power in the spousal relationship, in part because she now has demonstrable earning power and because she may feel more independent (Spitze, 1988). Such power or self-esteem also spills over into her interaction with her children, perhaps especially with a daughter. For example, Bronfenbrenner finds that working mothers give more positive descriptions of their young daughters than do nonworking mothers (Bronfenbrenner, Alvarez, & Henderson, 1984).

The mother's employment also forces changes in daily routines and in interaction patterns simply because she is not at home for as many hours. Fathers in dual-worker families spend somewhat more time in child care and household tasks than do fathers with homemaker wives, although it is still true that working mothers do about twice as much of this labor as do fathers (Blair & Johnson, 1992). This change in the division of

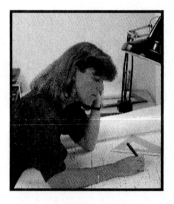

In the United States today, roughly half of women with children under age 3 and three-quarters of those with school-age or adolescent children work at least part time. In general, the effects seem to be beneficial for the children.

labor may have an effect on the quality of the parents' interaction with children and may alter the role model each parent provides for the child.

Finally, of course, when the mother works, it decreases the amount of time she has available for one-on-one interaction with the children, including supervision of the child's homework. These effects of employment on the woman and on her family are not automatic or uniform. The mother's attitude toward her work is an important intervening variable. Numerous studies show that the most negative outcomes are found among children in two subgroups: those with mothers who would prefer to work but are staying at home and those with working mothers who dislike their jobs or are unwilling workers (DeMeis, Hock, & McBride, 1986; Lerner & Galambos, 1986). The most positive outcomes occur when the mother wants to work and works at a job she likes. In such families, the mother's style of child rearing is more likely to be authoritative (Greenberger & Goldberg, 1989).

Fathers' Employment or Unemployment. I have already touched on the effects of a father's job loss when I talked about the McKenzie family at the beginning of this chapter. The research evidence tells us that when a man loses his job, it puts enormous strain on his marriage, so that marital conflict rises and both parents show more symptoms of depression. The resulting effects on family dynamics look much like what we see in divorcing families or in families facing other sorts of stresses: Both parents become less consistent in their behavior toward their children, less affectionate, and less good at monitoring (Conger, Patterson, & Ge, 1995). The children respond to this deterioration in their parents' behavior in the same way children do during a divorce: They show a variety of symptoms, including sometimes depression, aggression, or delinquency. Often their school performance declines (Conger et al., 1992; Conger et al., 1994; Flanagan & Eccles, 1993). The negative pattern can be softened if the unemployed father receives enough emotional support from his wife and is generally cured when the father again finds work. But the whole sequence illustrates nicely how an event outside the family affects the child through the impact on the parents' behavior toward one another and toward the child.

Quality of Parents' Work. The newer studies that examine the effects of the quality of the parents' work point to a similar conclusion. The now classic studies were done by Melvin Kohn and Carmi Schooler (Kohn, 1980; Kohn & Schooler, 1983), who found that men (or women) whose jobs require higher levels of self-direction and autonomy

In December of 1991, these General Motors workers had just heard that the company would be laying off 74,000 employees over the next few years. Such an upheaval affects the worker's family not only economically, but also psychologically. Adults typically become less authoritative in their child rearing in the face of such stress.

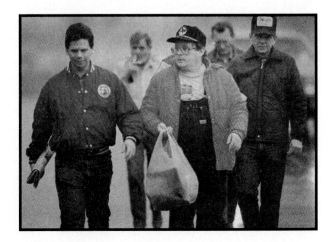

showed increases in intellectual flexibility over time. Routine, highly supervised jobs led to decreases in intellectual flexibility. Kohn's own work and that of several current researchers (Greenberger, O'Neil, & Nagel, 1994; Parcel & Menaghan, 1994) show that these differences spill over into family life. Men and women who work at routine jobs come to place greater emphasis on obedience from their children than is true for parents in more intellectually flexible jobs, a pattern that has been found among African-American parents as well as Euro-Americans (Mason et al., 1994). Furthermore, when a mother who has been at home with her children begins work at a job that is low in complexity, the child's home environment deteriorates, becoming less stimulating and supportive than it was before; however, beginning work at an intellectually complex job is linked to improvements in the child's environment (Menaghan & Parcel, 1995). In the terms I have been using in this chapter, complex jobs are linked to increases in authoritative and decreases in authoritarian child rearing. Thus, the character of a parent's job affects his (or her) way of thinking, particularly his thinking about authority, and he applies that thinking to his interactions with his children.

Social Support for Parents

A second aspect of parents' lives that affects the family microsystem is the quality of their network of relationships and their satisfaction with the social support they receive from that network. The general point is fairly easy to state: Parents who have access to adequate emotional and physical support—from each other or from friends and family—are able to respond to their children more warmly, more consistently, and with better control (Crnic et al., 1983; Taylor, Casten, & Flickinger, 1993). Their children, in turn, look better on a variety of measures (Melson, Ladd, & Hsu, 1993). For example, children whose parents have access to more assistance from friends complete more years of school than do children whose parents have less support of this type (Hofferth, Boisjoly, & Duncan, 1995).

The effect of social support on parents is particularly evident when they experience stress, such as job loss, chronic poverty, teenage childbirth, a temperamentally difficult or handicapped infant, divorce, or even just fatigue. You may recall the discussion in Chapter 9 of a study by Susan Crockenberg (1981) that illustrates the point nicely. She found that temperamentally irritable infants were very likely to end up with an insecure attachment to their mothers only when the mother *lacked* adequate social support. When the mother felt that she had enough support, similarly irritable children were later securely attached. There are many other examples of this "buffering effect" of social support:

- New mothers who lack good social and emotional support are more likely to suffer from postpartum depression than are those with adequate support (Cutrona & Troutman, 1986).

- Divorced parents who have help and emotional support from friends or family members are much more able to maintain a stable and affectionate environment for their children than are those who grapple with the problem in isolation (Hetherington, 1989).

- Among African-American single mothers, those who have enough aid and emotional support from kin show a more authoritative style of parenting than do single mothers lacking such aid (Taylor et al., 1993).

As a general rule, social support seems to allow parents to mobilize the best parenting skills they may have in their repertoire. Of course not all "help" from families or friends feels like support. (I'm sure you have all been given unwanted advice from your parents or in-laws or friends!) The key is not the objective amount of contact or advice received, but the parent's *satisfaction* with the level and quality of the support he or she is experiencing. The moral seems to be that at those times of greatest difficulty or stress—when a new child is born, when a child presents special difficulties, when the family moves or experiences major changes—you most need the emotional and physical support of others. But if you wait until that difficult moment to look around and see who is there to help, you may not find what you need. Social networks must be developed and nurtured over time. But they certainly seem to pay dividends for parents, and thus for children.

Summary

1 To understand children's development we must move beyond examination of the child alone or the mother-child pair. We must examine the total ecological system.

2 A system is understood as being more than the sum of its parts. It is also adaptive to change, and any change in any one part of the system affects every other part.

3 Bronfenbrenner conceives of the child's ecological system as composed of three types of elements: microsystems, such as the family or the school, in which the child is directly involved; exosystems, such as the parent's job, which affect the child indirectly by influencing some aspect of a microsystem; and macrosystems, such as the ethnic subculture, or the broader society or culture in which the family exists.

4 Within the family microsystem several dimensions of parental behavior toward children seem to be particularly significant, including the emotional tone of the family, the method of maintaining control, and the patterns of communication.

5 Families that provide high levels of warmth and affection, compared to those that are more cold or rejecting, have children with more secure attachments and better peer relationships.

6 Families that have clear rules and standards, and relatively high levels of expectation or maturity demands and that enforce those rules and expectations consistently have children with the greatest

self-esteem and the greatest competence across a broad range of situations.

7 Children who are talked to frequently, in complex sentences, and who are listened to in turn not only develop language more rapidly, but also have more-positive and less-conflicted relationships with their parents.

8 These elements of parental behavior occur in combinations or styles of child rearing. Four such styles, suggested by several theorists, are authoritarian, authoritative, permissive, and neglecting.

9 The authoritative style is high in nurturance, control, communication, and maturity demands; the authoritarian style is high in control and maturity demands but low in warmth and communication; the permissive style is high in warmth and low in communication, control, and maturity demands; the neglecting style is low on all dimensions.

10 The authoritative style appears to be the most generally effective for producing confident, competent, independent, and affectionate children. The most negative outcomes are found in neglecting families.

11 Research by Steinberg and Dornbusch suggests ethnic differences in the ways in which family styles affect children. In particular, Asian-American children do generally very well in school despite low rates of authoritative parenting, which may indicate that the categorization of family styles is culture-specific.

12   The family system is also affected by the child's characteristics, such as temperament, age, gender, and position in the family.

13   Siblings growing up in the same family nonetheless often turn out very differently. New research suggests that parents often behave quite differently toward different children.

14   Parental characteristics that affect the family system include depression and the parent's own internal working model of attachment.

15   The structure of the family also has an impact on family functioning, which in turn affects children's behavior. The majority of children born in the United States today will spend at least a portion of their childhood in one-parent families.

16   Children reared in single-parent families are at higher risk for a variety of negative outcomes, including school dropout, teen parenthood, and delinquency. Stepfamilies too are associated with heightened risks for the children.

17   Any change in family structure, such as after a divorce, is likely to produce short-term disruption (often including an increase in authoritarian or neglecting child-rearing style) before the system adapts to a new form.

18   A mother's employment affects the family system by changing the mother's self-image, increasing her power, and altering the distribution of labor. The effects on the children are generally positive, especially for girls.

19   A father's job loss disrupts the family system, increasing authoritative child rearing and reducing marital satisfaction. Children often show disrupted behavior.

20   The character of a parent's job also has an effect on family interactions. Complex jobs that demand greater independence are linked to increased authoritative parenting, while less complex, routine jobs are linked to increases in authoritarian control.

21   The impact of family change or stress is mitigated by the availability of a sufficient amount of social support from the parents' social network.

Key Terms

authoritarian parental style (p. 373)

authoritative parental style (p. 373)

neglecting parental style (p. 374)

permissive parental style (p. 373)

responsiveness (p. 368)

restrictiveness (p. 370)

warmth versus hostility (p. 367)

Suggested Readings

Boer, F., & Dunn, J. (Eds.). (1992). *Children's sibling relationships: Developmental and clinical issues.* Hillsdale, NJ: Erlbaum.

A first-rate collection of papers on a subject that is of growing interest to many psychologists. Each paper is relatively brief and reviews the available literature on one aspect of sibling relationships.

Furstenberg, F. F., Jr., & Cherlin, A. J. (1991). *Divided families: What happens to children when parents part.* Cambridge, MA: Harvard University Press.

A relatively brief, current review of this important subject, aimed at lay readers and decision makers rather than at other psychologists. The focus is on the impact of divorce on children.

Hernandez, D. J. (1993). *America's children: Resources from family, government, and the economy.* New York: Russell Sage Foundation.

A dense, difficult, but remarkable book based on U.S. Census data and exploring everything that we know about the status of children in the United States. He focuses particularly on the changing demographics of mother's employment, single parenthood, and family incomes as they affect children. Not easy reading, but fascinating.

McLanahan, S., & Sandefur, G. (1994). *Growing up with a single parent: What hurts, what helps.* Cambridge, MA: Harvard University Press.

A sobering book, based on a careful reading of five major national studies, several of them longitudinal in design. It is well worth a look, if only because it raises some crucial issues. It is also written in a not too technical style that I think you will find comprehensible.

Beyond the Family: The Impact of the Broader Culture

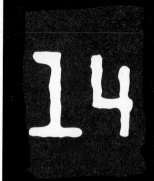

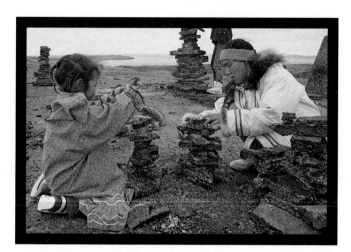

The ecological approach to studying the family's influence on the child's development has brought us many new insights. But of course we cannot stop at the edges of the family. To understand a child's development, we must also understand the impact of other institutions that affect the child directly. And as a final step, we need to try to understand the ways in which all these institutions are embedded in still broader subcultural and cultural contexts. In the best of all possible worlds, we would look at these beyond-the-family effects in many different cultural systems: in collectivist as well as individualist cultures, in nonindustrialized as well as highly industrialized systems, in stable cultures and those undergoing change, in cultures in which schooling is rare or brief as well as those in which it is a normal part of childhood, and so on and on. Ultimately, we will need such an analysis to understand the ways in which nonfamily influences shape the child's development. But not only is such an analysis beyond the scope of this book, it is also beyond the scope of our knowledge. So what I want to try to do here is to take our own complex culture as a kind of case study, looking at what we know about the ways in which nonfamily institutions affect the child, beginning with several institutions with which the child is likely to have direct experience: day care, schools, part-time jobs, and television.

Day Care

In virtually every industrialized country in the world, in the past two decades, women have gone into the workforce in great numbers. In the United States the change has been particularly rapid and massive: In 1972, only 24 percent of women with children under age 1 were in the labor force; by 1991 the *majority* of such women were working outside the home at least part time, a rate that appears to be higher than that for any other country in the world (Cherlin, 1992). It is now typical for infants as well as school-age children to spend a significant amount of time being cared for by someone other than a parent. Similar changes have occurred in other countries to a lesser degree, but in the discussion to follow I'm going to be talking almost exclusively about day care as it exists in the United States.

What effect does such nonparental care have on infants and young children? As you can easily imagine, this is *not* a simple question to answer, for a whole host of reasons:

- An enormous variety of different care arrangements are all lumped under the general title of "day care."

- Children enter these care arrangements at different ages and remain in them for varying lengths of time.

- Some children have the same alternate caregiver over many years; others shift often from one care setting to another.

- Day care varies hugely in quality.

- Families who place their children in day care are undoubtedly different in a whole host of ways from those who care for their children primarily at home. How can we be sure that effects attributed to day care are not the result of these other family differences instead?

Most of the research we have to draw on does not really take these complexities into account. Researchers have frequently compared children "in day care" with those "reared at home" and have assumed that any differences between the two groups were attributable to the day-care experience. Recent studies are often better, but we are still a long way from having clear or good answers to even the most basic questions about the impact of day care on children's development. Nonetheless, because the question is so critical, you need to be aware of what we know, as well as what we do not yet know.

Who Is Taking Care of the Children?

Let me begin at the descriptive level. Just who is taking care of all those children while their parents work? In some countries, such as France or Belgium, child care is organized and subsidized by the government and free to all parents. In the United States we have

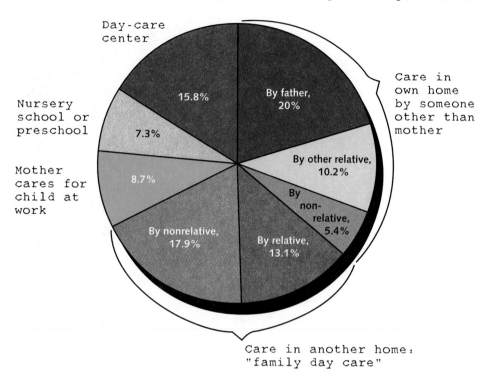

Day-care
center

Nursery
school or
preschool

Mother
cares for
child at
work

Care in
own home
by someone
other than
mother

Care in another home:
"family day care"

By father,
20%

By other relative,
10.2%

By non-relative,
5.4%

By nonrelative,
17.9%

By relative,
13.1%

15.8%

7.3%

8.7%

FIGURE 14.1 Child-care arrangements in the United States in 1991 for children 5 and under whose mothers worked outside the home at least part time. (*Source:* U.S. Bureau of the Census, 1994, Table 603.)

no such governmental system, and each family must make its own arrangements as best it can.

Figure 14.1 summarizes the solutions working parents have found. I'll bet these figures surprise you. When they think of "day care," most people think of a day-care center or perhaps someone caring for a group of children in a home (called **family day care**). But in fact, the most common pattern today is for a child to be cared for in his *own* home, by the father, by another relative, or by someone employed for that purpose. Family day care is a close second. Day-care centers are actually one of the least common arrangements, although this varies somewhat by age. Among 3- and 4-year-olds, center care or nursery school care is the most frequent choice; for infants under 1 year of age, care by a relative and family day care are much more common (U.S. Bureau of the Census, 1994).

But even the wide variability in the type of care illustrated in the figure does not begin to convey the enormous variety of solutions parents arrive at in seeking alternative care for their children. For example, a very popular combination is to have a child in a nursery school for part of each day, with the remainder of the child's care provided by some kind of in-home caregiver, sometimes the mother who is working only part time, a grandmother part of the time, or some other creative combination (Clarke-Stewart, Gruber, & Fitzgerald, 1994). For example, in one recent national survey, between a quarter and a third of employed mothers reported that their children are in some type of combined care, such as family day care combined with relative care (Folk & Yi, 1994)—arrangements that are often dictated by the fact that the parent works an evening or night shift, or at variable times.

High-quality care is possible in any of these settings, although they do differ from one another in systematic ways. For example, center care typically provides the most cognitive enrichment, while family day-care homes typically provide the least; both center

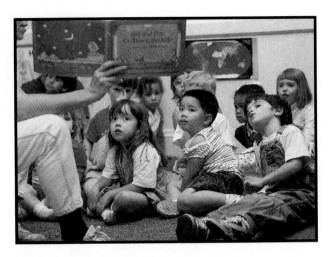

The majority of children in the U.S. have at least some experience with nonparental care, although group care like this day-care center is not at all the most common form.

care and family day care give the child an opportunity to play with same-age peers, while at-home care does not. Such variations make it very difficult to talk about global effects of day care, because the systems are quite different. Furthermore, the majority of researchers have studied exclusively children in center care, and we cannot be sure that these findings will generalize to children in family day care or with at-home care by someone other than a parent (let alone to some other culture altogether!). Still, let me tell you what the current evidence suggests.

Effects on Cognitive Development

Until fairly recently, the standard conclusion about the effects of day care on children's cognitive development was that such care has little effect on the cognitive development of children from advantaged families but that it often has a positive effect on children from disadvantaged families (Scarr & Eisenberg, 1993). When the child care is highly cognitively enriched, the beneficial effect for poor children is especially clear, as in the Ramey programs I talked about in Chapter 6 (see Figure 6.4).

Newer research, though, suggests that this apparently clear conclusion requires some qualification. On the positive side, a study in Sweden, where day care is typically of very high quality, suggests that even middle-class children may benefit intellectually from day care, especially when they begin such care in infancy. Andersson (1992) found that among a large group of 13-year-olds, those who had spent the most time in day-care centers had better school performance throughout elementary school compared to those totally home-reared or those with only minimal day-care experience. And in a study in the U.S., Alison Clarke-Stewart (Clarke-Stewart et al., 1994) finds that regardless of the economic situation of the child's parents, the more cognitively enriched the child's daytime experience—at home or in day care—the higher the child's later cognitive performance. Children who are read to, talked to, and explicitly taught show greater cognitive gains than do children who spend their days in less stimulating environments.

Ranged on the other side are several studies in the United States that point to possible negative effects of day-care experience on cognitive development in some children, perhaps particularly middle-class children. This is especially clear in two studies of the children of a large sample of young adults who have participated in a large longitudinal study called the National Longitudinal Study of Youth. One group of researchers (Baydar

& Brooks-Gunn, 1991) has studied the 3- and 4-year-old offspring of this group—a sample of more than 1000 children; another set of investigators (Caughy, DiPietro, & Strobino, 1994) has looked at the outcomes for the 5- and 6-year-olds. In both cases, they were able to compare results for children reared entirely at home with outcomes for kids who had been in day care for varying lengths of time and beginning at various ages. Among the white 3- and 4-year-olds—but *not* among the black children—those who began some kind of alternative care in the first year of life had the lowest vocabulary scores later in preschool, whether they were from advantaged or poverty-level families. No negative effects were found for those who entered day care after age 1. Among the 5- and 6-year-olds, the pattern of results was a bit different: Those from poor families who began day care before age 1 had *higher* reading or math scores at the start of school, while those from middle-class families who entered day care in infancy had *poorer* scores.

How can we reconcile these myriad findings? One fairly straightforward possibility is that the crucial issue is the discrepancy between the level of stimulation the child would receive at home and the quality of the child care. When the day-care setting for a child provides *more* enrichment than that child would normally receive at home, we see some beneficial cognitive effects. When day care is less stimulating than the child's home care would have been, it has negative effects. Most (but not all) of the results I've described are consistent with this hypothesis, but we don't yet have enough good, large studies to be confident that this is the right way to conceptualize the process.

Do you buy this argument? What other explanation(s) can you come up with?

Effects on Personality

When we look at the impact of day care on children's personality, we find yet another confusing story. A number of investigators have found that children in day care are more sociable and popular, and have better peer-play skills than do those reared primarily at home. Andersson found this in his longitudinal study in Sweden (1989; 1992), as have researchers in the United States (Scarr & Eisenberg, 1993). But this is by no means the consistent finding. Many other researchers find day-care attendance linked to subsequently heightened aggression with peers and lower compliance with teachers and parents. For example, in one very-well-designed large study, John Bates and his colleagues (Bates et al., 1994) find that among kindergarten children, those who had spent the most time in day care—in infancy, toddlerhood, or preschool years—were more aggressive and less popular with their peers at school age than were children who had been reared entirely at home or who had spent fewer years in day care. Bates did not find that those who had entered day care early in infancy were worse off; the critical variable was the total length of time in nonhome care, not the timing of that care.

I should hasten to add that these negative effects are fairly small. A child's level of aggressiveness in elementary school is influenced by a whole variety of things, including temperament and the effectiveness of the parents' disciplinary techniques. But the fact that day care is implicated in this equation certainly raises a cautionary note.

Confusing, isn't it? By some measures day-care children seem to be *more* socially competent; by other measures, they seem less so. One possible resolution is again to look at the relative quality of care at home or in day care. Consistent with this argument is a finding by Tiffany Field (1991) that the beneficial effects of day-care experience on the child's social competence holds only for *good-quality* care. Similarly, Alison Clarke-Stewart, in a study comparing various types of day care (Clarke-Stewart et al., 1994), finds that what is critical for the child's level of aggression is whether the child was spending his daytime hours in an organized, well-structured situation or in a messy, unstimulating one—whether the unstructured and messy setting was a home or a day-care setting. If this argument holds, then it is not day care per se that is at issue, but the child's daily experiences. But even if this turns out to be the best explanation of the observed negative effects, it is hardly cause for cheering. The children in Bates's study, for example, were in ordinary, everyday types of day-care situations. And if run-of-the-mill care is of such poor quality that it has even small negative effects on children's later behavior, we need to be concerned. Some psychologists, perhaps most notably Jay Belsky, take this pessimism a step further and argue that these hints of behavioral maladjustment among children who have been in day care may reflect more basic difficulties in the child, such as problems with attachment.

Effects on Children's Attachments to Parents

Can an infant or toddler develop a secure attachment to her mother or father if she is repeatedly separated from them? This question has been at the center of a hot debate. We know that the majority of infants develop secure attachments to their fathers, even though the father typically goes away every day to work, so it is clear that such regular separations do not *preclude* secure attachment. Still, perhaps separation from both parents on a daily basis adversely affects the security of the child's attachment.

We can narrow the window of uncertainty a good deal if we consider the child's age at the time she or he first enters day care. All parties to the current dispute agree that children who enter day care after the first year of life show *no* consistent loss of security of attachment to their parents. But the effects on infants who enter day care before 12 months of age are still hotly disputed.

Until about a decade ago, most psychologists reading the relevant research had concluded that there was no negative effect of infant day care. But then Belsky, in a series of papers and in testimony before a congressional committee, sounded an alarm (1985; 1992; Belsky & Rovine, 1988). Combining data from several studies, he concluded that there was a heightened risk of an insecure attachment among infants who enter day care before their first birthday. Controversy erupted. Since that time, a number of other researchers have analyzed the combined results from larger numbers of studies and confirmed Belsky's original conclusion.

Summing across the findings from 13 different studies involving 897 infants, Michael Lamb (Lamb, Sternberg, & Prodromidis, 1992) reported that 35 percent of infants who had experienced at least 5 hours per week of nonmaternal care were insecurely attached, compared to 29 percent of the infants with exclusively maternal care. He also found that the risk of an insecure attachment did *not* rise as the number of hours of the mother's employment increased. That is, babies whose mothers worked 40 hours a week, or 20 hours a week, were not more likely to be insecurely attached than those whose mothers worked 5 hours a week.

This is clearly not a huge difference, although it is statistically significant. The present controversy swirls around how to interpret or explain this difference.

Belsky has his supporters. Alan Sroufe, one of the major figures in studies of early attachment, points out that we know that security of attachment is fostered both by the child's sense of the responsiveness of care and by the opportunity for parent and child to fine-tune their interactive dance. Both of these may be disrupted by placing the child in

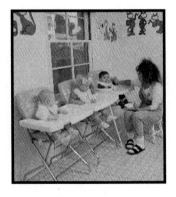

Only when babies enter day care before age 1, as some of these youngsters seem to have done, is there a slightly increased likelihood of an insecure attachment. But psychologists are still arguing about how to interpret this difference, or even whether we ought to worry about it at all.

day care, although clearly in the majority of cases, parents find ways to counteract such disruptions, because the majority of children in day care are nonetheless securely attached (Sroufe, 1990).

On the other side of the argument are ranged a group of researchers who either don't believe there is a serious problem to be dealt with or argue that there are so many confounding variables that it is impossible to draw any clear conclusion (e.g., Roggman et al., 1994). For one thing, a serious problem of self-selection is involved in any comparison of day-care and parent-reared infants. Mothers who work are different in other ways from mothers who do not. More are single mothers, more prefer to work or find child care onerous. So how can we be sure that any heightened probability of insecure attachment is due to the day-care experience and not to other factors?

For these and other reasons, Alison Clarke-Stewart (1990) concludes that "at the present time . . . it is not appropriate to interpret the difference, as Belsky appears to, as suggesting that these children are emotionally insecure" (p. 69). Others have concluded that there may indeed be a link between some aspect of day care and security of attachment but that we simply don't yet know what the link might be (Lamb et al., 1992).

One can also argue that Belsky is asking the wrong question. For the vast majority of families, the question is not "Should I put my child in day care?" but rather "Given that I have to work to help support my family, how do I find good-quality, affordable care for my child?"

Everything I have already said underlines the importance of the quality of the child's care. Good-quality care is generally linked with positive or neutral outcomes, while inconsistent or poor-quality custodial care can be actively detrimental to the child. In Table 14.1 I've listed the characteristics of good-quality programs, a list that might serve as a starting point in your evaluation of alternatives if and when you face this choice with your own children.

> What other differences might you expect to find between working and nonworking mothers of infants? How might those differences affect the likelihood that a child would be securely or insecurely attached?

Table 14.1
Ideal Characteristics of a Day-Care Setting

A low teacher/child ratio. For children younger than 2, the ratio should be no higher than 1:4; for 2- to 3-year-olds, ratios between 1:4 and 1:10 appear to be okay.

A small group size. The smaller the number of children cared for together—whether in one room in a day-care center or in a home—the better for the child. For infants, a maximum of 6 to 8 per group appears best; for 1- to 2-year-olds, between 6 and 12 per group; for older children, groups as large as 15 or 20 appear to be okay.

A clean, colorful space, adapted to child play. Lots of expensive toys are not critical, but there must be a variety of activities that children will find engaging, organized in a way that encourages play.

A daily plan with at least some structure, some specific teaching, some supervised activities. Too much regimentation is not ideal, but children are better off with *some* structure.

A caregiver who is positive, involved, and responsive to the child, not merely custodial.

A caregiver with some knowledge of child development.

Sources: Clarke-Stewart, 1992; Howes, Phillips, & Whitebook, 1992; Scarr & Eisenberg, 1993.

The Impact of Schools

Another vitally important "microsystem" experienced by virtually all children in the great majority of cultures is school. School normally begins between ages 5 and 7, and in industrialized countries typically continues through age 16 or older. During these 10 or more years, the child learns an enormous number of facts and develops new and much more complex forms of thinking, many of which I talked about in Chapter 7. But what role does schooling itself play in this set of cognitive changes? Is schooling the *cause* of the cognitive shifts Piaget referred to as concrete and formal operations?

Schooling and Cognitive Development

Researchers have attempted to test this hypothesis by studying children in societies or cultures in which schooling is not compulsory or is not universally available. By comparing similar groups of children, some of them in school and some of them not, it may be possible to discover the role that schooling plays in cognitive development. Alternatively, researchers in countries with compulsory schooling have compared children who are nearly the same age but who have different years of schooling, such as children whose birthdays are just before or just after the cutoff date for entry into first grade (e.g., Bisanz, Morrison, & Dunn, 1995).

A wide variety of such studies—in Mexico, Peru, Colombia, Liberia, Zambia, Nigeria, Uganda, Hong Kong, and many other countries—has led to the conclusion that school experiences are indeed causally linked to the emergence of advanced cognitive skills. Children who do not attend schools do not learn many complex concepts and strategies and are not as good at generalizing a learned concept or principle to some new setting. So attending school helps children learn to think, which is precisely what it is intended to do.

A good illustration of this effect comes from Harold Stevenson's study of the Quechua Indian children of Peru (Stevenson & Chen, 1989; Stevenson et al., 1991). He and his associates tested 6- to 8-year-old children in rural areas as well as in city barrios, and in each setting they tested some who had been in school for about six months and some who had not yet started school or who were living in an area where no school was available. Stevenson found that in both rural and urban areas, schooled children performed better on virtually all tasks, including a measure of seriation (putting things in serial order, such as by size or length) and a measure of concept formation. These differences remained even if the parents' level of education, the nutritional status of the child, and the amount of educational enrichment offered at home were taken into account. Only on measures of memory, such as the ability to repeat back a set of numbers that had been read to the child, were there no differences.

This does not mean that schooling is the only way for children to acquire complex forms of thinking. Specific experience in some area can also promote expertise. But schooling exposes children to many specific skills and classes of knowledge, and it appears to stimulate the development of more abstract, flexible, generalized strategies for remembering and solving problems.

Schooling may also have important cultural side effects. For example, in a study in rural Mexico, Medardo Uribe (Uribe, LeVine, & LeVine, 1994) noted that children who attended school showed a shift away from a more collectivist and toward a more individualist set of values, a change that can produce conflict in a home dominated by a collectivist perspective. Indeed, Uribe reports that in the community he studied, many parents chose not to send their children to school because they saw the school experience as undermining family and culture.

Fitting in and Adapting to School

School is not just a neutral setting for acquiring cognitive skills. It is a complex social environment, with its own rules and values, with intricate peer relationships, with new demands. Among children in the U.S., a key factor in the child's successful adaptation to this new environment is his readiness to learn to read. But it is not the only factor. Parent involvement in the school also matters, as do some aspects of the child's temperament.

When parents come regularly to parent-teacher conferences and open houses, attend school events, and get involved in supervising the child's homework, children are more strongly motivated, feel more competent, and adapt better to school. They learn to read more readily and get better grades through elementary school (Grolnick & Slowiaczek, 1994; Reynolds & Bezruczko, 1993). This effect of parent involvement has been found within groups of poor children as well as among the middle class, which tells us that the effect is not just a social class difference in disguise.

But it also matters whether the child's own personality or temperament matches the qualities valued and rewarded within the school setting. For example, Karl Alexander and his colleagues (Alexander, Entwisle, & Dauber, 1993) have found that children who are enthusiastic, interested in new things, cheerful, easygoing, and not restless do better in the early years of school than those who are more withdrawn, moody, or high-strung.

What all this research indicates is that the way a child starts out in the first few years of school has a highly significant effect on the rest of her school experience and success. To a considerable degree, the "rich get richer." Children who come to school with good skills clearly have an easier time. They then acquire more new skills and can thus adapt to later school demands more easily. Children who enter school with poor skills and less optimal temperamental qualities learn less in the early years. The trajectory is not inevitable. Parent involvement can make a difference; a particularly skillful first-grade teacher can make a difference. But the child does not enter school with a blank slate; she brings her history, her qualities with her.

The consequences of these different trajectories and of the different beliefs about their own abilities that students develop (and that I talked about in Chapter 10) are substantial. For instance, students who believe they can do well are more likely to choose classes that prepare them for college. Students who do not believe they can do well make quite different choices, or may drop out of school altogether. Let me say just a few words about these two ends of the achievement continuum.

Achievers. You'll remember from Chapter 6 that the best single predictor of a student's academic performance in high school is IQ and that this is true for every ethnic and social class group in U.S. society. Both adolescent IQ and school grades also predict adult job success to at least some degree (Barrett & Depinet, 1991). A myriad of studies of military jobs, for example, show correlations in the range of .45 to .55 between scores on IQ-like tests and the recruits' later proficiency and success at a wide range of jobs (Ree & Earles, 1992). Outside of the military, the same general relationship holds, although education plays a key intervening role. Students with higher IQ or better grades in high school tend to go on to more years of additional education, and this is as true among

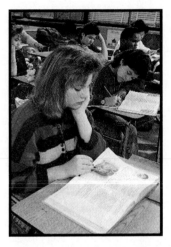

This Texas high school girl taking a weekly test in her biology class already has quite firmly developed beliefs about her abilities and potentials, based on her past school successes and failures. These beliefs will affect important life choices, such as whether to go to college or drop out of school altogether.

Research Report

Underachievers

Particularly puzzling and interesting are those students who achieve at consistently lower levels than you would predict, based on their IQ or other test scores: *under-achievers*. Two or three times as many boys as girls fall into this category, but underachievers come from families at every economic level and from every ethnic group.

A large and comprehensive study by Robert McCall and his colleagues (McCall, Evahn, & Kratzer, 1992) gives us a picture of this group. They studied 6720 teenagers who had completed an extensive questionnaire when they were juniors or seniors in high school during the middle 1960s. Thirteen years later, when the subjects were between 28 and 31 years old, nearly 5000 of them were interviewed on the phone about their adult lives.

Within this large group, McCall identified those whose school grades had been significantly lower than what would have been predicted by standardized test scores. He then compared these underachievers to several other subgroups, including some who had the same apparent ability but had achieved at a level commensurate with their ability and others who had achieved at about the same lower level as the underachievers but whose standardized scores were also low.

Several results stand out from these analyses. First, the underachievers had consistently low self-esteem. In high school they saw themselves as having less competence and less ability to do well in school, and they had lower aspirations for their future. Such low self-esteem and low expectations were not unique to underachievers. Other students who were getting poor grades in school expressed many of the same ideas, which underlines the general conclusion that students' perceptions of their abilities are strongly linked to the evaluations they are receiving in school.

What was unique about the underachievers, though, was their consistently poorer performance in adulthood—poorer even than low-ability students who had been receiving equivalently low grades in high school. The underachievers were less likely to complete college than any of the other groups, had lower-status jobs with lower income at age 30, and were 50 percent more likely to have divorced in the 13 years after high school.

A few underachievers "caught up" later in life. In particular, those few who, despite their relatively poor grades, nonetheless had high aspirations and saw themselves as able to complete college did catch up to their higher-achieving peers. But this was the exception. Most did not "get their act together" later on, and this was particularly true of those whose high school performance was substantially below expectations. In the end, McCall concludes that the most striking quality of underachievers is their "lack of persistence in the face of challenge and adversity" (p. 143). They lack the stick-to-itiveness needed to succeed in school, on a job, or in a marriage.

McCall's study doesn't tell us where such lack of persistence may have come from. Nor does it indicate what type of intervention, if any, would be successful in altering the pattern of underachievement and nonperseverence characteristic of these young people. But it does suggest that underachievement is a recognizable syndrome, one we need to know more about.

---

children reared in poverty as it is among the middle class (Barrett & Depinet, 1991). Those extra years of education, in turn, have a powerful effect on the career path a young person enters in early adulthood (Rosenbaum, 1984).

You are surely an achiever or you would not be reading this book. Does the profile of the achiever fit you?

These relationships exist not just because brighter kids have an easier time with schoolwork, but also because the cumulative effect of success over many years of schooling fosters a greater sense of self-efficacy in these intellectually more able students. Those who achieve, especially those who achieve despite poverty backgrounds or other daunting obstacles, also are more likely to have parents who have high aspirations for them (Brooks-Gunn, Guo, & Furstenberg, 1993b) or an authoritative family style. So as always, the effect of the family and the effect of the school interact.

Dropouts. At the other end of the continuum are those who drop out of school before completing high school—a rarer occurrence than you might guess. Roughly three-quarters of young adults in the U.S. have received a high school diploma, and another 12 percent receive a General Equivalency Diploma (GED) later. So only about 15 percent of current young adults failed to graduate from high school (McLanahan & Sandefur, 1994). Among students in the most recent high school classes, the rate is even lower. For example, among those students who entered high school in 1988, only 11 percent had failed to graduate by 1993. Hispanics had the highest dropout rates in this group at 32 percent, compared to 16 percent for African-Americans and 10 percent for Anglos (*New York Times,* 1994).

Despite these ethnic difference, social class is a better predictor than is ethnicity. Kids growing up in poor families—especially poor families with a single parent—are considerably more likely to drop out of high school than are those from more economically advantaged or intact families. When you hold social class constant, drop-out rates among blacks, whites, and Hispanics differ very little (Entwisle, 1990). But because minority youth in the United States are so much more likely to come from poor families or from families that do not provide psychological support for academic achievement, they are also more likely to drop out of school. When a teenager's peer group also puts a low value on achievement, as is true in many black and Hispanic teen groups in the United States, the risk of dropping out is even stronger (Takei & Dubas, 1993).

Teenagers who drop out of school list many reasons for such a decision, including not liking school, poor grades, being suspended, or needing to find work to support a family. For girls there are additional factors. They most often say that they dropped out because they planned to marry, were pregnant, or felt that school was simply not for them (Center for Health Statistics, 1987). Some of these same factors appear when we try to predict which kids will drop out. For example, in their longitudinal study of more than 500 children, Robert and Beverly Cairns (1994) find two strong predictors of subsequent dropout: whether the teenager had a history of low academic success, often including repeating a grade, and whether there was a pattern of aggressive behavior. More than 80 percent of boys and about 50 percent of girls who had shown *both* characteristics in seventh grade later dropped out of school before completing high school. For girls in this study, giving birth or getting married were also strongly linked to dropping out—although it was also true that early pregnancy was more likely among girls who had a history of poor school performance or high levels of aggression. So it is unclear what is cause and what is effect here.

Yet another factor for some adolescents is their perception that a high school diploma won't buy them much extra in the job world. Some of the young men in the Cairns study, for example, were already working part time at jobs that paid above the minimum wage and saw no rationale for staying in school when they could earn more by working full time. Here are two voices:

> *"[School] was boring, I felt like I knew all I had to know . . . was going to go back . . . , but I figure I was making $6 an hour and nothing in school, so . . ." (Chuck)*

> *"I just hate it. I said well if I could go to school 8 hours a day, I could get me a job 8 hours a day, 5 days a week. I said I'm going to school 40 hours a week and I said I'm not getting paid for it and I said well I'm gonna go get me a job and get paid" (Amy) (Cairns & Cairns, 1994, pp. 180, 181)*

Yet in the long term, teens who use such a rationale for dropping out of high school are wrong. Unemployment is higher among high school dropouts than in any other

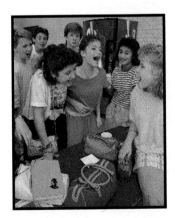

The odds tell us that out of these seven junior high schoolers, one will likely drop out of high school.

education group, and dropouts who do manage to find jobs earn lower wages than do those with a high school diploma. In 1984, for example, the average yearly income of young men (ages 25–44) with some high school education was $15,684, compared to $21,851 for those who had graduated from high school and $33,319 for those who had graduated from college (Crystal, Shae, & Krishnaswami, 1992). The difference between these two groups may be smaller today than it was in 1984; a man or woman with a high school diploma can no longer count on finding good-paying, skilled industrial jobs, as was the case even a decade ago. But a high school education still offers distinct advantages. Those who drop out enter a very different—and far less optimal—life trajectory.

School Quality

A very different set of questions about school experience has to do with variations in the quality of the schools themselves. Real estate agents have always touted a "good school district" as a reason for settling in one town or neighborhood rather than in another. Now we have research to show that the real estate agents were right: Specific characteristics of schools, and teachers, do affect children's development.

Researchers interested in possible effects of good and poor schools have most often approached the problem by identifying unusually "effective" or "successful" schools (Good & Weinstein, 1986; Rutter, 1983). In this research, an effective school is defined as one in which pupils show one or more of the following characteristics at higher rates than you would predict, knowing the kind of families or neighborhoods the pupils come from: high scores on standardized tests, good school attendance, low rates of disruptive classroom behavior or delinquency, a high rate of later college attendance, or high self-esteem. Some schools seem to achieve such good outcomes consistently, year after year, so the effect is unlikely to result from mere chance. When these successful schools are compared to others in similar neighborhoods that have less-impressive track records, certain common themes emerge, summarized in Table 14.2.

What strikes me when I read this list is how much effective schools sound like authoritative parenting. They have clear goals and rules, good control, good communication, and high nurturance. The same seems to be true of effective teachers: The pupils of "authoritative" teachers do best academically. Such teachers have clear goals, clear rules, effective management strategies, and personal and warm relationships with their pupils (Linney & Seidman, 1989). They also have high expectations for their students and make sure that virtually all the students in their classes complete the year's normal work in an age-appropriate text. They do not teach "down" to slower students (MacIver, Reuman, & Main, 1995).

But as with any system, the quality of the whole is more than the sum of the qualities of the teachers or classrooms. Each school also has an overall climate or ethos that makes a difference for the youngsters. The most positive school climate occurs when the principal provides clear and strong leadership, when goals are widely shared, when there is dedication to effective teaching, and when concrete assistance is provided for such teaching. In such schools, pupils and parents are respected, and parents participate in school activities at a high rate. If you are making a decision about a city or a neighborhood in which to rear your children, these are the qualities to look for.

Table 14.2
Characteristics of Unusually Effective Schools

Qualities of pupils	A *mixture* of backgrounds or abilities but with a reasonably large concentration of pupils who come to school with good academic skills. When too many children have poor skills, it is more difficult for the rest of the things on this list to occur.
Goals of the school	Effective schools have a strong emphasis on academic excellence, with high standards and high expectations, clearly stated by the administration and shared by the staff.
Organization of classrooms	Classes are focused on specific academic learning. Daily activities are structured, with a high percentage of time in actual group instruction.
Homework	Homework is assigned regularly, graded quickly.
Discipline	Most discipline is handled within the classroom, with relatively little fallback to "sending the child to the principal." In really effective schools not much class time is actually spent in discipline, because these teachers have very good control of the class. They intervene early in potentially difficult situations rather than imposing heavy discipline after the fact.
Praise	Pupils receive high doses of praise for good performance or for meeting stated expectations.
Teacher experience	Teacher *education* is not related to effectiveness of schools, but teacher *experience* is, presumably because it takes time to learn effective class management and instruction strategies.
Building surroundings	Age or general appearance of the school building is not critical, but maintenance of good order, cleanliness, and attractiveness do have an effect.
School leadership	Effective schools have strong principals who state their goals clearly and often and who back up their intentions with actions. They move ineffective teachers out of the school, arrange helpful staff assistance programs, and so on.
Responsibilities for children	In effective schools, children are more likely to be given real responsibilities—in individual classrooms and in the school as a whole.
Size	As a general rule, smaller schools are more effective, in part because in such schools children feel more involved and are given more responsibility. This effect is particularly clear in studies of high schools.
Money	Increasing the amount of money spent on schools (above the basic amount needed to provide a physically safe, clean environment, staffed with highly competent teachers) does not *automatically* improve quality, but if the added money is carefully spent, it can have positive effects. For example, reducing class size doesn't automatically result in better school performance, but if smaller classes are combined with new methods of instruction, it can be beneficial.

Sources: Rutter, 1983; Linney & Seidman, 1989; Sadowski, 1995; Stringfield, 1991.

Joining the Work World: The Impact of Jobs on Teenagers

In earlier historical eras (and in many cultures around the world today), teenagers already fulfilled normal adult work responsibilities. They worked in the mines and in the fields, herded animals, and fished. Child labor laws changed this picture drastically in the nineteenth century in most industrialized countries. Today adolescents are in school for many hours each day and are not available for adult work. Yet increasingly, adolescents have jobs. Beginning in about 1950 in the United States, teenage employment rates have risen steadily. Today roughly three-fifths of all high school juniors have some kind of formal part-time job during at least part of the school year, and the great majority of students have had at least some work experience before they graduate (Bachman & Schulenberg, 1993; Greenberger & Steinberg, 1986).

For some, such work is an economic necessity. Others work to earn money for college, or to support their favorite hobbies or habits—a car, pizza with friends, or whatever. Parents are frequently very supportive of such work on the grounds that it "builds character" and teaches young people about "real life." Here's one parental voice:

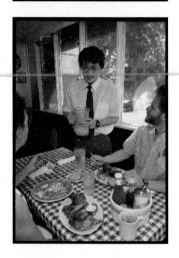

Most part-time teen jobs are low-skill and low-paying, like working in a fast food restaurant or selling clothing. Such jobs appear not to build character, but rather to have negative effects.

> *Let's face it . . . some time in life, someone is going to tell you what to do. . . . I think*
> *work is the only place to learn to deal with it. . . . Parents can give you a little discipline,*
> *but it isn't accepted. . . . You can't learn that in school, because there is another so-called*
> *tyrant, the teacher. But then they get . . . a boss, and you get out there and learn it.*
> *(Greenberger & Steinberg, 1986, p. 39)*

But are parents right about such beneficial effects of work? Does it really teach responsibility and reliability? Maybe, but maybe not. Results of several decades of research on students in the U.S. give us mixed answers.

The Pessimistic View

On the negative side, we find several major studies that suggest that the more hours adolescents work, the more *negative* the consequences are. In the largest single study, Jerald Bachman and John Schulenberg (1993) accumulated information from more than 70,000 students, seniors in the graduating classes of 1985 through 1989. Subjects were drawn each year from both private and public schools in every state in the country. Roughly four-fifths of the students—both males and females—worked at least a few hours per week, most of them for pay. Nearly half of the boys (46.5 percent) and more than a third of the girls (38.4 percent) worked more than 20 hours per week.

Bachman and Schulenberg found that the more hours a student worked, the more he or she used drugs (alcohol, cigarettes, marijuana, cocaine), the more aggression he or she showed toward peers, the more arguments he or she had with parents, the less sleep he or she got, the less often he or she ate breakfast, the less exercise he or she had, and the less satisfied he or she was with life. An impressive list of negatives, isn't it?

The second major piece of pessimistic evidence comes from a study with which you are very familiar by now—the Steinberg and Dornbusch study of Wisconsin and California teens I talked about at some length in the last chapter (1991; Steinberg, Fegley, & Dornbusch, 1993). They have employment information from 5300 of their sample of ninth to twelfth graders, data collected in 1987 and 1988. Like Bachman and Schulenberg, they find that work has a variety of negative effects on teenagers, including on their school grades and commitment to school.

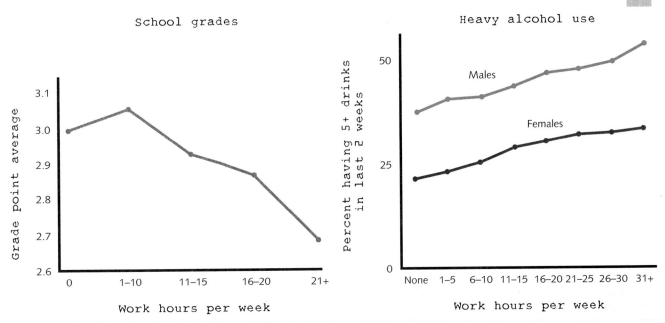

FIGURE 14.2 The data on the left come from Steinberg and Dornbusch's study; the data on the right come from Bachman and Schulenberg. (*Sources:* Steinberg & Dornbusch, 1991, upper section of Figure 1, p. 308; Bachman & Schulenberg, 1993, upper right section of Figure 1, p. 226.)

Figure 14.2 gives two findings from these two studies, the relationship between work and school grades from the Steinberg and Dornbusch study and the link between heavy alcohol use and work from the Bachman and Schulenberg study. I should note, by the way, that Steinberg and Dornbusch found essentially the same pattern of results for all the ethnic groups in their study, and for students from every economic level. So this is a widespread and significant effect.

Causal Effect or Self-selection? At this point, some of you are undoubtedly thinking that results like those in Figure 14.2 may not mean that working during the high school years *causes* bad effects. Instead, the findings might reflect self-selection: Those students who are least interested in school, who already hang out with others who smoke or drink more, may be the same ones who choose to work more. In fact, Bachman and Schulenberg's data are consistent with such an interpretation. They find that those high school seniors who are getting the best grades, who are planning to go on to college, are least likely to work. But that is still correlational evidence and doesn't solve the problem. Steinberg and his colleagues are able to help unravel these two factors because they have longitudinal data. They found that those who later worked 20 hours a week had indeed been less involved with or committed to school in earlier years, which illustrates the effect of self-selection. But these same students became even *more* withdrawn from school and showed not only increases in drug use and delinquency but a *decline* in self-reliance after they began working.

The Optimistic View

A quite different answer to the question comes from Jeylan Mortimer and her colleagues (1995), who have studied a group of more than 1000 students from Minnesota, following them from ninth through twelfth grades. She finds that over these years, teenagers work more and more hours, and that their work becomes somewhat more complex over time. She also finds no correlation between the number of hours students work and their school grades or risk for problem behavior—with the exception of alcohol use, which is higher among those students who work more. What matters more than work per se, in this group of young people, is the quality of work they are doing. Students who have positive work experiences developed increased feelings of competence and efficacy; those students who see themselves gaining useful skills through their work also seem to develop that constellation of work-related values and attitudes that most adults mean when they say that work is "character building."

It is not clear how we should add up the results of these several studies. One possible resolution is suggested by Kristelle Miller (Miller & Pedersen-Randall, 1995), who finds that only work on weekdays, and *not* weekend work, has a detrimental effect on high school students' grades. This suggests the hypothesis that work is academically detrimental to the extent that it distracts young people from academic tasks. Even Mortimer's findings are consistent with this. The employed eleventh and twelfth graders in her study often said that the time on the job made it hard to get homework done and meant they often came to school tired. On the other hand, Mortimer is probably right that the quality of work is a critical ingredient in the equation. Low-skilled work that affords little opportunity for independence and little chance to learn long-term job skills is much more likely to be associated with poor outcomes than is complex, skilled work.

Collectively, these findings are a good illustration of why it is so very difficult to arrive at clear social policy recommendations. At the very least, however, this mixture of results should make parents think twice before they (we) encourage teenagers to work 15 or 20 hours a week.

In light of your own experience and the results of these studies, would you want your own children to work when they are teenagers?

The Impact of the Mass Media

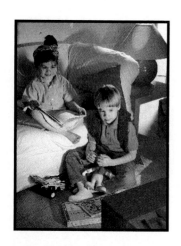

In the United States, children the age of these two watch an average of four hours of TV every day. Amazing.

Another direct influence on children coming from outside the family is the mass media, particularly television. Ninety-eight percent of U.S. homes have a television set, which young children (between 2 and 11) watch an average of 28 hours a week. Adolescents watch about 23 hours a week (American Psychological Association, 1993). Indeed, "By the time American children are 18 years old, they have spent more time watching television than in any other activity except sleep" (Huston et al., 1990). High levels of viewing are more common among African-American children than among whites or Hispanics, and more common in families in which the parents are less well educated (Anderson et al., 1986).

Viewing rates are not as high in most other countries, but TV ownership is above 50 percent of households in most of Eastern and Western Europe and in Latin America, so this is not an exclusively U.S. phenomenon (Comstock, 1991).

Just what are children seeing during all those hours? Preschoolers see many programs designed specifically to be educational or informative, such as "Sesame Street" or "Mr. Rogers' Neighborhood." As they get older, however, children increasingly watch cartoons, comedies, and adult entertainment programs (Huston et al., 1990).

I can give you only a few tidbits from the vast amount of research designed to detect any effects such viewing may have on children and on adults. Still, a taste is better than no meal at all.

Research Report
Family Viewing Patterns

The mythical "average child" in the U.S. watches three or four hours of TV a day. But such averages obviously disguise very large variations among families in both viewing patterns and attitudes about television. To a considerable extent, parents control their children's TV through explicit rules and through attitudes—an example of the way in which broad cultural forces interact with individual family styles. Nearly half of families have consistent rules about what type or which programs a child may view. About 40 percent restrict the number of hours a child can watch, while another 40 percent encourage the child's viewing at least some of the time (Comstock, 1991).

Michelle St. Peters (St. Peters et al., 1991) found that she could classify families into one of four types, on the basis of the degree of regulation and degree of encouragement of TV viewing parents imposed: *Laissez-faire* parents had few regulations but did not specifically encourage viewing; *restrictive* parents had high regulations and little encouragement; *promotive* parents had few regulations and high levels of encouragement for TV viewing; and *selective* parents had high regulations but encouraged some types of viewing.

In a two-year longitudinal study of 5-year-olds and their parents, St. Peters found that children in restrictive families watched the least TV (11.9 hours per week). When they watched, it was most likely to be entertainment or educational programs aimed specifically at children (such as "Sesame Street," "Mr. Rogers' Neighborhood," or Walt Disney). The heaviest viewers were children with parents classed as promotive, who watched an average of 21.1 hours per week. They watched not only children's programs but also adult comedy, drama, game shows, and action adventure. Both laissez-faire families (16.7 hours) and selective families (19.2 hours) watched an intermediate number of hours each week.

The key point here is that families create the conditions for children's viewing and thus for what children learn from TV. Not only do parents establish a degree of regulation, but they may also watch with the child and interpret what the child sees. A family that wishes to do so can take advantage of the beneficial things TV has to offer and minimize exposure to programs with aggressive, violent, or sexist content. The difficulty for many families, however, is that such a planned approach to TV may mean that the parents will have to give up their own favorite programs.

Positive Educational Effects of TV

Programs specifically designed to be educational or to teach children positive values do indeed have demonstrable effects. This is particularly clear among preschoolers, for whom most such programming is designed. Children who watch "Sesame Street" more regularly, for example, develop larger vocabularies than do children who do not watch or watch less often (Rice et al., 1990). Moreover, those who watch programs that emphasize sharing, kindness, and helpfulness, such as "Mr. Rogers' Neighborhood," "Sesame Street," or even "Lassie," show more kind and helpful behavior (Murray, 1980). Results like these show that, as Huston and Wright say, "Television can be an ally, not an enemy, for parents. Parents can use television programs for their children's benefit just as they use books and toys" (1994, p. 80).

Negative Effects of TV on Cognitive Skills

However, among elementary and high school students, heavy TV viewing is associated with *lower* scores on achievement tests, including measures of such basic skills as reading, arithmetic, and writing. This is particularly clear in the results of an enormous study in

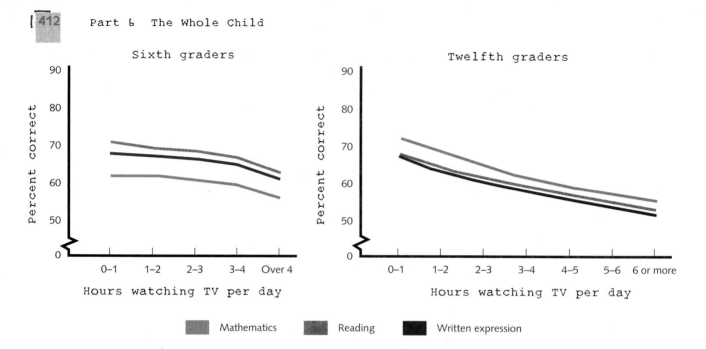

FIGURE 14.3 This large California survey showed links between hours of TV watched and children's academic performance among both sixth graders and twelfth graders. (*Source:* Comstock, 1991, from Figure 3.1, p. 88, and Figure 3.2, p. 89.)

How many different explanations can you think of for the relationship between amount of TV watching and school performance? What kind of data would you need to check the plausibility of each of your explanations?

California that included more than 500,000 sixth and twelfth graders (California Assessment Program, 1980). In this very large sample, the more hours the students watched TV, the lower their scores on standardized tests—as you can see in Figure 14.3. This relationship was actually *stronger* among children from well-educated families, so this result is not an artifact of the fact that working-class or low-education families watch more TV. However, among children with limited English fluency, high levels of viewing were associated with somewhat higher school achievement. Thus, television can help to teach children things they did not already know (including language), but among children with basic skills at the start of school, TV viewing time appears to have a negative effect on school performance.

Television and Aggression

By far the largest body of research has focused on the potential impact of TV on children's aggressiveness. On U.S. television, the level of violence is remarkably high and has remained high over the past two decades (despite many congressional investigations and cries of alarm). In prime-time programs, a violent act occurs five or six times per hour; on Saturday morning cartoons, the rate is 20 to 25 times per hour. Cable TV, now available in roughly 60 percent of homes in the U.S., adds to this diet of violence. The most violent periods are between 6:00 and 9:00 in the morning and between 2:00 and 5:00 in the afternoon—both times when young children are likely to be watching (Donnerstein, Slaby, & Eron, 1994).

Observers also agree that the "good guys" are just as likely to be violent as the "bad guys" and that violence on most TV programs is rewarded: People who are violent get what they want. In fact, violence is usually portrayed as a successful way of solving problems. Furthermore, the consequences of violence—pain, blood, and damage—are seldom shown, so the child is protected from seeing the painful and negative consequences of aggression and thus receives an unrealistic portrayal of those consequences.

Does the viewing of such a barrage of violence *cause* higher rates of aggression or violence in children? Demonstrating such a causal link is a bit like demonstrating a causal link between smoking and lung cancer. Unequivocal findings would require an experimental design—a strategy ruled out for obvious ethical reasons. One cannot assign some people randomly to smoke for 30 years, or assign some children to watch years of violent TV while others watch none. But we have three other types of research evidence that all point strongly toward the existence of a causal link.

Several dozen short-term experiments have been done in which one group of children is exposed to a few episodes of moderately aggressive TV while others watch neutral programs. Collectively, these studies show a significant short-term increase in aggression among those who watched the aggressive programs—a finding that has been repeated in studies of preschoolers and of school-age and adolescent subjects (Paik & Comstock, 1994). For example, in a recent version of this type of study, Chris Boyatzis (1995) found that early-elementary-school-age children who were randomly assigned to watch episodes of a currently popular (and highly violent) children's program, "The Mighty Morphin Power Rangers," showed seven times as many aggressive episodes during subsequent free play with peers as did comparable children who had not just viewed the violent program.

A second type of research relies on correlational evidence. Children who watch a lot of TV in their normal lives are compared with those who watch less. The almost universal finding is that those who watch more TV are more aggressive than their low-TV peers. Of course this leaves us with a problem of interpretation. In particular, children who already behave aggressively may *choose* to watch more TV and more violent TV. And families in which TV is watched a great deal may also be more likely to use patterns of discipline that will foster aggressiveness in the child. One partial solution to this dilemma is to study children longitudinally, such as Leonard Eron did in a 22-year study of aggressiveness from age 8 to age 30 (1987).

Eron has found that the best predictor of a young man's aggressiveness at age 19 was the violence of television programs he watched when he was 8. Twelve years later, when the men were 30, Eron found that the seriousness of criminal behavior was strongly related to the frequency of TV viewing at age 8, a set of results shown in Figure 14.4. The pattern is the same for women, by the way, but the level of criminal offenses is far lower, just as the level of aggression is lower among girls in childhood.

The results shown in the figure, of course, are still a form of correlation. They don't prove that the TV viewing contributed in any causal way to the later criminality, because those children who chose to watch a lot of violent TV at age 8 may already have been the most violent children. Indeed, Eron found just such a pattern: Eight-year-old boys who watched a lot of violent television were already more aggressive with their peers, indicating that aggressive boys choose to watch more violent TV. However, the longitudinal design allows Eron to tease out some additional patterns. In particular, he finds that among the *already*-aggressive 8-year-olds, those who watched the most TV were more delinquent or aggressive as teenagers and as adults (Eron, 1987; Huesmann, Lagerspetz, & Eron, 1984). Shorter-term longitudinal studies in Poland, Finland, Israel, and Australia show similar links between TV viewing and later increased aggression among children (Eron, Huesmann, & Zelli, 1991), which further strengthens the point. Evidence like this

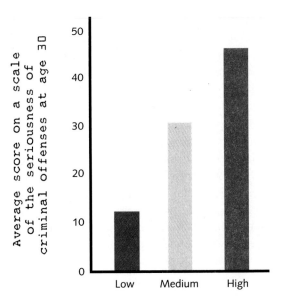

FIGURE 14.4 These data from Leonard Eron's 22-year longitudinal study show the relationships between the amount of TV a group of boys watched when they were 8 and the average severity of criminal offenses they had committed by the age of 30. (*Source:* Eron, 1987, Figure 3, p. 440.)

suggests that the causality runs both ways: "Aggressive children prefer violent television, and the violence on television causes them to be more aggressive" (Eron, 1987, p. 438).

The newest type of evidence, perhaps the most persuasive of all, comes from epidemiology. Brandon Centerwall (1989; 1992) proposed that if we think of societal violence as an epidemic disease, we could use exactly the same strategy to study it that an epidemiologist would use in trying to trace the causal factors in any other epidemic. In his study, Centerwall looked at the homicide rate in Canada, and among whites in both the United States and South Africa, as a function of the time since television was introduced into each country.

TV was introduced in both the United States and Canada in about 1950; in South Africa, about 25 years later. In each of these three countries, the homicide rate began to rise rapidly 10 to 15 years after TV viewing became widespread. That is, as soon as the first generation of children who had grown up watching TV became adults, homicide rates soared. Figure 14.5 shows the results for both Canada and the United States, as well as the homicide rates for whites in South Africa, which remained low over the same years.

Naturally, this is *also* correlational evidence. You might well argue that lots of changes other than the introduction of TV in these three societies in the same years might have caused the rise in violence in Canada and the U.S. To try to rule out such alternative explanations, Centerwall checked out a number of the more obvious possibilities, such as possible parallel changes in the age distribution of the populations (since young people are more violent), in urbanization, in economic conditions, in alcohol consumption, in civil unrest, or in the availability of firearms. He found that the pattern of changes on each of these dimensions in the three countries did *not* match the shifts in the homicide rates. That doesn't mean that there still might not be some other explanation of the epidemiological data, but it considerably strengthens Centerwall's basic argument.

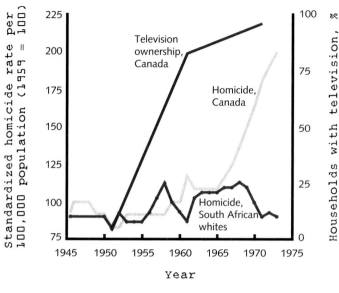

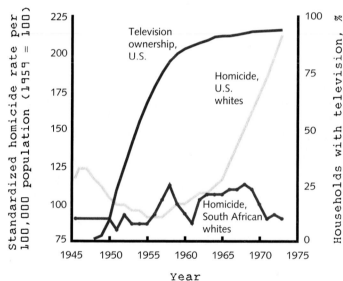

FIGURE 14.5 Centerwall looked at societal violence as if it were a disease and asked what relationship the introduction of TV in each culture had to the rate of such violence. You can see that in both the U.S. and Canada, homicide rates rose dramatically about 15 years after TV was introduced; in South Africa, where TV was not widely available until quite recently, homicide rates remained low. (*Source:* Centerwall, 1989, Figure 1, p. 6, and Figure 2, p. 7.)

Virtually all psychologists, after reviewing the combined evidence, would agree with Eron's testimony before a Senate committee:

> *There can no longer be any doubt that heavy exposure to televised violence is one of the causes of aggressive behavior, crime and violence in society. The evidence comes from both the laboratory and real-life studies. Television violence affects youngsters of all ages, of both genders, at all socioeconomic levels and all levels of intelligence. The effect is not limited to children who are already disposed to being aggressive and is not restricted to this country. (1992, p. S8539)*

Other evidence suggests that repeated viewing of TV violence leads to emotional desensitization toward violence, to a belief that aggression is a good way to solve prob-

Given all of what you have now read about television and children's development, how could you as a parent maximize the benefits and limit the negative effects? Would you be willing to give up having a television altogether if you thought that was necessary for your child's optimum development?

lems, and to a reduction in prosocial behavior (Donnerstein et al., 1994). Violent television is clearly not the only, or even the major, cause of aggressiveness among children or adults. But it is a significant influence, both individually and at the broader cultural level.

Macrosystem Effects: The Impact of the Larger Culture

Finally, we come explicitly to the question of contexts and cultures. Each family, and thus each child, is embedded in a series of overlapping contexts, each of which affects the way the family itself interacts and each of which affects all other parts of the system. These contexts include the overall economic position of the family, the ethnic group to which the family belongs, and the larger culture in which all this exists. These days one should probably also think about the global culture, because the global marketplace affects job opportunities and standards of living in individual countries. But that is a level of complexity I cannot yet begin to grasp.

Economic Variations: Social Class and Poverty

Every society is made up of social layers, usually called **social classes,** with each layer having a different degree of access to goods or status. In Western societies, the social class of a given family is most often defined in terms of the income and education of the adults in that family. In the United States, three social classes are usually identified: middle-class, working-class, and poverty-level families. Members of each of these social layers tend to share certain values or styles of interaction, with the largest differences found between families living in poverty and those in higher social class groups. For children it is clear that the disadvantages of poverty are enormous—and these disadvantages are not equally distributed across ethnic groups in the U.S.

Figure 14.6 shows the percentages of children in the United States who live below the poverty line—defined in 1992 as an income for a family of four of $14,335 per year or less. *Proportionately more children in the United States live in poverty than in any other*

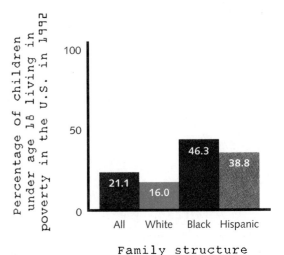

FIGURE 14.6 The percentage of children under age 18 living in poverty in the United States in 1992. (*Source:* U.S. Bureau of the Census, 1994, Table 728, p. 475.)

industrialized country in the world. By way of specific contrast, the poverty rate for children in Canada is roughly 9 percent; in Sweden it is 2 percent.

Figure 14.6 also makes clear that poverty is unequally distributed across ethnic groups in the U.S. It is also unequally distributed across family structures: Roughly 60 percent of black and Hispanic children, and 40 percent of white children reared by single mothers in the U.S. live in poverty (Zill & Nord, 1994). Many of these mothers have jobs, but the jobs pay too little to raise the family out of poverty (Lichter & Eggebeen, 1994).

Data like those in Figure 14.6 can give us only a slice in time. Perhaps more important for the child is the overall family history of poverty. Such an analysis points to even greater disadvantage for minority children. Greg Duncan (Duncan, Brooks-Gunn, & Klebanov, 1994) notes that two-fifths of black children but only 6 percent of white grow up in families that are poor for all the child's first five or six years. Half of white children grow up in families that are never poor and never live in a poor neighborhood, while this is true for only 5 percent of blacks. Thus, even those black families that do not fall below the poverty line at any one moment are likely to have fallen below it at some time and/or to spend some time living in a poor neighborhood.

The Effects of Poverty on Families and Children. Among many other things, poverty reduces options for parents. They may not be able to afford prenatal care, so their children are more likely to be born with some sort of disability. When the mother works, she is likely to have fewer choices of affordable child care. Such children spend more time in poor-quality care, and they shift more from one care arrangement to another. Poor families also live in smaller and less-adequate housing, frequently in decaying neighborhoods with high rates of violence, and many of them move frequently, which means their children change schools often. The parents are less likely to feel they have adequate social support, and the children frequently lack a stable group of playmates (Dodge, Pettit, & Bates, 1994). Overall, poverty environments are more chaotic, more highly stressed, with fewer resources (McLoyd & Wilson, 1991).

Mothers and fathers living in poverty also treat their children quite differently than do mothers and fathers in working-class or middle-class families in the United States. They talk to them less, provide fewer age-appropriate toys, spend less time with them in intellectually stimulating activities, explain things less often and less fully, are less warm, and are stricter and more physical in their discipline (Dodge et al., 1994; Sampson & Laub, 1994). In the terms I introduced in the last chapter, poor parents are more likely to be either neglecting or authoritarian and less likely to be authoritative.

Some of this pattern of parental behavior is undoubtedly a response to the extraordinary stresses and special demands of the poverty environment—a point buttressed by the repeated observation that those parents living in poverty who nonetheless feel they have enough social support are much less likely to be harshly punitive or unsupportive toward their children (Hashima & Amato, 1994). Some of the stricter discipline and emphasis on obedience may also be thought of as a logical response to the realities of life in a very poor neighborhood. Parents in this kind of situation need to keep control of their children, and mild physical discipline may actually help in some cases—a point I made in the box on spanking in the last chapter. Some of the differences in child-rearing patterns between poor and nonpoor parents may also result from straightforward modeling of the way these same parents were brought up in their own childhood; some may be a product of ignorance of children's needs. Poor parents with relatively more education, for example, typically talk to their children more, are more responsive, and provide more intellectual stimulation than do equally poor parents with lower levels of education (Kelley, Sanches-Hucles, & Walker, 1993). But whatever the cause, children reared in poverty experience not only different physical conditions but quite different interactions with their parents.

Not surprisingly, such children turn out differently, as I have pointed out repeatedly in earlier chapters. Children from poverty environments have higher rates of birth defects and early disabilities; they recover less well from early problems; they are more often ill and malnourished throughout their childhood years (Klerman, 1991). Typically, they also have lower IQs and move through the sequences of cognitive development described by Piaget more slowly. The more years they have lived in poverty, the larger the observed IQ decrement, even when family structure and the mother's level of education are taken into account (Duncan et al., 1994). They come to school less ready to learn to read, and from that early point they consistently do less well in school and are less likely to go on to college (Huston, 1994)—a pattern that is particularly true of children who change schools often (Mehana & Reynolds, 1995). Such children, in turn, are more likely to be poor as adults, thus continuing the cycle through another generation.

Figure 14.7 shows one of these effects, drawn from research by Greg Duncan and his colleagues (Duncan et al., 1994). Duncan has information on family income for a large sample of families over the years from the child's birth to age 5. He looked at the child's IQ at age 5 as a function of whether she had been poor in every one of those five years or only some of those years. The figure compares the IQ scores of each of these groups to the benchmark IQ of children who never lived in poverty. It's clear that constant poverty has a greater negative effect than sometime poverty, and both are worse than nonpoverty. In this analysis, Duncan has controlled for the mother's education and the structure of the household (single mother versus two parents, for example), so these differences seem to be real effects of poverty.

The Special Case of Inner-City Poverty. All these effects are probably much worse for children growing up in poverty-ravaged urban areas. They are exposed to street gangs and street violence, to drug pushers, to overcrowded homes and abuse. Whole communities have become like war zones.

In the United States, almost 13 million children live in such urban poverty (Garbarino, Kostelny, & Dubrow, 1991). More than 1.5 million of these live in public

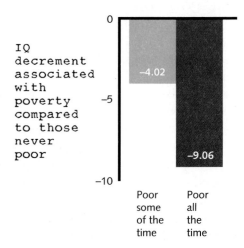

FIGURE 14.7 Duncan's analysis shows that children who have spent all their first five years living in poverty have considerably lower IQs than those who have lived in poverty only part of the time, and both groups are significantly lower than the benchmark group—those who never lived in poverty. (*Source:* Duncan, Brooks-Gunn, & Klebanov, 1994, from Table 3, p. 306.)

IQ decrement associated with poverty compared to those never poor

-4.02

-9.06

Poor some of the time

Poor all the time

housing developments, including some with the highest crime rates in the country. Surveys in Chicago, Washington, DC, New Orleans, and elsewhere find that nearly half of inner-city elementary school children have witnessed muggings, and a third have seen shootings or dead bodies. Among high school students in the inner city, 42 percent had witnessed a shooting and a third had seen a stabbing (Hammond & Yung, 1994). Guns are common in schools as well as on the streets. I was stunned to read that in Seattle (a city with a rate of urban poverty well below that of Chicago, New York, or Los Angeles), 11.4 percent of teen males reported owning a handgun and a third of these gun owners had fired at someone (Callahan & Rivara, 1992). Nationally, about 15 percent of teenagers carry some kind of weapon, either a gun or a knife (U.S. Department of Health and Human Services, 1994).

Are you also shocked by such statistics? What do you think we ought to do about it?

In the early years of childhood, when youngsters spend most of their time with a parent or other caregiver, or with siblings, it may be possible for parents to protect children from some of the dangers inherent in such poverty environments. But in middle childhood, when children pass through the streets to travel to and from school and to play with their peers, they experience the impact of urban poverty and decay far more keenly. Many show all the symptoms of posttraumatic stress disorder (Garbarino et al., 1992), including sleep disturbances, irritability, inability to concentrate, angry outbursts, and hypervigilance. Many experience flashbacks or intrusive memories of traumatic events. And because they are likely to have missed out on many of the forms of intellectual stimulation and consistent family support that would allow them to succeed in school, they have high rates of behavior problems and academic failures. Less than half of urban poor children graduate from high school (Garbarino et al., 1991). The reasons for such school failures are complex, as I have already pointed out, but there is little doubt that the chronic stress experienced by poor children is one highly significant component.

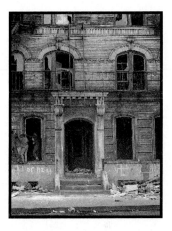

When you look at scenes of urban poverty like this, you can see why some refer to them as war zones.

The Role of Stress and Protective Factors. Arnold Sameroff and his colleagues have argued that the effects of various different kinds of stresses accumulate. A child may be able to handle one or two, but as the stresses and risks pile up, the probability that a child will thrive intellectually, emotionally, or socially declines steadily (Sameroff et al., 1987). For a child growing up in poverty, perhaps especially urban poverty, the chances of experiencing multiple separate types of stress are very high indeed.

At the same time, studies of resilient and vulnerable children (Easterbrooks, Davidson, & Chazan, 1993; Garmezy & Masten, 1991; Masten, Best, & Garmezy, 1990) suggest that certain characteristics or circumstances may help to protect some children from the detrimental effects of repeated stresses and upheavals, including the following:

- High IQ in the child
- Competent adult parenting, such as an authoritative style
- Effective schools
- A secure initial attachment of the child to the parent

For example, in a major longitudinal study in Kauai, Hawaii, Emmy Werner (Werner & Smith, 1992) has found that a subset of those children reared in poverty nonetheless became competent, able, autonomous adults. The families of these resilient children were clearly more authoritative, more cohesive, and more loving than were the equivalently poor families whose children had worse outcomes. Similarly, studies of boys

The Real World

Children in Danger

I cannot leave the subject of urban poverty—so common now in America—without quoting some of James Garbarino's eloquent words.

What is truly needed in America's urban war zones is restoration of a safe environment where children can have a childhood, and where parents can exert less energy on protecting children from random gunfire and more on helping children to grow. No one can eliminate all risk from the lives of families. But America does have the resources to make a real childhood a real possibility even for the children of the urban poor. But sometimes the war close to home is the most difficult to see. (Garbarino et al., 1991, p. 148)

reared in high-crime inner-city neighborhoods show that high intelligence and at least a minimum level of family cohesion are key ingredients affecting a boy's chance of creating a successful adult life pattern (Long & Vaillant, 1984; McCord, 1982; Sampson & Laub, 1994). Boys reared in poverty-level families in which there was alcoholism or who had parents with strong antisocial tendencies or low IQ were much less likely to develop the competence needed to bootstrap themselves out of their difficult circumstances.

Thus, the outcome depends on some joint effect of the number of stresses the child must cope with and the range of competencies or advantages the child brings to the situation. Poverty does not guarantee bad outcomes, but it stacks the deck against most children. As Judith Musick puts it, these environments are "densely layered with risk" (1994, p. 1).

Ethnicity

In the United States, social class and ethnic group membership are strongly linked to one another, because poverty status is so much more common among some ethnic groups than among others. But if we are to gain an understanding of children's development, we need to understand the separate effects of ethnic group membership. For example, what difference does it make to a child to grow up in a family whose cultural roots emphasize collectivism rather than individualism? Of course I have touched on these questions throughout the book. But let me take one final look at what we know at this point about ethnic effects, using the several major ethnic groups in the United States as illustration.

First, though, we need a better definition of ethnicity than I have given so far. Porter and Washington (1993) define it this way:

> An **ethnic group** *is a subgroup whose members are perceived by themselves and others to have a common origin and culture, and shared activities in which the common origin or culture is an essential ingredient. (p. 140, emphasis added)*

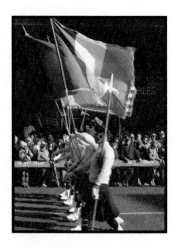

These Irish-Americans marching in a St. Patrick's Day parade would fit the definition of an ethnic group but are not a race.

Note that race and ethnicity are not the same. *Ethnicity* refers primarily to social and cultural characteristics, while *race* normally designates a group with specific physical characteristics. Thus, Hispanic-, African-, and Asian-Americans may be viewed as both ethnic and racial categories, while Polish-Americans or Italian-Americans would be regarded only as ethnic groups.

African-Americans. African-Americans, the largest ethnic minority group in the United States, including roughly 12 percent of the total population, have a culture that has been shaped by their African heritage, their experience of slavery, and a continuing experience of discrimination and segregation. The central values of this ethnic culture include the following (Hill et al., 1994):

- Collectivism or communalism as opposed to individualism; identity is collective as well as personal

- Person centered rather than object centered; relationships with people are more important than material possessions

- Mutuality and reciprocity; a belief that "what goes around comes around," that each person's actions will eventually have repercussions for that individual

- A strong religious or spiritual orientation, involving acknowledgment of a higher power

- An emphasis on the importance of children for family continuity

- Harmony and a sense of connection with nature, including a belief in the "oneness of being" of all humanity

- Role flexibility

These values, especially the emphasis on collectivism or communalism and the importance of children, have contributed to a pattern of family structures that is quite different from what exists within the majority Euro-American culture. Euro-Americans think of "the family" as (normatively) a father, a mother, and several children. But within the African-American culture, "family" has a much broader definition, including many

Cultures and Contexts
Child Rearing and Family Values in West Africa

The emphasis on collectivism that we see in the African-American subculture naturally enough has its roots in African cultural traditions. In many West African cultures, for example (Ivory Coast, Cameroon, and other countries), adults clearly distinguish between social intelligence and "book learning" intelligence. They say that a person can read and write but be quite dumb or that a person can be wise without having book learning (Dasen, 1984; Nsamenang & Lamb, 1994). In rearing their children, adults in these cultures pay more attention to the child's social knowledge or skill than to his biological age. A child is given new responsibilities or tasks when he seems ready for them, not when he reaches some arbitrary age.

In one study of these cultures, Bame Nsamenang and Michael Lamb (1994) interviewed 389 adults of the Nso tribe in Cameroon. These adults defined a "good child" as one who showed obedience and respect, filial service, hard work, helpfulness, honesty, and intelligence. Although many children in this setting attend school (a training system that is an artifact of colonial rule), adult Nsos see the primary training of children as occurring both through apprenticeships, in which adults act as role models, and through training of younger children by their older sibs or by peers. This is a very different model of child rearing and child development than what we see in the U.S. and most Western cultures.

variations of extended family structures. Martin and Martin, in their book *The Black Extended Family*, defined it this way:

> *a multigenerational, interdependent kinship system which is welded together by a sense of obligation to relatives, is organized around a dominant figure; extends across geographic boundaries to connect family units to an extended family network; and has a built-in mutual aid system for the welfare of its members and the maintenance of the family as a whole. (1978, p. 1)*

Thus, the key is not just that three or more generations often live in the same household, but also that contact with nonresident kin is frequent and integral to the functioning of the family unit. When asked, African-Americans overwhelmingly report a strong sense of family solidarity (Hatchett & Jackson, 1993; Wilson, 1986; 1989).

Within this subculture, marriage does not play the dominant role in family formation that it does among Euro-Americans. Far fewer black adults marry, they are less likely to be satisfied with their marriages, and divorce is more common (Broman, 1993). One result is that a much larger percentage of black children are born to or reared by unmarried mothers. But because of the cultural emphasis on the importance of children and on communalism, these single mothers occupy a different niche within the African-American culture than is true for single Euro-American mothers. The latter are more likely to receive financial help from their parents but to live independently; African-American single mothers are more likely to live in an extended family with their own mother or grandmother (Wilson, 1986).

These extended family structures allow individuals to combine their economic resources, and they provide social and emotional support to the members of the household. The presence of the grandmother seems to provide especially helpful support for the young single mother; black children in such three-generation families do better in school and show fewer behavior problems than do black children reared in single-mother households. There is also some evidence that the presence of the grandmother increases the chance that an infant will develop a secure rather than an insecure attachment (Egeland & Sroufe, 1981). Thus, the extended family has not only a cultural history, it also seems to be a successful adaptive strategy for many black families.

Religion also appears to play a special, positive role within the African-American community. The church is a place for participation and belonging, a structure in which prestige and status can be conferred on those who take on specific roles. For black children, participation in church activities seems to be a plus as well; a few studies suggest that those who are more active in a church are more likely to be successful in other arenas, such as school or on the job (Lee, 1985).

The culture of African-American families is also profoundly shaped by the persistence of prejudice and discriminatory housing practices, the difficulty in finding good jobs, the (often accurate) perception that hard work will not necessarily yield good results. African-American adolescents who are most aware of such prejudice are most likely to see school achievement as irrelevant (Taylor et al., 1994). In many inner cities, the combined effect of these forces has been to create a subculture in which illegal activity or idleness become the norm for African-American teenagers, especially teenage boys (Spencer & Dornbusch, 1990). And among adult black men, "economic marginality" appears to be a significant precursor to divorce or family strain—a pattern that is not unique to the black subculture but that is particularly relevant for this group precisely because job opportunities are more limited.

Because so many black families and children live in or near poverty, it is very difficult to sort out which patterns are due to economic conditions and which to distinctive African-American cultural processes. The two obviously interact and are further embedded within the larger culture in which prejudice and discrimination against blacks are still a part of everyday life.

Hispanic-Americans. The same is true of Hispanic-Americans, for whom poverty is also endemic. The term *Hispanic* actually covers a wide range of separate groups, all with some historical link to Spain but differing somewhat in values and cultural traditions. Of the present-day 22.7 million Hispanic-Americans (9 percent of the total U.S. population), 14.6 million are Mexican-Americans (also called Chicanos), 2.4 million are Puerto Rican, about a million are Cuban, and the rest are from other Central and South American countries (U.S. Bureau of the Census, 1994). Within this diverse group, Puerto Ricans have the highest poverty rates, and divorce rates comparable to those of African-Americans. Both Chicanos and Cubans have divorce rates more like the dominant Euro-American culture.

All these subgroups, however, share a number of cultural values, all of which are aspects of a basic collectivist world view (Hill et al., 1994):

- Preference for group participation or work rather than individual effort (allocentrism)

- Strong commitment to and adherence to family; the family comes before the individual (familism)

- Avoidance of personal conflict; keeping the peace at all costs (*simpatia*)

- Respect for and deference to authority, such as parents, elders, teachers, or government officials (*respeto*)

- Maximal value on personal relationships, seen as more important than reputation or material gain (*personalismo*)

In addition, of course, there is the common thread of the Spanish language. The great majority of Hispanics in the United States today are either monolingual in Spanish or bilingual. Because of rapid recent immigration, more than half of Hispanic-American school-age children have only limited English proficiency; a shift toward English as the dominant language generally occurs among second- or third-generation Hispanic-Americans, but many, if not most, continue to speak Spanish in the home (Chapa & Valencia, 1993; Grenier, 1985). Many Hispanic communities also have Spanish-language newspapers and radio and TV stations; in many neighborhoods, Spanish is the dominant tongue.

The significance of family life within the Hispanic culture is hard to exaggerate. The nuclear family is the core of this kin system, although contact with extended family members and with "fictive kin" is frequent. Fictive kin, who are also a common part of the extended family system within African-American families, might include a child's godparents or other friends who take on a long-term connection with the family and with each child (Keefe & Padilla, 1987).

Are there any "fictive kin" in your own family network? What is their role within the family?

This Hispanic family has obviously assimilated some of the larger American culture: They are celebrating Thanksgiving. At the same time, they have doubtless retained many features of Hispanic culture, including the centrality of family loyalty.

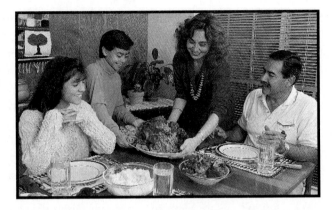

In general, Hispanics see frequent contacts with kin as not only enjoyable but also as vital signs of the closeness of kin relationships. It is not enough to write or talk on the phone; to maintain close ties you need to see and touch your relatives and friends. Among Hispanics, an individual's self-esteem may also be more strongly related to the valuation given by the kin group. William Madsen described the difference this way:

> When an Anglo fails, he thinks first of how this failure will affect him and his status in society. When a Chicano fails, his first evaluation of the failure is in terms of what it will do to his family and how it will affect his relationship to other family members. (1969, p. 224)

This pattern seems to be stronger in first-generation immigrants, who rely almost exclusively on family members for emotional support and problem solving. Second-generation immigrants seem to have more extensive nonkin networks, and many have shifted somewhat toward an individualist set of values (Delgado-Gaitan, 1994). But in both generations, the extended family clearly plays a more central role in the daily life of Hispanics than it does in the Anglo culture.

This emphasis on the central role of the family is reflected in the values taught to children. In Chicano parlance, the relevant set of values is called *bien educado* and includes politeness, respect, loyalty, and attachment to the extended family and cooperation with others. Hispanic mothers emphasize the importance of a child showing proper demeanor in public; an Anglo mother, in contrast, is likely to be pleased or even proud when her child behaves in some independent but slightly naughty way (Harwood, 1992).

These values are taught in the home through all the mechanisms I have described throughout the book: modeling, direct reinforcement, and style of family interaction. A number of studies suggest that the more fully the parents identify with their Hispanic ethnic heritage, the more likely it is that the child will show these valued qualities, such as concern for others (Knight, Cota, & Bernal, 1993).

The collectivist Hispanic values often conflict with the strong individualism and competitiveness of the dominant Anglo culture. Where the values of the minority and majority cultures overlap is in the value placed on education. Hispanic parents, like both African-American and Anglo parents, place a strong value on doing well in school. Yet Hispanic youth are even more likely to drop out of school or to get poor grades in school than are African-American teens. This pattern has been difficult to explain. It is certainly linked partially to poverty, doubtless also to persisting language difficulties. It may also arise in part from the emphasis on deference and respect that are part of *bien educado,* because such an emphasis means that Hispanic parents are quite likely to show an authoritarian rearing style. We know that such a rearing style is associated with poorer school performance, so it may be that the very aspect of Hispanic culture that is one of its greatest strengths may also contribute to less-optimal school outcomes for children—at least within the larger Anglo cultural system.

Asian-Americans.   But wait a minute. That can't be all the explanation either, because Asian-American families *also* place great stress on obedience to family, on respect for elders, on family honor. Their family style is rarely authoritative, yet Asian-American children do extremely well in school—in American schools as well as in Asian schools. So how do the Asian-American values or family systems differ from what we see in Hispanic families?

If you look at a list of key values of Asian-American culture, you can see that some of the ingredients are similar, but the whole is distinct. These values include the following (American Psychological Association, 1993, p. 39):

- Pacifism, self-discipline, and self-control—all values linked to Confucianism, and thus common for those Asian groups with a strong Confucian heritage (Chinese, Korean, Vietnamese, and Japanese)

- An emphasis on hierarchy and respect in social systems and personal relationships (parents are superior to children; men are superior to women)

- Strong family links; young people are expected to obey elders; family solidarity and harmonious relationships are highly valued

- A strong belief that each person controls his or her own destiny

- A powerful work ethic and belief in the importance of achievement

Asian-American families resemble Hispanic families in some respects. They often include three generations in the same household; they are generally hierarchically organized with the father as the clear head, with a strong emphasis on the interdependence of family members. But the mixture of values is distinct, and expressed differently. The Asian family model includes a striking combination of indulgence, physical contact, comfort, and care, on the one side, along with high expectations for both obedience and achievement. Children are taught that empathy with others is highly important, and yet that respecting the privacy of others is also critical (Lebra, 1994). Overall, children are highly valued, yet the family's collective needs normally take precedence over the child's individual needs (Rothbaum, Pott, & Morelli, 1995).

Asian-American families also believe in *effort* as one of the primary roads to success (Harrison et al., 1990; Stevenson, 1988). In contrast, in the Euro-American culture, *ability* rather than hard work is seen as the key to success. This difference is not trivial. If you believe in ability as the key ingredient, then there is not much point in pressing for greater effort, and you will accept mediocre performance from your child. But an Asian parent, believing in the centrality of effort, takes a very different attitude toward both success and failure. He takes success more or less for granted but responds to failure by insisting on more effort. As a result of these different belief systems, Asian-American parents spend more time tutoring their children and have higher standards for the child's achievement. They are also less likely to be satisfied with the schools, believing that the schools too can always do better. Yet, despite what (to Euro-American eyes) seems like

Think about your own beliefs for a moment. Do you think of effort or ability as the most significant element in an individual's success? Has your belief about this affected your own choices or behavior at any point in your life?

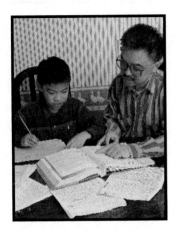

Nine-year-old Brian gets help with his homework from his dad—a common activity in Asian-American households, where parents typically place great emphasis on the importance of hard work to reach academic goals.

Imagine a largish group of Euro-Americans set down in the midst of some quite different culture, such as perhaps China or Japan. What cultural conflicts would the children of this subgroup be likely to experience?

strong pressure to achieve, Asian students do not report high feelings of stress or anxiety, while high-achieving Euro-American adolescents *do* report frequent feelings of stress (Crystal et al., 1994)

Given all these differences, we shouldn't be surprised that Asian-American children as a group do achieve at higher levels in schools, just as Asian children from Japan, China, Taiwan, and Korea regularly outperform American children and teenagers on standardized tests of math and science. Asian-Americans have the highest rate of high school completion and the highest rate of college completion of any group in the United States, including Anglos.

Asian families are also more stable and more upwardly mobile than other groups and quite unlikely to involve single parents. Collectively, all of these factors mean that Asian-Americans are least likely to live in poverty of any of the minority groups I have described here.

Ethnicity in Perspective. What conclusions can we draw about the role of ethnicity (or culture, more broadly) in children's development from these three brief (and necessarily simplistic) sketches? Sadly, not many. First and foremost, of course, I have been talking almost entirely about subgroups within U.S. culture, which tells us little about other cultural systems. And even within these limits, we are working mostly with research that involves comparisons of each ethnic group with children or families in the Anglo culture. Until recently, most of this research assumed that the Anglo culture was right or best and that all other variations were inferior or "deviations" from the standard. That assumption has faded, but we rarely have information about all these groups at the same time, and even less often do we have data about whether the same *processes* operate in each subgroup. What we are left with is a kind of snapshot of each group, without being able to tell which characteristics are the most crucial, which attitudes or values the most significant.

For example, if we look for reasons for good or poor school performance in different subcultural experiences, what conclusions can we draw? Bilingualism cannot be the sole answer, because both Asian-Americans and Hispanics are typically bilingual; child-rearing style cannot be the sole answer because Asian-American parents are most likely to be authoritarian, yet their children do well in school. Doubtless it is the *pattern* of values and parental behavior that is crucial, and not any one variable operating at once. Cultures and subcultures are incredibly complex systems, and their effects come from the combination and not merely from the adding up of a set of separate variables. In addition, of course, because we are talking about subcultures here, we must try to understand how each culture, each set of values, combines or conflicts with the values of the majority culture. For a child growing up with a foot in each culture, these are highly important issues.

The Culture as a Whole

The culture as a whole is also a system, made up of values, assumptions, and beliefs; a political and an economic system; a pattern of personal relationships; and so forth. Each piece of that system affects all the other parts; changing one part changes the whole. The wide cultural consequences of the rapid increase of women in the labor force in the U.S. and other industrialized countries is a very good example. It has led, among many other things, to a huge new demand for day care (with consequent changes in children's lives), to changes in male-female relationships, to new political alignments, and to shifts in patterns of interactions within families, which in turn affect children in still other ways.

Research Report

Asian and U.S. Teenagers and Their Parents Define a "Bad Kid"

If I asked you to think about and describe some specific teenager you consider to be a "bad kid," what qualities would define "badness" for you? It turns out that this is a useful question to ask in different cultures as a way to uncover differences in values and expectations for children.

David Crystal and Harold Stevenson asked this question of nearly 600 eleventh graders in the U.S., in Taiwan, and in Japan (1995). The U.S. teens, more than either Asian group, described a "bad" kid as someone who lacked self-control—someone who was "childish" or "immature." Taiwanese teens, more than the other groups, emphasized society-related conduct, such as "makes trouble for society" or "rebels against society," while Japanese students most often referred to lack of interper-

sonal harmony, such as "hurting other people's feelings," "being argumentative and starting fights," or "not caring about others." Both American and Taiwanese children also mentioned disruptions of interpersonal harmony as being part of "badness," but this was almost the only category the Japanese students mentioned.

Crystal and Stevenson also interviewed the mothers of these students, asking them the same question, with similar results. In simple terms, these results suggest that for the U.S. teens, failure to achieve an appropriate individuality defines badness, while in both Asian cultures badness occurs when the child fails to have a proper respect for the collective. It would be interesting to see what the responses of Hispanic students and their parents would be to this same question.

Throughout the book, I have pointed to a variety of patterns or sequences of children's development that seem to occur regardless of cultural context. The stages of moral judgment, the early stages of language development, the creation of internal models of attachment, physical maturation, the development of a theory of mind—all of these and many other patterns appear to be universal aspects of development.

But examples of cultural differences are also easy to come by. At the most visible and measurable level are variations in children's specific beliefs, the social scripts that they learn, and the pattern of family and kin relationships they experience.

An interesting example comes from the work of Giyoo Hatano and his colleagues (Hatano et al., 1993), who compared beliefs about the nature of plants and animals among Japanese, Israeli, and American kindergarten, second-grade, and fourth-grade children. Piaget noted, and others have confirmed, that children typically begin with the idea of *animism,* in which they attribute not only life but also feelings and self-awareness to inanimate objects, to plants, and to animals. Later they differentiate among these several facets of life and understand that plants are alive but have no self-awareness. Hatano's study confirms the broad features of this shift: Younger children in all three cultures had much stronger beliefs in animism. But Hatano also found differences in the developmental pattern, depending on the specific cultural beliefs about life.

Japanese culture includes the belief that plants are much like humans; in the Buddhist system, even a blade of grass is thought to have a mind. In contrast, in Israeli culture, plants are put into a quite different category from animals and humans. When children in these two countries, along with U.S. children, were asked if a tree or a tulip were alive, 91 percent of the Japanese but only 60 percent of the Israeli fourth graders said that it was. In contrast, a fifth of Japanese fourth graders still attributed sensory properties to plants, saying that a tree or a tulip could feel that it is cold or could feel pain if it is hit with a stick. Overall, because of their stronger distinction between plants and animals, Israeli children were much slower than either Japanese or American children to come to the understanding that people, animals, and plants are all alive. This study thus illustrates both an underlying developmental pattern that seems to be shared across cultures (or at least across these three cultures) and cultural variations on that basic pattern.

It is not hard to generate similar examples. Cultures may vary in the proportion of securely and insecurely attached children because of variations in their typical child-rearing styles or beliefs, even while the *process* by which a child becomes securely or insecurely attached is much the same from one culture to another: Adolescents in all cultures need to change their identity to at least some extent in order to move into the adult world, but cultures that provide initiation rituals at puberty may make the process much simpler and less confusing.

Certainly we need to know a great deal more about how such cultural variations affect development. But as I pointed out in Chapter 1, we also must ask a more subtle set of questions. In particular, we need to know whether the *relationship* between environmental events or child characteristics and some outcome for the child is the same in every culture. Is authoritative child rearing optimal in all cultures, or is some other style better to prepare children for adult life in some settings? Are aggressive children unpopular in every culture, or are there some settings in which this quality would be highly valued? Indeed, is unpopularity in childhood a major risk factor for adult dysfunction in every culture?

As yet we do not have answers, although researchers are beginning to ask the questions. Steinberg and Dornbusch, for example, asked whether authoritative parental style had the same effects in each of several ethnic groups in the United States. They found that it did not; this finding forces us to reexamine our assumptions about the way parental style operates to affect children's development.

It is extremely difficult to conceptualize the developmental process as part of a complex system, and even harder to design research that allows us to look at all the pieces of the puzzle at the same time. But it is precisely that kind of research we need if we are to understand the full impact of the ecology of the child's development, including cultural and subcultural influences.

Summary

1   Children's development is influenced by institutions beyond the family that affect them directly, including day care, school, jobs, and television. It is also affected by the subculture and culture in which they grow up.

2   The majority of children in the United States now spend some part of their infancy or preschool years in some form of nonparental care. Currently, the most common forms of such care are care in the child's own home by someone other than the mother and family day care.

3   Day care often has positive effects on the cognitive development of less advantaged children, but it may have negative effects on advantaged children if the discrepancy between the home environment and the level of stimulation in day care is large.

4   The impact of day care on children's personality is unclear. Some studies show children with a history of day care to be more aggressive; others show them to be more socially skillful.

5   Numerous studies show a small difference in security of attachment between children in day care and those reared at home. Interpreting this difference has proven difficult and contentious.

6   The quality of care appears to be a highly significant element. Good-quality care involves small groups of children, in clean spaces designed for children's play, with responsive caregivers trained in child development.

7   Experience with school appears to be causally linked to some aspects of cognitive development, such as the ability to generalize strategies from one situation to another.

8   Children's adaptation to school is affected by their readiness to learn to read, and by the parent's involvement in the school and in the child's educational attainment.

9   School experience shapes a sense of self-efficacy. By adolescence, children have a clearly developed idea of their comparative skills and abilities. These beliefs are a significant element in decisions about high school completion or dropping out.

10 Unusually effective schools have features much like an authoritative parenting style: clear rules and control, high expectations, good communication, and high nurturance.

11 The majority of teenagers in the United States work at part-time jobs. Most research shows that the more hours a student works, the lower his school grades, the more drugs or alcohol he uses, and the more aggression he shows.

12 The average American child watches four hours of television per day. Preschoolers can learn vocabulary, politeness, or other skills. Among schoolchildren, the more TV watched, the lower the grades.

13 Experts agree that watching violence on TV also increases the level of personal aggression or violence shown by a child.

14 Children growing up in poverty, perhaps especially urban poverty, are markedly disadvantaged in many ways, including lower access to medical care and exposure to multiple stresses. They do worse in school and drop out of school at far higher rates.

15 Some protective factors, including a secure attachment, higher IQ, authoritative parenting, and effective schools, can counterbalance poverty effects for some children.

16 The African-American subculture includes a strong emphasis on extended family households and contact and on religion, but a weaker emphasis on marriage as the vehicle for household formation. Because a large fraction of African-Americans live in poverty, it is difficult to sort out the separate effects of ethnic culture and poverty.

17 Hispanic-Americans place great emphasis on family ties, on family honor and solidarity, heightened by the use of a shared language. In this collectivist cultural system, kin contact is frequent and central to daily life. Values taught to children include politeness, respect, and loyalty, an emphasis somewhat at odds with the individualism of the larger society.

18 Asian-Americans also emphasize respect and loyalty to family but stress the central importance of effort (rather than inherent ability) as the path to achievement. Asian-American families are more stable, with lower divorce rates and fewer single-parent families; their children achieve in school at a higher rate than any other ethnic group.

19 As yet we know far too little about the ways in which these varying mixtures of values and family patterns interact to affect children's development.

20 When we compare whole cultures, our ignorance also exceeds our knowledge. Some patterns of development appear to be independent of culture, such as perhaps moral judgment reasoning. Others are affected by cultural variation, but many basic processes appear to be the same across cultures, such as the importance fostering a secure attachment.

21 Finally, there are some aspects of development in which both the observed pattern of development and the process by which it occurs vary as a function of cultural or subcultural patterns.

Key Terms

ethnic group **(p. 420)**

family day care **(p. 397)**

social class **(p. 416)**

Suggested Readings

Booth, A. (Ed.). (1992). *Child care in the 1990s: Trends and consequences.* Hillsdale, NJ: Erlbaum.

If you want to get the day-care debate from the horses' mouths, this is an excellent source. It includes a summary of the effects of day care on children by Alison Clarke-Stewart, along with a reply by Belsky and others. If nothing else, this book will persuade you that academic arguments are not always dry and dull. There is plenty of heat here!

Eron, L. D., Gentry, J. H., & Schlegel, P. (Eds.). (1994). *Reason to hope: A psychological perspective on violence and youth.* Washington, DC: American Psychological Association.

The chapter on the effect of TV on violence is a good current review of this material. But there are many other fascinating chapters here as well.

Garbarino, J., Dubrow, N., Kostelny, K., & Pardo, C. (1992). *Children in danger: Coping with the consequences of community violence.* San Francisco: Jossey-Bass.

A striking, frightening book about children growing up in "war zones," including urban poverty in the United States, as well as in literal war zones in other countries.

Huston, A. C. (Ed.). (1991). *Children in poverty: Child development and public policy.* Cambridge, England: Cambridge University Press.

An excellent collection of papers on all aspects of poverty.

McAdoo, H. P. (Ed.). (1993). *Family ethnicity: Strength in diversity.* Newbury Park, CA: Sage.

A very helpful collection of papers describing the family life and experiences of African-Americans, Hispanic-Americans, Native Americans, Asian-Americans, and Muslim families.

Atypical Development

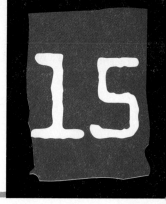

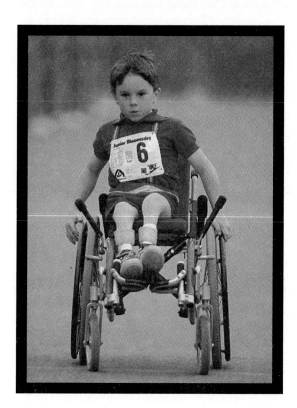

When Jeffrey was 4, he couldn't walk or talk and spent most of his time in a crib. His parents fed him pureed baby food through a bottle. After six years with a loving foster family, at age 10 Jeffrey is now in a special class in a regular elementary school and is learning to print and read.

Nine-year-old Archie seemed "different from other children even when he started school." Often he was "disoriented" or "distractible." Although he scored in the normal range on an IQ test, he had great difficulty learning to read. Even after several years of special tutoring he could read only by sounding out the words each time; he didn't recognize even familiar words by sight (Cole & Traupmann, 1981).

Janice's parents are worried about her. Right about the time that she turned 13 she seemed to change in disturbing ways. She's lost weight, even though she's growing fast; she doesn't seem to call up her friends anymore and is listless and gloomy. This has been going on for about six months now, and her parents think this is just not normal; they're going to talk to the school counselor about her and will consider family therapy if it will help.

Each of these children is "atypical" in some way. In each, the developmental processes I have been describing in the past 13 chapters haven't quite worked in the normal way. Jeffrey is a Down syndrome child and is mentally retarded. Archie has some kind of learning disability, while Janice shows many signs of a clinical depression.

How Common Are Such Problems?

How common are such problems? Given the critical practical relevance of this question, you'd think that psychologists and epidemiologists would long ago have come to some agreement. But we haven't, in large part because the line between typical and atypical is very much a matter of degree rather than of kind. *Most* children show at least some kinds of "problem behavior" at one time or another. For example, parents in the United States report that 10 to 20 percent of 7-year-olds still wet their beds at least occasionally, 30 percent have nightmares, 20 percent bite their fingernails, 10 percent suck their thumbs, and 10 percent swear enough for it to be considered a problem. Another 30 percent or so have temper tantrums (Achenbach & Edelbrock, 1981). Problems like these, especially if they last only a few months, should more properly be considered part of "normal" development. Usually, we label a child's development "atypical" or deviant only if a problem persists for six months or longer, or if the problem is at the extreme end of the continuum for that behavior.

When we count only such extreme or persisting problems, the incidence is much lower—although higher than most of you will have guessed. Table 15.1 gives some current estimates for each of a series of deviant patterns. Some of these numbers are based on extensive data and are widely accepted, such as the 3.5 percent rate of mental retardation. Others are still in some dispute, such as the rate of depression in adolescence. Where the findings are not in agreement, I have given the range of current estimates.

We might also want to combine all these individual rates in some way, to give us an idea of the total percentage of children with some type of problem. Unfortunately, this is not a simple matter of addition, since the categories overlap a good deal. For example, many children with serious learning disabilities also show an attention-deficit disorder or conduct disorders. Still, even if we allow for some overlap, the totals are astonishing: Between 14 and 20 percent of children and teenagers show at least *some* form of significant psychopathology (Costello & Angold, 1995). If we add in cognitive disorders, the total is at least 20 percent. That is, at least one in five, and maybe as many as one in four, children will show at least one form of significantly deviant or abnormal behavior *at some time in their early years.* The majority of these children will require some type of special help in school, in a child guidance clinic, or the equivalent. When you think of these figures in terms of the demands on the school system and on other social agencies, the prospect is somewhat staggering.

Do you think that such high rates of problems would be found in every culture? Why or why not?

Table 15.1

Estimated Incidence of Various Types of Atypical Development in the United States and Other Developed Countries

Type of Problem	Percentage of Children 0–18 with That Problem
Psychopathologies	
Externalizing Problems	
1. Attention-deficit disorder (hyperactivity)	3–5
2. Conduct disorders	5–7
3. Arrest by police (delinquency)	3
Internalizing Problems	
1. Significant anxiety and fear	2.5
2. Serious or severe depression	
Elementary-school-age children	1–2
Adolescents	3–10
Intellectually Atypical Development	
IQ below 70 (mentally retarded)	3.5
Speech and language problems, including delayed language, articulation problems, and stuttering	3.5
Serious learning disability	4.0
Physical Problems	
Autism	0.04
Significant hearing impairment	0.3
All other problems, including blindness, cerebral palsy, epilepsy, etc.	0.2

Sources: Barkley, 1990; Brandenburg et al., 1990; Broman et al., 1987; Cantwell, 1990; Chalfant, 1989; Kopp & Kaler, 1989; Marschark, 1993; Merikangas & Angst, 1995; Nolen-Hoeksema, 1994; Rutter, 1989; Rutter & Garmezy, 1983; Tuna, 1989.

If we are going to meet those needs, we must obviously understand the origins of such atypical patterns. In this chapter I can give you only a glimpse of our current knowledge, but I can at least alert you to the issues and remaining questions about the most common forms of deviance.

Developmental Psychopathology: A New Approach

Our knowledge about the dynamics of deviant development in general and of psychopathology in particular has been enormously enhanced in the past few years by the emergence of a new theoretical and empirical approach, called **developmental psychopathology,** pioneered by such researchers as Norman Garmezy, Michael Rutter,

Cultures and Contexts
Problem Behaviors Among Children in Kenya and Thailand

A growing body of information links particular cultural values and the type of emotional or behavioral problem children may show. In one recent study, John Weisz and his colleagues (1993) compared the incidence of externalizing and internalizing problems among teenagers in a rural Kenyan group (the Embu) and in a rural Thailand group with the rates among rural black and white youth in the United States. Both the Thai and Embu cultures place great emphasis on obedience and politeness, a pattern of cultural values that appears to be linked to higher rates of "overcontrolled" or internalizing problems, such as shyness, fearfulness, or depression. In contrast, the United States culture, with its greater emphasis on individual freedom, appears to foster higher rates of "undercontrolled" or externalizing problems, such as fighting, showing off, or hyperactivity.

In each of the three cultures, parents were asked a series of questions about specific behaviors or symptoms their child showed. Weisz found that the Embu teens had the highest rates of internalizing and the lowest rate of externalizing problems, while American white teens had the highest rates of undercontrol, followed by African-American teens. Interestingly, the Thai group showed low rates of both types of problems, although other studies in Thailand have shown high levels of overcontrol problems in this culture.

The fact that the Embu and Thai patterns are not the same certainly reminds us yet again that cultural effects are not going to be as simple as a difference between an emphasis on obedience versus personal freedom. But the results also remind us that the pattern of frequencies of various types of problems that we note in U.S. populations is at least in part a product of our culture.

Dante Cicchetti, Alan Sroufe, and others (e.g., Cicchetti & Cohen, 1995; Rutter & Garmezy, 1983). These theorists have emphasized several key points.

First, normal and abnormal development both emerge from the same basic processes. To understand either we must understand both and how they interact. The task of a developmental psychopathologist is to uncover those basic processes—both to see how they work "correctly," in the case of normal development, and to identify the *developmental deviations* and their causes (Sroufe, 1989). Alan Sroufe's studies of the consequences of secure or insecure attachment, which I talked about in Chapter 6, are good examples of research based on such assumptions.

Second, the approach is *developmental.* Theorists in this new tradition are interested in the *pathways* leading to both deviant and normal development, from earliest infancy through childhood and into adult life. What are the sequences of experiences that lead to increased risk of depression in adolescence? What pathways lead to delinquency or other antisocial behavior, or to peer rejection? And what factors may inhibit or exacerbate an early deviation or turn an initially normal developmental trajectory into a deviant pattern?

One of the potentially exacerbating factors may be the underlying developmental pathway itself. Each age has special tasks, special stresses that interact with the child's ongoing patterns and internal models to produce either normal or deviant behavior. For example, it is now very clear that rates of depression among young people rise markedly at adolescence (e.g., Nolen-Hoeksema, 1994). A developmental psychopathologist would ask what is unique about adolescence that would contribute to such heightened depression rates.

He or she would also want to know what special qualities or early experiences a child may bring to the experience of puberty that might increase or decrease her risk of developing a pathological pattern such as depression. One of the unexpected results of many recent studies of children thought to be "at risk" for particular kinds of problems, such as children reared by depressed parents, children in divorcing families, or abused children, has been that some children seem to be unexpectedly resilient in the face of what appear to be disturbing circumstances. The obverse has also been found repeatedly: Some children seem to be unexpectedly vulnerable, despite what appear to be supportive life circumstances. Developmental psychopathologists such as Rutter and Garmezy have not only taken the lead in studying resilient children, but have insisted that these "exceptions" to the general rules offer us crucial information about the basic processes of both normal and abnormal development.

A growing body of research, cast in this framework, can help us examine the origins and manifestations of the array of psychopathologies.

The Psychopathologies of Childhood

Experts in childhood psychopathology now agree that there are two main categories of such disorders: **externalizing problems** (also described as *disturbances of conduct*), in which the deviant behavior is directed outward, such as hyperactivity, excessive aggressiveness or defiance, and delinquency; and **internalizing problems** (also called *emotional disturbances*), such as depression, anxiety, or eating disorders, in which the deviance is largely internal to the individual.

Externalizing Problems

One of the most obvious types of externalizing problems is what in layman's terms we might call *antisocial behavior*. In the most recent revision of the American Psychiatric Association's *Diagnostic and Statistical Manual of Mental Disorders* (called DSM-IV) (American Psychiatric Association, 1994), this is called a **conduct disorder** and includes high levels of aggression, argumentativeness, bullying, disobedience, irritability, and threatening and loud behavior.

It has been clear for a long while that there are a number of subvarieties of conduct disorders, although developmental psychopathologists have not yet reached agreement on the best way to characterize the variations. Achenbach (1993) argues for two subtypes: *aggressive behavior,* which includes arguing, being mean to others, destruction of objects, fighting, attacking, showing off, sudden mood changes, temper tantrums, and loudness; and *delinquent behavior,* which includes specific law-breaking, such as setting fires and stealing, but also a lack of guilt, lying, running away from home, swearing and obscenity, and use of alcohol and drugs.

In contrast, Hinshaw (Hinshaw, Lahey & Hart, 1993) argues that the crucial issue is when the deviant behavior began. *Childhood-onset conduct disorders* are more serious, with high levels of aggression, and are far more likely to persist to adult criminality; *adolescent-onset* problems appear to be milder, more transitory, more a function of hanging about with bad companions than a deeply ingrained behavior problem.

These two category systems overlap a good deal. The cluster of problems Achenbach calls aggressive behavior typically begins early and is much more persistent. Thus, it fits within Hinshaw's childhood-onset group, while delinquent behavior most often begins in adolescence and is less persisting and serious. But the fit between the two taxonomies is

Why does it matter what kind (or how good) of a category system we use?

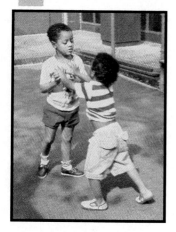

We can't tell from one picture whether these preschool boys are consistently aggressive or defiant. But we know that those who do show high levels of such behavior at this early age are far more likely to have long-term problems than are those who only develop conduct disorders or delinquency at later ages.

What kind of social policy implications (if any) do you see in the fact that early-onset conduct disorders are most likely to persist and be followed by adult criminality or violence?

not perfect. In particular, many children with early-onset conduct problems show both aggressive and delinquent behaviors. But both of these category systems may turn out to be helpful in aiming researchers toward clearer questions about the origins of the various types of conduct disorders.

The developmental pathway for early-onset conduct disorders is one you are familiar with by now from all I have said about Patterson's research on aggressive children. In early life, these are children who throw tantrums and defy parents; indeed, they may also develop insecure attachments (Greenberg, Speltz, & DeKlyen, 1993). Once the defiance appears, if the parents are not up to the task of controlling the child, the child's behavior worsens to overt aggression toward others, who then reject the child, which aggravates the problem, pushing the seriously aggressive child in the direction of other children with similar problems, who become the child's only supportive peer group (Shaw, Kennan, & Vondra, 1994). Such children are not friendless, but their friends are almost always other problem children. By adolescence, these youngsters are firmly established in antisocial behavior, and in adulthood they are highly likely to continue with aggression, crime, or—at the least—a chaotic life.

The degree of continuity of this form of deviant behavior is striking. The correlation between aggression in childhood and aggression in adulthood averages .60 to .70—very high correlations for data of this kind, and replicated in studies in both England and the United States (Farrington, 1991). One example, which you may remember from Chapter 14, is Leonard Eron's longitudinal study of aggressive boys. Those who were most aggressive at age 8 were much more likely to show antisocial or damaging aggressive behavior as adults than were those who had been less aggressive at age 8 (Eron et al., 1987).

There is also some indication that the early-onset/aggressive syndrome has a much stronger genetic component than is true for the later-onset/delinquent pattern (Achenbach, 1993). Thus, the preschooler who already shows defiant and oppositional behavior as well as aggressiveness may have strong inborn propensities for such behavior. But if Patterson is correct—and I think he is—then whether that propensity will develop into a full-fledged, persisting conduct disorder will depend on the unfolding sequence of events, including the parents' ability to handle the child's early defiance as well as the general environment in which the child lives, such as inner city versus small town (Gottesman & Goldsmith, 1994).

Delinquency. Let me also say just a word about **delinquency,** a term that is likely to be more familiar to you. Delinquency is a narrower category than conduct disorders, referring only to specific law-breaking. Some lawless behavior, such as lying or stealing, is fairly common in children as young as 4 or 5. But it is in adolescence that we see a significant increase in the number of youngsters who display such behaviors and in the seriousness and consistency of delinquent behavior.

It is extremely difficult to estimate how many teenagers engage in such behavior. One window on the problem is to look at the number of arrests—although arrest rates are arguably only the tip of the iceberg. More than 1 million juveniles in the U.S. are arrested each year, which is 3 to 4 percent of all youngsters between ages 10 and 17. Among those 15 to 17, the arrest rate is roughly 11 percent (Dryfoos, 1990). In fact, the rate of arrests among these older teens is higher than in any other age group across the entire life span. Many of these arrests are for relatively minor infractions: shoplifting, vandalism, liquor law violations, or the like. But about a third are for serious crimes, including murder, burglary, rape, and arson.

Self-reports of delinquency by U.S. adolescents suggest even higher rates. Four-fifths of youngsters between ages 11 and 17 say that they have been delinquent at some time or another. One-third admit truancy and disorderly conduct, and a fifth say they have committed criminal acts, most often physical assaults or thefts (Dryfoos, 1990).

Just as conduct disorders are much more common among preschool and elementary-school-age boys than girls, delinquent acts and arrests are far more common among teenage males than females. Among those actually arrested, the ratio is more than 4:1; in self-reports the ratios vary, but the more physically violent the act, the more common it is among boys.

Although there are many subvarieties of delinquents, as a group they tend to have deficits in *social* understanding: They have poor skills in reading others' cues and poor understanding of many social rules (Schonfeld et al., 1988). Delinquents are also likely to have parents (especially fathers) who are antisocial or criminal and to show high levels of many other types of deviant behavior, including drug and alcohol use, truancy or dropping out of school, and other high-risk behaviors. For example, in one longitudinal study of a sample of high school students from Colorado, Donovan and Jessor (1985) found correlations of .54 between delinquent behavior and marijuana usage, .41 between delinquent behavior and drunken episodes, and .36 between delinquent acts and frequency of sexual experience among the boys in the study. The correlations were similar for girls but somewhat lower.

However, unlike the broader category of conduct disorders, which are quite stable from childhood to adulthood, delinquency does not necessarily persist into adulthood. Many teens commit only occasional delinquent acts and show no further problem in adulthood. For them, mild delinquent behavior is merely a phase. It is those who show a syndrome of delinquent acts plus high-risk behavior, and who come from families with low warmth and ineffective control, who are quite likely to show criminality in their adult lives.

At the risk of repeating something I said in Chapter 11, one other point deserves emphasis: Many adults, observing the high rate of delinquent behavior or substance abuse among teenagers, attribute the problem to the "bad influence" of the peer group. Somehow, we think, the kids would be okay if they hadn't somehow fallen in with "bad companions." But the evidence provides little support for such a belief. Certainly, teenage peer groups do sometimes seduce youngsters into riskier, less-approved behavior than they might otherwise engage in. But the crucial factor seems to be that a young person is drawn to such a group of peers in the first place, rather than any subsequent behavioral contamination by the group. Delinquency, drug and alcohol use or abuse, risky sexual behavior—all these are most often symptoms of deeper forms of deviance, many of which have their roots in earlier developmental periods.

Attention-Deficit/Hyperactivity Disorder. A second important category of externalizing psychopathology has been given a rather long-winded name in DSM-IV: **attention-deficit/hyperactivity disorder (ADD).** The briefer and more common name is simply **hyperactivity.** A glance at the diagnostic criteria, which I've listed in Table 15.2, will tell you quickly that the hallmarks of this disorder are physical restlessness and problems with attention—precisely as the label implies (Barkley, 1990).

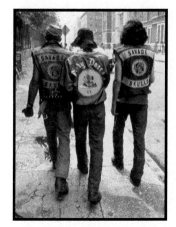

Teenage gangs or delinquent groups may strengthen tendencies toward illegal or high-risk behaviors. But young people drawn to such groups are likely to have a history of misbehavior or peer rejection, and/or to have ineffective parents.

Research Report

Delinquency Among Girls

When we use the term *delinquent*, most of us think immediately of teenage boys. But although the incidence of delinquency or criminality in girls is much lower, it is not zero. Girls are much less likely to be involved in forms of delinquency that involve violence, just as girls are consistently less aggressive at every age. But girls do get involved in delinquent behaviors, such as shoplifting or the use of illegal drugs (Zoccolillo, 1993).

An interesting study in New Zealand by Avshalom Caspi and his colleagues (Caspi et al., 1993) provides some interesting insights into the possible origins of such delinquent behavior. The sample of students involved in this study included all the children born in one town in one year (1972–1973), a group of more than 1000 (the same large sample, by the way, that is represented in the Moffitt data shown in Figure 15.1, page 440). The children were tested and assessed repeatedly, at ages 3, 5, 7, 9, 11, 13, and 15. In one analysis, Caspi looked at rates of delinquency among the girls as a function of the earliness or lateness of their menarche and of whether they went to an all-girls or a mixed-sex high school. Caspi's hypothesis was that girls who attended a mixed-sex secondary school would be more likely to be involved in delinquent activities because they would have more rule-breaking models (delinquent boys) among their peers. He also expected to find that girls with early puberty would be more likely to become delinquent, especially in mixed-sex schools.

These hypotheses were generally confirmed, although there are some interesting wrinkles. At age 13, the girls were asked to report on "norm violations," which included a variety of mild delinquent acts, such as breaking windows, stealing from schoolmates, getting drunk, swearing loudly in public, or making prank telephone calls. As you can see in the figure below, such norm violations were most common among early-maturing girls attending coed schools. Further analysis shows that this difference is almost entirely contributed by a small group of girls who had had a history of high levels of aggression earlier in childhood *and* who had early puberty. Early-maturing girls in coed schools who had no such history of early problems showed no heightened rate of delinquency.

To make it still more complicated, Caspi found that at age 15, early-developing girls in co-ed schools continued to have high rates of delinquency, but at this age the highest rate of delinquency was found among *on-time-puberty* girls attending coed schools. Puberty, whether early or on-time, thus seems to increase the likelihood that vulnerable girls will get involved with antisocial peers. But this is only true of girls in coed schools.

I find this study fascinating not only because it points to the complex relationships between physical maturation and social relationships, but also because it offers an interesting argument in favor of all-girls schools.

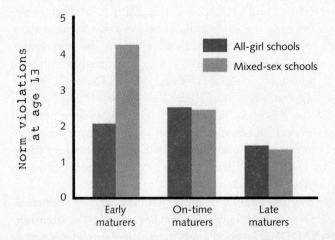

Table 15.2
Diagnostic Criteria for Attention-Deficit/Hyperactivity Disorder

The child must show either significant *inattention* **or** significant *hyperactivity-impulsivity* (or both).

Inattention would be indicated by any six or more of the following:
1. Often fails to give close attention to details or makes careless mistakes in schoolwork or other activities
2. Often has difficulty sustaining attention in tasks or play
3. Often does not seem to listen when spoken to directly
4. Often does not follow through on instructions and fails to finish chores, homework, or duties
5. Often has difficulty organizing tasks and activities
6. Often avoids, dislikes, or is reluctant to engage in tasks that require sustained mental effort
7. Often loses things necessary for tasks or activities (e.g., toys, pencils, books, tools)
8. Often is easily distracted by extraneous stimuli
9. Often is forgetful in daily activities

Hyperactivity-impulsivity is indicated by the presence of six of the following, persisting over a period of at least six months:
1. Often fidgets with hands or feet or squirms in seat
2. Often leaves seat in classroom or in other situations in which remaining seated is expected
3. Often runs about or climbs excessively or reports feelings of restlessness
4. Often has difficulty playing quietly
5. Often is "on the go" or acts as if "driven by a motor"
6. Often talks excessively
7. Often blurts out answers before questions are completed
8. Often has difficulty waiting for a turn
9. Often interrupts or intrudes on others

The onset of the problem must be before age 7.

At least some of the symptoms must be present in at least two settings, such as home and school, or school and play with peers.

The behavior must interfere with developmentally appropriate social, academic, or occupational functioning.

Source: Paraphrased from *Diagnostic and Statistical Manual of Mental Disorders* (4th ed.), 1994. Washington, D.C.: American Psychiatric Association, pp. 83–85. Copyright © 1994 by the American Psychiatric Association.

Many children show a few of these behaviors, and it is tempting—for both teachers and parents—to label a boisterous or obstreperous child as ADD. There is no doubt that some mislabeling of this kind does occur. But in fact the full syndrome is quite distinctive. ADD children's interactions with their peers are so strikingly different that novice observers need to watch videotapes for only a few minutes before they can reliably distinguish between a child diagnosed as hyperactive and a normally behaving child—even when the hyperactive child displays no aggression and the sound is turned off (Henker & Whalen, 1989). The body language is distinctive, the level of activity is different, and the child's social behavior is often inappropriate. About half of such children *also* show conduct disorders, and most do poorly in school.

By definition, this is an early-developing disorder. It is also a persistent problem in the majority of cases, lasting well into adulthood for at least half of those diagnosed as having this disorder (Henker & Whalen, 1989). But the severity of the long-term problem seems to be strongly influenced by whether or not the child also develops a conduct disorder. It is the combination of hyperactivity and aggressiveness or delinquency that is especially deadly (Barkley et al., 1990). You can see one facet of this effect in the results of a longitudinal study by Terrie Moffitt (1990) of a group of 434 boys in New Zealand, including all boys born in a particular town over a one-year period. When the boys were 13 they were classed in one of four groups based on the presence or absence of two factors: attention-deficit disorder and delinquency. Moffitt then traced backward for each of these groups, looking at scores at earlier ages on measures of antisocial behavior, intelligence, and family adversity. You can see the results for antisocial behavior in Figure 15.1.

It is clear that the boys who showed *both* hyperactivity and delinquency as adolescents had been the most antisocial at every earlier age. Hyperactivity that was not accompanied by antisocial behavior at early ages was also not linked to delinquency at 13. Other research tells us that this same group of hyperactive *and* delinquent boys is also the most likely to have continued serious problems in adulthood, including criminal behavior.

Where might hyperactivity come from? Because the pattern begins so early and has such a strong physical component, most clinicians have assumed that this problem has a biological origin. Surprisingly, early research failed to confirm such a biological hypothesis. Investigators could find no sign of overt brain damage, and typical neurological tests revealed no underlying physical problem. But three converging lines of evidence have revived the biological hypothesis.

First, physicians and psychologists have known for some time that a biological *treatment* is very often effective in reducing or eliminating the deviant behavior. Many (but not all) hyperactive children treated with a stimulant medication (most commonly Ritalin) show decreases in demanding, disruptive, and noncompliant behaviors, and more attentiveness in the classroom (Henker & Whalen, 1989). This type of evidence is consistent with a biological explanation of ADD, although naturally it does not prove that the root cause of ADD is biological. More persuasive evidence for an underlying bio-

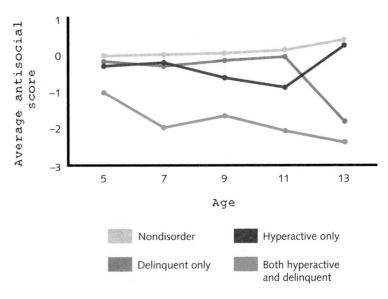

FIGURE 15.1 The boys in Moffitt's study had been studied every two years from the time they were 5. When they were 13, they were assigned to one of four hyperactivity/delinquency categories, and then Moffitt backtracked from that age. You can see that those who were *both* delinquent and hyperactive at 13 had shown markedly higher rates of antisocial behavior from the time they were 5, while those who were only hyperactive at 13 had been much less socially deviant at earlier ages. (*Source:* Moffitt, 1990, Figure 1, p. 899.)

logical cause comes from behavior genetic research, which suggests that a pattern of hyperactivity is inherited, at least in certain families. About a quarter of the parents of hyperactive children themselves have a history of hyperactivity (Biederman et al., 1990). Studies of twins also show a genetic contribution. Among identical twins, if one is diagnosed as hyperactive, the other is highly likely to have the same diagnosis; among fraternal twins this "concordance rate" is much lower (Deutsch & Kinsbourne, 1990).

Finally, newer methods of assessing brain function have begun to reveal differences between the brains of hyperactive and nonhyperactive individuals. In one widely publicized study, Alan Zametkin and his colleagues (1990) used positron emission tomography (PET) scans to examine the glucose (sugar) metabolism in the brains of hyperactive and normal adults. All the hyperactive adults reported that they had also been hyperactive as children, and all had at least one offspring with the same diagnosis. Each subject was injected with a concentrated dose of glucose; then repeated PET scans were done to look at how the brain metabolized the sugar. Zametkin found that the hyperactive adults had significantly slower brain metabolism of the glucose, and this was especially so in the portions of the brain that are known to be involved in attentiveness and the ability to inhibit inappropriate responses. Results like this may represent a real breakthrough, not only in helping us to understand the origins of hyperactivity, but also conceivably in devising better treatments. At the very least, they greatly strengthen the argument that this disorder has biological origins.

But being more sure about the origins does not settle all the important questions. From the point of view of developmental psychopathology we also need to understand how such an initially deviant biological pattern affects the child's interactions with parents and peers to produce the common combination of hyperactivity and antisocial behavior. For many hyperactive children, the pathway is very like the one Patterson has described for defiant or aggressive children. These kids are just plain hard to raise. And those parents whose child management skills are not up to the task of dealing with the hyperactive toddler's typically higher rates of noncompliance or who face major family stresses that prevent them from maintaining good child care routines may find that their child's behavior becomes more and more disruptive, which in turn adversely affects the child's emerging social skills. By school age, parent-child conflict is high, as is child-peer conflict. Poor school performance makes it worse by lowering the child's self-esteem. Such children are then on a pathway that is highly likely to lead to continued problems in adolescence and adulthood (Campbell, 1990). In Moffitt's New Zealand study, for example, those boys who eventually showed the combination of hyperactivity and delinquency came from families with much higher than average levels of stress and fewer resources. The hyperactive boys who did not develop the accompanying antisocial behavior came from families with lower than average levels of stress and more resources. Thus, once again we find that the key for long-term problems or for recovery from difficulties lies in the interaction between the child's inborn or early-developed qualities and the capacity of the family and the environment more generally to support the child's optimum behavior.

Internalizing Problems: The Example of Depression

A different set of antecedents, and a different pathway, is found among children who show internalizing forms of psychopathology. The particular form of deviance that has been most often addressed within the framework of developmental psychopathology has been **depression,** so let me use that as an example.

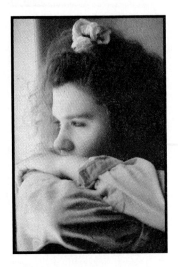

We can't know for sure what has caused this teenager's dejected look, but we do know that both depressed mood and significant clinical depressions are common in the adolescent years.

For many years, psychiatrists took the position that significant depression could not occur in children or adolescents. But we now have abundant evidence that depression is actually quite common in adolescence and occurs at least occasionally among younger children. Both Thomas Achenbach and Michael Rutter, in separate large studies, have found that approximately 10 percent of preadolescent children and 40 percent of adolescents are described by parents or teachers as appearing miserable, unhappy, sad, or depressed (Achenbach & Edelbrock, 1981; Rutter, Tizard, & Whitmore, 1981). When teenagers themselves are asked about their state of mind, a third describe at least moderate levels of depressed mood (Petersen et al., 1993).

When depressive episodes last six months or longer and are accompanied by other symptoms such as disturbances of sleeping and eating and difficulty concentrating, they are usually referred to as *clinical depression* or a *depressive disorder.* Recent epidemiological studies tell us that such severe forms of depression occur in perhaps 1 to 2 percent of preadolescents and in something like 10 percent of adolescents. Perhaps twice that many will experience a serious depression at some time in their adolescent years (Compas, Ey, & Grant, 1993; Petersen et al., 1993).

Interestingly, among preadolescents, boys appear to be slightly more likely than girls to be unhappy or depressed; but beginning at about age 13, girls are twice as likely to report high or chronic levels of depression, a sex difference that exists throughout adulthood and that has been found in a number of industrialized countries and among African-Americans, Hispanic-Americans, and Anglo-Americans (Nolen-Hoeksema, 1994; Nolen-Hoeksema & Girgus, 1994; Petersen et al., 1993; Roberts & Sobhan, 1992).

Although teenagers and preadolescents who describe themselves as depressed do not invariably display all the symptoms of a full-blown clinical depression as seen in adulthood, depressed youngsters do show the same kind of hormonal and other endocrine changes during their depressed episodes as are observed in depressed adults, so we know that depression in children is a real and potentially serious clinical state, not just a "normal" or transitory unhappiness—a conclusion further buttressed by the fact that a significant portion of depressed teens say they think about suicide. In one longitudinal study of youth growing up in a working-class neighborhood in the U.S., a fifth of those who had had a serious depression by age 18 had also attempted suicide (Reinherz et al., 1993).

The search for the developmental pathways leading to later depression begins with the clear finding that children growing up with depressed parents are much more likely than are those growing up with nondepressed parents to develop depression themselves (Downey & Coyne, 1990). Of course this could indicate a genetic factor at work here, a possibility supported by at least a few studies of twins and adopted children (Petersen et al., 1993). Or we could understand this link between parental and child depression in terms of the changes in the parent-child interaction that are caused by the parent's depression.

I mentioned in Chapter 11 that depressed mothers are much more likely than are nondepressed mothers to have children who are insecurely attached. In particular, their behavior with their child is often so nonresponsive that it seems to foster in the child a kind of helpless resignation. Such a sense of helplessness has been found to be strongly related to depression in both adults and adolescents (Dodge, 1990).

Of course not all children of depressed parents are themselves depressed. About 60 percent show no abnormality at all. Whether a child moves along a pathway toward depression or not seems to be a function of a whole series of protective or disruptive factors (Billings & Moos, 1985):

- If the parent's depression is short-lived or is medically treated so that the symptoms are less severe, the child has a much better chance of avoiding depression herself.

- The more other forms of stress the family experiences in addition to one parent's depression—such as an illness, family arguments, work stress, loss of income, job loss, or marital separation—the more likely the child is to show depressive symptoms.

- The more emotional and logistical support the family receives from others, the less likely the child is to show depressive symptoms.

Thus, the family system can buffer the child from the effects of a parent's depression far more effectively if the adults have adequate social supports and not too many other stresses. But when stresses accumulate, the effect is magnified.

In fact, this detrimental role of stress in the emergence of depression is just as clear among children whose parent or parents are not depressed. Any combination of stresses has a similar effect, such as the parents' divorce, the death of a parent or another loved person, the father's loss of job, a move, a change of schools, or whatever (Compas et al., 1993). Indeed, the role of such individual life stresses may help to explain the sex differences in depression among adolescents. Anne Petersen (Petersen, Sarigiani, & Kennedy, 1991) has proposed that girls are more likely to experience simultaneous stressful experiences in adolescence, such as pubertal changes combined with a shift in schools. In her own longitudinal study, Peterson finds that when such synchronous stresses are taken into account, the sex difference in adolescent depression disappears. That is, in this study, depression was *not* more common among girls than among boys when both groups had encountered equal levels of life stress or simultaneous stressful experiences.

Susan Nolen-Hoeksema agrees with Petersen that one of the keys is that teenage girls face more stresses than do teenage boys (1994; Nolen-Hoeksema & Girgus, 1994). But she also argues that girls respond to their "down" moods quite differently than do boys. Girls (and women) are more likely to *ruminate* about their sadness or distress, a coping strategy that actually accentuates the depression ("What does it mean that I feel this way?"; "I just don't feel like doing anything") and produces longer-lasting episodes. Boys (and men), on the other hand, are more likely to use distraction to deal with their blue moods—exercising, playing a game, or working—a coping strategy that tends to reduce depression.

Yet another possible pathway is through lowered self-esteem. Susan Harter's studies tell us that a young person who feels she (or he) does not measure up to her own standards is much more likely to show symptoms of a clinical depression. The fact that depression increases markedly in adolescence makes good sense from this point of view. We know that in adolescence, children are much more likely to define themselves and others in *comparative* terms—to judge against some standard, or to see themselves as "less than" or "more than" some other person. We also know that at adolescence, appearance becomes highly salient, and that a great many teenagers are convinced that they do not live up to the culturally defined appearance standards. Self-esteem thus drops in early adolescence and depression rises. Girls in current Western cultures seem especially vulnerable to this process too, because the increase in body fat that is typical for girls in adolescence runs counter to the desired slim body type.

All this research has taken us a fair distance in our efforts to understand both the rise in depression in adolescence and the marked gender difference in rates of depression. But

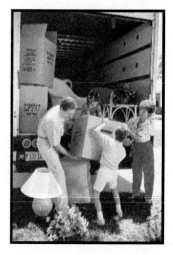

Whether a child will show a behavior problem at a stressful time like moving will depend in part on whether he faces several other stresses or life changes at the same time—such as perhaps his parents' divorce.

Do you recall having been significantly depressed during adolescence? If so, do any of these explanations or causal factors fit your own experience?

The Real World
Adolescent Suicide and Its Prevention

One possible accompaniment of depression is suicide. Suicide is very uncommon in children before adolescence. Even among children between 10 and 14, less than 1 child in 100,000 in the United States commits suicide each year. But among those between 15 and 19, the rate is considerably higher, and rising, as I pointed out in Chapter 4.

The likelihood of suicide is almost five times as high among adolescent boys as among girls, and nearly twice as high among whites as among nonwhites *except* for Native-American youth, who attempt and commit suicide at higher rates than any other group (Centers for Disease Control, 1994e). The rate among Native-Americans is 26.3 per 100,000 per year, compared to about 20 per 100,000 among white teen males.

In contrast, suicide *attempts* are estimated to be three times more common in girls than in boys (Garland & Zigler, 1993). Girls, more often than boys, use less-"successful" methods, such as self-poisoning. In one study in England, for example, the rate of hospital admissions for self-poisoning among girls rose from 4 per 10,000 among 12-year-olds to over 50 per 10,000 at age 16. Among boys, the rate at age 16 was one fifth that level (Hawton & Goldacre, 1982).

It is obviously very difficult to uncover the contributing factors in successful or completed suicides, because the crucial individual is no longer available to be interviewed. Researchers and clinicians are forced to rely on second-hand reports by parents or others about the mental state of the suicide before the act—reports that are bound to be at least partially invalid, because in many cases the parents or friends had no suspicion that a suicide attempt was imminent. Nonetheless, it does seem clear that some kind of significant psychopathology is virtually a universal ingredient, including but not restricted to depression. Behavior problems such as aggression are also common in the histories of completed suicides, as is a family history of psychiatric disorder or suicide, or a pattern of drug or alcohol abuse (Garland & Zigler, 1993).

But these factors alone are not enough to explain suicidal behavior. After all, many teenagers (or adults) display one or more of these risk factors, and very few actually commit suicide. David Shaffer (Shaffer, et al., 1988) suggests at least three other important elements:

1. Some triggering stressful event. Studies of suicides suggest that among adolescents, this triggering event is often a disciplinary crisis with the parents, or some rejection or humiliation, such as breaking up with a girlfriend or boyfriend, or failure in a valued activity.
2. An altered mental state, which might be an attitude of hopelessness, reduced inhibitions from alcohol consumption, or rage (Swedo et al., 1991). Among girls, in particular, the sense of hopelessness seems to be common: a feeling that the world is against them *and that they can't do anything about it.*
3. There must be an opportunity—a loaded gun available in the house, a bottle of sleeping pills in the parents' medicine cabinet, or the like.

Attempts to prevent teen suicide have not been notably successful. Despite the fact that most suicides and suicide attempters have displayed significantly deviant behavior for some time before the event, most do not find their way to mental health clinics or other professionals, and increasing the availability of such clinics, of hot lines, or crisis phones has not proven effective in reducing suicide rates.

Other prevention efforts have focused on education, such as providing training to teachers or to teenagers on how to identify students who are at risk for suicide, in the hope that vulnerable individuals might be reached before they attempt suicide. Special training in coping abilities has also been offered to students, so that teenagers might be able to find a nonlethal solution to their problems. Unfortunately, most such programs appear to be ineffective in changing student attitudes or knowledge (Shaffer et al., 1991).

These discouraging results are not likely to change until we know a great deal more about the developmental pathways that lead to this particular form of psychopathology. What makes one teenager particularly vulnerable and another able to resist the temptation? What combination of stressful circumstances is most likely to trigger a suicide attempt, and how do those stressful circumstances interact with the teenager's personal resources? Only when we can answer questions of this kind will we be on the road to understanding teenage suicide.

teenagers still vary widely in their responses to what appear to be the same levels of stress. Not every teenager who faces multiple stresses, fails to live up to some standard, is inclined to ruminate rather than use distraction, or is temperamentally shy ends up being clinically depressed. These are all risk factors, but even with these risk factors, some are more vulnerable than others.

Vulnerability and Resilience

This question of vulnerability or resilience has been a persistent theme among developmental psychopathologists. The research findings suggest that the same kinds of protective factors that help poor children rise above their negative circumstances (listed in Chapter 14) also mitigate the effect of other kinds of stresses. Children who are securely attached to someone (whether it be a parent or someone else), who have good cognitive skills, and who have sufficient social skills to make connections with peers are better able to weather the stresses they encounter.

For example, in her studies of resilience among school-age children, Ann Masten (1989) has found that when children have experienced a year with high levels of life stresses, those with higher IQs are much less likely to respond to that stress by becoming disruptive. Masten speculates that this may be due to the fact that such children, who have a history of successful problem solving, have a stronger sense of self-efficacy, which may help them resist frustration.

On the other side of the coin are the vulnerable children, who are far more likely to show significant psychopathology in the face of stress. Some kinds of vulnerabilities are inborn, such as physical abnormalities, prenatal trauma or preterm birth, prenatal malnutrition, or exposure to disease *in utero*. A tendency toward "difficult" temperament, which also seems to be inborn, is another significant vulnerability, not only because, by definition, such children have greater difficulty adapting to new experiences, but because such children are harder to raise. Their parents may be less able to establish regular discipline patterns.

Other vulnerabilities emerge during infancy or early childhood. An insecure early attachment, and the internal working model that accompanies it, seems to make a child more vulnerable to stress at later ages, particularly to stresses that involve losses or severe strains on key relationships. And any combination of circumstances that results in a high rate of aggressive or disruptive behavior with peers makes a child more vulnerable to a whole variety of stresses in the elementary and high school years (Masten, 1989).

Kenneth Rubin (Rubin et al., 1994) has proposed a model of the origins of internalizing disorders that combines many of these elements. He argues that one important pathway begins with an infant who shows high levels of behavioral inhibition (a temperamental pattern you'll recall from Chapter 9). Among infants with such a tendency, those who become securely attached to their parents appear to be okay. But those who become insecurely attached tend to move down a path that includes anxiety and fearfulness in the preschool years and anxiety and perhaps victimization by bullies in early school years. This results in more anxiety and withdrawal from peers, and a failure to develop helpful social skills. By adolescence, these children are at high risk for depression.

Overall, it seems very helpful to think of each child as possessing some inborn *vulnerabilities;* some *protective factors,* such as a secure attachment or a middle-class family; and some *resources,* such as higher IQ, an array of friends, or good peer interaction skills. How any given child will react to stressful life circumstances or to normal developmental

How would you describe your own vulnerabilities, protective factors, and resources?

passages like school entry or adolescence will depend on the relative weight of these three elements—*and* on how many separate stresses the child must face at the same time. No matter how fundamentally resilient he may be, any child is more likely to show at least a short-term behavior problem when multiple stresses pile up at once.

Developmental Psychopathology: A Reprise

I think that even this brief foray into research on psychopathology makes clear that a developmental framework is the only one that is going to yield real understanding of the emergence of deviant behavior. Even for a disorder such as hyperactivity, which appears to be rooted in an inborn biological dysfunction, the severity and persistence of the disorder can be best understood in terms of the child's cumulative patterns of interaction and the child's own internal models of relationships. Ultimately, studies within this emerging tradition of developmental psychopathology may end up telling us as much about normal development as about the emergence of pathology.

Intellectually Atypical Development

If you go back and look at Table 15.1 you'll see that the frequency of the various forms of intellectually atypical development among children ranks right up there with that of the various psychopathologies. Roughly one in ten children shows at least some form of intellectual abnormality, including learning disabilities, speech problems, and mental retardation.

Mental Retardation

Mental retardation is normally diagnosed when a child has an IQ below 70 *and* has significant problems in *adaptive behavior*—such as an inability to dress or eat alone or a problem getting along with others or adjusting to the demands of a regular school classroom. Thus, a low IQ score is a necessary but not sufficient condition for an individual to be classed as retarded. As Thomas Achenbach (1982) says, "Children doing well in school are unlikely to be considered retarded no matter what their IQ scores" (p. 214).

Low IQ scores are customarily divided up into several ranges, with different labels attached to each, as you can see in Table 15.3. I've given both the labels used by psycholo-

Table 15.3
IQ Scores and Labels for Children Classed as Retarded

Approximate IQ Score Range	Label Used by Psychologists	Label Used in Schools
68–83	Borderline retarded	(No special label)
52–67	Mildly retarded	Educable mentally retarded (EMR)
36–51	Moderately retarded	Trainable mentally retarded
19–35	Severely retarded	(No special label)
Below 19	Profoundly retarded	(No special label)

gists, and those that may be more common in the school system. (There are no school system labels for children with IQs below about 35 because schools very rarely deal with children functioning at this level.)

The farther down the IQ scale you go, the fewer children there are. More than 80 percent of all children with IQs below 70 are in the "mild" range; only about 2 percent of low-IQ youngsters (perhaps 3500 children in the U.S.) are profoundly retarded (Broman et al., 1987).

Cognitive Functioning in Retarded Children.   In Chapter 7 I mentioned that some researchers interested in information processing have tried to understand normal intellectual processing by looking at the ways in which retarded children think or approach problems differently than do normal-IQ children (Campione, Brown, & Ferrara, 1982; DeLoache & Brown, 1987). The major conclusions from this research are that retarded children:

1. Think and react more slowly.

2. Require much more complete and repeated instruction to learn new information or a new strategy (compared to normal-IQ children, who may discover a strategy for themselves, or profit from incomplete instruction).

3. Do not generalize or transfer something they have learned in one situation to a new problem or task. They thus appear to lack those "executive" functions that enable older, higher-IQ children (or adults) to compare a new problem to familiar ones or to scan through a repertoire of strategies until they find one that works.

On simple tasks, retarded children learn in ways and at rates that are similar to younger normal-IQ children. The more significant deficit lies in higher-order processing. These children *can* learn, but they do so more slowly and require far more exhaustive and task-specific instruction.

Causes of Retardation.   About 15 to 25 percent of mentally retarded children have an identifiable physical problem (Broman et al., 1987). **Chromosomal anomalies** such as Down syndrome or the Fragile X syndrome are one major culprit. As Scarr and Kidd put it, "Having too much or too little [genetic material] will affect intelligence, always for the worse" (1983, p. 380). A child may also inherit a specific disease or **inborn error of metabolism** that can cause retardation if not treated. The best-known inherited metabolism error is phenylketonuria (PKU), which I described in Chapter 2 (Table 2.2).

A third physical cause of retardation is **brain damage,** which can result from a large number of causes, including prenatal maternal diseases like syphilis or cytomegalovirus, prenatal malnutrition, or alcoholism. Brain damage may also occur during birth or be caused by an accident later (e.g., an auto accident or falling out of a tree house on your head).

The remaining three-quarters of retarded children show no signs of brain damage or other physical disorder. In almost all such cases, these children come from families in which the parents have low IQs, family life is highly disorganized, the parents are mentally ill, or emotional or cognitive deprivation exists. Often both genetic and environmental influences operate simultaneously.

Large-scale studies have now shown quite conclusively that these several causes of retardation are not distributed evenly across the range of low IQ scores. The lower the IQ, the more likely it is that the cause is physical rather than environmental. This is especially

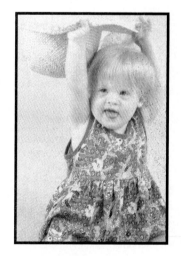

About 15 percent of mentally retarded children have clear physical abnormalities, such as Down syndrome.

clear from the results of the Collaborative Perinatal Project, which involved nearly 40,000 American children studied from before birth to age 7. In this sample, 71.7 percent of white and 53.9 percent of black children with IQs *below* 50 had an identifiable physical abnormality. In contrast, among those with IQs between 50 and 70, only 13.9 percent of whites and 6.3 percent of blacks had any recognizable physical problem (Broman et al., 1987).

You can see this difference even more vividly in another set of data from the same study. It happened that in a fair number of cases the sample included several children from the same family. So Broman and her colleagues were able to look at the IQs of the *siblings* of retarded children. The results for white children are shown in Figure 15.2.

The siblings of those with IQs below 50 had normal IQs; none was retarded. But the siblings of the mildly retarded were themselves fairly likely to be mildly retarded as well, a pattern that suggests quite different causes in the two groups. Among black children, whose families are more likely to be impoverished, the results are less clear: Siblings of both IQ groups are about equally likely to be retarded themselves. But the findings as a whole strongly support the conclusion that there are really two distinct types of retardation, each with its own set of causes.

One implication of this conclusion is that interventions like the enriched day care and preschool Ramey devised (recall Figure 6.4) are more likely to be effective in preventing or ameliorating milder retardation that has familial-cultural causes. This is not to say that we should ignore environmental enrichment or specific early training for children with physically caused retardation. Greater breadth of experience would enrich their lives and may help to bring their level of functioning closer to the top end of their "reaction range." But even massive early interventions are not going to make most brain-damaged or genetically anomalous children intellectually normal, although they can help the child to function much more independently (Spiker, 1990).

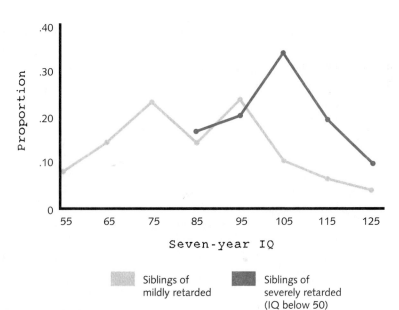

FIGURE 15.2 These data suggest that there are really two quite different kinds of retarded individuals: those whose retardation is caused by physical abnormalities, who usually have IQs below 50 and have *normal-IQ* siblings, and those whose retardation is cultural-familial in origin, usually with IQs in the mildly retarded range, whose siblings are also likely to be retarded. (*Source:* Broman et al., 1987, Figure 10-1, p. 269.)

Learning Disorders

Some children with normal IQs and essentially good adaptive functioning nonetheless have difficulty learning to read, write, or do arithmetic. The typical label for this problem is **learning disability,** although you will also hear terms like *dyslexia* (literally "nonreading") or *minimal brain damage.* The official definition of this problem includes the presumption that the difficulty arises from some type of central nervous system dysfunction or damage.

How *many* such children there are and how they should be characterized are still a matter of considerable dispute. Sylvia Farnham-Diggory (1992), one of the leading experts in the field, argues that up to 80 percent of all children classified by school systems as learning-disabled (LD) are misclassified. She claims that only about 5 out of every 1000 children are genuinely learning-disabled. The remainder are more appropriately called slow learners, or they may suffer from another difficulty, perhaps temporary emotional distress, poor teaching, or whatever.

Practically speaking, however, the term *learning disability* is used very broadly within school systems (at least within the United States) to label a grab bag of children who have unexpected or otherwise unexplainable difficulty with schoolwork, particularly reading. Nearly 5 percent of all children in the U.S. are currently labeled in this way (Farnham-Diggory, 1992).

There are good reasons why schools identify so many children as learning-disabled. For one thing, the diagnostic problem is extremely difficult. The designation of a learning disability is basically a *residual* diagnosis. It is the label normally applied to a child who does not learn some school task, who is *not* generally retarded, and does *not* show persistent or obvious emotional disturbance or a hearing or vision problem. Thus, we can say what learning disability is *not*; what we cannot say is what it *is.*

The identification problem is complicated still further by the fact that among children identified as LD, the specific form of the problem varies widely, with some displaying difficulties in reading only, some having trouble with reading and spelling (such as the boy whose writing sample is shown in Figure 15.3), and others having more difficulty with arithmetic.

Furthermore, school districts receive federal funds to pay for special education for children identified as learning disabled, but they do *not* receive such funds for education of children labeled as "slow learners." Thus, schools have a strong financial incentive to label almost any kind of delayed or slow learning a "learning disability."

For all of these reasons, I cannot give you a precise estimate of the frequency of the problem, although I am inclined to believe Farnham-Diggory's 5 out of 1000.

The Nature of the Problem. Given such problems with definition, we shouldn't be surprised that the search for causes has been fraught with difficulties. As Farnham-Diggory says, "We are trying to find out what's wrong with children whom we won't be able to accurately identify until after we know what's wrong with them" (1986, p. 153).

The most central problem has been with the basic assumption that learning disability has a neurological basis. The difficulty is that children so labeled (like hyperactive children) rarely show signs of major brain damage on any standard tests—perhaps because many children are mislabeled or perhaps because the brain dysfunction is more subtle than what can be measured with standard tests.

The most promising current view is that a large number of small abnormalities develop in the brain during prenatal life, such as some irregularity of neuron arrangement,

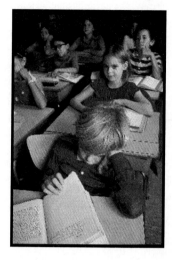

School can surely be a discouraging and frustrating place for a child with a learning disability.

Can you think of any way out of this dilemma? Should schools be given additional funds for those labeled as "slow learners" too? What might be the effects of such a policy?

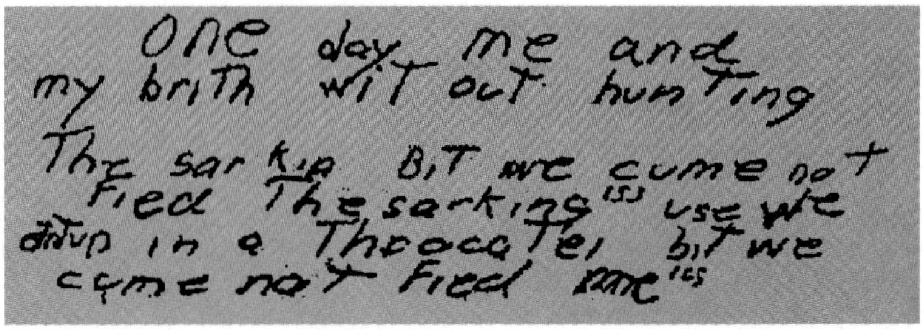

FIGURE 15.3 This is part of a story written by 13-year-old Luke, who has a significant and persistent learning disability. The little numbers next to some of the words are Luke's word counts. They show that despite his severe writing handicap, his counting abilities were intact (*Source:* Farnham-Diggory, 1992, p. 61. Reprinted by permission of the President and Fellows of Harvard College.)

clumps of immature brain cells, or scars or congenital tumors. The growing brain compensates for these problems by "rewiring" around the problem areas. These rewirings, in turn, may scramble normal information-processing procedures just enough to make reading, calculation, or some other specific task very difficult (Farnham-Diggory, 1992).

Another explanation of the problem, one you may recall from Chapter 8, is that reading disability may reflect a more general problem with understanding the sound and structure of language. The research findings supporting this conclusion have been very helpful in pointing educators toward possible remedial programs for children with reading difficulties. But they do not tell us why a child might have such language deficits in the first place. The problem may indeed lie in some type of brain dysfunction, or it may be that children whose reading problem has a linguistic origin are among the 80 percent Farnham-Diggory says are misclassified. They do indeed have a reading problem, but a neurological problem may not be responsible for it.

I want to emphasize that the continuing confusions and disagreements about identification and explanation of learning disability occur despite thousands of research studies and a great deal of theorizing by thoughtful and capable people. Not surprisingly, the uncertainty at the theoretical level is reflected in confusion at the practical level. Children are labeled "learning disabled" and assigned to special classes, but whether the child will be helped by a particular type of intervention program will depend on whether that specific program (1) is any good and (2) happens to match his or her type of disability or problem. Remediation does seem possible, but it is *not* simple, and a program that works well for one child may not work at all for another. Of course this is not good news for parents whose child is having difficulty with some aspect of schooling, whose only recourse is trial and error and eternal vigilance. But it reflects the disordered state of our knowledge.

Giftedness

For parents whose children lie at the other end of the intellectual continuum, the gifted, the problem is almost as tough. Finding good programs for such children is a continuing dilemma. Let me give you an extreme example, a child named Michael described by Halbert Robinson (1981):

> When Michael was 2 years and 3 months old, the family visited our laboratory. At that time, they described a youngster who had begun speaking at age 5 months and by 6 months had exhibited a vocabulary of more than 50 words. He started to read English when he was 13 months old. In our laboratory he spoke five languages and could read in

three of them. He understood addition, subtraction, multiplication, division, and square root, and he was fascinated by a broad range of scientific constructs. He loved to make puns, frequently bilingual ones. (p. 63)

Michael's IQ on the Stanford Binet was in excess of 180 at age 2; two years later, when Michael was 4½, he performed on the test like a 12-year-old and was listed as having an IQ beyond 220.

Definitions and Labels. We can certainly all agree that Michael should be labeled as **gifted.** But defining the term precisely is more difficult (Sternberg & Davidson, 1986). Giftedness includes those with exceptional specific talents, such as musical or artistic skills, or specific mathematical or spatial ability, as well as those with very high IQs. This broadening of the definition of giftedness has been widely accepted among theorists, who agree that there are many kinds of exceptional ability, each of which may reflect unusual speed or efficiency with one or another type of cognitive function.

Within school systems, however, giftedness is still typically defined entirely by IQ test scores, such as all scores above 130 or 140. Robinson suggested that it may be useful to divide the group of high-IQ children into two sets, the "garden variety gifted," with high IQs (perhaps 130 to 150) but without extraordinary ability in any one area, and the "highly gifted" (like Michael), with extremely high IQ scores and/or remarkable skill in one or more areas. These two groups of children may have quite different experiences at home and in school.

Cognitive and Social Functioning in Gifted Children. Just as retarded children show slower and less efficient information processing, the gifted show speedy and efficient processing on simple tasks, and flexible use of strategies on more complex tasks. They learn quickly and transfer that learning broadly (Sternberg & Davidson, 1985). Further, they seem to have unusually good *metacognitive* skills: They know what they know and what they don't know, and they spend *more* time than do average-IQ children in planning how to go about solving a problem (Dark & Benbow, 1993).

Whether such advanced intellectual abilities transfer to *social* situations is not so well established. Many parents are concerned about placing their gifted child in a higher grade because of fears that the child will be unable to cope socially; others have assumed that rapid development in one area should be linked to rapid development in all areas.

One famous and remarkable early study of gifted children, by Lewis Terman, pointed to the latter conclusion. Terman selected about 1500 children with high IQs from the California school system in the 1920s. These children—now adults in their seventies and eighties—have been followed regularly throughout their lives (e.g., Holahan, 1988; Terman, 1925; Terman & Oden, 1959). Terman found that the gifted children he studied were better off than their less-gifted classmates in many ways other than school performance. They were healthier; they were interested in many things, such as hobbies and games; and they were successful in later life. Both the boys and the girls in this study went on to complete many more years of education than was typical of children of their era and had successful careers as adults.

More recent research suggests a more neutral conclusion: Gifted children appear to have about the same risk of social or emotional problems as do normal-IQ children. Most are well adjusted and socially adept (Gottfried et al., 1994). Furthermore, good social development seems to be just as likely for gifted children who have been accelerated through school as for those who have been kept with their age mates but provided with "enrichment" programs (Robinson & Janos, 1986).

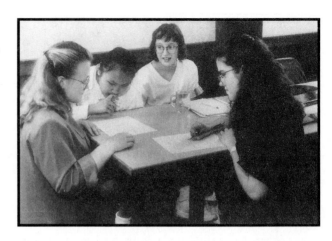

Elizabeth Lovance of Hartland, Wisconsin, on the right, skipped several grades and graduated from high school at age 14. She said of her experience of being accelerated through school: "I would have had a mental breakdown if I had remained where I was."

Are you persuaded by my arguments in favor of encouraging grade skipping by gifted children? If you were a parent of a gifted child, what kind of data would you want to have to help make a decision on this question?

Such optimism about the social robustness of gifted children may have to be tempered somewhat, however, in the case of the highly gifted subgroup, such as those with IQs above 180. These children are *so* different from their peers that they are likely to be seen as strange or disturbing. And these highly gifted children do show higher rates of emotional problems than do nongifted children (Janos & Robinson, 1985).

Also on the negative side of the ledger is the fact that many gifted children are so bored by school that they drop out, often because their school district does not allow acceleration in grade or has no special programs for the gifted. Given the fact that grade skipping does not seem to be linked to social maladjustment, it seems to make very good sense to encourage accelerated schooling, if only to help ward off terminal boredom for the gifted child.

Physically Atypical Development

The last group of children I want to talk about, albeit briefly, is that made up of children with clear physical problems, such as blindness or deafness. Such children experience very substantial difficulties in everyday living; most require special schooling or special facilities in school.

The Deaf Child

Most children with hearing loss can function adequately with the assistance of a hearing aid. In fact, many physicians are now fitting **hearing-impaired** children with hearing aids during infancy rather than waiting until the child is of preschool age. The situation is quite different, though, for the profoundly deaf—the child whose sense of hearing is essentially nonfunctional, even with mechanical assistance. There are approximately 23,000 such children in the U.S. today. Another 45,000 children have less total hearing loss but nonetheless require special education programs in school (Marschark, 1993). Here are a few facts about this deaf or severely hearing-impaired group:

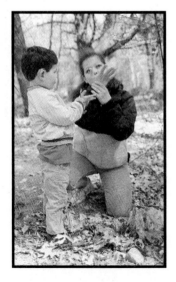

This hearing mother has learned to use sign language so that she can communicate with her deaf child.

1. The vast majority of deaf children (about 90 percent) are born to *hearing* parents and thus grow up in a world dominated by spoken language.

2. Most profoundly deaf children have major deficits in both spoken and written language. They have difficulty speaking, most do not lip-read well, and most read at only the most basic level—although deaf children and adults show essentially no decrement on nonverbal IQ or other measures of overall cognitive development (Braden, 1994).

3. Among the deaf, those with deaf parents usually do as well or *better* on measures of written and spoken language than do those with hearing parents (Marschark, 1993).

It is this last fact that is the most surprising and that raises key practical and theoretical questions. Why would children raised by deaf parents have a better prognosis? Schlesinger and Meadow (1972), in an early and influential book, argued that the major reason is that these children are learning a language—in this case sign language—at the normal time. Deaf parents use sign language with each other and with their children, so the children learn that language. But a deaf child of hearing parents, unless the parents learn to sign, will learn no language. Such children do develop their own gestures, even stringing two gestures together into a kind of simple sentence. But beyond this level, the child needs language input.

Not all the existing research is consistent with this hypothesis. Early learning of sign language may not be as vital as Schlesinger and Meadow thought. But *some* exposure to signing does seem to be critical. If the emphasis is placed exclusively on *oral* language, the deaf child has much more difficulty developing either speech or reading than if the child is taught sign language, lipreading, and oral language at the same time (Marschark, 1993). Some children with good combined training can function in a normal school environment, but even with good early training, most deaf or severely hearing-impaired children require special schooling.

The Blind Child

If I had asked you, before you read this chapter, to tell me which would be worse, to have been blind or deaf from birth, most of you would have said it would be far worse to be blind. Yet from the point of view of the child's ability to function in most normal settings, including school, blindness is a smaller handicap. The blind child can learn to read (with braille), can talk with others, can listen to tapes and to a teacher, and so on. Because of this greater academic potential and because of the enormous role of language in forming and maintaining social relationships, more options are open to the blind child or adult than to the deaf.

Still, there are obviously important limitations for the blind, and important potential pitfalls. One of these lies in the earliest relationship with the parent, which I've discussed in the *Research Report* on page 454. Later relationships may be impaired for the same reasons.

The long-term consequences of either deafness or blindness seem to depend in part on how early intervention is begun. Early intervention that involves the family seems especially helpful, which is precisely what we should expect from the perspective of developmental psychopathology. If family interventions, such as Fraiberg's (described in the *Research Report*), can help families to form secure attachments and to establish more optimum patterns of interaction, then some of the second- and third-order effects of the child's physical problem may be avoided.

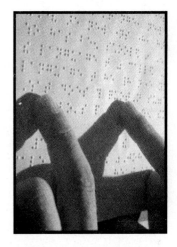

With the advent of small audiotape machines and books-on-tape, braille is not taught or learned by the blind as often as before. But signs in braille are still used in a variety of public places, such as elevators.

Sex Differences in Atypical Development

One of the most fascinating facts about atypical development is that virtually all forms of disorder are more common in boys than in girls. The major exception to this statement is depression, which as I've already mentioned, is about twice as common among adolescent girls and among adult women. I've put some of the comparisons in Table

Research Report

Basic Attachments Between Blind Babies and Their Mothers

In Chapter 11, I briefly mentioned Selma Fraiberg's work with blind infants as part of the discussion of the parents' attachment to the child. Because Fraiberg's work is so fascinating, I want to expand on the point.

Fraiberg (1974; 1975; 1977) found that blind babies begin to smile at about the same age as sighted babies (about 4 weeks) but that they smile less often. And at about 2 months, when the sighted baby begins to smile regularly at the sight of either parent's face, the blind baby's smiles become less and less frequent. The blind infant's smile is also less intense, more fleeting.

The other thing blind babies don't do is enter into mutual gaze. They don't look right at their parents, and everything we know about parents' responses to their babies underlines the importance of mutual gaze for the parents' feeling of attachment to the baby. Furthermore, the facial expressions of the blind infant are muted and sober. Many observers, including parents, conclude that the baby is depressed or indifferent. The combination of these circumstances often leaves the parents feeling as if the baby had rejected them.

Fraiberg found that most of the mothers of the blind babies in her studies gradually withdrew from their infants. They provided the needed physical care, but they stopped playing with the baby and gave up trying to elicit smiles or other social interactions. They often said they didn't "love" this baby.

Fortunately, it's possible to solve this particular problem. Fraiberg found that these mothers could be helped to form a strong bond with their infant if they could be shown how to "read" the baby's other signals. The blind child's face may be sober and relatively expressionless, but her hands and body move a lot and express a great deal. When the child *stops* moving when you come into the room, this means she is listening to your footsteps. Or she may move her hands when she hears your voice rather than smiling as a sighted child would do.

When parents of blind children learn to respond to these alternative "attachment behaviors" in their babies, then the mutuality of the relationship can be reestablished. And when this happens, and the parents can provide more varied stimulation, blind children develop more normal behavior in other ways. In particular, they don't show the "blindisms" so often observed in blind youngsters, such as rocking, sucking, head banging, and other repetitive actions.

Here, then, is a clear example of how psychological research can lead to very practical applications with families.

15.4 (p. 455), but even this list does not convey the extent of the difference. With very few exceptions, studies of the impact of environmental stresses show that boys are more adversely affected. This is true in studies of divorce, parental discord, parental mental illness, parental job loss, and many others. In these situations boys are more likely to show disturbed behavior, a decline in school performance, or some other indication of problem (Zaslow & Hayes, 1986).

How are we to explain differences like this? One possibility is that the double-X chromosome gives the girl protection from any form of inherited disorder or anomaly. Girls are obviously less likely to inherit any recessive disease that is carried on the sex chromosomes. We also have some hints that there may be a gene on the X chromosome that affects the individual's ability to respond effectively to stress. Since girls have two X chromosomes, they are less likely to suffer from a disorder in that gene. If this explanation is valid, then the appropriate conclusion is not that *all* boys are more vulnerable, but that *more* boys than girls have some minor neurological dysfunction, or high vulnerability to stressors of various kinds.

Two other physiological factors may also be important, each potentially explaining one or two of the differences listed in Table 15.4. First, hormonal differences may be important contributors. Since it is possible to construct a persuasive argument for the role of

Table 15.4
Sex Differences in the Incidence of Atypical Development

Type of Problem	Approximate Ratio of Males to Females
Psychopathologies	
Attention-deficit/hyperactivity disorder	4:1–9:1
Conduct disorders, including delinquency	5:1
Anxiety and depression: preadolescence	1:1
Anxiety and depression: adolescence	1:2
Estimated number of all children with all diagnoses seen in psychiatric clinics	2:1
Intellectually Atypical Development	
Mental retardation	3:2
Learning disabilities	3:1
Physical Problems	
Blindness or significant visual problems	1:1
Hearing impairment	5:4

Sources: Achenbach, 1982; Anthony, 1970; Eme, 1979; Nolen-Hoeksema & Girgus, 1994; Rutter, 1989; Rutter & Garmezy, 1983; Todd et al., 1995; Zoccolillo, 1993.

male hormones in aggressive behavior (as I attempted to do in Chapter 11), it is not a very great leap to the hypothesis that the higher incidence of conduct disorders among boys may also be related in some way to hormone variations.

A second possible physiological contributor is the comparative level of physical maturity of boys and girls. Because girls of any age are more physically mature than are boys of the same age, they may have more resources with which to meet various problems. For example, researchers have frequently observed that infant boys are more irritable and less able to achieve physical or emotional equilibrium after being upset than are infant girls (Haviland & Malatesta, 1981). Since such fussiness is also common in *younger* babies, the problem may not be maleness, but immaturity.

Experiences after birth may also contribute to the differing rates of deviance. One hypothesis is that adults are simply more tolerant of disruptive or difficult behavior in boys than in girls. By this argument, boys and girls initially respond similarly to stressful situations, but boys learn early that various forms of acting-out, tantrums, or defiance are tolerated or not punished severely. Girls learn to inhibit these responses—perhaps even to internalize them—because adults respond quite differently to them. We have only fragments of support for such a hypothesis (e.g., Eme, 1979). Studies of cultures in which *both* boys and girls are discouraged from behaving aggressively or assertively would provide very useful data to test such an explanation.

Can you think of any other explanations?

Whatever the explanation—and none of the existing explanations seems very satisfactory to me—it is nonetheless extremely interesting that girls do seem to be less vulnerable, less likely to show virtually any type of atypical development. Equally fascinating is the exception to this statement: depression among girls in adolescence. If girls are generally more robust, more able to handle stress, why should the stresses of puberty and adolescence be linked to such a significant rise in depression for girls? Is this a purely cultural phenomenon? Again, cross-cultural research would be very helpful in sorting out the possible causes.

The Impact of an Atypical Child on the Family

How does a family deal with an atypical child? In some instances of course, deficiencies or inadequacies in the family are part of the *cause* of the child's atypical development. But whether the original cause lies in the family or not, once a child does show some form of deviant development the family is inevitably affected, often adversely.

Grief. One of the first reactions is often a form of grief, almost as if the child had died. This reaction makes sense if you think about the fact that the *fantasy* "perfect child" did die or was never born. The parents grieve for the child-that-never-will-be, expressed poignantly by one parent:

> I wept for the perfect baby I had lost, for the sunsets he would never see, for the 4-year-old who would never be able to play outside unsupervised. (Featherstone, 1980, p. 26)

As with other forms of grief, denial, depression, and anger are all natural elements. Many parents also feel some guilt (e.g., "If only I hadn't had those drinks at that party while I was pregnant").

In some cases this process may result in an emotional rejection of the infant, aggravated by the difficulty many atypical infants have in entering fully into the mutually adaptive parent-child process. Such rejection seems to be particularly common when the marital relationship is conflicted, or when the family lacks adequate social support (Howard, 1978).

Adaptation by the Family. Once the initial shock and grief are dealt with as well as possible, the family must work toward an ongoing adaptive system with the atypical child. There are often massive financial burdens, problems of finding appropriate schooling, endless daily adjustments to the child's special needs.

> I look at the people down the street. Their kids are 15 and 18 and now they can just get in the car and take off when they want to . . . and then I think, "When will that happen for us? We'll always have to be thinking of Christopher. . . . We'll never have that freedom." (Featherstone, 1980, p. 17)

The system that evolves most often leaves the mother primarily in charge of the atypical child; fathers of physically handicapped children quite often seem to withdraw from interaction with or care of the child (Bristol, Gallagher, & Schopler, 1988). This is not a general withdrawal of the father from the family system, since such fathers continue to be involved with their other children. But the father's selective withdrawal leaves the mother with added burdens. One predictable response, among both mothers and fathers, is depression. Parents of atypical children are also more likely to have low self-esteem and to have lower feelings of personal competence (Howard, 1978). Where the marital relationship was poor before the birth of the atypical child, the presence of the handicapped child in the family system seems to increase the likelihood of further discord. However, there is no consistent indication that having an atypical child results in an average increase in marital disharmony or risk of divorce (Longo & Bond, 1984).

The fact that many (even most) parents manage to adapt effectively to the presence of an atypical child is testimony to the devotion and immense effort expended. But we cannot evade the fact that rearing such a child is very hard work and that it strains the family system in ways that rearing a normal child does not.

A Final Point

As a final point, I think it is crucial for me to state clearly what has been only implicit throughout this chapter: Children whose development is atypical in some respect are much more *like* normally developing children in other respects than they are unlike them. Blind, deaf, and retarded children all form attachments in much the same way that physically and mentally normal children do (Lederberg & Mobley, 1990); children with conduct disorders go through the same sequences of cognitive development that more adjusted children show. It is very easy, when dealing with an atypical child, to be overwhelmed by the sense of differentness. But as Sroufe and Rutter and all the other developmental psychopathologists are beginning to say so persuasively, the same basic processes are involved.

Summary

1 Approximately 20 percent of all children in the United States will need some form of special assistance because of atypical development at some time in childhood or adolescence.

2 Studies of psychopathology are more and more being cast in a *developmental* framework, with emphasis on the complex pathways that lead to deviance or normality. Such a framework also emphasizes the importance of the child's own resilience or vulnerability to stress.

3 Psychopathologies are divided into two broad groups: externalizing and internalizing.

4 One type of externalizing problem is conduct disorders, including patterns of both excess aggressiveness and delinquency. Conduct disorders can also be divided into early- and late-onset problems. The former are more serious and persistent.

5 Early-onset conduct disorders appear to have a genetic component and to be exacerbated by poor family interactions and subsequent poor peer relations.

6 Delinquent (law-breaking) acts increase in adolescence and may be found not only among children with early-onset conduct disorders, but also among some teens who show a brief period of delinquency without long-term negative consequences.

7 Attention-deficit/hyperactivity disorder is another type of externalizing problem, beginning in early childhood and typically persisting. The problems encountered by such children are much more acute if they also display conduct disorders.

8 Hyperactivity appears to have an initial biological cause, but deviant patterns are aggravated or ameliorated by subsequent experience.

9 Depression is one form of internalizing problem, relatively uncommon in childhood but common in adolescence. Depressed youngsters are more likely to have a family history of parental depression, to have developed low self-esteem, or to have a history of being ignored by peers.

10 Depression in adolescence is about twice as common among girls as among boys. No consensus has yet been reached on the explanation for this sex difference.

11 Family stress or stress experienced directly by the child, especially multiple simultaneous stresses, exacerbate any existing or underlying tendency toward pathology.

12 Children with inborn vulnerabilities (difficult temperament or physical problems), few protective factors, and few resources are more likely to respond to stressful circumstances with pathology.

13 Children with mental retardation, normally defined as IQ below 70 combined with significant problems of adaptation, show slower development and more immature or less efficient forms of information-processing strategies.

14 Two groups of retarded can be identified: those with clear physical abnormalities, overrepresented among the severely retarded, and those without physical abnormalities but with low-IQ parents and/or deprived environments, who are overrepresented among the mildly retarded.

15 Roughly 4 percent of the school population in the United States are labeled as learning-disabled. There is still considerable dispute about how to identify genuine learning disability, and many may be misclassified.

16 Learning disability may be caused by small anomalies in brain function; alternatively, they may reflect broader language or cognitive deficits, or both.

17 *Gifted* is a term applied to children with very high IQ or with unusual creativity or special skill. Their information processing is unusually flexible and generalized. Socially, they appear to be well adjusted, except for the small group of unusually highly gifted students.

18 Deaf children show significant deficits in reading and language, although those who are fully trained in signing and then learn English as a second language do somewhat better.

19 Blind children may have difficulty with early relationships because their interpersonal signals are quite different. However, they adapt much more readily to school than do the deaf.

20 Except for adolescent depression, boys show almost all forms of atypical development more often than do girls. This may reflect genetic differences, hormone differences, or differences in cultural expectations.

21 Families with atypical children experience chronically heightened stress and demands for adaptation. This is frequently accompanied by depression or other disturbance in the parents.

Key Terms

attention-deficit/hyperactivity disorder (ADD) (**p. 437**)

brain damage (**p. 447**)

chromosomal anomalies (**p. 447**)

conduct disorder (**p. 435**)

delinquency (**p. 436**)

depression (**p. 441**)

developmental psychopathology (**p. 433**)

externalizing problems (**p. 435**)

gifted (**p. 451**)

hearing-impaired (**p. 452**)

hyperactivity (**p. 437**)

inborn errors of metabolism (**p. 447**)

internalizing problems (**p. 435**)

learning disability (**p. 449**)

mental retardation (**p. 446**)

Suggested Readings

Farnham-Diggory, S. (1992). *The learning-disabled child.* Cambridge, MA: Harvard University Press.

This revision of an excellent book will give you an up-to-date source, pitched at the level of the lay reader.

Lewis, M., & Miller, S. M. (Eds.). (1990). *Handbook of developmental psychopathology.* New York: Plenum Press.

This book is definitely written for fellow professionals, so it is often very dense and technical. But if you are interested in any aspect of psychopathology, this is a highly valuable source.

Marschark, M. (1993). *Psychological development of deaf children.* New York: Oxford University Press.

A thoughtful, highly detailed, current discussion of what psychologists and linguists now know about deaf children.

Petersen, A. C., Compas, B. C., Brooks-Gunn, J., Stemmler, M., Ey, S., & Grant, K. E. (1993). Depression in adolescence. *American Psychologist, 48,* 155–168.

A brief, fairly dense review of the most current information on this important subject.

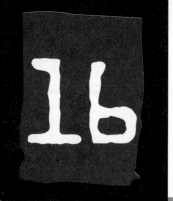

16 Putting It All Together: The Developing Child

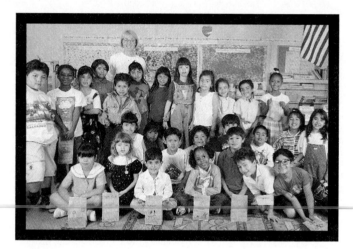

I remember the sense of unfairness I had in a world history class in high school when, after I had carefully learned all the kings of England in order and all the kings of France in order, I was asked on a test to say who had been king of France at the same time that Henry VIII had ruled England. I hadn't the foggiest idea; we had never studied it that way.

You may have something of the same feeling about the developing child. For example, you know a good deal about the sequence of development of language and about the sequential changes in cognitive functioning and in attachments, but you probably have not hooked these different developmental sequences to one another very well. If I asked you now what was happening at the same time that the child first used two-word sentences, you would probably have a difficult time answering. So what I want to do in this brief chapter is to put the child back together a bit by looking at the things that are happening at the same time.

I also want to take another look at some of the key questions I raised in Chapter 1: What are the major influences on development? Does the timing of experience matter? What is the nature of developmental change? Are there stages or sequences? And how best can we understand individual differences in development?

Think about it. What else is going on when the child first uses two-word sentences?

Transitions, Consolidations, and Systems

I see the process of development as being made up of a series of alternating periods of rapid growth (accompanied by disruption or disequilibrium) and periods of relative calm or consolidation. Change is obviously going on all the time, from conception to death. But I am persuaded that there are particular times when the changes pile up or when one highly significant change occurs. This might be a major physiological development like puberty; a highly significant cognitive change, such as the beginning of symbol usage at about 18 months, or some other major shift.

When such a significant change occurs, it has two related effects. First, in systems theory terms, any one change inevitably affects the entire system. So a rapid increase of skill in one area, like language, demands adaptation in all parts of the developing system. Because the child can now talk, her social interactions change, her thinking changes, no doubt even her nervous system changes as new synapses are created and redundant ones are pruned. Similarly, the child's early attachment may affect her cognitive development by altering the way she approaches new situations; the hormonal changes of puberty affect parent-child relations.

Second, when the system changes in such a major way, the child sometimes seems to come "unglued" for a while. The old patterns of relationships, of thinking, or of talking don't work very well any more, and it takes a while to work out new patterns. Erikson frequently uses the word *dilemma* to label such periods of semiupheaval. Klaus Riegel (1975) once suggested the phrase "developmental leaps," which conveys nicely the sense of excitement and blooming opportunity that often accompany these pivotal periods. I'm going to use the more pedestrian term *transition* to describe the times of change or upheaval and the term *consolidation* to describe the in-between times, when change is more gradual. Collectively, these concepts may help us examine what is happening during each of the major age periods.

Age Periods in Perspective

From Birth to 18 Months

Figure 16.1 shows the various changes during the first 18 months of life. The rows of the figure roughly correspond to the chapters of this book; what we need to do now is read up and down the figure rather than just across the rows.

The overriding impression one gets of the newborn infant—despite her remarkable skills and capacities—is that she is very much on automatic pilot. There seem to be built-in rules or schemas that govern the way the infant looks, listens, explores the world, and relates to others.

One of the really remarkable things about these rules, as I pointed out in Chapters 3 and 5, is how well designed they are to lead both the child and the caregivers into the

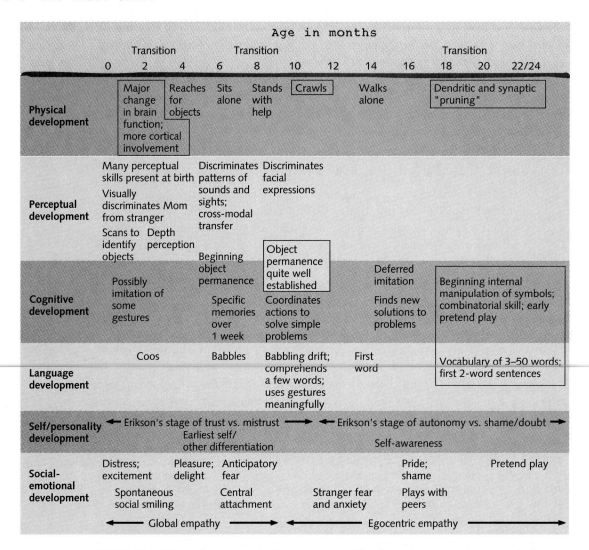

	Age in months											
	Transition				Transition					Transition		
	0	2	4	6	8	10	12	14	16	18	20	22/24
Physical development		Major change in brain function; more cortical involvement	Reaches for objects	Sits alone	Stands with help	Crawls		Walks alone		Dendritic and synaptic "pruning"		
Perceptual development		Many perceptual skills present at birth; Visually discriminates Mom from stranger; Scans to identify objects	Depth perception	Discriminates patterns of sounds and sights; cross-modal transfer	Discriminates facial expressions							
Cognitive development		Possibly imitation of some gestures		Beginning object permanence; Specific memories over 1 week	Object permanence quite well established; Coordinates actions to solve simple problems			Deferred imitation; Finds new solutions to problems		Beginning internal manipulation of symbols; combinatorial skill; early pretend play		
Language development		Coos		Babbles	Babbling drift; comprehends a few words; uses gestures meaningfully		First word			Vocabulary of 3–50 words; first 2-word sentences		
Self/personality development	← Erikson's stage of trust vs. mistrust →		Earliest self/other differentiation			← Erikson's stage of autonomy vs. shame/doubt →; Self-awareness						
Social-emotional development		Distress; excitement; Spontaneous social smiling	Pleasure; delight	Anticipatory fear; Central attachment			Stranger fear and anxiety		Pride; shame; Plays with peers		Pretend play	
	← Global empathy →				← Egocentric empathy →							

FIGURE 16.1 This brief summary chart shows some of the simultaneous developments during infancy. I have outlined the several developmental changes that seem to me to be pivotal.

"dance" of interaction and attachment. Think of an infant being breast-fed. The baby has the needed rooting, sucking, and swallowing reflexes to take in the milk; in this position, the mother's face is at just about the optimum distance from the baby's eyes for the infant's best focusing; the mother's facial features, particularly her eyes and mouth, are just the sort of visual stimuli that the baby is most likely to look at; the baby is particularly sensitive to the range of sounds of the human voice, particularly the upper register, so the higher-pitched, lilting voice most mothers use is easily heard by the infant; and during breast-feeding the release of a hormone called *cortisol* in the mother has the effect of relaxing her and making her more alert to the baby's signals. Both the adult and the infant are thus primed to interact with one another.

Sometime around 6 to 8 weeks there seems to be a change, with these automatic, reflexive responses giving way to behavior that looks more volitional. The child now looks at objects differently, apparently trying to identify what an object is rather than merely where it is; at this age she also begins to reliably discriminate one face from another, smiles more, sleeps through the night, and generally becomes a more responsive creature.

Because of these changes in the baby, and because it takes most mothers six to eight weeks to recover physically from the delivery (and for the mother and father jointly to begin to adjust to the immense change in their routine), we also see big changes in mother-infant interaction patterns at this time. The need for routine caretaking continues, of course (ah, the joys of diapers!), but as the child stays awake for longer periods and smiles and makes eye contact more, exchanges between parent and child become more playful and smoother-paced.

Once this transition has occurred there seems to be a brief period of consolidation lasting perhaps five or six months. Of course change continues during this consolidation period. Neurological change, in particular, is rapid, with the motor and perceptual areas of the cortex continuing to develop. The child's perceptual skills also show major changes in these months, with depth perception, clear cross-modal transfer, and identification of patterns of sounds and sights all emerging. Despite all these changes, a kind of equilibrium nonetheless exists in this period—an equilibrium that is altered by a series of changes that occur between about 7 and 9 months: (1) The baby forms a strong central attachment, followed a few months later by separation anxiety and fear of strangers; (2) the infant begins to move around independently (albeit very slowly and haltingly at first); (3) communication between infant and parents changes substantially, as the baby begins to use meaningful gestures and to comprehend individual words; (4) object permanence is grasped at a new level; the baby now understands that objects and people can continue to exist even when they are out of sight. At the very least, these changes profoundly alter the parent-child interactive system, requiring the establishment of a new equilibrium, a new consolidation, a new system.

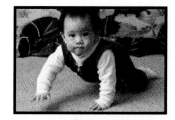

Eight-month-old Brandon not only can crawl, but undoubtedly also has a firm attachment to either or both parents, can perhaps understand a few words, and has a beginning understanding of object permanence. All these more or less simultaneous changes alter the system profoundly.

The baby continues to build gradually on this set of new skills—learning a few spoken words, learning to walk, consolidating the basic attachment—until 18 or 20 months of age, at which point the child's language and cognitive development appear to take another major leap forward—a set of changes I'll describe shortly.

So what is causing these patterns of development? Any short list of such causes is inevitably going to be a gross oversimplification. Still, undaunted, let me suggest four key processes that seem to me to be shaping the patterns shown in the summary table.

Physical Maturation. First and most obviously, the biological clock is ticking very loudly indeed during these early few months. Only at adolescence and again in old age do we see such an obvious maturational pattern at work. In infancy, it is the prepatterned growth of neural dendrites and synapses that appears to be the key. The shift in behavior we see at 2 months, for example, seems to be governed by just such built-in changes, as synapses in the cortex develop sufficiently to control behavior more fully.

Important as this built-in program is, it nonetheless *depends on* the presence of a minimum "expectable" environment (Greenough, Black, & Wallace, 1987). The brain may be wired to create certain synapses, but the process has to be triggered by exposure to particular kinds of experience. Because such a minimum environment exists for virtually all infants, the perceptual, motor, and cognitive developments we see are virtually identical from one baby to the next. But that does not mean that the environment is unimportant.

The Child's Explorations. A second key process is the child's own exploration of the world around her. She is born *ready* to explore, to learn from her experience, but she still has to learn the specific connections between seeing and hearing, to tell the differences between Mom's face and someone else's, to pay attention to the sounds emphasized in the language she is hearing, to discover that her actions have consequences, and so on.

Clearly, physiological maturation and the child's own exploration are intimately linked in a kind of perpetual feedback loop. The rapid changes in the nervous system, bones, and muscles permit more and more exploration, which in turn affects the child's perceptual and cognitive skills, which in turn affects the architecture of the brain. For example, we now have a good deal of evidence that the ability to crawl—a skill that rests on a whole host of maturationally based physical changes—profoundly affects the baby's understanding of the world. Before the baby can move independently, he seems to locate objects only in relation to his own body; after he can crawl, he begins to locate objects with reference to fixed landmarks (Bertenthal, Campos, & Kermoian, 1994). This shift, in turn, probably contributes to the infant's growing understanding of himself as an object in space.

Attachment. A third key process seems obviously to be the relationship between the infant and the caregiver(s). I am convinced that Bowlby is right about the built-in *readiness* of all infants to create an attachment. But in this domain, the quality of the specific experience the child encounters seems to have a more formative effect than is true for other aspects of development. A wide range of environments is "good enough" to support physical, perceptual, and cognitive growth in these early months. But for the establishment of a secure central attachment, the acceptable range seems to be narrower. Still, attachment does not develop along an independent track. Its emergence is linked both to maturational change and to the child's own exploration. For example, the child's understanding of object permanence may be a necessary precondition for the development of a basic attachment. As John Flavell puts it, "How ever could a child persistently yearn and search for a specific other person if the child were still cognitively incapable of mentally representing that person in the person's absence?" (1985, p. 135).

We might also turn this hypothesis on its head and argue that the process of establishing a clear attachment may cause, or at least affect, the child's cognitive development. For example, securely attached youngsters appear to persist longer in their play and develop the object concept more rapidly (Bates et al., 1982). Such a connection might exist because the securely attached child is simply more comfortable exploring the world around him from the safe base of his secure person. He thus has a richer and more varied set of experiences, which may stimulate more rapid cognitive (and neurological) development.

Internal Working Models. We could also think of attachment as a subcategory of a broader process, namely, the creation of internal working models. Seymour Epstein (1991) proposes that what the baby is doing is nothing less than beginning to create a "theory of reality." In Epstein's view, such a theory includes at least four elements:

- A belief about the degree to which the world is a place of pleasure or pain

- A belief about the extent to which the world is meaningful—predictable, controllable, and just versus capricious, chaotic, or uncontrollable

- A belief about whether people are desirable or threatening to relate to

- A belief about the worthiness or unworthiness of the self.

The roots of this theory of reality, so Epstein and others argue (Bretherton, 1991), lie in the experiences of infancy, particularly the experiences with caregivers and other humans. Indeed, Epstein suggests that the beliefs created in infancy are likely to be the most basic, and therefore the most durable and resistant to change at later ages. Not all psychologists would agree with Epstein about the broadness of the infant's "theory" of reality. But virtually all would now agree that the baby begins to create at least two significant internal models, one of the self and one of relationships with others (attachment). Of the two, the attachment model seems to be the most fully developed at 18 or 24 months; the model of the self undergoes many elaborations in the years that follow. You'll recall from Chapter 10 that it is only at about age 7 or 8 that the child seems to have a sense of his *global* worth (Harter, 1987; 1990).

Influences on These Basic Processes. These four basic processes are quite robust (Masten, Best, & Garmezy, 1990). Nonetheless, infants can be deflected from the common trajectory by several kinds of influences:

1. *Organic Damage.* The most obvious potential influence is some kind of damage to the physical organism, either from genetic anomalies, inherited disease, or teratogenic effects *in utero*. But even here, nature and nurture interact: The long-term consequences of such damage may be more or less severe, depending on the richness and supportiveness of the environment the baby grows up in.

2. *Family Environment.* The specific family environment in which the child is reared also affects the trajectory. On one end of the continuum we can see beneficial effects from an optimal environment that includes a variety of objects for the baby to explore, at least some free opportunity to explore, and loving, responsive, and sensitive adults who talk to the infant often and respond to the infant's cues (Bradley et al., 1989). On the other end of the continuum, some environments can be so poor that they fall outside the "good enough" range and thus fail to support the child's most basic development. Severe neglect or abuse would fall into this category, as might deep or lasting depression in a parent or persisting upheaval or stress in family life. In between these extremes are many variations in enrichment, in responsiveness, in loving support—all of which seem to have at least some impact on the child's pattern of attachment, his motivation, the content of his self-concept, his willingness to explore, and his specific knowledge. We see the consequences of such differences further down the developmental road, when the child is facing the challenging tasks of school and the demands of relating to other children.

Overall Impressions of Infancy. One of the strongest impressions one gets from so much of the current research on babies is that they are far more capable than we had thought. They appear to be born with many more skills, many more templates for handling their experiences. But they are not 6-year-olds, and we need to be careful not to get too carried away with our statements about how much the baby can do.

The Preschool Years

The sense one gets of this period, summarized in Figure 16.2, is that the child is making a slow but immensely important shift from dependent baby to independent child. The toddler and preschooler can now move around easily, can communicate more and more clearly, has a sense of himself as a separate person with specific qualities, and has the beginning cognitive and social skills that allow him to interact more fully and successfully with playmates. At the same time, to use Piaget's term, the child's thinking is *decentering*: She is shifting from using herself as the only frame of reference and has become less tied to the outside appearances of things.

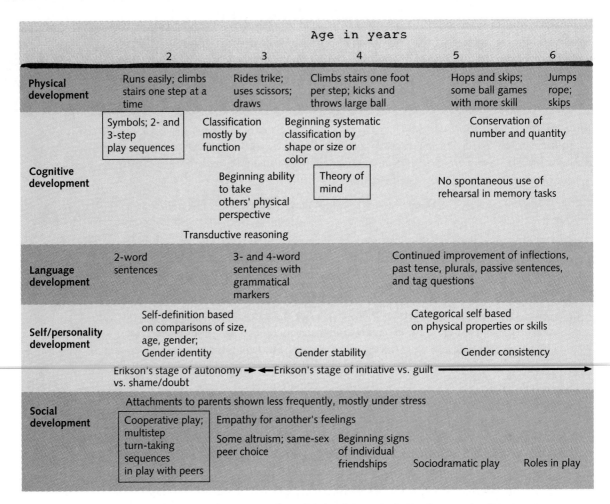

	Age in years				
	2	3	4	5	6
Physical development	Runs easily; climbs stairs one step at a time	Rides trike; uses scissors; draws	Climbs stairs one foot per step; kicks and throws large ball	Hops and skips; some ball games with more skill	Jumps rope; skips
Cognitive development	Symbols; 2- and 3-step play sequences	Classification mostly by function	Beginning systematic classification by shape or size or color	Conservation of number and quantity	
		Beginning ability to take others' physical perspective	Theory of mind	No spontaneous use of rehearsal in memory tasks	
		Transductive reasoning			
Language development	2-word sentences	3- and 4-word sentences with grammatical markers	Continued improvement of inflections, past tense, plurals, passive sentences, and tag questions		
Self/personality development	Self-definition based on comparisons of size, age, gender; Gender identity		Gender stability	Categorical self based on physical properties or skills	
				Gender consistency	
	Erikson's stage of autonomy ➔ ◄─ Erikson's stage of initiative vs. guilt ──────────────➤				
	vs. shame/doubt				
Social development	Attachments to parents shown less frequently, mostly under stress				
	Cooperative play; multistep turn-taking sequences in play with peers	Empathy for another's feelings			
		Some altruism; same-sex peer choice	Beginning signs of individual friendships	Sociodramatic play	Roles in play

FIGURE 16.2 A brief summary of parallel developments during the preschool years.

In the beginning, these newfound skills and new independence are not accompanied by much impulse control. Two-year-olds are pretty good at doing; it is *not* doing that gives them trouble. A large part of the conflict parents experience with children at this age comes about because the parent *must* limit the child, not only for the child's own survival, but to help teach the child impulse control (Escalona, 1981).

The preschool years also stand out as the period in which the seeds are sown for the child's enduring social skills and personality. The attachment process in infancy continues to be formative because it helps to shape the internal working model of social relationships the child creates. But in the years from 2 to 6, this early model is revised, consolidated, and established more firmly. The resultant interactive patterns tend to persist into elementary school and beyond. The 3-, 4-, or 5-year-old who develops the ability to share, to read others' cues well, to respond positively to others, and to control aggression and impulsiveness is likely to be a socially successful, popular 8-year-old. In contrast, the noncompliant, hostile preschooler is far more likely to become an unpopular, aggressive schoolchild (Campbell et al., 1991; Patterson, Capaldi, & Bank, 1991).

Many forces are at play in creating these changes, beginning with two immense cognitive advances in this period: the 18- or 24-month-old child's new ability to use symbols, and the rapid development, between ages 3 and 5, of a more sophisticated theory of mind.

Symbol Use. The development of symbol use is reflected in many different aspects of the child's life. We see it in the rapid surge of language development, in the child's approach to cognitive tasks, and in play, where the child now pretends, having an object *stand for* something else. The ability to use language more skillfully, in turn, affects social behavior in highly significant ways, such as the increasing use of verbal rather than physical aggression and the use of negotiation with parents in place of tantrums or defiant behavior.

Theory of Mind. The emergence of the child's more sophisticated theory of mind has equally broad effects, especially in the social arena, where the child's newfound abilities to read and understand others' behaviors form the foundation for new levels of interactions with peers and parents. It is probably not accidental that individual friendships between children are first visible at about the time that they also show the sharp drop in egocentrism that occurs with the emergence of the theory of mind.

We also see the seminal role of cognitive changes in the growing importance of several basic schemes. Not only does the 2- or 3-year-old have a more and more generalized internal model of attachment, but she also develops a self-scheme and a gender-scheme, each of which forms part of the foundation of both social behavior and personality.

Social Contacts. Important as these cognitive changes are, they are clearly not the only causal factors. Equally important are the child's contacts with adults and peers. When children play together, they expand each other's experience with objects and suggest new ways of pretending to one another, thus fostering still further cognitive growth. When two children disagree about how to explain something or insist on their own different views, it enhances each child's awareness that there *are* other ways of thinking or playing, thus creating opportunities to learn about others' mental processes (Bearison, Magzamen, & Filardo, 1986). Thus, social interactions are the arena in which much cognitive growth occurs. For example, in one recent study, Charles Lewis finds that children who have many siblings or who interact regularly with a variety of adult relatives show more rapid understanding of other people's thinking and acting than do children with fewer social partners (Lewis, Freeman, & Maridaki-Kassotaki, 1995). Some new research also shows that children with secure attachments show a more rapid shift to understanding false belief and other aspects of a representational theory of mind than do children with insecure attachments (Charman, Redfern, & Fonagy, 1995; Steele, Holder, & Fonagy, 1995)—a result that points to the importance of the *quality* as well as the quantity of social interactions for the child's cognitive development.

Play with other children also forms the foundation of the child's emerging gender schema. Noticing whether other people are boys or girls and what toys boys and girls play with, is itself the first step in the long chain of sex role learning.

Naturally enough, it is also in social interactions, especially those with parents, that the child's pattern of social behaviors are modified or reinforced. The parents' style of discipline becomes critical here. Gerald Patterson's work shows clearly that parents who lack the skills to control the toddler's impulsivity and demands for independence are likely to end up strengthening noncompliant and disruptive behavior, even if the parent's intention is the reverse (Patterson et al., 1991).

Family Dynamics. The family's ability to support the child's development in these years is affected not only by the skills and knowledge the parents bring to the process, but also by the amount of stress they are experiencing from outside forces and the quality of

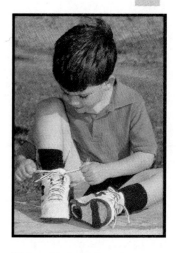

Pride and independence!

support they have in their personal lives (Crockenberg & Litman, 1990). In particular, mothers who are experiencing high levels of stress are more likely to be punitive and negative toward their children, with resulting increases in the child's defiant and noncompliant behavior (Webster-Stratton & Hammond, 1988). And maternal negativity, in turn, is implicated in the persistence of noncompliant behavior into elementary school. This link is clear, for example, in a longitudinal study of a group of such noncompliant children by Susan Campbell (Campbell & Ewing, 1990; Campbell et al., 1991). She finds that among a group of 3-year-olds who were labeled as "hard-to-manage," those who improved by age 6 had mothers who had been less negative.

The mother's stress is obviously not the only factor in her level of negativity toward the child. Depressed mothers are also more likely to show such behavior (Conrad & Hammen, 1989), as are mothers from working-class or poverty-level families, who may well have experienced such negativity and harsh discipline in their own childhoods. But stress and lack of personal social support are both part of the equation. Thus, the preschooler, like children of every age, is affected by broader social forces outside the family as well as by the family interaction itself.

The Elementary School Years

Figure 16.3 summarizes the changes and continuities of middle childhood. There are obviously many gradual changes: greater and greater physical skill, less and less reliance on appearance and more and more attention to underlying qualities and attributes, greater

> If a parent of a 2-year-old complained to you about the "terrible twoness" of his child, what comments might you make, in light of what you have just read? How could you explain the child's behavior to the parent in a way that might make it easier to deal with?

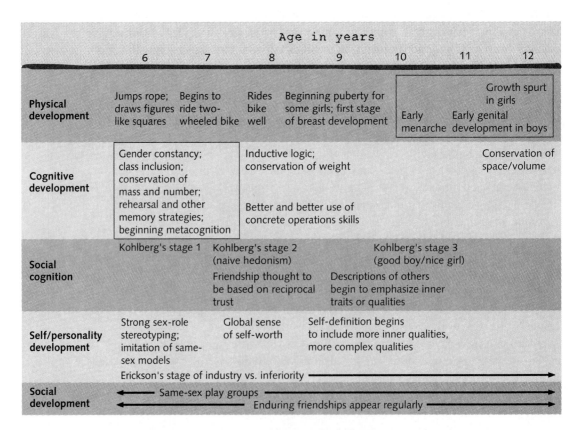

FIGURE 16.3 A summary of parallel changes during the elementary school years.

and greater role of peers. The one age at which there seems to be a more rapid change is right at the beginning of middle childhood, at the point of transition from the preschooler to the schoolchild.

Some kind of a transition into middle childhood has been noted in a great many cultures. There seems to be widespread recognition that a 6-year-old is somehow qualitatively different from a 5-year-old: more responsible, more able to understand complex ideas. Among the Kipsigis of Kenya, for example, the age of 6 is said to be the first point at which the child has *ngomnotet,* translated as *intelligence* (Harkness & Super, 1985). The fact that schooling begins at this age seems to reflect an implicit or explicit recognition of this fundamental shift.

Psychologists who have studied development across this transition have pointed to a whole series of changes.

- Cognitively, there is a shift to what Piaget calls concrete operational thinking. The child now understands conservation problems, seriation, and class inclusion. More generally, the child seems to pay less attention to surface properties of objects and more to underlying continuities and patterns, to be captured less by appearance and to focus on the underlying reality. We see this not only in children's understanding of physical objects but also in their understanding of others, of relationships, and of themselves. In studies of information processing, we see a parallel rapid increase in the child's use of executive strategies.

- In the self-concept, we first see a global judgment of self-worth at about age 7 or 8.

- In peer relationships, gender segregation becomes virtually complete by age 6 or 7, especially in individual friendships.

The apparent confluence of these changes is impressive and seems to provide some support for the existence of a Piaget-like stage. On the surface, at least, there seems to be some kind of change in the basic structure of the child's thinking that is reflected in all aspects of the child's functioning. But impressive as these changes are, it is not so clear that what is going on here is a rapid, pervasive, structural change to a whole new way of thinking and relating. Children don't make this shift all at once in every area of their thinking or relationships. For example, while the shift from a concrete to a more abstract self-concept may become noticeable at 6 or 7, it occurs quite gradually and is still going on at ages 11 and 12. Similarly, a child may grasp conservation of quantity at age 5 or 6 but typically does not understand conservation of weight until several years later.

Furthermore, expertise, or the lack of it, strongly affects the pattern of the child's cognitive progress. Thus, while I think most psychologists would agree that a set of important changes normally emerges together at about this age, most would also agree that no rapid or abrupt reorganization of the child's whole mode of operating is occurring.

Explaining the Changes. In trying to account for the developmental shifts we see during middle childhood, my bias has been to see the cognitive changes as most central, the necessary but not sufficient condition for the alterations in relationships and in the self-scheme during this period. A good illustration is the emergence of a global sense of self-worth, which seems to require not only a tendency to look beyond or behind surface characteristics but also the use of inductive logic. The child appears to arrive at a global sense of self-worth by some summative, inductive process.

Similarly, the quality of the child's relationships with peers and parents seems to rest in part on a basic cognitive understanding of reciprocity and perspective taking. The child now understands that others read him as much as he reads them. Children of 7 or 8 will now say of their friends that they "trust each other," something you would be very unlikely to hear from a 5-year-old.

Such a cognitive bias dominated theories and research on middle childhood for many decades, largely as a result of the powerful influence of Piaget's theory. This imbalance has begun to be redressed in recent years, as the central importance of the peer group and the child's social experience have been better understood. There are two aspects to this revision of thinking. First, we have reawakened to the (obvious) fact that a great deal of the experience on which the child's cognitive progress is based occurs in social interactions. Second, we have realized that social relationships make a unique set of demands, both cognitive and interactive, and have unique consequences for the child's social and emotional functioning. It is in these elementary school years, for example, that patterns of peer rejection or acceptance are consolidated, with reverberations through adolescence and into adult life.

Just what role physical change plays in this collection of developments I do not know. Clearly, physical changes *are* going on. Girls, in particular, begin the early stages of puberty during elementary school. But we simply don't know whether the rate of physical development in these years is connected in any way to the rate of the child's progress through the sequence of cognitive or social understandings. The one thing we know is that bigger, more coordinated, early-developing children are likely to have slightly faster cognitive development and be somewhat more popular with peers. Obviously, this is an area in which we need far more knowledge.

The Role of Culture. Most of what I have said about middle childhood—and about other ages as well—is almost entirely based on research on children growing up in Western cultures. I've tried to balance the scales a bit as I've gone along, but we must still ask, again and again, whether the patterns we see are specific to particular cultures or whether they reflect underlying developmental processes common to all children everywhere.

In the case of middle childhood, there are some obvious differences in the experiences of children in Western cultures versus those growing up in villages in Africa, in Polynesia, or in other parts of the world where families live by subsistence agriculture and schooling is not a dominant force in children's lives (Weisner, 1984). In many such cultures, children of 6 or 7 are thought of as "intelligent" and responsible and are given almost adultlike roles. They are highly likely to be given the task of caring for younger siblings and to begin their apprenticeships in the skills they will need as adults, such as agricultural skills or animal husbandry, learning alongside the adult. In some west African and Polynesian cultures, it is also common for children this age to be sent out to foster care, either with relatives, or as apprentices with a skilled tradesperson.

Such children obviously have a very different set of social tasks to learn in the middle-childhood years than do children growing up in industrialized countries. They do not need to learn how to relate to or make friends with strangers in a new school environment. Instead, from an early age they need to learn their place in an existing network of roles and relationships. For the Western child, the roles are less prescribed, the choices for adult life are far more varied.

Yet the differences in the lives of Western and non-Western children should not obscure the very real similarities. In all cultures, children this age develop individual friend-

As a way to grasp the importance of social contacts, try to imagine a child who grew up without ever playing with another child. How would such a child be different? What kind of adult would he or she become?

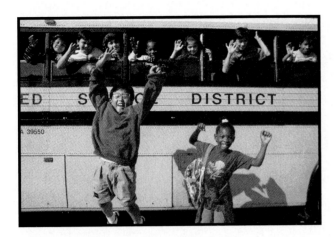

Going to school may not always be as filled with joy as this, but there is no doubt that it is a hugely formative experience for children in these ages.

ships, segregate their play groups by gender, develop the cognitive underpinnings of reciprocity, learn the beginnings of what Piaget calls concrete operations, and acquire some of the basic skills that will be required for adult life. These are not trivial similarities. They speak to the power of the common process of development, even in the midst of obvious variation in experience.

Adolescence

A number of experts on adolescence argue that it makes sense to divide the years between 12 and 20 into two subperiods, one beginning at 11 or 12, the other starting at perhaps 16 or 17. Some label these as *adolescence* and *youth* (Keniston, 1970), others as *early* and *late* adolescence (Brooks-Gunn, 1988). However we label them, there are distinct differences.

Early adolescence is, almost by definition, a time of transition, a time of significant change in virtually every aspect of the child's functioning. Late adolescence is more a time of consolidation, when the young person establishes a cohesive new identity, with clearer goals and role commitments. Norma Haan (1981), borrowing Piaget's concepts, suggests that early adolescence is a time dominated by assimilation, while late adolescence is primarily a time of accommodation.

The 12- or 13-year-old is assimilating an enormous number of new physical, social, and intellectual experiences. While all this absorption is going on, but before it is digested, the young person is in a more or less perpetual state of disequilibrium. Old patterns, old schemes no longer work very well, but new ones have not been established. It is during this early period that the peer group is so centrally important. Ultimately, the 16-, 17-, or 18-year-old begins to make the needed accommodations, pulls the threads together, and establishes a new identity, new patterns of social relationships, new goals and roles. Figure 16.4 presents a brief summary of the changes during adolescence.

Early Adolescence. In some ways the early years of adolescence have a lot in common with the early years of toddlerhood. Two-year-olds are famous for their negativism and for their constant push for more independence. At the same time, they are struggling to learn a vast array of new skills. Teenagers show many of these same qualities, albeit at much more abstract levels. Many of them go through a period of negativism, particularly with parents, right at the beginning of the pubertal changes. And many of the conflicts with parents center on issues of independence—they want to come and go when they

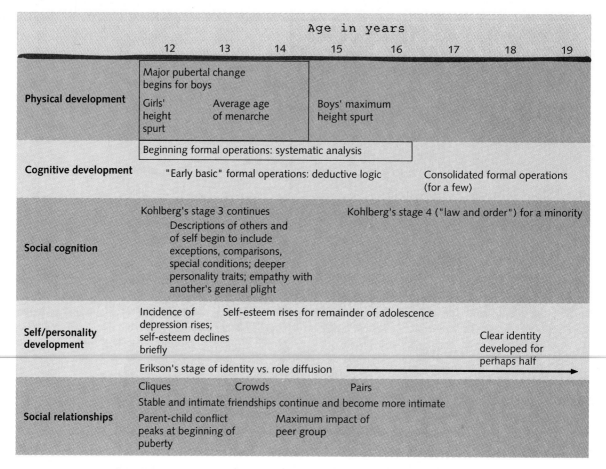

	Age in years							
	12	13	14	15	16	17	18	19
Physical development	Major pubertal change begins for boys Girls' height spurt Average age of menarche			Boys' maximum height spurt				
Cognitive development	Beginning formal operations: systematic analysis "Early basic" formal operations: deductive logic						Consolidated formal operations (for a few)	
Social cognition	Kohlberg's stage 3 continues Descriptions of others and of self begin to include exceptions, comparisons, special conditions; deeper personality traits; empathy with another's general plight				Kohlberg's stage 4 ("law and order") for a minority			
Self/personality development	Incidence of depression rises; self-esteem declines briefly Self-esteem rises for remainder of adolescence						Clear identity developed for perhaps half	
	Erikson's stage of identity vs. role diffusion ⟶							
Social relationships	Cliques Crowds Pairs Stable and intimate friendships continue and become more intimate Parent-child conflict peaks at beginning of puberty Maximum impact of peer group							

FIGURE 16.4 A brief summary of parallel developments during adolescence.

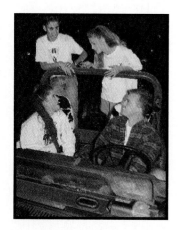

"Cruising" up and down the main streets of town, popular among teenagers in many parts of the United States, represents independence in a new form.

please, listen to the music they prefer at maximum volume, and wear the clothing and hairstyles that are currently "in."

As is true of the negativism of the 2-year-old, it is easy to overstate the depth or breadth of the conflict between young teenagers and their parents. For the great majority of teenagers, there is no major turmoil, only a temporary increase in disagreements or disputes. The depiction of adolescence as full of *Sturm und Drang* is as much an exaggeration as is the phrase *terrible twos*. But both ages are characterized by a new push for independence, which is inevitably accompanied by more confrontations with parents over limits.

While this push for independence is going on, young adolescents are also facing a whole new set of demands and skills to be learned—new social skills, new and more complex school tasks, a need to form an adult identity. The sharp increases in the rate of depression (especially among girls) and the drop in self-esteem we see at the beginning of adolescence seem to be linked to this surplus of new demands and changes. A number of investigators have found that those adolescents who have the greatest number of simultaneous changes at the beginning of puberty—changing to junior high school, moving to a new town or new house, perhaps a parental separation or divorce—also show the greatest loss in self-esteem, the largest rise in problem behavior, and the biggest drop in grade point average (Simmons, Burgeson, & Reef, 1988). Young adolescents who can cope with these changes one at a time, as when the youngster remains in the same school through eighth or ninth grade before shifting to junior or senior high school, show fewer symptoms of stress.

Facing major stressful demands, the 2-year-old uses Mom (or some other central attachment figure) as a safe base for exploring the world, returning for reassurance when fearful. Young adolescents seem to do the same with the family, using it as a safe base from which to explore the rest of the world, including the world of peer relationships. Parents of young adolescents must try to find a difficult balance between providing the needed security, often in the form of clear rules and limits, and still allowing independence—just as the parent of a 2-year-old must walk the fine line between allowing exploration and keeping the child safe. Among teenagers, as among toddlers, the most confident and successful are those whose families manage this balancing act well.

Still a third way in which theorists have likened the young teenager to the 2-year-old is in egocentrism. David Elkind (1967) suggested some years ago that egocentrism rises in adolescence. This new egocentrism, according to Elkind, has two facets: (1) the belief that "others in our immediate vicinity are as concerned with our thoughts and behavior as we ourselves are" (Elkind & Bowen, 1979, p. 38), which Elkind describes as having an *imaginary audience,* and (2) the possession of a *personal fable,* a tendency to consider their own ideas and feelings unique and singularly important. This is typically accompanied by a sense of invulnerability—a feeling that may lie behind the adolescent's apparent attraction to high-risk behavior, such as unprotected sex, drugs, drinking, high-speed driving, and the like.

Elkind's own research (Elkind & Bowen, 1979) shows that the preoccupation with others' views of the self (imaginary audience behavior) peaks at about ages 13 to 14. Teenagers this age are most likely to say that if they went to a party where they did not know most of the kids, they would wonder *a lot* about what the other kids were thinking of them. They also report that they worry a lot when someone is watching them work and feel desperately embarrassed if they discover a grease spot on their clothes or have newly erupted pimples. Of course younger children and adults may also worry about these things, but they seem to be much less disturbed or immobilized by these worries than are 13- and 14-year-olds—an age when the dominance of the peer crowd or clique is at its peak.

Drawing a parallel between the early adolescent and the toddler also makes sense in that both age groups face the task of establishing a separate identity. The toddler must separate herself from the symbiotic relationship with Mom or central caregiver. She must figure out not only that she is separate but also that she has abilities and qualities. Physical maturation also allows her new levels of independent exploration. The young adolescent must separate himself from his family, and from his identity as a child, and begin to form a new identity as an adult.

Late Adolescence. To carry the basic analogy further, late adolescence is more like the preschool years. Major changes have been weathered and a new balance has been achieved. The physical upheavals of puberty are mostly complete, the family system has changed to allow the teenager more independence and freedom, and the beginnings of a new identity have been created. This period is not without its strains. For most young people, a clear identity is not achieved until college age, if then, so the identity process continues. And the task of forming emotionally intimate sexual or presexual partnerships

Does the comparison of early adolescence and toddlerhood make sense to you? If it is a valid comparison, then does that suggest that development is somehow like a spiral, returning to the same issues repeatedly, but at levels of ever greater complexity?

is a key task of late adolescence. Nonetheless, I think Haan is correct that this later period is more one of accommodation than of assimilation. At the very least, we know that it is accompanied by rising levels of self-esteem and declining levels of family confrontation or conflict.

Possible Causal Links. How might all these simultaneous changes be connected to one another? There has been a good deal of interest in this set of questions in recent years, but we are still a long way from clear answers.

The obvious place to begin is with the role of puberty itself. Puberty not only defines the beginning of early adolescence, it also clearly affects all other facets of the young person's development, either directly or indirectly.

Direct effects might be seen in several ways. Most clearly, the surges of pubertal hormones stimulate sexual interest while they also trigger body changes that make adult sexuality and fertility possible. It seems inescapable that these changes are causally linked to the gradual shift from same-sex peer groupings to heterosexual crowds and finally to heterosexual pair relationships.

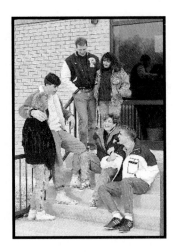

By late adolescence, the form of peer interaction has shifted from crowds and cliques to pairs.

Hormone changes may also be directly implicated in the increases in confrontation or conflict between parents and children, and the rise in various kinds of aggressive or delinquent behavior. Steinberg's research suggests such a direct link because he finds pubertal stage and not age to be the critical variable in predicting the level of adolescent-parent conflict. Other investigators have found that in girls, the rise in estradiol at the beginning of puberty is associated with increases in verbal aggression and a loss of impulse control, while in boys, increases in testosterone are correlated with increases in irritability and impatience (Paikoff & Brooks-Gunn, 1990). But there are also many studies in which no such connection is found. This has led most theorists to conclude that the connections between pubertal hormones and changes in adolescent social behavior are considerably more complicated than we had first imagined.

One of the complications is that the physical changes of puberty have highly significant indirect effects as well. When the child's body grows and becomes more like that of an adult, the parents begin to treat the child differently and the child begins to see himself as a soon-to-be-adult. Both of these changes may be linked to the brief rise in parent-adolescent confrontation and may help to trigger some of the searching self-examinations that are part of this period of life.

Physiological changes may also play some role in the shift to formal operations. We have some indication, for example, that a second major synaptic and dendritic "pruning" occurs at adolescence. At the same time, any link between formal operational thinking and pubertal change cannot be inevitable, because we know that all adolescents experience puberty but not all make the transition to formal operations. The best guess at the moment is that neurological or hormonal changes at adolescence may be *necessary* for further cognitive gains, but they cannot be *sufficient* conditions for such developments.

An equally attractive possibility is that cognitive changes are the most central. The cognitive shift from concrete to formal operations obviously does not cause pubertal changes, but cognitive development may be central to many of the other changes we see at adolescence, including changes in the self-concept, the process of identity formation, increases in level of moral reasoning, and changes in peer relationship.

There is ample evidence, for example, that the greater abstractness of the child's self-concept and of his descriptions of others are intimately connected to the broader changes in cognitive functioning (Harter, 1990). You will also remember from Chapter 12 that the shift in the child's thinking from concrete operations to at least beginning formal operations seems to be a necessary precondition for the emergence of more advanced forms of social cognition and moral judgment. Finally, some ability to use formal operations may also be necessary but not sufficient for the formation of a clear identity. One of the characteristics of formal operations thinking is the ability to imagine possibilities that you have never experienced and to manipulate ideas in your head. These new skills may help to foster the broad questioning of old ways, old values, old patterns that is a central part of the identity formation process. For example, several studies show that among high school and college students, those in Marcia's identity achievement or moratorium statuses are much more likely also to be using formal operations reasoning than are those in the diffusion or foreclosure statuses. In Rowe and Marcia's study (Rowe & Marcia, 1980), the *only* individuals who showed full identity achievement were those who were also using full formal operations. But the converse was not true. That is, there were a number of subjects who used formal operations who had not yet established a clear identity. Thus, formal operations thinking may *enable* the young person to rethink many aspects of his life, but it does not guarantee that he will do so.

Overall, we are left with the impression that both the physical changes of puberty and the potential cognitive changes of formal operations are central to the phenomena of adolescence, but the connections between them, and their impact on social behavior, remain unclear.

Returning to Some Basic Questions

With this brief overview in mind, let me now go back to some of the questions I raised in Chapter 1 and see if the answers can be made any clearer.

What Are the Major Influences on Development?

In Chapter 1 and throughout the book I have contrasted nature and nurture, nativism and empiricism, as basic explanations of developmental patterns. In every instance I have also said that the real answer lies in the interaction between the two. I certainly hope that it is this interactive message that you will take away with you. I can perhaps make the point clearest by going back to Aslin's five models of environmental/internal influences on development I showed in Figure 1.1. You'll recall that he is proposing one purely physical model (which he calls maturation), in which a particular development would occur regardless of environmental input, and one purely environmental pattern (which he calls induction), in which some development is entirely a function of experience. These two "pure" alternatives make logical sense, but in fact, probably neither of them occurs at all. *All* development is a product of various forms of interaction between internal and external influences.

Even in those areas of development that appear to be the most clearly biologically determined or influenced, such as physical development or early perceptual development, normal development can occur *only* if the child is growing in an environment that falls within the range of adequate or sufficient environments. The fact that the vast majority of environments fall within that range in no way reduces the crucial importance of the environment. John Flavell puts it this way: "Environmental elements do not become any less

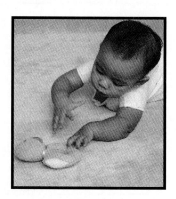

The fact that virtually all babies have some chance to reach for and examine objects does not mean that such experience is unimportant in the child's emerging perceptual or motor skills. Most (if not all) so-called maturational sequences require particular kinds of environmental inputs if they are to occur at all.

essential to a particular form of development just because they are virtually certain to be available for its use" (1985, p. 284).

Similarly, even those aspects of development that seem most obviously to be a product of environment, such as the quality of the child's first attachment, rest on a physiological substrate and on instinctive patterns of attachment behaviors. The fact that all intact children possess that substrate and those instincts makes them no less essential for development.

At the same time, it is not enough merely to say that all development is a product of interaction of nature and nurture. We need to be able to specify much more clearly just how that interaction operates. Aslin's models illustrate three of the many alternatives, but in most cases what we see is doubtless a subtle combination of many interactive patterns.

Furthermore, the form and extent of the interaction may well vary as a function of the aspect of development we are talking about. It may help to think of different facets of development along a continuum, with those most fully internally programmed on one end and those most externally influenced on the other.

Physical development defines one end of this continuum, since it is very strongly shaped by internal forces. *Given the minimum necessary environment,* maturational timetables are extremely powerful and robust, particularly during infancy and adolescence. Next along the continuum is probably language (although some experts will argue with this conclusion, given the possible dependence of language development upon prior cognitive developments). Language seems to emerge with only minimal environmental support—though here too the environment must fall within an acceptable range. At the very least, the child must hear language spoken (or see it signed). Still, specific features of the environment seem to matter a bit more here than is true for physical development. For example, parents who respond contingently to their children's vocalizations seem to be able to speed up the process, an example of what Aslin calls facilitation.

Cognitive development falls somewhere in the middle of the continuum. Clearly, powerful internal forces are at work. Let me quote John Flavell once again:

> *There is an impetus to childhood cognitive growth that is not ultimately explainable by this environmental push or that experiential shove. (1985, p. 283)*

Whether the impressive regularity of the sequences of cognitive development arises from built-in processes like assimilation and accommodation, whether physiological changes in information-processing capacity are the critical factor, or whether some combination of the two is involved we don't yet know. But it is clear that this engine is moving along a shared track. At the same time, we know that the specific qualities of the environment affect both cognitive power and structure. Children with varied and age-appropriate toys, with encouragement for exploration and achievement, with parents who are responsive to the child's overtures show faster cognitive development and higher eventual IQ scores— not just facilitation in Aslin's models, but actual attunement.

Social and emotional development lie at the other end of the continuum, where the impact of the environment seems to be the greatest, although even here genetic factors are obviously at work. Some aspects of temperament seem clearly to be built in genetically, and attachment behaviors may be instinctive; both of these inborn factors certainly shape the child's earliest encounters with others. But the balance of nature/nurture seems to lean more toward nurture in this area. In particular, the security of the child's attachment and the quality of the child's relationships with others outside of the family seem to be powerfully affected by the specific quality of the interactions within the family.

Even this fairly complex analysis, however, only begins to scratch the surface. For one thing, many of the statements I have just made need to be modified in terms of *when* a particular environmental event takes place.

Does Timing Matter?

You've encountered many variations of the timing hypothesis through the chapters of this book but the most pervasive question has been whether the early years of life are a critical or sensitive period, establishing many of the trajectories of the child's later development. To borrow Clarke's analogy (Clarke & Clarke, 1976): When we construct a house, does the shape of the foundation determine the final structure partially or completely, or can many final structures be built on the original foundation? Are any flaws or weaknesses in the original foundation permanent, or can they be corrected later, after the house is completed?

There are arguments on both sides. Some psychologists, such as Sandra Scarr (Scarr-Salapatek, 1976), point to the fact that virtually all children successfully complete the sensorimotor period; and even mild and moderately retarded children achieve some form of what Piaget called concrete operations. The term that has been widely used to describe such developmental patterns is **canalization,** a notion borrowed from an embryologist named Waddington (1957). He suggested that we think of development metaphorically as a marble rolling down a gully on a hillside, as in Figure 16.5. Where the gully is narrow and deep, development is said to be "highly canalized." The marble will roll down that gully with little deviation. Other aspects of development, in contrast, might be better depicted with much flatter or wider gullies, with many side branches. Thus, Scarr and others argue that in the early years of life, development is highly canalized, with strong "self-righting" tendencies. If deflected, the baby rapidly returns to the bottom of the gully and proceeds along the normal track. Such self-righting is illustrated, for example, by the large percentage of low-birth-weight or other initially vulnerable babies who nonetheless catch up to their normal-birth peers in physical and cognitive development by the time they are 2 or 3.

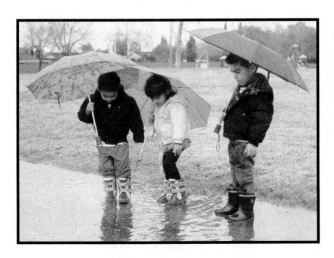

If infancy is a critical period for some aspects of personality development, then these preschoolers' characters are already well formed. Whether this is true or not remains one of the most crucial theoretical and practical issues in developmental psychology.

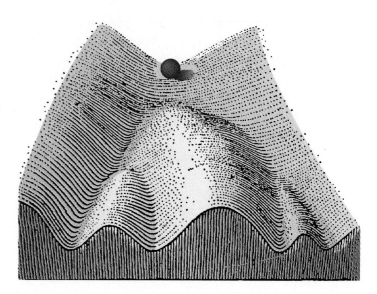

FIGURE 16.5 Waddington's visual depiction of the concept of canalization. A narrow and deep gully depicts strong canalization. If infancy is highly canalized, it means that almost any environment will support or sustain that development. (*Source:* Waddington, 1974.)

On the other side of the argument are the obvious cases in which an early experience has been highly formative. Some prenatal influences are permanent; some effects of early cognitive impoverishment, malnutrition, or abuse may also be long-lasting.

Thus, the early years of life seem both to be a sensitive period for some kinds of development and at the same time seem to be highly canalized. How can we resolve this paradox? Two possible resolutions occur to me. First, we might think of such canalization not just as a product of powerful built-in programming, but as the result of such programming *occurring in a sufficiently supportive environment.* When we do that, much of the apparent dispute disappears (Turkheimer & Gottesman, 1991). It is only when a child's particular environment falls outside of the range of sufficiently supportive environments that we see a so-called environmental effect, such as a child reared in an extremely impoverished orphanage setting or a child who is regularly physically abused. In these conditions, environmental effects can be strongly negative and long-lasting. The earlier such a deviation occurs, the more pervasive the effects seem to be. In this way of looking at critical periods versus canalization, infancy may be less *frequently* pivotal in the pattern of the child's development than are more minor deviations in toddlerhood or the preschool years. But *if* the deviations in infancy are extreme enough to deflect the infant from the normal developmental path—as in the case of severe abuse or malnutrition— the effect is larger than at any other age.

Robert Cairns (1991) offers a second resolution to the paradox when he points out that in any given period, some facets of development may be highly canalized while other facets may be strongly responsive to environmental variation. In infancy, for example, physical, perceptual, and perhaps linguistic development may be strongly canalized, but the development of internal working models of attachment is clearly affected by the child's specific family experiences. Indeed, I would argue that all internal working models—of attachment, of gender identity and self-concept, of peer relations—are likely to be more powerfully affected by early than by later experiences, simply because the model, once formed, affects and filters all later experience.

A particularly nice example of this kind of early effect comes from one of Alan Sroufe's studies of the long-term consequences of attachment security. He and his col-

Does either of these resolutions of the paradox persuade you? If not, why not?

leagues (Sroufe, Egeland, & Kreutzer, 1990) compared two groups of elementary school children. One group had had a good adaptation in infancy, with a secure attachment, but for various reasons had not functioned well in the preschool years. The second group had shown poor adaptation at both ages. When these two groups of children were assessed at elementary school age, Sroufe found that those who had had a good early start "rebounded" better. They had better emotional health and peer competence at school age than did those who had had a poor adaptation in infancy, even though both groups had functioned poorly as preschoolers. The infancy experience is not totally formative; the child's current circumstances also have a major impact. But at least in this domain, early experience leaves a lingering trace.

Timing and internal models interact in yet another way when we look at the effect of earliness or lateness of some experience such as puberty. What matters in this case seems not to be the actual timing, but the child's interpretation of that timing, the child's internal model.

Still a third way to think about timing is to emphasize the importance of specific psychological tasks at different ages. Erikson's theory, for example, emphasizes each of a series of psychological dilemmas. Any experience that affects the way a child resolves a particular task will be formative at that time; at an earlier or later time the same experience might have much less effect. Alan Sroufe and Michael Rutter (1984) have offered a broader list of age-graded tasks, given in Table 16.1. In this way of looking at things, the child is seen as *focusing* on different aspects of the environment at different times. Thus, during the period from 1 to 2½, when the child is focused on mastery of the object world, the quality and range of inanimate experiences the child has access to may be of special importance.

Table 16.1
Tasks or Issues in Each of Several Age Periods

Age in Years	Issues or Tasks
0–1	Biological regulation; harmonious dyadic interaction; formation of an effective attachment relationship
1–2½	Exploration, experimentation, and mastery of the object world (caregiver as secure base); individuation and autonomy; responding to external control of impulses
3–5	Flexible self-control; self-reliance; initiative; identification and gender concept; establishing effective peer contacts (empathy)
6–12	Social understanding (equity, fairness); gender constancy; same-sex chumships; sense of "industry" (competence); school adjustment
13+	"Formal operations" (flexible perspective taking; "as if" thinking); loyal friendships (same-sex); beginning heterosexual relationships; emancipation; identity

Source: Sroufe & Rutter, 1984, adapted from Sroufe, 1979.

Overall, I do not think that any specific age is "critical" for all aspects of development; I do think that for any aspect of development, some ages are more central than others and that during those times, patterns are set that affect later experience. As Alan Sroufe says, "Development is hierarchical; it is not a blackboard to be erased and written upon again. Even when children change rather markedly, the shadows of the earlier adaptation remain" (1983, pp. 73–74).

What Is the Nature of Developmental Change?

My bias has no doubt been apparent throughout the book, so you can predict my conclusion that developmental change is more qualitative than quantitative. Certainly, the child acquires more vocabulary words, more information-processing strategies, but these are used in different ways by older children than by younger ones. Further, it seems clear that these qualitative changes occur in sequences. Such sequences are apparent in physical development, in cognitive development, in social and moral development.

Stages. Whether it is meaningful to speak of stages, however, is still an open question. Some hierarchically organized stages have certainly been observed, Kohlberg's stages of moral reasoning being the most obvious example. And we can certainly find examples of apparently stagelike changes across domains, such as what happens at about ages 18 to 24 months when the child seems to discover the ability to combine symbols, which shows up in two-word sentences, in thinking, and in multistep play with other children. There also appears to be a quite stagelike shift between ages 3 and 4, of which the new theory of mind is the centerpiece. But the majority of the evidence has not supported the notion of pervasive changes in structure. More commonly, each new skill, each new understanding seems to be acquired in a fairly narrow area first and is only later generalized more fully. In fact, one of the things that differentiates the gifted or higher-IQ child from the lower-IQ or retarded child is how quickly and broadly the child generalizes some new concept or strategy to new instances.

Despite this nonstagelike quality of most developmental change, it is still true that if you compare the patterns of relationship, of thinking, of problem solving of two children of widely differing ages—say a 5-year-old and an 11-year-old—they will differ in almost every respect. So there is certainly orderliness in the sequences, and some linkages between them, but probably not major stages quite like those Piaget proposed.

Continuities. In the midst of all this change, all these sequences, all the new forms of relating and thinking, we also see continuity. Each child carries forward some core of individuality. The notion of temperament certainly implies such a core, as does the concept of an internal working model. Alan Sroufe once again offers an elegant way of thinking about this central core. Continuity in development, he says, "takes the form of coherence across transformations" (1983, p. 51). Thus, the specific behavior that we see in the child may change; the clinging toddler may not be a clinging 9-year-old. But the underlying attachment model or the temperament that led to the clinging will still be at least partially present, manifesting itself in new ways. In particular, it has become increasingly clear that *mal*adaptations often persist over time, as seen in the consistency of high levels of aggression or tantrum behavior and in the persistence of some of the maladaptive social interactions that flow from insecure attachments. Our task as psychologists is to understand both coherence or consistency and the underlying patterns of development or transformation.

Individual Differences

The whole issue of individual continuities emphasizes the fact that development is individual as well as collective. I have talked about individual differences in virtually every chapter, so you know that both inborn differences and emergent or environmentally produced variations are present among children in every aspect of development. This is all familiar stuff by now and bears little repeating. But I want to try to tie together many of the threads I have been weaving in this chapter by returning to a dimension of individual differences I have talked about several times, namely, vulnerability and resilience.

I think it is useful to define these concepts somewhat differently than usual, in terms of the *range of environments that will be sufficiently supportive for optimal development.* By this definition, a vulnerable infant is one with a narrow range of potentially supportive environments. For such a child, only the most stimulating, the most responsive, the most adaptive environment will do. When the child's environment falls outside of that range, the probability of a poor outcome is greatly increased. A resilient child, in contrast, is one for whom any of a very wide range of environments will support optimum development. A resilient child may thus be more strongly canalized, a vulnerable child less so.

Some kinds of vulnerabilities are inborn, such as genetic abnormalities, prenatal trauma or stress, preterm birth, or malnutrition. Any such child will thrive only in a highly supportive environment. You've encountered this pattern again and again through the chapters of this book.

- Low-birth-weight infants typically have normal IQs if they are reared in middle-class homes but have a high risk of serious retardation if they are reared in non-stimulating poverty-level homes (Bradley et al., 1994).

- Prenatally malnourished infants, or those with other complications during pregnancy or delivery, look normal if reared in highly stimulating special preschools but have significantly lower IQs if reared at home by low-education mothers (Breitmayer & Ramey, 1986; Zeskind & Ramey, 1981).

- Children born with cytomegalovirus are much more likely to have learning problems in school if they are reared in poverty-level environments than if they are reared in middle-class families (Hanshaw et al., 1976).

So far that's fairly straightforward. But let me propose a further, more speculative, theoretical step: I think that "vulnerability" in this sense does not remain constant throughout life. A more general proposition, which I suggest as a working hypothesis, is that each time the child's environment falls outside of the range of acceptably supporting environments *for that child* (i.e., each time a mismatch occurs between the child's needs and what is available), the child becomes *more vulnerable,* while each period during which the child's needs are met makes the child more resilient. For example, I would predict that a temperamentally difficult child whose family environment was nonetheless sufficient to foster a secure attachment will become more resilient, more able to handle the next set of tasks, while a temperamentally easy child who nonetheless developed an insecure attachment would become more vulnerable to later stress or environmental insufficiency.

Furthermore, the qualities of the environment that are critical for a child's optimum development no doubt change as the child passes from one age to another. Responsive and warm interactions with parents seem particularly central in the period from perhaps

What I am suggesting is that resilience or vulnerability is a little like a bank account. Vulnerable children start out with little in the account, while resilient children have a lot. Experience then adds to or subtracts from the account. Does this make sense to you? Can you think of any other implications of this concept than those I have suggested here?

6 months to 18 months; richness of cognitive stimulation seems particularly central between perhaps 1 year and 4 years; opportunity for practicing social skills with peers may be especially central at a later age. Thus, as the tasks change with age, the optimum environment will change also. Among other things, this means that the same family may be very good with a child of one age and not so good with a child of another age.

Most generally, this model leads to the conclusion that even the most "vulnerable" child can show improvement if her environment improves markedly. Because some congenitally vulnerable children do not encounter sufficiently supportive environments, their vulnerability will continue to increase. In this way, early problems will often persist. But at the same time, improvement is possible, even likely. *Most* children manage to survive and thrive, despite stresses and vulnerabilities. As Emmy Werner puts it, "We could not help being deeply impressed by the resilience of most children and youth and their capacity for positive change and personal growth" (1986, p. 5).

A Final Point: The Joy of Development

On a similarly optimistic note, I want to end both this chapter and the book by pointing out that in the midst of all the "crises" and "transitions" and "vulnerabilities," development has a special *joyous* quality. When a child masters a new skill, she is not just pleased, she is delighted and will repeat that new skill at length, quite obviously getting vast satisfaction from it. A 5-year-old I once knew learned to draw stars and drew them on everything in sight, including paper, walls, clothes, and napkins. It was so much *fun* to draw stars. A 10-year-old who learns to do cartwheels will delightedly display this new talent to anyone who will watch and will practice endlessly.

The same joyous quality can be part of the family's development as well. Confronting and moving successfully through one of the periodic (and inevitable) upheavals in family life can be immensely pleasing. Watching your child progress, liking your child, enjoying walking or talking together are all deeply satisfying parts of rearing children. When parents cry at their son's or daughter's high school graduation or wedding, it is not merely sentiment. It is an expression of that sense of love, pride, and wonderment that you have gotten this far.

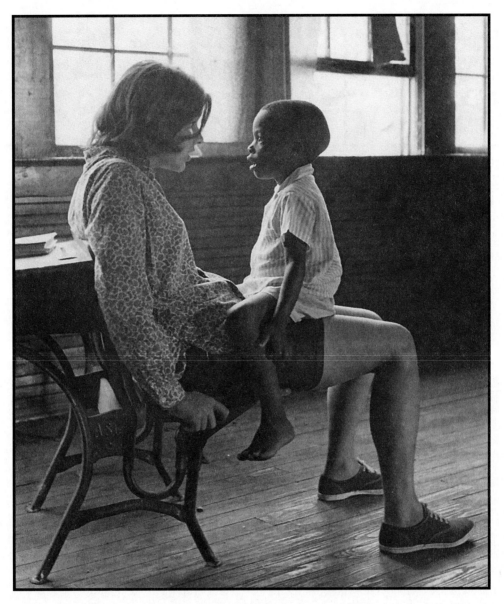

I have used this photo at the end of every edition of this book because it speaks to me so eloquently of the quality of joy, of discovery, that is so much a part of development.

Summary

1 The child's development may be thought of as a series of alternating periods of transition and consolidation. The transitions occur when there are individual major changes or pileups of smaller change.

2 To understand development we must understand the system, not just the individual parts. A change in any part of the system affects all the other facets.

3 Within infancy, there appear to be at least two transition periods, one at about 2 months and the other at roughly 8 months.

4 Four key processes appear to underlie the changes we see in infancy: physical maturation, including changes in the nervous system; the child's own explorations of the environment; the process of attachment; and perhaps most broadly, the emergence of the early forms of internal working models.

5 The transition at 18 months is marked by the remarkable emergence of symbolic activity, evidenced in language, in thinking, in play. A general combinatorial ability also appears at about this time, with a more sophisticated theory of mind several years later.

6 These cognitive accomplishments combine with major new motor skills to allow the child significantly greater independence, which in turn fosters further cognitive growth.

7 The preschool child basically shifts from dependent to independent, and from poor to better impulse control.

8 The transition at ages 5 to 7 is marked both by the beginning emergence of still-more-powerful cognitive skills and by the beginning of school, and by the emergence of a global sense of self-worth.

9 Peer relationships become central for the child's emerging social skills and for the development of skillful social cognition. These relationships are largely gender segregated.

10 The transition at adolescence is triggered primarily by the physical changes of puberty but is accompanied by still further cognitive changes, major alterations in patterns of peer interaction, increases in family disruption, and increases in depression.

11 A shift toward formal operations at adolescence may be one contributor to a rise in self-questioning; pubertal changes may have both direct and indirect effects on the other developments of this period.

12 All facets of development are the product of some combination or interaction of internal and external influences.

13 Nonetheless, the various facets of development can be arrayed along a continuum from those most affected by internal influences to those most affected by external influences, in the following order: physical development, language, cognition, and social/personality development.

14 Paradoxically, development in the early years of life appears to be both highly canalized and (at extremes of environment) highly sensitive to environmental variation.

15 The early years of life may also be especially important for all children because internal working models are established in that period.

16 Each age period can also be thought of as having a set of central tasks; experiences that are especially important for the successful completion of those tasks will thus be "critical" for that age.

17 Development seems clearly to be made up of a large number of widely shared (if not universal) sequences. But whether broad, structurally different stages occur is less clear.

18 The dimension of vulnerability/resilience is one way to think about individual differences. The dimension may be defined in terms of the range of environments that will support optimal development for a particular child. A large range implies resilience; a narrow range defines vulnerability.

19 Vulnerability may be increased or decreased over time, depending on the adequacy or inadequacy of environments at each of a series of points in development. Children may thus recover from, or surmount, even very poor starts.

20 For both the child and the parent, development is full of joy as well as travail.

Key Terms

canalization (**p. 477**)

Suggested Readings

Many of the books I have suggested in earlier chapters are relevant here as well, including the Rosenblith (1992) and Osofsky (1987) books on infancy, and Flavell's book on cognitive development (1985), which includes an elegant discussion of many of the basic issues I have been talking about in this chapter. Let me also suggest several other books that give the flavor of particular ages.

Collins, W. A. (Ed.). (1984). *Development during middle childhood: The years from six to twelve.* Washington, DC: National Academy Press.

This collection of papers touches on all facets of school-age children: biology, cognition, self-understanding, family and peer relationships, school, and atypical development. An excellent source of information about this often-neglected age period.

Feldman, S. S., & Elliott, G. R. (Eds.). (1990). *At the threshold: The developing adolescent.* Cambridge, MA: Harvard University Press.

An especially good and helpful collection of papers on adolescence—an age period that has been "discovered" by psychologists in the past decade.

Glossary

accommodation That part of the adaptation process proposed by Piaget by which a person modifies existing schemes to fit new experiences or creates new schemes when old ones no longer handle the data.

achievement test Test designed to assess a child's learning of specific material taught in school, such as spelling or arithmetic computation, typically given to all children in designated grades.

acuity Sharpness of perceptual ability—how well or clearly one can see, hear, or use other senses.

affectional bond A "relatively long-enduring tie in which the partner is important as a unique individual and is interchangeable with none other."

aggression Behavior with the apparent intent to injure some other person or object.

alpha-fetoprotein test A prenatal diagnostic test frequently used to screen for the risk of neural tube defects. May also be used in combination with other tests to diagnose Down syndrome and other chromosomal anomalies.

altruism Giving or sharing objects, time, or goods with others, with no obvious self-gain.

amniocentesis A medical test for genetic abnormalities in the embryo/fetus that may be done at about 15 weeks of gestation.

amnion The sac or bag, filled with liquid, in which the embryo and fetus floats during prenatal life.

androgyny A self-concept including, and behavior expressing, high levels of both masculine and feminine qualities.

anorexia nervosa A serious eating disorder characterized by extreme dieting, intense fear of gaining weight, and distorted body image.

anoxia A shortage of oxygen. If it is prolonged it can result in brain damage. This is one of the potential risks at birth.

Apgar score An assessment of the newborn completed by the physician or midwife at one minute and again at five minutes after birth, assessing five characteristics: heart rate, respiratory rate, muscle tone, response to stimulation, and color.

assimilation That part of the adaptation process proposed by Piaget that involves the "taking in" of new experiences or information into existing schemes. Experience is not taken in "as is," however, but is modified (or interpreted) somewhat so as to fit the preexisting schemes.

attachment An especially intense and central subtype of affectional bond in which the presence of the partner adds a special sense of security, a "safe base," for the individual. Characteristic of the child's bond with the parent.

attachment behavior The collection of (probably) instinctive behaviors of one person toward another that bring about or maintain proximity and caregiving, such as the smile of the young infant; behaviors that reflect an attachment.

attention-deficit/hyperactivity disorder (ADD) The technical term for what is more normally called hyperactivity, characterized by significant problems with attention, distractibility, and heightened levels of physical activity.

authoritarian parental style One of the three styles described by Baumrind, characterized by high levels of control and maturity demands and low levels of nurturance and communication.

authoritative parental style One of the three styles described by Baumrind, characterized by high levels of control, nurturance, maturity demands, and communication.

autosomes The 22 pairs of chromosomes in which both members of the pair are the same shape and carry parallel information.

axon The long appendage-like part of a neuron; the terminal fibers of the axon serve as transmitters in the synaptic connection with the dendrites of other neurons.

babbling The frequently repetitive vocalizing of consonant-vowel combinations by an infant, typically beginning at about 6 months of age.

Bayley Scales of Infant Development The best-known and most widely used test of infant "intelligence," revised most recently in 1993.

behavior genetics The study of the genetic basis of behavior, such as intelligence or personality.

Big Five personality dimensions Five dimensions of personality variation found in studies of adults and widely perceived to describe the core facets of personality, including extraversion, agreeableness, conscientiousness, neuroticism, and openness/intellect.

brain damage Some injury to the brain, either during prenatal development or later, that results in improper functioning of the brain.

bulimia An eating disorder characterized by an intense concern about weight combined with binge eating followed by purging, either through self-induced vomiting, excessive use of laxatives, or excessive exercise.

canalization Term used to describe the degree to which development during any given period follows some clear, shared "canal" or "channel," difficult to disrupt except by extreme environmental variation.

cephalocaudal From the head downward. Describes one recurrent pattern of physical development in infancy.

cesarean section Delivery of the child through an incision in the mother's abdomen.

chorionic villus sampling A technique for prenatal genetic diagnosis involving taking a sample of cells from the placenta. Can be performed earlier in the pregnancy than amniocentesis but carries slightly higher risks.

chromosomal anomalies Variations in the number or configuration of the normal set of 23 pairs of chromosomes, almost always resulting in physical or mental abnormalities in the affected child. Down syndrome is an example of a chromosomal anomaly.

chromosome The structures in each cell in the body that contain genetic information. Each cell contains 23 pairs of chromosomes, each of which is made up of many segments called genes.

classical conditioning One of three major types of learning. An automatic unconditioned response, such as an emotion or a reflex, comes to be triggered by a new cue, called the conditioned stimulus (CS), after the CS has been paired several times with the original unconditioned stimulus.

clique Defined by Dunphy as a group of six to eight friends with strong affectional bonds and high levels of group solidarity and loyalty; currently used by researchers to describe a self-chosen group of friends, in contrast to reputation-based crowds.

cohort A group of persons of approximately the same age who have shared similar major life experiences, such as cultural training, historical events, or general economic conditions.

collectivism A cultural perspective or belief system (contrasted with individualism) in which the emphasis is on collective rather than individual identity and on group solidarity, decision making, duties, and obligations. Characteristic of most Asian, Hispanic, and African cultures.

color constancy The ability to see the color of an object as remaining the same despite changes in illumination or shadow. One of the basic perceptual constancies that make up "object constancy."

competence The behavior of a person as it would be under ideal or perfect circumstances. It is not possible to measure competence directly.

componential intelligence One of three types of intelligence in Sternberg's triarchic theory of intelligence; that type of intelligence typically measured on IQ tests, including analytic thinking, remembering facts, and organizing information.

concrete operations The stage of development between ages 6 and 12 proposed by Piaget, in which mental operations such as subtraction, reversibility, and multiple classification are acquired.

conditioned stimulus In classical conditioning, the stimulus that, after being paired a number of times with an unconditioned stimulus, comes to trigger the unconditioned response. For example, the sound of the mother's footsteps may become a conditioned stimulus for the baby's turning his head as if to suck.

conduct disorder Diagnostic term for a pattern of deviant behavior, including high levels of aggressive, antisocial, or delinquent acts.

conservation The concept that objects remain the same in fundamental ways, such as weight or number, even when there are external changes in shape or arrangement. Typically understood by children after age 5.

contextual intelligence One of three types of intelligence in Sternberg's triarchic theory of intelligence; often also called "street smarts," this type of intelligence includes skills in adapting to an environment and in adapting an environment to one's own needs.

control group The group of subjects in an experiment that receives either no special treatment or some neutral treatment.

conventional morality The second level of moral judgment proposed by Kohlberg, in which the person's judgments are dominated by considerations of group values and laws.

cooing An early phase of the prelinguistic period, from about 1 to 4 months of age, when vowel sounds are repeated, particularly the *uuu* sound.

correlation A statistic used to describe the degree or strength of a relationship between two variables. It can range from +1.00 to −1.00. The closer it is to 1.00, the stronger the relationship being described.

cortex The convoluted gray portion of the brain that governs most complex thought, language, and memory.

critical period Any time period during development when the organism is especially responsive to and learns from a specific type of stimulation. The same stimulation at other points in development has little or no effect.

cross-cultural research Research involving in-depth study of non-Western cultures, or research involving comparisons of several cultures or subcultures.

cross-modal transfer The ability to transfer information gained through one sense to another sense at a later time; for example, identifying visually something you had previously explored only tactually.

cross-sectional design A form of research in which samples of subjects from several different age groups are studied at the same time.

crowd Defined by Dunphy as a larger and looser group of friends than a clique, normally made up of several cliques joined together; defined by current researchers as a reputation-based group, common in adolescent subculture, with widely agreed-upon characteristics (e.g., "brains," "jocks," or "druggies").

culture A system of meanings and customs shared by some identifiable group or subgroup and transmitted from one generation of that group to the next.

cumulative deficit Any difference between groups in IQ (or achievement test) scores that becomes larger over time.

deductive logic Reasoning from the general to the particular, from a rule to an expected instance, or from a theory to a hypothesis. Characteristic of formal operational thought.

delinquency A subcategory of conduct disorders involving explicit lawbreaking.

dendrites The branchlike parts of a neuron that serve as the receptors in synaptic connections with the axons of other neurons.

deoxyribonucleic acid Called DNA for short, this is the chemical of which genes are composed.

dependent variable The variable in an experiment that is expected to show the impact of manipulations of the independent variable; also called the *outcome variable*.

depression A combination of sad mood, sleep and eating disturbances, and difficulty concentrating. When all these symptoms are present, it is usually called *clinical depression*.

developmental psychopathology A relatively new approach to the study of deviance that emphasizes that normal and abnormal development have common roots and that pathology can arise from many different pathways or systems.

dilation A key process in the first stage of childbirth, when the cervix widens sufficiently to allow the infant's head to pass into the birth canal. Full dilation is 10 centimeters.

Down syndrome A genetic anomaly in which every cell contains three rather than two copies of chromosome 21. Children born with this genetic pattern are usually mentally retarded and have characteristic physical features.

effacement The flattening of the cervix that, along with dilation, is a key process of the first stage of childbirth.

ego In Freudian theory, that portion of the personality that organizes, plans, and keeps the person in touch with reality. Language and thought are both ego functions.

egocentrism A cognitive state in which the individual (typically a child) sees the world only from his own perspective, without awareness that there are other perspectives.

embryo The name given to the organism during the period of prenatal development from about two to eight weeks after conception, beginning with implantation of the blastocyst into the uterine wall.

empathy As defined by Hoffman, it is a "vicarious affective response that does not necessarily match another's affective state but is more appropriate to the other's situation than to one's own" (Hoffman, 1984, p. 285).

empiricism Opposite of *nativism*. The theoretical point of view that all perceptual skill arises from experience.

endocrine glands These glands—including the adrenals, the thyroid, the pituitary, the testes, and the ovaries—secrete hormones governing overall physical growth and sexual maturing.

equilibration The third part of the adaptation process, as proposed by Piaget, involving a periodic restructuring of schemes into new structures.

estrogen The female sex hormone secreted by the ovaries.

ethnic group "A subgroup whose members are perceived by themselves and others to have a common origin and culture, and shared activities in which the common origin or culture is an essential ingredient" (Porter & Washington, 1993, p. 140).

ethnography A detailed description of a single culture or context, based on extensive observation by a resident observer.

executive processes Proposed subset of information processes involving organizing and planning strategies. Similar in meaning to metacognition.

experiential intelligence One of three types of intelligence described by Sternberg in his triarchic theory of intelligence; includes creativity, insight, and seeing new relationships among experiences.

experiment A research strategy in which subjects are assigned randomly to experimental and control groups. The experimental group is then provided with a designated experience that is expected to alter behavior in some specified fashion.

experimental group The group (or groups) of subjects in an experiment that is given a special treatment intended to produce some specific outcome.

expressive language The term used to describe the child's skill in speaking and communicating orally.

expressive style One of two styles of early language proposed by Nelson, characterized by low rates of nounlike terms and high use of personal-social words and phrases.

externalizing problems One of two major categories of psychopathologies, including any deviant behavior primarily directed away from the individual, such as conduct disorders or hyperactivity.

fallopian tube The tube between the ovary and the uterus down which the ovum travels and in which conception usually occurs.

family day care Nonparental care in which the child is cared for in someone else's home, usually with a small group of other children.

fetal alcohol syndrome (FAS) A pattern of physical and mental abnormalities, including mental retardation and minor physical anomalies, found often in children born to alcoholic mothers.

fetus The name given to the developing organism from about eight weeks after conception until birth.

fontanels The "soft spots" in the skull present at birth. These disappear when the several bones of the skull grow together.

foreclosure One of four identity statuses proposed by Marcia, involving an ideological or occupational commitment without having gone through a reevaluation.

formal operations Piaget's name for the fourth and final major stage of cognitive development, occurring during adolescence, when the child becomes able to manipulate and organize ideas as well as objects.

gametes Sperm and ova. These cells, unlike all other cells of the body, contain only 23 chromosomes rather than 23 pairs.

gender concept The understanding of one's own gender, including the permanence and constancy of gender.

gender constancy The final step in developing a gender concept, in which the child understands that gender doesn't change even though there are external changes in things like clothing or hair length.

gender identity The first step in gender concept development, in which the child labels herself correctly and categorizes others correctly as male or female.

gender schema A fundamental schema created by children beginning at age 18 months or younger by which the child categorizes people, objects, activities, and qualities by gender.

gender stability The second step in gender concept development, in which the child understands that a person's gender continues to be stable throughout the lifetime.

gene A uniquely coded segment of DNA on a chromosome that affects one or more specific body processes or developments.

genotype The pattern of characteristics and developmental sequences mapped in the genes of any specific individual. Will be modified by individual experience into the phenotype.

gifted Normally defined in terms of very high IQ (above 140 or 150) but may also be defined in terms of remarkable skill in one or more specific areas, such as mathematics or memory.

glial cells One of two major classes of cells making up the nervous system, glial cells provide the firmness and structure, the "glue," to hold the system together.

gonadotropic hormones Hormones produced in the pituitary gland that stimulate the sex organs to develop.

habituation An automatic decrease in the intensity of a response to a repeated stimulus, enabling a child or adult to ignore the familiar and to focus attention on the novel.

hearing-impaired The phrase currently used in place of "hard of hearing" to describe children or adults with significant hearing loss. The term *deaf* refers to the most extreme end of this continuum of impairment.

holophrases The expression of a whole idea in a single word combined with gesture. Characteristic of the child's language from about 12 to 18 months.

hyperactivity The common term for attention deficit hyperactivity disorder.

id In Freudian theory, the first, primitive portion of the personality; the storehouse of basic energy, continually pushing for immediate gratification.

identification The process of taking into oneself ("incorporating") the qualities and ideas of another person, which Freud thought was the result of the Oedipus conflict at ages 3 to 5. The child attempts to make himself like his parent of the same sex.

identity achievement One of four identity statuses proposed by Marcia, involving the successful resolution of an identity "crisis," resulting in a new commitment.

identity diffusion One of four identity statuses proposed by Marcia, involving neither a current reevaluation nor a firm personal commitment.

inborn errors of metabolism Inherited patterns of physical dysfunction in which the infant or child fails to metabolize one or more amino acids in the normal fashion. Phenylketonuria is the best-known such error.

independent variable A condition or event an experimenter varies in some systematic way in order to observe the impact of that variation on the subjects' behavior.

individualism A cultural perspective or belief system (contrasted with collectivism), in which the emphasis is placed on the separateness and independence of individual development and behavior. Characteristic of most Western cultures.

inductive logic Reasoning from the particular to the general, from experience to broad rules. Characteristic of concrete operational thinking.

infant-directed speech The formal scientific term for "motherese," that special form of simplified, higher-pitched speech adults use with infants and young children.

inflections The various grammatical "markers" such as the *s* for plurals or the *ed* for past tenses, auxiliary verbs such as *is,* and the equivalent.

information processing Phrase used to refer to a new, third approach to the study of intellectual development that focuses on changes with age, and individual differences, in fundamental intellectual skills.

insecure attachment Internal working model of relationship in which the child does not readily use the parent as a safe base and is not readily consoled by the parent if upset. Includes three subtypes of attachment: ambivalent, avoidant, and disorganized/disoriented.

internalizing problems One of two major categories of psychopathology, in which the deviant behavior is directed inward, including anxiety and depression.

internal working model Bolby's phrase for the child's cognitive model of relationships, for which the earliest relationships may form the template. The model includes such things as expectations of support or affection, trustworthiness, and so on.

intelligence quotient (IQ) Originally defined in terms of a child's mental age and chronological age, IQs are now computed by comparing a child's performance with that of other children of the same chronological age.

intrinsic reinforcements Those inner sources of pleasure, pride, or satisfaction that serve to increase the likelihood that an individual will repeat the behavior that led to the feeling.

learning disability (LD) Term broadly used to describe any child with an unexpected or unexplained problem in learning to read, spell, or calculate. More precisely used to refer to a subgroup of such children who have some neurological dysfunction.

libido The term used by Freud to describe the pool of sexual energy in each individual.

longitudinal design A research design in which the same subjects are observed or assessed repeatedly over a period of months or years.

low birth weight (LBW) The phrase now used (in place of the word *premature*) to describe infants whose weight is below the optimum range at birth. Includes infants born too early (preterm or short-gestation infants) and those who are small for date.

maturation The sequential unfolding of physical characteristics, governed by instructions contained in the genetic code and shared by all members of a species.

mean length of utterance The average number of meaningful units in a sentence (usually abbreviated MLU). Each basic word is one meaningful unit, as is each inflection, such as the *s* for plural or the *ed* for a past tense.

medulla A portion of the brain that lies immediately above the spinal cord; largely developed at birth.

menarche Onset of menstruation in girls.

mental retardation Defined as an IQ below 70 combined with poor adaptive behavior.

metacognition General and rather loosely used term describing an individual's knowledge of his own thinking processes. Knowing what you know and how you go about learning or remembering.

metamemory A subcategory of metacognition; knowledge about your own memory processes.

midbrain A section of the brain lying above the medulla and below the cortex that regulates attention, sleeping, waking, and other "automatic" functions. Largely developed at birth.

modeling A term used by Bandura and others to describe observational learning.

moratorium One of four identity statuses proposed by Marcia, involving an ongoing reexamination but without a new commitment as yet.

motherese *See* **infant-directed speech.**

motor development Growth and change in ability to do physical activities, such as walking, running, or riding a bike.

myelin Material making up an insulating sheath that develops around most axons. This sheath is not completely developed at birth.

myelinization The process by which myelin is added.

nativism *See also* **empiricism.** The view that perceptual skills are inborn and do not require experience to develop.

negative reinforcement The strengthening of a behavior because of the removal or cessation of an unpleasant stimulus.

neglecting parental style Fourth major parenting style suggested by Maccoby and Martin, involving low levels of both acceptance and control.

neuron The second major class of cells in the nervous system, neurons are responsible for transmission and reception of nerve impulses.

object constancy The general phrase describing the ability to see objects as remaining the same despite changes in retinal image.

objective self Second major step in the development of the self-concept; awareness of the self as an object with properties.

object permanence Part of the object concept. The recognition that an object continues to exist even when it is temporarily out of sight.

observational learning Learning of motor skills, attitudes, or other behaviors through observing someone else perform them.

Oedipus conflict The pattern of events Freud believed occurred between ages 3 and 5 when the child experiences a "sexual" desire for the parent of the opposite sex; the resulting fear of possible reprisal from the parent of the same sex is resolved when the child "identifies" with the parent of the same sex.

operant conditioning That type of learning in which the probability of a person performing some behavior is strengthened by positive or negative reinforcements.

operation Term used by Piaget for complex, internal, abstract, reversible schemes, first seen at about age 6.

ossification The process of hardening by which soft tissue becomes bone.

overregularization The tendency on the part of children to make the language regular by creating regularized versions of irregular past tenses or plurals.

ovum The gamete produced in a woman's ovaries. If fertilized by a sperm from the male, it forms the basis for the developing organism.

partial reinforcement Reinforcement of behavior on some schedule less frequent than every occasion.

perceptual constancies A collection of constancies, including shape, size, and color constancy.

performance The behavior shown by a person under actual circumstances. Even when we are interested in competence, all we can ever measure is performance.

performance tests A new category of criterion-referenced tests used in some school systems today, in which students are required to demonstrate some actual skills, such as writing, performing experiments, or explaining mathematical reasoning, with performance assessed against some specified criterion.

permissive parental style One of the three styles described by Baumrind, characterized by high levels of nurturance and low levels of control, maturity demands, and communication.

personality The collection of individual, relatively enduring patterns of reacting to and interacting with others that distinguishes each child or adult.

phenotype The expression of a particular set of genetic information in a specific environment; the observable result of the joint operation of genetic and environmental influences.

placenta An organ that develops during gestation between the fetus and the wall of the uterus. The placenta filters nutrients from the mother's blood, acting as liver, lungs, and kidneys for the fetus.

positive reinforcement Strengthening of a behavior by the presentation of some pleasurable or positive stimulus.

postpartum depression A severe form of the common experience of postpartum blues. Affecting perhaps 20 percent of women, this form of clinical depression typically lasts six to eight weeks.

pragmatics The rules for the use of language in communicative interaction, such as the rules for taking turns, the style of speech appropriate for varying listeners, and the equivalent.

preconventional morality The first level of morality proposed by Kohlberg, in which moral judgments are dominated by consideration of what will be punished and what feels good.

prelinguistic phase The period before the child speaks his first words.

preoperational stage Piaget's term for the second major stage of cognitive development, from age 2 to age 6, marked at the beginning by the ability to use symbols and by the development of basic classification and logical abilities.

preterm infant Descriptive phrase now widely used to label infants born before 37 weeks of gestational age.

principled morality The third level of morality proposed by Kohlberg, in which considerations of justice, individual rights, and contracts dominate moral judgment.

prosocial behavior See **altruism.**

proximodistal From the center outward. With *cephalocaudal*, describes the pattern of physical changes in infancy.

psychosexual stages The stages of personality development suggested by Freud, including the oral, anal, phallic, latency, and genital stages.

psychosocial stages The stages of personality development suggested by Erikson, including trust, autonomy, initiative, industry, identity, intimacy, generativity, and ego integrity.

puberty The collection of hormonal and physical changes at adolescence that brings about sexual maturity.

punishment Unpleasant consequences, administered after some undesired behavior by a child or adult, with the intent of extinguishing the behavior.

receptive language Term used to describe the child's ability to understand (receive) language, as contrasted to his ability to express language.

referential style Second style of early language proposed by Nelson, characterized by emphasis on objects and their naming and description.

reflexes Automatic body reactions to specific stimulation, such as the knee jerk or the Moro reflex. Adults retain many reflexes, but the newborn also has some "primitive" reflexes that disappear as the cortex is fully developed.

responsiveness An aspect of parent-child interaction. A responsive parent is sensitive to the child's cues and reacts appropriately, following the child's lead.

restrictiveness Term used to describe a particular pattern of parental control, involving limitation of the child's movements or options, such as by the use of playpens or harnesses in a young child, or strict rules about play areas or free choices in an older child.

rubella A form of measles that if contracted during the first few weeks of a pregnancy is likely to have severe effects on the developing baby.

scheme Piaget's word for the basic actions of knowing, including both physical actions (sensorimotor schemes, such as looking or reaching) and mental actions, such as classifying or comparing or reversing. An experience is assimilated to a scheme, and the scheme is modified or created through accommodation.

secular trends Patterns of change in some characteristic over several cohorts, such as systematic changes in the average timing of menarche or average height or weight.

secure attachment Postulated internal working model of relationship, fostered by responsive parenting, in which the child readily uses the parent as a safe base and is consoled after separation, when fearful, or when otherwise stressed.

self-concept The broad idea of "who I am," including the subjective self and the objective self.

self-esteem A global judgment of self-worth; how well you like who you perceive yourself to be.

semantics The rules for conveying meaning in language.

sensitive period Similar to a critical period except broader and less specific. A time in development when a particular type of stimulation is especially important or effective.

sensorimotor stage Piaget's term for the first major stage of cognitive development, from birth to about 18 months, when the child moves from reflexive to voluntary action.

sequential design A family of research designs involving multiple cross-sectional or multiple longitudinal studies, or a combination of the two.

sex chromosomes The X and Y chromosomes, which determine the sex of the child. In humans, XX is the female pattern, XY is the male pattern.

sex role The set of behaviors, attitudes, rights, duties, and obligations that are part of the "role" of being a boy or a girl, a male or a female in any given culture.

sex-role behavior The performance of behavior that matches the culturally defined sex role, such as choosing "sex-appropriate" toys or playing with same-sex children.

sex typing See **sex-role behavior.**

shape constancy The ability to see an object's shape as remaining the same despite changes in the shape of the retinal image. A basic perceptual constancy.

size constancy The ability to see an object's size as remaining the same despite changes in size of the retinal image. A key element in this constancy is the ability to judge depth.

small-for-date infant An infant who weighs less than is normal for the number of weeks of gestation completed.

social class Widely used term to describe broad variations in economic and social positions within any given society. Four broad groups are most often described: upper class, middle class, working class, and lower class (also called poverty level). For an individual family, the designation is based on the income, occupation, and education of the adults in the household.

social cognition Term used to describe an area of research and theory focused on the child's *understanding* of social relationships.

social referencing Using another person's emotional reaction to some situation as a basis for deciding one's own reaction. A baby does this when she checks her parent's facial expression or body language before responding positively or negatively to something new.

Stanford-Binet The best-known American intelligence test. It was written by Louis Terman and his associates on the basis of the first tests by Binet and Simon.

Strange Situation A series of episodes used by Mary Ainsworth and others in studies of attachment. The child is observed with the mother, with a stranger, alone, and then reunited with stranger and mother.

subjective self The first major step in the development of the self-concept; the initial awareness that "I exist" separate from others.

sudden infant death syndrome (SIDS) Unexpected death of an infant who otherwise appears healthy. Also called *crib death*. Cause is unknown.

superego In Freudian theory, the "conscience" part of personality that develops as a result of the identification process. The superego contains the parental and societal values, and attitudes incorporated by the child.

synapse The point of communication between two neurons, where nerve impulses are passed from one neuron to another by means of chemicals called neurotransmitters.

syntax The rules for forming sentences; also called *grammar*.

telegraphic speech A characteristic of early child sentences in nearly all languages in which everything but the crucial words is omitted, as if for a telegram.

temperament Term sometimes used interchangeably with *personality* but best thought of as the emotional substrate of personality, at least partially genetically determined.

teratogen Any outside agent, such as a disease or a chemical, whose presence significantly increases the risk of deviations or abnormalities in prenatal development.

theory of mind The theory a child or adult has about the way his own and other people's minds work, and how others are affected by their beliefs and feelings. By 4 or 5, children have a well-developed theory of mind.

tracking Also called *smooth pursuit*. The smooth movements of the eye used to follow the track of some moving object.

triarchic theory of intelligence A theory advanced by Sternberg, proposing the existence of three types of intelligence, the componential, the contextual, and the experiential.

ultrasound A form of prenatal diagnosis in which high-frequency sound waves are used to provide a picture of the moving fetus. Can be used to detect many physical deformities, such as neural tube defects, as well as multiple pregnancies and gestational age.

unconditioned response In classical conditioning, the basic unlearned response that is triggered by the unconditioned stimulus. A baby's turning of his head when touched on the cheek is an unconditioned response.

unconditioned stimulus In classical conditioning, the cue or signal that automatically triggers the unconditioned response. A touch on a baby's cheek, triggering head turning, is an unconditioned stimulus.

uterus The female organ in which the blastocyst implants itself and within which the embryo/fetus develops. (Popularly referred to as the womb.)

warmth versus hostility The key dimension of emotional tone used to describe family interactions.

WISC-III The most recent revision of the Wechsler Intelligence Scale for Children, a well-known American IQ test that includes both verbal and performance (nonverbal) subtests.

References

Achenbach, T. M. (1982). *Developmental psychopathology* (2nd ed.). New York: Wiley.

Achenbach, T. M. (1993). Taxonomy and comorbidity of conduct problems: Evidence from empirically based approaches. *Development and Psychopathology, 5,* 51–64.

Achenbach, T. M., & Edelbrock, C. S. (1981). Behavioral problems and competencies reported by parents of normal and disturbed children aged 4 through 16. *Monographs of the Society for Research in Child Development, 46* (1, Whole No. 188).

Adams, M. J. (1990). *Beginning to read: Thinking and learning about print.* Cambridge, MA: MIT Press.

Adashek, J. A., Peaceman, A. M., Lopez-Zeno, J. A., Minogue, J. P., & Socol, M. L. (1993). Factors contributing to the increased cesarean birth rate in older parturient women. *American Journal of Obstetrics and Gynecology, 169,* 936–940.

Adler, A. (1948). *Studies in analytical psychology.* New York: Norton.

Ahadi, S. A., & Rothbart, M. K. (1994). Temperament, development, and the big five. In C. F. Halverson, Jr., G. A. Kohnstamm, & R. P. Martin (Eds.), *The developing structure of temperament and personality from infancy to adulthood* (pp. 189–207). Hillsdale, NJ: Erlbaum.

Ahlsten, G., Cnattingius, S., & Lindmark, G. (1993). Cessation of smoking during pregnancy improves foetal growth and reduces infant morbidity in the neonatal period: A population-based prospective study. *Acta Paediatrica, 82,* 177–182.

Ainsworth, M. D. S. (1972). Attachment and dependency: A comparison. In J. L. Gewirtz (Ed.), *Attachment and dependency* (pp. 97–138). Washington, DC: V. H. Winston.

Ainsworth, M. D. S. (1982). Attachment: Retrospect and prospect. In C. M. Parkes & J. Stevenson-Hinde (Eds.), *The place of attachment in human behavior* (pp. 3–30). New York: Basic Books.

Ainsworth, M. D. S. (1989). Attachments beyond infancy. *American Psychologist, 44,* 709–716.

Ainsworth, M. D. S., Blehar, M., Waters, E., & Wall, S. (1978). *Patterns of attachment.* Hillsdale, NJ: Erlbaum.

Aksu-Koc, A. A., & Slobin, D. I. (1985). The acquisition of Turkish. In D. I. Slobin (Ed.), *The crosslinguistic study of language acquisition: Vol. 1. The data* (pp. 839–878). Hillsdale, NJ: Erlbaum.

Al Awad, A. M. E. L., & Sonuga-Barke, E. J. S. (1992). Childhood problems in a Sudanese city: A comparison of extended and nuclear families. *Child Development, 63,* 906–914.

Albrecht, S. L., Miller, M. K., & Clarke, L. L. (1994). Assessing the importance of family structure in understanding birth outcomes. *Journal of Marriage and the Family, 56,* 987–1003.

Alexander, J. M., & Schwanenflugel, P. J. (1994). Strategy regulation: The role of intelligence, metacognitive attributions, and knowledge base. *Developmental Psychology, 30,* 709–723.

Alexander, K. L., Entwisle, D. R., & Dauber, S. L. (1993). First-grade classroom behavior: Its short and long-term consequences for school performance. *Child Development, 64,* 801–814.

Allen, M. C., Donohue, P. K., & Dusman, A. E. (1993). The limit of viability—neonatal outcome of infants born at 22 to 25 weeks' gestation. *New England Journal of Medicine, 329,* 1597–1601.

Alsaker, F. D., & Olweus, D. (1992). Stability of global self-evaluations in early adolescence: A cohort longitudinal study. *Journal of Research on Adolescence, 2,* 123–145.

Amato, P. R. (1993). Children's adjustment to divorce: Theories, hypotheses, and empirical support. *Journal of Marriage and the Family, 55,* 23–38.

Ambert, A. (1994). An international perspective on parenting: Social change and social constructs. *Journal of Marriage and the Family, 56,* 529–543.

Ambuel, B. (1995). Adolescents, unintended pregnancy, and abortion: The struggle for a compassionate social policy. *Current Directions in Psychological Science, 4,* 1–5.

American Psychiatric Association (1994). *Diagnostic and statistical manual of mental disorders* (4th ed.). Washington, DC: American Psychiatric Association.

American Psychological Association (1993). *Violence and youth: Psychology's response: Vol. 1. Summary report of the American Psychological Association Commission on Violence and Youth.* Washington, DC: American Psychological Association.

Anderson, D. R., Lorch, E. P., Field, D. E., Collins, P. A., & Nathan, J. G. (1986). Television viewing at home: Age trends in visual attention and time with TV. *Child Development, 57,* 1024–1033.

Andersson, B. (1989). Effects of public day-care: A longitudinal study. *Child Development, 60,* 857–886.

Andersson, B. (1992). Effects of day-care on cognitive and socioemotional competence of thirteen-year-old Swedish school children. *Child Development, 63,* 20–36.

Anglin, J. M. (1993). Vocabulary development: A morphological analysis. *Monographs of the Society for Research in Child Development, 58* (Serial No. 238).

Anisfeld, M. (1991). Neonatal imitation. *Developmental Review, 11,* 60–97.

Annunziato, P. W., & Frenkel, L. M. (1993). The epidemiology of pediatric HIV–1 infection. *Pediatric Annals, 22,* 401–405.

Anthony, E. J. (1970). The behavior disorders of childhood. In P. H. Mussen (Ed.), *Carmichael's manual of child psychology* (3rd ed., Vol. 2) (pp. 667–764). New York: Wiley.

Apgar, V. A. (1953). A proposal for a new method of evaluation of the newborn infant. *Current Research in Anesthesia and Analgesia, 32,* 260–267.

Arn, P., Chen, H., Tuck-Muller, C. M., Mankinen, C., Wachtel, G., Li, S., Shen, C.-C., & Wachtel, S. S. (1994). SRVX, a sex reversing locus in Xp21.2 → p22.11. *Human Genetics, 93,* 389–393.

Arnett, J. (1992). Reckless behavior in adolescence: A developmental perspective. *Developmental Review, 12,* 339–373.

Aslin, R. N. (1981a). Experiential influences and sensitive periods in perceptual development: A unified model. In R. N. Aslin, J. R. Alberts, & M. R. Petersen (Eds.), *Development of perception: Psychobiological perspectives: Vol. 2. The visual system* (pp. 45–93). New York: Academic Press.

Aslin, R. N. (1981b). Development of smooth pursuit in human infants. In D. F. Fisher, R. A. Monty, & J. W. Senders (Eds.), *Eye movements: Cognition and visual perception* (pp. 31–51). Hillsdale, NJ: Erlbaum.

Aslin, R. N. (1987a). Motor aspects of visual development in infancy. In P. Salapatek & L. Cohen (Eds.), *Handbook of infant perception: Vol. 1. From sensation to perception* (pp. 43–113). Orlando, FL: Academic Press.

Aslin, R. N. (1987b). Visual and auditory development in infancy. In J. D. Osofsky (Ed.), *Handbook of infant development* (2nd ed.) (pp. 5–97). New York: Wiley-Interscience.

Astbury, J., Orgill, A. A., Bajuk, B., & Yu, V. Y. H. (1990). Neurodevelopmental outcome, growth and health of extremely low-birthweight survivors: How soon can we tell? *Developmental Medicine and Child Neurology, 32,* 582–589.

Astington, J. W., & Gopnik, A. (1991). Theoretical explanations of children's understanding of the mind. In G. E. Butterworth, P. L. Harris, A. M. Leslie, & H. M. Wellman (Eds.), *Perspectives on the child's theory of mind* (pp. 7–31). New York: Oxford University Press.

Astone, N. M. (1993). Are adolescent mothers just single mothers? *Journal of Research on Adolescence, 3,* 353–371.

Attie, I., & Brooks-Gunn, J. (1989). Development of eating problems in adolescent girls: A longitudinal study. *Developmental Psychology, 25,* 70–79.

Attie, I., & Brooks-Gunn, J. (1995). The development of eating regulation across the life span. In D. Cicchetti & D. J. Cohen (Eds.), *Developmental psychopathology: Vol. 2. Risk, disorder, and adaptation* (pp. 332–368). New York: Wiley.

Attie, I., Brooks-Gunn, J., & Petersen, A. (1990). A developmental perspective on eating disorders and eating problems. In M. Lewis & S. M. Miller (Eds.), *Handbook of developmental psychopathology* (pp. 409–420). New York: Plenum Press.

Avis, J., & Harris, P. L. (1991). Belief-desire reasoning among Baka children: Evidence for a universal conception of mind. *Child Development, 62,* 460–467.

Bachman, J. G., & Schulenberg, J. (1993). How part-time work intensity relates to drug use, problem behavior, time use, and satisfaction among high school seniors: Are these consequences or merely correlates? *Developmental Psychology, 29,* 220–235.

Bailey, J. M., & Pillard, R. C. (1991). A genetic study of male sexual orientation. *Archives of General Psychiatry, 48,* 1089–1096.

Bailey, J. M., Pillard, R. C., Neale, M. C., & Agyei, Y. (1993). Heritable factors influence sexual orientation in women. *Archives of General Psychiatry, 50,* 217–223.

Baillargeon, R. (1994). How do infants learn about the physical world? *Current Directions in Psychological Science, 3,* 133–140.

Baird, P. A., Sadovnick, A. D., & Yee, I. M. L. (1991). Maternal age and birth defects: A population study. *Lancet, 337,* 527–530.

Baker-Ward, L., Gordon, B. N., Ornstein, P. A., Larus, D. M., & Clubb, P. A. (1993). Young children's long-term retention of a pediatric examination. *Child Development, 64,* 1519–1533.

Bakketeig, L. S., Cnattingius, S., & Knudsen, L. B. (1993). Socioeconomic differences in fetal and infant mortality in Scandinavia. *Journal of Public Health Policy, 14*(Spring), 82–90.

Balaban, M. T. (1995). Affective influences on startle in five-month-old infants: Reactions to facial expressions of emotion. *Child Development, 66,* 28–36.

Baldwin, D. A. (1993). Early referential understanding: Infants' ability to recognize referential acts for what they are. *Developmental Psychology, 29,* 832–843.

Bamford, F. N., Bannister, R. P., Benjamin, C. M., Hillier, V. F., Ward, B. S., & Moore, W. M. O. (1990). Sleep in the first year of life. *Developmental Medicine and Child Neurology, 32,* 718–724.

Bandini, L. G., & Dietz, W. H. (1992). Myths about childhood obesity. *Pediatric Annals, 21,* 647–652.

Bandura, A. (1973). *Aggression: A social learning analysis.* Englewood Cliffs, NJ: Prentice Hall.

Bandura, A. (1977). *Social learning theory.* Englewood Cliffs, NJ: Prentice Hall.

Bandura, A. (1982). The self and mechanisms of agency. In J. Suls (Ed.), *Psychological perspectives on the self* (pp. 3–40). Hillsdale, NJ: Erlbaum.

Bandura, A. (1986). *Social foundations of thought and action: A social cognitive theory.* Englewood Cliffs, NJ: Prentice Hall.

Bandura, A. (1989). Social cognitive theory. *Annals of Child Development, 6,* 1–60.

Bardoni, B., Zanaria, E., Guioli, S., Floridia, G., Worley, K. C., Tonini, G., Ferrante, E., Chiumello, G., McCabe, E. R. B., Fraccaro, M., Zuffardi, O., & Camerino, G. (1994). A dosage sensitive locus at chromosome Xp21 is involved in male to female sex reversal. *Nature Genetics, 7,* 497–501.

Barenboim, C. (1977). Developmental changes in the interpersonal cognitive system from middle childhood to adolescence. *Child Development, 48,* 1467–1474.

Barenboim, C. (1981). The development of person perception in childhood and adolescence: From behavioral comparisons to psychological constructs to psychological comparisons. *Child Development, 52,* 129–144.

Barkley, R. A. (1990). Attention deficit disorders: History, definition, and diagnosis. In M. Lewis & S. M. Miller (Eds.), *Handbook of developmental psychopathology* (pp. 65–76). New York: Plenum Press.

Barkley, R. A., Fischer, M., Edelbrock, C. S., & Smallish, L. (1990). The adolescent outcome of hyperactive children diagnosed by research criteria: I. An 8-year prospective follow-up study. *Journal of the American Academy of Child and Adolescent Psychiatry, 29,* 546–557.

Barnard, K. E., & Bee, H. L. (1983). The impact of temporally patterned stimulation on the development of preterm infants. *Child Development, 54,* 1156–1167.

Barnard, K. E., & Eyres, S. J. (1979). *Child health assessment: Part 2. The first year of life.* (DHEW Publication No. HRA 79–25) Washington, DC: U.S. Government Printing Office.

Barnard, K. E., Hammond, M. A., Booth, C. L., Bee, H. L., Mitchell, S. K., & Spieker, S. J. (1989). Measurement and meaning of parent–child interaction. In J. J. Morrison, C. Lord, & D. P. Keating (Eds.), *Applied developmental psychology* (Vol. 3, pp. 40–81). San Diego: Academic Press.

Barnes, H. L., & Olson, D. H. (1985). Parent-adolescent communication and the circumplex model. *Child Development, 56,* 438–447.

Barnett, W. S. (1993). Benefit–cost analysis of preschool education: Findings from a 25-year follow-up. *American Journal of Orthopsychiatry, 63,* 500–508.

Barr, H. M., Streissguth, A. P., Darby, B. L., & Sampson, P. D. (1990). Prenatal exposure to alcohol, caffeine, tobacco, and aspirin: Effects on fine and gross motor performance in 4-year-old children. *Developmental Psychology, 26,* 339–348.

Barrett, G. V., & Depinet, R. L. (1991). A reconsideration of testing for competence rather than for intelligence. *American Psychologist, 46,* 1012–1024.

Bartsch, K. (1993). Adolescents' theoretical thinking. In R. M. Lerner (Ed.), *Early adolescence: Perspectives on research, policy, and intervention* (pp. 143–157). Hillsdale, NJ: Erlbaum.

Bates, E. (1993). Commentary: Comprehension and production in early language development. *Monographs of the Society for Research in Child Development, 58*(3–4, Serial No. 233), 222–242.

Bates, E., Bretherton, I., Beeghly-Smith, M., & McNew, S. (1982). Social bases of language development: A reassessment. In H. W. Reese & L. P. Lipsitt (Eds.), *Advances in child development and behavior* (Vol. 16, pp. 8–68). New York: Academic Press.

Bates, E., Bretherton, I., & Snyder, L. (1988). *From first words to grammar: Individual differences and dissociable mechanisms.* Cambridge, England: Cambridge University Press.

Bates, E., O'Connell, B., & Shore, C. (1987). Language and communication in infancy. In J. D. Osofsky (Ed.), *Handbook of infant development* (2nd ed.) (pp. 149–203). New York: Wiley.

Bates, J. E. (1987). Temperament in infancy. In J. D. Osofsky (Ed.), *Handbook of infant development* (2nd ed.) (pp. 1101–1149). New York: Wiley-Interscience.

Bates, J. E. (1989). Applications of temperament concepts. In G. A. Kohnstamm, J. E. Bates, & M. K. Rothbart (Eds.), *Temperament in childhood* (pp. 321–356). Chichester, England: Wiley.

Bates, J. E., Marvinney, D., Kelly, T., Dodge, K. A., Bennett, D. S., & Pettit, G. S. (1994). Child-care history and kindergarten adjustment. *Developmental Psychology, 30,* 690–700.

Bates, J. E., Maslin, C. A., & Frankel, K. A. (1985). Attachment security, mother-child interaction, and temperament as predictors of behavior problem ratings at age three years. In I. Bretherton & E. Waters (Eds.), Growing points of attachment theory and research. *Monographs of the Society for Research in Child Development, 50*(1–2, Serial No. 209), 167–193.

Baumgartner, R. N., Roche, A. F., & Himes, J. H. (1986). Incremental growth tables: Supplementary to previously published charts. *American Journal of Clinical Nutrition, 43,* 711–722.

Baumrind, D. (1971). Current patterns of parental authority. *Developmental Psychology Monograph, 4*(1, Part 2).

Baumrind, D. (1972). Socialization and instrumental competence in young children. In W. W. Hartup (Ed.), *The young child: Reviews of research* (Vol. 2, pp. 202–224). Washington, DC: National Association for the Education of Young Children.

Baydar, N., & Brooks-Gunn, J. (1991). Effects of maternal employment and child-care arrangements on preschoolers' cognitive and behavioral outcomes: Evidence from the children of the National Longitudinal Survey of Youth. *Developmental Psychology, 27,* 932–945.

Baydar, N., Brooks-Gunn, J., & Furstenberg, F. F. (1993). Early warning signs of functional illiteracy: Predictors in childhood and adolescence. *Child Development, 64,* 815–829.

Bayley, N. (1969). *Bayley scales of infant development.* New York: Psychological Corporation.

Bear, G. G., & Rys, G. S. (1994). Moral reasoning, classroom behavior, and sociometric status among elementary school children. *Developmental Psychology, 30,* 633–638.

Bearison, D. J., Magzamen, S., & Filardo, E. K. (1986). Sociocognitive conflict and cognitive growth in young children. *Merrill-Palmer Quarterly, 32,* 51–72.

Bedard, J., & Chi, M. T. H. (1992). Expertise. *Current Directions in Psychological Science, 1,* 135–139.

Bee, H. L., Barnard, K. E., Eyres, S. J., Gray, C. A., Hammond, M. A., Spietz, A. L., Snyder, C., & Clark, B. (1982). Prediction of IQ and language skill from perinatal status, child performance, family characteristics, and mother-infant interaction. *Child Development, 53,* 1135–1156.

Bell, L. G., & Bell, D. C. (1982). Family climate and the role of the female adolescent: Determinants of adolescent functioning. *Family Relations, 31,* 519–527.

Bellinger, D. C., Stiles, K. M., & Needleman, H. L. (1992). Low-level lead exposure, intelligence and academic achievement: A long-term follow-up study. *Pediatrics, 90,* 855–861.

Belsky, J. (1985). Prepared statement on the effects of day care. In Select Committee on Children, Youth, and Families, House of Representatives, 98th Congress, Second Session, *Improving child care services: What can be done?* Washington, DC: U.S. Government Printing Office.

Belsky, J. (1992). Consequences of child care for children's development: A deconstructionist view. In A. Booth (Ed.), *Child care in the 1990s: Trends and consequences* (pp. 83–94). Hillsdale, NJ: Erlbaum.

Belsky, J. (1993). Etiology of child maltreatment: A developmental-ecological analysis. *Psychological Bulletin, 114,* 413–434.

Belsky, J., Lang, M. E., & Rovine, M. (1985). Stability and change in marriage across the transition to parenthood: A second study. *Journal of Marriage and the Family, 47,* 855–865.

Belsky, J., & Rovine, M. (1988). Nonmaternal care in the first year of life and the security of infant-parent attachment. *Child Development, 59,* 157–167.

Bem, S. L. (1974). The measurement of psychological androgyny. *Journal of Consulting and Clinical Psychology, 42,* 155–162.

Benbow, C. P. (1988). Sex differences in mathematical reasoning ability in intellectually talented preadolescents: Their nature, effects, and possible causes. *Behavioral and Brain Sciences, 11,* 169–232.

Bendersky, M., & Lewis, M. (1994). Environmental risk, biological risk, and developmental outcome. *Developmental Psychology, 30,* 484–494.

Benenson, J. F. (1994). Ages four to six years: Changes in the structures of play networks of girls and boys. *Merrill-Palmer Quarterly, 40,* 478–487.

Benoit, D., & Parker, K. C. H. (1994). Stability and transmission of attachment across three generations. *Child Development, 65,* 1444–1456.

Berch, D. B., & Bender, B. G. (1987). Margins of sexuality. *Psychology Today, 21*(December), 54–57.

Bergeman, C. S., Chipuer, H. M., Plomin, R., Pedersen, N. L., McClearn, G. E., Nesselroade, J. R., Costa, P. T., & McCrae, R. R. (1993). Genetic and environmental effects on openness to experience, agreeableness, and conscientiousness: An adoption/twin study. *Journal of Personality, 61,* 159–179.

Berkowitz, G. S., Skovron, M. L., Lapinski, R. H., & Berkowitz, R. L. (1990). Delayed childbearing and the outcome of pregnancy. *New England Journal of Medicine, 322,* 659–664.

Berndt, T. J. (1983). Social cognition, social behavior, and children's friendships. In E. T. Higgins, D. N. Ruble, & W. W. Hartup (Eds.), *Social cognition and social development: A sociocultural perspective* (pp. 158–192). Cambridge, England: Cambridge University Press.

Berndt, T. J. (1986). Children's comments about their friendships. In M. Perlmutter (Ed.), *The Minnesota Symposia on Child Psychology* (Vol. 18, pp. 189–212). Hillsdale, NJ: Erlbaum.

Berndt, T. J. (1992). Friendship and friends' influence in adolescence. *Current Directions in Psychological Science, 1,* 156–159.

Berndt, T. J., & Keefe, K. (1995). *Friends' influence on school adjustment: A motivational analysis.* Paper presented at the biennial meetings of the Society for Research in Child Development, Indianapolis.

Bertenthal, B. I., & Campos, J. J. (1987). New directions in the study of early experience. *Child Development, 58,* 560–567.

Bertenthal, B. I., Campos, J. J., & Kermoian, R. (1994). An epigenetic perspective on the development of self-produced locomotion and its consequences. *Current Directions in Psychological Science, 3,* 140–145.

Betancourt, H., & Lopez, S. R. (1993). The study of culture, ethnicity, and race in American psychology. *American Psychologist, 48,* 629–637.

Bettes, B. A. (1988). Maternal depression and motherese: Temporal and intonational features. *Child Development, 59,* 1089–1096.

Biederman, J., Faraone, S., Keenan, K., Knee, D., & Tsuang, M. (1990). Family-genetic and psychosocial risk factors in DSM-III attention deficit disorder. *Journal of the American Academy of Child and Adolescent Psychiatry, 29,* 526–533.

Bigelow, B. J., & La Gaipa, J. J. (1975). Children's written descriptions of friendships: A multidimensional analysis. *Developmental Psychology, 11,* 857–858.

Billings, A. G., & Moos, R. H. (1985). Children of parents with unipolar depression: A controlled 1-year follow-up. *Journal of Abnormal Child Psychology, 14,* 149–166.

Billy, J. O. G., Brewster, K. L., & Grady, W. R. (1994). Contextual effects on the sexual behavior of adolescent women. *Journal of Marriage and the Family, 56,* 387–404.

Bingham, C. R., Miller, B. C., & Adams, G. R. (1990). Correlates of age at first sexual intercourse in a national sample of young women. *Journal of Adolescent Research, 5,* 18–33.

Bisanz, J., Morrison, F. J., & Dunn, M. (1995). Effects of age and schooling on the acquisition of elementary quantitative skills. *Developmental Psychology, 31,* 221–236.

Biswas, M. K., & Craigo, S. D. (1994). The course and conduct of normal labor and delivery. In A. H. DeCherney & M. L. Pernoll (Eds.), *Current obstetric and gynecologic diagnosis & treatment* (pp. 202–227). Norwalk, CT: Appleton & Lange.

Bivens, J. A., & Berk, L. E. (1990). A longitudinal study of the development of elementary school children's private speech. *Merrill-Palmer Quarterly, 36,* 443–463.

Bjorklund, D. F., & Muir, J. E. (1988). Remembering on their own: Children's development of free recall memory. In R. Vasta (Ed.), *Annals of child development* (Vol. 5, pp. 79–124). Greenwich, CT: JAI Press.

Black, K. A., & McCartney, K. (1995). *Associations between adolescent attachment to parents and peer interactions.* Paper presented at the biennial meetings of the Society for Research in Child Development, Indianapolis.

Blackman, J. A. (1990). Update on AIDS, CMV, and herpes in young children: Health, developmental, and educational issues. In M. Wolraich & D. K. Routh (Eds.), *Advances in de-velopmental and behavioral pediatrics* (Vol. 9, pp. 33–58). London: Jessica Kingsley Publishers.

Blair, S. L., & Johnson, M. P. (1992). Wives' perceptions of the fairness of the division of household labor: The intersection of housework and ideology. *Journal of Marriage and the Family, 54,* 570–581.

Blake, I. K. (1994). Language development and socialization in young African-American children. In P. M. Greenfield & R. R. Cocking (Eds.), *Cross-cultural roots of minority child development* (pp. 167–195). Hillsdale, NJ: Erlbaum.

Block, J. (1971). *Lives through time.* Berkeley, CA: Bancroft.

Block, J., & Robins, R. W. (1993). A longitudinal study of consistency and change in self-esteem from early adolescence to early adulthood. *Child Development, 64,* 909–923.

Bloom, L. (1973). *One word at a time.* The Hague: Mouton.

Bloom, L. (1991). *Language development from two to three.* Cambridge, England: Cambridge University Press.

Bloom, L. (1993). *The transition from infancy to language: Acquiring the power of expression.* Cambridge, England: Cambridge University Press.

Bloom, L., Tinker, E., & Margulis, C. (1993). The words children learn: Evidence against a noun bias in early vocabularies. *Cognitive Development, 8,* 431–450.

Boer, F., & Dunn, J. (Eds.). (1992). *Children's sibling relationships: Developmental and clinical issues.* Hillsdale, NJ: Erlbaum.

Boer, F., Godhart, A. W., & Treffers, P. D. A. (1992). Siblings and their parents. In F. Boer & J. Dunn (Eds.), *Children's sibling relationships. Developmental and clinical issues* (pp. 41–54). Hillsdale, NJ: Erlbaum.

Bond, M. H., Nakazato, H., & Shiraishi, D. (1975). Universality and distinctiveness in dimensions of Japanese person perception. *Journal of Cross-Cultural Psychology, 6,* 346–357.

Booth, A. (Ed.). (1992). *Child care in the 1990s: Trends and consequences.* Hillsdale, NJ: Erlbaum.

Borkenau, P., & Ostendorf, F. (1990). Comparing exploratory and confirmatory factor analysis: A study on the five-factor model of personality. *Personality and Individual Differences, 11,* 515–524.

Bornstein, M. H. (1987). Sensitive periods in development: Definition, existence, utility, and meaning. In M. H. Bornstein (Ed.), *Sensitive periods in development: Interdisciplinary perspectives* (pp. 3–18). Hillsdale, NJ: Erlbaum.

Bornstein, M. H. (Ed.). (1989). *Maternal responsiveness: Characteristics and consequences.* San Francisco: Jossey-Bass.

Bornstein, M. H. (1992). Perception across the life span. In M. H. Bornstein & M. E. Lamb (Eds.), *Developmental psychology: An advanced textbook* (3rd ed.) (pp. 155–210). Hillsdale, NJ: Erlbaum.

Bornstein, M. H., Tal, J., & Tamis-LeMonda, C. S. (1991). Parenting in cross-cultural perspective: The United States, France, and Japan. In M. H. Bornstein (Ed.), *Cultural approaches to parenting* (pp. 69–90). Hillsdale, NJ: Erlbaum.

Bornstein, M. H., Tamis-LeMonda, C. S., Tal, J., Ludemann, P., Toda, S., Rahn, C. W., Pecheux, M., Azuma, H., & Vardi, D. (1992). Maternal responsiveness to infants in three societies: The United States, France, and Japan. *Child Development, 63,* 808–821.

The Boston Women's Health Collective (1992). *The new our bodies, ourselves: A book by and for women.* New York: Simon & Schuster.

Bouchard, T. J., Jr. (1984). Twins reared apart and together: What they tell us about human diversity. In S. Fox (Ed.), *The chemical and biological bases of individuality.* New York: Plenum Press.

Bouchard, T. J., Jr., & McGue, M. (1981). Familial studies of intelligence: A review. *Science, 212,* 1055–1059.

Bower, T. G. R. (1966). The visual world of infants. *Scientific American, 215,* 80–92.

Bower, T. G. R. (1989). *The rational infant.* New York: Freeman.

Bowerman, M. (1985). Beyond communicative adequacy: From piecemeal knowledge to an integrated system in the child's acquisition of language. In K. E. Nelson (Ed.), *Children's language* (Vol. 5, pp. 369–398). Hillsdale, NJ: Erlbaum.

Bowlby, J. (1969). *Attachment and loss: Vol. 1. Attachment.* New York: Basic Books.

Bowlby, J. (1973). *Attachment and loss: Vol. 2. Separation, anxiety, and anger.* New York: Basic Books.

Bowlby, J. (1980). *Attachment and loss: Vol. 3. Loss, sadness, and depression.* New York: Basic Books.

Bowlby, J. (1988a). Developmental psychiatry comes of age. *American Journal of Psychiatry, 145,* 1–10.

Bowlby, J. (1988b). *A secure base.* New York: Basic Books.

Boyatzis, C. J., Matillo, G., Nesbitt, K., & Cathey, G. (1995). *Effects of "The Mighty Morphin Power Rangers" on children's aggression and prosocial behavior.* Paper presented at the biennial meetings of the Society for Research in Child Development, Indianapolis.

Boyes, M. C., & Allen, S. G. (1993). Styles of parent-child interactions and moral reasoning in adolescence. *Merrill-Palmer Quarterly, 39,* 551–570.

Bradbard, M. R., Martin, C. L., Endsley, R. C., & Halverson, C. F., Jr. (1986). Influence of sex stereotypes on children's exploration and memory: A competence versus performance distinction. *Developmental Psychology, 22,* 481–486.

Braden, J. P. (1994). *Deafness, deprivation, and IQ.* New York: Plenum Press.

Bradley, R. H., Caldwell, B. M., Rock, S. L., Barnard, K. E., Gray, C., Hammond, M. A., Mitchell, S., Siegel, L., Ramey, C. D., Gottfried, A. W., & Johnson, D. L. (1989). Home environment and cognitive development in the first 3 years of life: A collaborative study involving six sites and three ethnic groups in North America. *Developmental Psychology, 25,* 217–235.

Bradley, R. H., Whiteside, L., Mundfrom, D. J., Casey, P. H., Kelleher, K. J., & Pope, S. K. (1994). Early indications of resilience and their relation to experiences in the home environments of low birthweight, premature children living in poverty. *Child Development, 65,* 346–360.

Brand, E., Clingempeel, W. E., & Bowen-Woodward, K. (1988). Family relationships and children's psychological adjustment in stepmother and stepfather families: Findings and conclusions from the Philadelphia Stepfamily Research Project. In E. M. Hetherington & J. D. Arasteh (Eds.), *Impact of divorce, single parenting, stepparenting on children* (pp. 299–324). Hillsdale, NJ: Erlbaum.

Brandenburg, N. A., Friedman, R. M., & Silver, S. E. (1990). The epidemiology of childhood psychiatric disorders: Prevalence findings from recent studies. *Journal of the American Academy of Child and Adolescent Psychiatry, 29,* 76–83.

Breitmayer, B. J., & Ramey, C. T. (1986). Biological nonoptimality and quality of postnatal environment as codeterminants of intellectual development. *Child Development, 57,* 1151–1165.

Breland, H. M. (1974). Birth order, family configuration, and verbal achievement. *Child Development, 45,* 1011–1019.

Breslau, N., DelDotto, J. E., Brown, G. G., Kumar, S., Ezhuthachan, S., Hufnagle, K. G., & Peterson, E. L. (1994). A gradient relationship between low birth weight and IQ at age 6 years. *Archives of Pediatric and Adolescent Medicine, 148,* 377–383.

Bretherton, I. (1991). Pouring new wine into old bottles: The social self as internal working model. In M. R. Gunnar & L. A. Sroufe (Eds.), *The Minnesota Symposia on Child Development* (Vol. 23, pp. 1–42). Hillsdale, NJ: Erlbaum.

Bretherton, I. (1992a). The origins of attachment theory: John Bowlby and Mary Ainsworth. *Developmental Psychology, 28,* 759–775.

Bretherton, I. (1992b). Attachment and bonding. In V. B. Van Hasselt & M. Hersen (Eds.), *Handbook of social development: A lifespan perspective* (pp. 133–155). New York: Plenum Press.

Bretherton, I. (1993). From dialogue to internal working models: The co-construction of self in relationships. In C. A. Nelson (Ed.), *The Minnesota Symposia on Child Psychology* (Vol. 26, pp. 237–264). Hillsdale, NJ: Erlbaum.

Bristol, M. M., Gallagher, J. J., & Schopler, E. (1988). Mothers and fathers of young developmentally disabled and nondisabled boys: Adaptation and spousal support. *Developmental Psychology, 24,* 441–451.

Brody, G. H., Stoneman, Z., McCoy, J. K., & Forehand, R. (1992). Contemporaneous and longitudinal associations of sibling conflict with family relationship assessments and family discussions about sibling problems. *Child Development, 63,* 391–400.

Brody, N. (1992). *Intelligence* (2nd ed.). San Diego: Academic Press.

Broman, C. L. (1993). Race differences in marital well-being. *Journal of Marriage and the Family, 55,* 724–732.

Broman, S. H., Nichols, P. L., & Kennedy, W. A. (1975). *Preschool IQ: Prenatal and early developmental correlates.* Hillsdale, NJ: Erlbaum.

Broman, S. H., Nichols, P. L., Shaughnessy, P., & Kennedy, W. (1987). *Retardation in young children.* Hillsdale, NJ: Erlbaum.

Bronfenbrenner, U. (1979). *The ecology of human development.* Cambridge, MA: Harvard University Press.

Bronfenbrenner, U. (1989). Ecological systems theory. *Annals of Child Development, 6,* 187–249.

Bronfenbrenner, U., Alvarez, W. F., & Henderson, C. R., Jr. (1984). Working and watching: Maternal employment status and parents' perceptions of their three-year-old children. *Child Development, 55,* 1362–1378.

Bronson, G. W. (1991). Infant differences in rate of visual encoding. *Child Development, 62,* 44–45.

Bronson, G. W. (1994). Infants' transitions toward adult-like scanning. *Child Development, 65,* 1253–1261.

Brooks-Gunn, J. (1987). Pubertal processes and girls' psychological adaptation. In R. M. Lerner & T. T. Foch (Eds.), *Biological-psychosocial interactions in early adolescence* (pp. 123–154). Hillsdale, NJ: Erlbaum.

Brooks-Gunn, J. (1988). Commentary: Developmental issues in the transition to early adolescence. In M. R. Gunnar & W. A. Collins (Eds.), *The Minnesota Symposia on Child Psychology* (Vol. 21, pp. 189–208). Hillsdale, NJ: Erlbaum.

Brooks-Gunn, J., Klebanov, P. K., Liaw, F., & Spiker, D. (1993a). Enhancing the development of low-birthweight, premature infants: Changes in cognition and behavior over the first three years. *Child Development, 64,* 736–753.

Brooks-Gunn, J., Guo, G., & Furstenberg, F. F., Jr. (1993b). Who drops out of and who continues beyond high school? A 20-year follow-up of black urban youth. *Journal of Research on Adolescence, 3,* 271–294.

Brooks-Gunn, J., & Matthews, W. S. (1979). *He and she: How children develop their sex-role identity.* Englewood Cliffs, NJ: Prentice Hall.

Brooks-Gunn, J., & Reiter, E. O. (1990). The role of pubertal processes. In S. S. Feldman & G. R. Elliott (Eds.), *At the threshold. The developing adolescent* (pp. 16–53). Cambridge, MA: Harvard University Press.

Brooks-Gunn, J., & Warren, M. P. (1985). The effects of delayed menarche in different contexts: Dance and nondance students. *Journal of Youth and Adolescence, 13,* 285–300.

Broverman, I. K., Broverman, D., Clarkson, F. E., Rosenkrantz, P. S., & Vogel, S. R. (1970). Sex-role stereotypes and clinical judgments of mental health. *Journal of Consulting and Clinical Psychology, 34,* 1–7.

Brown, B. B. (1990). Peer groups and peer cultures. In S. S. Feldman & G. R. Elliott (Eds.), *At the threshold: The developing adolescent* (pp. 171–196). Cambridge, MA: Harvard University Press.

Brown, B. B., Dolcini, M. M., & Leventhal, A. (1995). *The emergence of peer crowds: Friend or foe to adolescent health?* Paper presented at the biennial meetings of the Society for Research in Child Development, Indianapolis.

Brown, B. B., Mory, M. S., & Kinney, D. (1994). Casting adolescent crowds in a relational perspective: Caricature, channel, and context. In R. Montemayor, G. R. Adams, & T. P. Gullotta (Eds.), *Personal relationships during adolescence* (pp. 123–167). Thousand Oaks, CA: Sage.

Brown, L., Karrison, T., & Cibils, L. A. (1994). Mode of delivery and perinatal results in breech presentation. *American Journal of Obstetrics and Gynecology, 171,* 28–34.

Brown, R. (1965). *Social psychology.* New York: Free Press.

Brown, R. (1973). *A first language: The early stages.* Cambridge, MA: Harvard University Press.

Brown, R., & Bellugi, U. (1964). Three processes in the acquisition of syntax. *Harvard Educational Review, 334,* 133–151.

Brown, R., & Hanlon, C. (1970). Derivational complexity and order of acquisition. In J. R. Hayes (Ed.), *Cognition and the development of language* (pp. 155–207). New York: Wiley.

Brownell, C. A. (1988). Combinatorial skills: Converging developments over the second year. *Child Development, 59,* 675–685.

Brownell, C. A. (1990). Peer social skills in toddlers: Competencies and constraints illustrated by same-age and mixed-age interaction. *Child Development, 61,* 836–848.

Bruck, M., Ceci, S. J., Francoeur, E., & Barr, R. (1995). "I hardly cried when I got my shot!" Influencing children's reports about a visit to their pediatrician. *Child Development, 66,* 193–208.

Bryant, P. E., MacLean, M., Bradley, L. L., & Crossland, J. (1990). Rhyme and alliteration, phoneme detection, and learning to read. *Developmental Psychology, 26,* 429–438.

Buchanan, C. M., Maccoby, E. E., & Dornbusch, S. M. (1991). Caught between parents: Adolescents' experience in divorced homes. *Child Development, 62,* 1008–1029.

Buchanan, C. M., Maccoby, E. E., & Dornbusch, S. M. (1992). Adolescents and their families after divorce: Three residential arrangements compared. *Journal of Research on Adolescence, 2,* 261–292.

Buehler, J. W., Kaunitz, A. M., Hogue, C. J. R., Hughes, J. M., Smith, J. C., & Rochat, R. W. (1986). Maternal mortality in women aged 35 years or older: United States. *Journal of the American Medical Association, 255,* 53–57.

Bullock, M., & Lütkenhaus, P. (1990). Who am I? Self-understanding in toddlers. *Merrill-Palmer Quarterly, 36,* 217–238.

Burchinal, M., Lee, M., & Ramey, C. (1989). Type of day-care and preschool intellectual development in disadvantaged children. *Child Development, 60,* 128–137.

Burns, A. (1992). Mother-headed families: An international perspective and the case of Australia. *Social Policy Report, Society for Research in Child Development, 6*(1), 1–22.

Buss, A. (1989). Temperaments as personality traits. In G. A. Kohnstamm, J. E. Bates, & M. K. Rothbart (Eds.), *Temperament in childhood* (pp. 49–58). Chichester, England: Wiley.

Buss, A. H., & Plomin, R. (1984). *Temperament: Early developing personality traits.* Hillsdale, NJ: Erlbaum.

Buss, A. H., & Plomin, R. (1986). The EAS approach to temperament. In R. Plomin & J. Dunn (Eds.), *The study of temperament: Changes, continuities and challenges* (pp. 67–80). Hillsdale, NJ: Erlbaum.

Bussey, K., & Bandura, A. (1992). Self-regulatory mechanisms governing gender development. *Child Development, 63,* 1236–1250.

Byrnes, J. P., & Takahira, S. (1993). Explaining gender differences on SAT-Math items. *Developmental Psychology, 29,* 805–810.

Cairns, R. B. (1991). Multiple metaphors for a singular idea. *Developmental Psychology, 27,* 23–26.

Cairns, R. B., & Cairns, B. D. (1994). *Lifelines and risks. Pathways of youth in our time.* Cambridge, England: Cambridge University Press.

California Assessment Program (1980). *Student achievement in California schools: 1979–1980 annual report. Television and student achievement.* Sacramento: California State Department of Education.

Callahan, C. M., & Rivara, F. P. (1992). Urban high school youth and handguns: A school-based survey. *Journal of the American Medical Association, 267*(22), 3038–3042.

Calvert, S. L., & Huston, A. C. (1987). Television and children's gender schemata. *New Directions for Child Development, 38,* 75–88.

Campbell, F. A., & Ramey, C. T. (1994). Effects of early intervention on intellectual and academic achievement: A follow-up study of children from low-income families. *Child Development, 65,* 684–698.

Campbell, R. L., & Bickhard, M. H. (1992). Types of constraints on development: An interactionist approach. *Developmental Review, 12,* 311–338.

Campbell, S. B. (1990). The socialization and social development of hyperactive children. In M. Lewis & S. M. Miller (Eds.), *Handbook of developmental psychopathology* (pp. 77–92). New York: Plenum Press.

Campbell, S. B., Cohn, J. F., Flanagan, C., Popper, S., & Meyers, T. (1992). Course and correlates of postpartum depression during the transition to parenthood. *Development and Psychopathology, 4,* 29–47.

Campbell, S. B., & Ewing, L. J. (1990). Follow-up of hard-to-manage preschoolers: Adjustment at age 9 and predictors of continuing symptoms. *Journal of Child Psychology and Psychiatry, 31,* 871–889.

Campbell, S. B., Pierce, E. W., March, C. L., & Ewing, L. J. (1991). Noncompliant behavior, overactivity, and family stress as predictors of negative maternal control with preschool children. *Development and Psychopathology, 3,* 175–190.

Campione, J. C., & Brown, A. L. (1984). Learning ability and transfer propensity as sources of individual differences in intelligence. In P. H. Brooks, C. McCauley, & R. Sperber (Eds.), *Learning and cognition in the mentally retarded.* Hillsdale, NJ: Erlbaum.

Campione, J. C., Brown, A. L., & Ferrara, R. A. (1982). Mental retardation and intelligence. In J. R. Sternberg (Ed.), *Handbook of human intelligence* (pp. 392–492). Cambridge, England: Cambridge University Press.

Campione, J. C., Brown, A. L., Ferrara, R. A., Jones, R. S., & Steinberg, E. (1985). Breakdowns in flexible use of information: Intelligence-related differences in transfer following equivalent learning performance. *Intelligence, 9,* 297–315.

Cantwell, D. P. (1990). Depression across the early life span. In M. Lewis & S. M. Miller (Eds.), *Handbook of developmental psychopathology* (pp. 293–310). New York: Plenum Press.

Capron, C., & Duyme, M. (1989). Assessment of effects of socio-economic status on IQ in a full cross-fostering study. *Nature, 340,* 552–554.

Capute, A. J., Palmer, F. B., Shapiro, B. K., Wachtel, R. C., Ross, A., & Accardo, P. J. (1984). Primitive reflex profile: A quantification of primitive reflexes in infancy. *Developmental Medicine and Child Neurology, 26,* 375–383.

Carey, S., & Bartlett, E. (1978). Acquiring a single new word. *Papers and Reports on Child Language Development, 15,* 17–29.

Carlson, E. A., & Sroufe, L. A. (1995). Contribution of attachment theory to developmental psychopathology. In D. Cicchetti & D. J. Conen (Eds.), *Developmental psychopathology: Vol. 1. Theory and methods* (pp. 581–617). New York: Wiley.

Caron, A. J., & Caron, R. F. (1981). Processing of relational information as an index of infant risk. In S. Friedman & M. Sigman (Eds.), *Preterm birth and psychological development* (pp. 219–240). New York: Academic Press.

Perspectives on research, policy, and intervention (pp. 71–91). Hillsdale, NJ: Erlbaum.

Crystal, D. S., Chen, C., Fuligni, A. J., Stevenson, H. W., Hsu, C., Ko, H., Kitamura, S., & Kimura, S. (1994). Psychological maladjustment and academic achievement: A cross-cultural study of Japanese, Chinese, and American high school students. *Child Development, 65,* 738–753.

Crystal, D. S., & Stevenson, H. W. (1995). What is a bad kid? Answers of adolescents and their mothers in three cultures. *Journal of Research on Adolescence, 5,* 71–91.

Crystal, S., Shae, D., & Krishnaswami, S. (1992). Educational attainment, occupational history, and stratification: Determinants of later-life economic outcomes. *Journal of Gerontology: SOCIAL SCIENCES, 47,* S213–S221.

Cummings, E. M., & Davies, P. T. (1994). Maternal depression and child development. *Journal of Child Psychology and Psychiatry, 35,* 73–112.

Cunningham, A. S., Jelliffe, D. B., & Jelliffe, E. F. P. (1991). Breast-feeding and health in the 1980s: A global epidemiologic review. *Journal of Pediatrics, 118,* 659–666.

Cutrona, C. E., & Troutman, B. R. (1986). Social support, infant temperament, and parenting self-efficacy: A mediational model of postpartum depression. *Child Development, 57,* 1507–1518.

D'Alton, M. E., & DeCherney, A. H. (1993). Prenatal diagnosis. *New England Journal of Medicine, 328,* 114–118.

Damon, W. (1977). *The social world of the child.* San Francisco: Jossey-Bass.

Damon, W. (1983). The nature of social-cognitive change in the developing child. In W. F. Overton (Ed.), *The relationship between social and cognitive development* (pp. 103–142). Hillsdale, NJ: Erlbaum.

Danner, F. W., & Day, M. C. (1977). Eliciting formal operations. *Child Development, 48,* 1600–1606.

Dark, V. J., & Benbow, C. P. (1993). Cognitive differences among the gifted: A review and new data. In D. K. Detterman (Ed.), *Current topics in human intelligence: Vol. 3. Individual differences and cognition* (pp. 85–120). Norwood, NJ: Ablex.

Darling, N., & Steinberg, L. (1993). Parenting style as context: An integrative model. *Psychological Bulletin, 113,* 487–496.

Darlington, R. B. (1991). The long-term effects of model preschool programs. In L. Okagaki & R. J. Sternberg (Eds.), *Directors of development* (pp. 203–215). Hillsdale, NJ: Erlbaum.

Dasen, P. R. (1984). The cross-cultural study of intelligence: Piaget and the Baoule. *International Journal of Psychology, 19,* 407–434.

Davidson, E. S., Yasuna, A., & Tower, A. (1979). The effect of television cartoons on sex-role stereotyping in young girls. *Child Development, 50,* 597–600.

Davies, G. M. (1993). Children's memory for other people: An integrative review. In C. A. Nelson (Ed.), *The Minnesota Symposia on Child Psychology* (Vol. 26, pp. 123–157). Hillsdale, NJ: Erlbaum.

Davies, P. T., & Cummings, E. M. (1994). Marital conflict and child adjustment: An emotional security hypothesis. *Psychological Bulletin, 116,* 387–411.

Dawson, D. A. (1991). Family structure and children's health and well-being: Data from the 1988 National Health Interview Survey on child health. *Journal of Marriage and the Family, 53,* 573–584.

de Chateau, P. (1980). Effects of hospital practices on synchrony in the development of the infant-parent relationship. In P. M. Taylor (Ed.), *Parent-infant relationships* (pp. 137–168). New York: Grune & Stratton.

de Haan, M., Luciana, M., Maslone, S. M., Matheny, L. S., & Richards, M. L. M. (1994). Development, plasticity, and risk: Commentary on Huttenlocher, Pollit and Gorman, and Gottesman and Goldsmith. In C. A. Nelson (Ed.), *The Minnesota Symposia on Child Psychology* (Vol. 27, pp. 161–178). Hillsdale, NJ: Erlbaum.

de Jong-van den Berg, L. T. W., Waardenburg, C. M., Haaijer-Ruskamp, F. M., Dukes, M. N. G., & Wesseling, H. (1993). Drug use in pregnancy: A comparative appraisal of data collection methods. *European Journal of Clinical Pharmacology, 45,* 9–14.

de Villiers, P. A., & de Villiers, J. G. (1992). Language development. In M. H. Bornstein & M. E. Lamb (Eds.), *Developmental psychology: An advanced textbook* (3rd ed., pp. 337–418). Hillsdale, NJ: Erlbaum.

DeCasper, A. J., & Fifer, W. P. (1980). Of human bonding: Newborns prefer their mothers' voices. *Science, 208,* 1174–1176.

DeCasper, A. J., Lecaneut, J., Busnel, M., Granier-Deferre, C., Maugeais, R. (1994). Fetal reactions to recurrent maternal speech. *Infant Behavior and Development, 17,* 159–164.

DeCasper, A. J., & Spence, M. J. (1986). Prenatal maternal speech influences newborns' perception of speech sounds. *Infant Behavior and Development, 9,* 133–150.

Delgado-Gaitan, C. (1994). Socializing young children in Mexican-American families: An intergenerational perspective. In P. M. Greenfield & R. R. Cocking (Eds.), *Cross-cultural roots of minority child development* (pp. 55–86). Hillsdale, NJ: Erlbaum.

DeLoache, J. S. (1989). The development of representation in young children. In H. W. Reese (Ed.), *Advances in child development and behavior* (Vol. 22, pp. 2–37). San Diego: Academic Press.

DeLoache, J. S., & Brown, A. L. (1987). Differences in the memory-based searching of delayed and normally developing young children. *Intelligence, 11,* 277–289.

Carver, R. P. (1990). Intelligence and reading ability in grades 2–12. *Intelligence, 14,* 449–455.

Casas, J. F., & Mosher, M. (1995). *Relational and overt aggression in preschool: "You can't come to my birthday party unless. . . ."* Paper presented at the biennial meetings of the Society for Research in Child Development, Indianapolis.

Case, R. (1985). *Intellectual development: Birth to adulthood.* New York: Academic Press.

Casey, M. B. (1986). Individual differences in selective attention among prereaders: A key to mirror-image confusions. *Developmental Psychology, 22,* 58–66.

Caspi, A., Henry, B., McGee, R. O., Moffitt, T. E., & Silva, P. A. (1995). Temperamental origins of child and adolescent behavior problems: From age three to age fifteen. *Child Development, 66,* 55–68.

Caspi, A., Lynam, D., Moffitt, T. E., & Silva, P. A. (1993). Unraveling girls' delinquency: Biological, dispositional, and contextual contributions to adolescent misbehavior. *Developmental Psychology, 29,* 19–30.

Cassidy, J., & Berlin, L. J. (1994). The insecure/ambivalent pattern of attachment: Theory and research. *Child Development, 65,* 971–991.

Caughy, M. O., DiPietro, J. A., & Strobino, D. M. (1994). Daycare participation as a protective factor in the cognitive development of low-income children. *Child Development, 65,* 457–471.

Ceci, S. J., & Bruck, M. (1993). Suggestibility of the child witness: A historical review and synthesis. *Psychological Bulletin, 113,* 403–439.

Center for Educational Statistics (1987). *Who drops out of high school? From high school and beyond.* Washington, DC: Office of Educational Research and Improvement, U.S. Department of Education.

Centers for Disease Control (1992a). Selected behaviors that increase risk for HIV infection among high school students—United States, 1990. *Morbidity and Mortality Weekly Report, 41*(231), 237–240.

Centers for Disease Control (1992b). Sexual behavior among high school students—United States, 1990. *Morbidity and Mortality Weekly Report, 40,* 885–888.

Centers for Disease Control (1992c). Recommendations for the use of folic acid to reduce the number of cases of spina bifida and other neural tube defects. *Morbidity and Mortality Weekly Report, 41,* 1–7.

Centers for Disease Control (1992d). Pregnancy risks determined from birth certificate data—United States, 1989. *Morbidity and Mortality Weekly Report, 41*(30), 556–563.

Centers for Disease Control (1993). Rates of cesarean delivery—United States, 1991. *Journal of the American Medical Association, 269*(18), 2360.

Centers for Disease Control (1993a). Childbearing patterns among selected racial/ethnic minority groups—United States, 1990. *Morbidity and Mortality Weekly Reports, 42,* 399–403.

Centers for Disease Control (1993b). Mortality trends and leading causes of death among adolescents and young adults—United States, 1979–1988. *Morbidity and Mortality Weekly Reports, 42,* 459–461.

Centers for Disease Control (1994a). Recommendations of the U.S. Public Health Service task force on the use of zidovudine to reduce perinatal transmission of human immunodeficiency virus. *Morbidity and Mortality Weekly Report, 43*(August 5), 1–20.

Centers for Disease Control (1994b). Preventing tobacco use among young people: A report of the Surgeon General. Executive summary. *Morbidity and Mortality Weekly Report, 43*(RR-4), 2–10.

Centers for Disease Control (1994c). Health-risk behaviors among persons aged 12–21 years—United States, 1992. *Morbidity and Mortality Weekly Report, 43,* 231–235.

Centers for Disease Control (1994d). Prevalence of overweight among adolescents—United States, 1988–91. *Morbidity and Mortality Weekly Reports, 43,* 818–811.

Centers for Disease Control (1994e). Programs for the prevention of suicide among adolescents and young adults. *Morbidity and Mortality Weekly Reports, 43*(RR-6, April 22), 3–7.

Centerwall, B. S. (1989). Exposure to television as a cause of violence. In G. Comstock (Ed.), *Public communication and behavior* (pp. 1–58). San Diego: Academic Press.

Centerwall, B. S. (1992). Television and violence: The scale of the problem and where to go from here. *Journal of the American Medical Association, 267*(22), 3059–3063.

Cernoch, J. M., & Porter, R. H. (1985). Recognition of maternal axillary odors by infants. *Child Development, 56,* 1593–1598.

Chalfant, J. C. (1989). Learning disabilities: Policy issues and promising approaches. *American Psychologist, 44,* 392–398.

Chang, L., & Murray, A. (1995). *Math performance of 5- and 6-year-olds in Taiwan and the U.S.: Maternal beliefs, expectations, and tutorial assistance.* Paper presented at the biennial meetings of the Society for Research in Child Development, Indianapolis.

Chao, R. K. (1994). Beyond parental control and authoritarian parenting style: Understanding Chinese parenting through the cultural notion of training. *Child Development, 65,* 1111–1119.

Chapa, J., & Valencia, R. R. (1993). Latino population growth, demographic characteristics, and educational stagnation: An examination of recent trends. *Hispanic Journal of Behavioral Sciences, 15,* 165–187.

Charman, T., Redfern, S., & Fonagy, P. (1995). *Individual differences in theory of mind acquisition: The role of attachment security.* Paper presented at the biennial meetings of the Society for Research in Child Development, Indianapolis.

Chen, X., Rubin, K. H., & Sun, Y. (1992). Social reputation and peer relationships in Chinese and Canadian children: A cross-cultural study. *Child Development, 63,* 1336–1343.

Cheng, M., & Hannah, M. (1993). Breech delivery at term: A critical review of the literature. *Obstetrics and Gynecology, 82,* 605–618.

Cherlin, A. J. (1992a). *Marriage, divorce, remarriage.* Cambridge, MA: Harvard University Press.

Cherlin, A. J. (1992b). Infant care and full-time employment. In A. Booth (Ed.), *Child care in the 1990s: Trends and consequences* (pp. 209–214). Hillsdale, NJ: Erlbaum.

Chess, S., & Korn, S. J. (1980). Temperament and behavior disorder in mentally retarded children. *Journal of Special Education, 23,* 122–130.

Chess, S., & Thomas, A. (1984). *Origins and evolution of behavior disorders: Infancy to early adult life.* New York: Brunner/Mazel.

Chi, M. T. (1978). Knowledge structure and memory development. In R. S. Siegler (Ed.), *Children's thinking: What develops?* (pp. 73–96). Hillsdale, NJ: Erlbaum.

Chi, M. T. H., & Ceci, S. J. (1987). Content knowledge: Its role, representation, and restructuring in memory development. In H. W. Reese (Ed.), *Advances in child development and behavior* (Vol. 20, pp. 91–142). Orlando, FL: Academic Press.

Chi, M. T. H., Hutchinson, J. E., & Robin, A. F. (1989). How inferences about novel domain-related concepts can be constrained by structured knowledge. *Merrill-Palmer Quarterly, 35,* 27–62.

Chisholm, J. S. (1989). Biology, culture, and the development of temperament: A Navaho example. In J. K. Nugent, B. M. Lester, & T. B. Brazelton (Eds.), *The cultural context of infancy: Vol. 1. Biology, culture, and infant development.* Norwood, NJ: Ablex.

Chomsky, N. (1965). *Aspects of a theory of syntax.* Cambridge, MA: MIT Press.

Chomsky, N. (1975). *Reflections on language.* New York: Pantheon Books.

Chomsky, N. (1986). *Knowledge of language: Its nature, origin, and use.* New York: Praeger.

Chomsky, N. (1988). *Language and problems of knowledge.* Cambridge, MA: MIT Press.

Christophersen, E. R. (1989). Injury control. *American Psychologist, 44,* 237–241.

Chumlea, W. C. (1982). Physical growth in adolescence. In B. B. Wolman (Ed.), *Handbook of developmental psychology* (pp. 471–485). Englewood Cliffs, NJ: Prentice Hall.

Cicchetti, D., & Barnett, D. (1991). Attachment organization in maltreated preschoolers. *Development and Psychopathology, 3,* 397–411.

Cicchetti, D., & Cohen, D. J. (1995). Perspectives on developmental psychopathology. In D. Cicchetti & D. J. Cohen (Eds.), *Developmental psychopathology: Vol. 1. Theory and methods* (pp. 3–20). New York: Wiley.

Cillessen, A. H. N., van IJzendoorn, H. W., van Lieshout, C. F. M., & Hartup, W. W. (1992). Heterogeneity among peer-rejected boys: Subtypes and stabilities. *Child Development, 63,* 893–905.

Clark, E. V. (1975). Knowledge, context, and strategy in the acquisition of meaning. In D. P. Date (Ed.), *Georgetown University round table on language and linguistics.* Washington, DC: Georgetown University Press.

Clark, E. V. (1983). Meanings and concepts. In J. H. Flavell & E. M. Markman (Eds.), *Handbook of child psychology: Cognitive development* (Vol. 3, pp. 787–840). New York: Wiley.

Clark, E. V. (1987). The principle of contrast: A constraint on language acquisition. In B. MacWhinney (Ed.), *Mechanisms of language acquisition* (pp. 1–34). Hillsdale, NJ: Erlbaum.

Clark, E. V. (1990). On the pragmatics of contrast. *Journal of Child Language, 41,* 417–431.

Clarke, A. M., & Clarke, A. D. B. (1976). *Early experience: Myth and evidence.* New York: Free Press.

Clarke-Stewart, A. (1990). "The 'effects' of infant day care reconsidered" reconsidered: Risks for parents, children, and researchers. In N. Fox & G. G. Fein (Eds.), *Infant day care: The current debate* (pp. 61–86). Norwood, NJ: Ablex.

Clarke-Stewart, A. (1992). Consequences of child care for children's development. In A. Booth (Ed.), *Child care in the 1990s: Trends and consequences* (pp. 63–82). Hillsdale, NJ: Erlbaum.

Clarke-Stewart, K. A., Gruber, C. P., & Fitzgerald, L. M. (1994). *Children at home and in day care.* Hillsdale, NJ: Erlbaum.

Cnattingius, S., Berendes, H. W., & Forman, M. R. (1993). Do delayed childbearers face increased risks of adverse pregnancy outcomes after the first birth? *Obstetrics and Gynecology, 81,* 512–516.

Cohen, Y. A. (1964). *The transition from childhood to adolescence.* Chicago: Aldine.

Coie, J. D., & Cillessen, A. H. N. (1993). Peer rejection: Origins and effects on children's development. *Current Directions in Psychological Science, 2,* 89–92.

Colby, A., Kohlberg, L., Gibbs, J., & Lieberman, M. (1983). A longitudinal study of moral judgment. *Monographs of the Society for Research in Child Development, 48*(1–2, Serial No. 200).

Cole, D. A. (1991). Change in self-perceived competence as a function of peer and teacher evaluation. *Developmental Psychology, 27,* 682–688.

Cole, M. (1992). Culture in development. In M. H. Bornstein & M. E. Lamb (Eds.), *Developmental psychology: An advanced textbook* (pp. 731–789). Hillsdale, NJ: Erlbaum.

Cole, M., & Traupmann, K. (1981). Comparative cognitive research: Learning from a learning disabled child. In W. A. Collins (Ed.), *The Minnesota Symposia on Child Psychology* (Vol. 14, pp. 125–154). Hillsdale, NJ: Erlbaum.

Collins, W. A. (Ed.). (1984). *Development during middle childhood: The years from six to twelve.* Washington, DC: National Academy Press.

Colombo, J. (1993). *Infant cognition: Predicting later intellectual functioning.* Newbury Park, CA: Sage.

Colton, M., Buss, K., Mangelsdorf, S., Brooks, C., Sorenson, D., Stansbury, K., Harris, M., & Gunnar, M. (1992). *Relations between toddler coping strategies, temperament, attachment and adrenocortical stress responses.* Poster presented at the 8th International Conference on Infant Studies, Miami.

Compas, B. E., Ey, S., & Grant, K. E. (1993). Taxonomy, assessment, and diagnosis of depression during adolescence. *Psychological Bulletin, 114,* 323–344.

Comstock, G. (1991). *Television and the American child.* San Diego: Academic Press.

Conger, R. D., Conger, K. J., Elder, G. H., Jr., Lorenz, F. O., Simons, R. L., & Whitbeck, L. B. (1992). A family process model of economic hardship and adjustment of early adolescent boys. *Child Development, 63,* 526–541.

Conger, R. D., Ge, X., Elder, G. H., Jr., Lorenz, F. O., & Simons, R. L. (1994). Economic stress, coercive family process, and developmental problems of adolescence. *Child Development, 65,* 541–561.

Conger, R. D., Patterson, G. R., & Ge, X. (1995). It takes two to replicate: A mediational model for the impact of parents' stress on adolescent adjustment. *Child Development, 66,* 80–97.

Connolly, K., & Dalgleish, M. (1989). The emergence of a tool-using skill in infancy. *Developmental Psychology, 25,* 894–912.

Conrad, M., & Hammen, C. (1989). Role of maternal depression in perceptions of child maladjustment. *Journal of Consulting and Clinical Psychology, 57,* 663–667.

Cooper, R. P., & Aslin, R. N. (1994). Developmental differences in infant attention to the spectral properties of infant-directed speech. *Child Development, 65,* 1663–1677.

Costa, P. T., Jr., & McCrae, R. R. (1984). Personality as a lifelong determinant of wellbeing. In C. Z. Malatesta & C. E. Izard (Eds.), *Emotion in adult development* (pp. 141–158). Beverly Hills, CA: Sage.

Costa, P. T., Jr., & McCrae, R. R. (1994). Set like plaster? Evidence for the stability of adult personality. In T. F. Hetherton & J. L. Weinberger (Eds.), *Can personality change?* (pp. 21–40). Washington, DC: American Psychological Association.

Costello, E. J., & Angold, A. (1995). Developmental epidemiology. In D. Cicchetti & D. J. Cohen (Eds.), *Developmental psychopathology: Vol. 1. Theory and methods* (pp. 23–56). New York: Wiley.

Cowan, B. R., & Underwood, M. K. (1995). *Sugar and spice and everything nice? A developmental investigation of social aggression among girls.* Paper presented at the biennial meetings of the Society for Research in Child Development, Indianapolis.

Crain-Thoreson, C., & Dale, P. S. (1995). *Parent vs. staff storybook reading as an intervention for language delay.* Paper presented at the biennial meetings of the Society for Research in Child Development, Indianapolis.

Crick, N. R., & Grotpeter, J. K. (1995). Relational aggression, gender, and social-psychological adjustment. *Child Development, 66,* 710–722.

Crisafi, M. A., & Brown, A. L. (1986). Analogical transfer in very young children: Combining two separately learned solutions to reach a goal. *Child Development, 57,* 953–968.

Crittenden, P. M., Partridge, M. F., & Claussen, A. H. (1991). Family patterns of relationship in normative and dysfunctional families. *Development and Psychopathology, 3,* 491–512.

Crnic, K. A., Greenberg, M. T., Ragozin, A. S., Robinson, N. M., & Basham, R. B. (1983). Effects of stress and social support on mothers and premature and full-term infants. *Child Development, 54,* 209–217.

Crockenberg, S. B. (1981). Infant irritability, mother responsiveness, and social support influences on the security of infant-mother attachment. *Child Development, 52,* 857–865.

Crockenberg, S. B. (1987). Predictors and correlates of anger toward and punitive control of toddlers by adolescent mothers. *Child Development, 58,* 964–975.

Crockenberg, S. B., & Litman, C. (1990). Autonomy as competence in 2-year-olds: Maternal correlates of child defiance, compliance, and self-assertion. *Developmental Psychology, 26,* 961–971.

Cromer, R. F. (1991). *Language and thought in normal and handicapped children.* Oxford, England: Basil Blackwell.

Crook, C. (1987). Taste and olfaction. In P. Salapatek & L. Cohen (Eds.), *Handbook of infant perception: Vol. 1. From sensation to perception* (pp. 237–264). Orlando, FL: Academic Press.

Crouter, A. C., & McHale, S. M. (1993). Familial economic circumstances: Implications for adjustment and development in early adolescence. In R. M. Lerner (Ed.), *Early adolescence:*

Carver, R. P. (1990). Intelligence and reading ability in grades 2–12. *Intelligence, 14,* 449–455.

Casas, J. F., & Mosher, M. (1995). *Relational and overt aggression in preschool: "You can't come to my birthday party unless . . . ."* Paper presented at the biennial meetings of the Society for Research in Child Development, Indianapolis.

Case, R. (1985). *Intellectual development: Birth to adulthood.* New York: Academic Press.

Casey, M. B. (1986). Individual differences in selective attention among prereaders: A key to mirror-image confusions. *Developmental Psychology, 22,* 58–66.

Caspi, A., Henry, B., McGee, R. O., Moffitt, T. E., & Silva, P. A. (1995). Temperamental origins of child and adolescent behavior problems: From age three to age fifteen. *Child Development, 66,* 55–68.

Caspi, A., Lynam, D., Moffitt, T. E., & Silva, P. A. (1993). Unraveling girls' delinquency: Biological, dispositional, and contextual contributions to adolescent misbehavior. *Developmental Psychology, 29,* 19–30.

Cassidy, J., & Berlin, L. J. (1994). The insecure/ambivalent pattern of attachment: Theory and research. *Child Development, 65,* 971–991.

Caughy, M. O., DiPietro, J. A., & Strobino, D. M. (1994). Daycare participation as a protective factor in the cognitive development of low-income children. *Child Development, 65,* 457–471.

Ceci, S. J., & Bruck, M. (1993). Suggestibility of the child witness: A historical review and synthesis. *Psychological Bulletin, 113,* 403–439.

Center for Educational Statistics (1987). *Who drops out of high school? From high school and beyond.* Washington, DC: Office of Educational Research and Improvement, U.S. Department of Education.

Centers for Disease Control (1992a). Selected behaviors that increase risk for HIV infection among high school students—United States, 1990. *Morbidity and Mortality Weekly Report, 41*(231), 237–240.

Centers for Disease Control (1992b). Sexual behavior among high school students—United States, 1990. *Morbidity and Mortality Weekly Report, 40,* 885–888.

Centers for Disease Control (1992c). Recommendations for the use of folic acid to reduce the number of cases of spina bifida and other neural tube defects. *Morbidity and Mortality Weekly Report, 41,* 1–7.

Centers for Disease Control (1992d). Pregnancy risks determined from birth certificate data—United States, 1989. *Morbidity and Mortality Weekly Report, 41*(30), 556–563.

Centers for Disease Control (1993). Rates of cesarean delivery—United States, 1991. *Journal of the American Medical Association, 269*(18), 2360.

Centers for Disease Control (1993a). Childbearing patterns among selected racial/ethnic minority groups—United States, 1990. *Morbidity and Mortality Weekly Reports, 42,* 399–403.

Centers for Disease Control (1993b). Mortality trends and leading causes of death among adolescents and young adults—United States, 1979–1988. *Morbidity and Mortality Weekly Reports, 42,* 459–461.

Centers for Disease Control (1994a). Recommendations of the U.S. Public Health Service task force on the use of zidovudine to reduce perinatal transmission of human immunodeficiency virus. *Morbidity and Mortality Weekly Report, 43*(August 5), 1–20.

Centers for Disease Control (1994b). Preventing tobacco use among young people: A report of the Surgeon General. Executive summary. *Morbidity and Mortality Weekly Report, 43*(RR–4), 2–10.

Centers for Disease Control (1994c). Health-risk behaviors among persons aged 12–21 years—United States, 1992. *Morbidity and Mortality Weekly Report, 43,* 231–235.

Centers for Disease Control (1994d). Prevalence of overweight among adolescents—United States, 1988–91. *Morbidity and Mortality Weekly Reports, 43,* 818–811.

Centers for Disease Control (1994e). Programs for the prevention of suicide among adolescents and young adults. *Morbidity and Mortality Weekly Reports, 43*(RR–6, April 22), 3–7.

Centerwall, B. S. (1989). Exposure to television as a cause of violence. In G. Comstock (Ed.), *Public communication and behavior* (pp. 1–58). San Diego: Academic Press.

Centerwall, B. S. (1992). Television and violence: The scale of the problem and where to go from here. *Journal of the American Medical Association, 267*(22), 3059–3063.

Cernoch, J. M., & Porter, R. H. (1985). Recognition of maternal axillary odors by infants. *Child Development, 56,* 1593–1598.

Chalfant, J. C. (1989). Learning disabilities: Policy issues and promising approaches. *American Psychologist, 44,* 392–398.

Chang, L., & Murray, A. (1995). *Math performance of 5- and 6-year-olds in Taiwan and the U.S.: Maternal beliefs, expectations, and tutorial assistance.* Paper presented at the biennial meetings of the Society for Research in Child Development, Indianapolis.

Chao, R. K. (1994). Beyond parental control and authoritarian parenting style: Understanding Chinese parenting through the cultural notion of training. *Child Development, 65,* 1111–1119.

Chapa, J., & Valencia, R. R. (1993). Latino population growth, demographic characteristics, and educational stagnation: An examination of recent trends. *Hispanic Journal of Behavioral Sciences, 15,* 165–187.

Charman, T., Redfern, S., & Fonagy, P. (1995). *Individual differences in theory of mind acquisition: The role of attachment security.* Paper presented at the biennial meetings of the Society for Research in Child Development, Indianapolis.

Chen, X., Rubin, K. H., & Sun, Y. (1992). Social reputation and peer relationships in Chinese and Canadian children: A cross-cultural study. *Child Development, 63,* 1336–1343.

Cheng, M., & Hannah, M. (1993). Breech delivery at term: A critical review of the literature. *Obstetrics and Gynecology, 82,* 605–618.

Cherlin, A. J. (1992a). *Marriage, divorce, remarriage.* Cambridge, MA: Harvard University Press.

Cherlin, A. J. (1992b). Infant care and full-time employment. In A. Booth (Ed.), *Child care in the 1990s: Trends and consequences* (pp. 209–214). Hillsdale, NJ: Erlbaum.

Chess, S., & Korn, S. J. (1980). Temperament and behavior disorder in mentally retarded children. *Journal of Special Education, 23,* 122–130.

Chess, S., & Thomas, A. (1984). *Origins and evolution of behavior disorders: Infancy to early adult life.* New York: Brunner/Mazel.

Chi, M. T. (1978). Knowledge structure and memory development. In R. S. Siegler (Ed.), *Children's thinking: What develops?* (pp. 73–96). Hillsdale, NJ: Erlbaum.

Chi, M. T. H., & Ceci, S. J. (1987). Content knowledge: Its role, representation, and restructuring in memory development. In H. W. Reese (Ed.), *Advances in child development and behavior* (Vol. 20, pp. 91–142). Orlando, FL: Academic Press.

Chi, M. T. H., Hutchinson, J. E., & Robin, A. F. (1989). How inferences about novel domain-related concepts can be constrained by structured knowledge. *Merrill-Palmer Quarterly, 35,* 27–62.

Chisholm, J. S. (1989). Biology, culture, and the development of temperament: A Navaho example. In J. K. Nugent, B. M. Lester, & T. B. Brazelton (Eds.), *The cultural context of infancy: Vol. 1. Biology, culture, and infant development.* Norwood, NJ: Ablex.

Chomsky, N. (1965). *Aspects of a theory of syntax.* Cambridge, MA: MIT Press.

Chomsky, N. (1975). *Reflections on language.* New York: Pantheon Books.

Chomsky, N. (1986). *Knowledge of language: Its nature, origin, and use.* New York: Praeger.

Chomsky, N. (1988). *Language and problems of knowledge.* Cambridge, MA: MIT Press.

Christophersen, E. R. (1989). Injury control. *American Psychologist, 44,* 237–241.

Chumlea, W. C. (1982). Physical growth in adolescence. In B. B. Wolman (Ed.), *Handbook of developmental psychology* (pp. 471–485). Englewood Cliffs, NJ: Prentice Hall.

Cicchetti, D., & Barnett, D. (1991). Attachment organization in maltreated preschoolers. *Development and Psychopathology, 3,* 397–411.

Cicchetti, D., & Cohen, D. J. (1995). Perspectives on developmental psychopathology. In D. Cicchetti & D. J. Cohen (Eds.), *Developmental psychopathology: Vol. 1. Theory and methods* (pp. 3–20). New York: Wiley.

Cillessen, A. H. N., van IJzendoorn, H. W., van Lieshout, C. F. M., & Hartup, W. W. (1992). Heterogeneity among peer-rejected boys: Subtypes and stabilities. *Child Development, 63,* 893–905.

Clark, E. V. (1975). Knowledge, context, and strategy in the acquisition of meaning. In D. P. Date (Ed.), *Georgetown University round table on language and linguistics.* Washington, DC: Georgetown University Press.

Clark, E. V. (1983). Meanings and concepts. In J. H. Flavell & E. M. Markman (Eds.), *Handbook of child psychology: Cognitive development* (Vol. 3, pp. 787–840). New York: Wiley.

Clark, E. V. (1987). The principle of contrast: A constraint on language acquisition. In B. MacWhinney (Ed.), *Mechanisms of language acquisition* (pp. 1–34). Hillsdale, NJ: Erlbaum.

Clark, E. V. (1990). On the pragmatics of contrast. *Journal of Child Language, 41,* 417–431.

Clarke, A. M., & Clarke, A. D. B. (1976). *Early experience: Myth and evidence.* New York: Free Press.

Clarke-Stewart, A. (1990). "The 'effects' of infant day care reconsidered" reconsidered: Risks for parents, children, and researchers. In N. Fox & G. G. Fein (Eds.), *Infant day care: The current debate* (pp. 61–86). Norwood, NJ: Ablex.

Clarke-Stewart, A. (1992). Consequences of child care for children's development. In A. Booth (Ed.), *Child care in the 1990s: Trends and consequences* (pp. 63–82). Hillsdale, NJ: Erlbaum.

Clarke-Stewart, K. A., Gruber, C. P., & Fitzgerald, L. M. (1994). *Children at home and in day care.* Hillsdale, NJ: Erlbaum.

Cnattingius, S., Berendes, H. W., & Forman, M. R. (1993). Do delayed childbearers face increased risks of adverse pregnancy outcomes after the first birth? *Obstetrics and Gynecology, 81,* 512–516.

Cohen, Y. A. (1964). *The transition from childhood to adolescence.* Chicago: Aldine.

Coie, J. D., & Cillessen, A. H. N. (1993). Peer rejection: Origins and effects on children's development. *Current Directions in Psychological Science, 2,* 89–92.

Colby, A., Kohlberg, L., Gibbs, J., & Lieberman, M. (1983). A longitudinal study of moral judgment. *Monographs of the Society for Research in Child Development, 48*(1–2, Serial No. 200).

Cole, D. A. (1991). Change in self-perceived competence as a function of peer and teacher evaluation. *Developmental Psychology, 27,* 682–688.

Cole, M. (1992). Culture in development. In M. H. Bornstein & M. E. Lamb (Eds.), *Developmental psychology: An advanced textbook* (pp. 731–789). Hillsdale, NJ: Erlbaum.

Cole, M., & Traupmann, K. (1981). Comparative cognitive research: Learning from a learning disabled child. In W. A. Collins (Ed.), *The Minnesota Symposia on Child Psychology* (Vol. 14, pp. 125–154). Hillsdale, NJ: Erlbaum.

Collins, W. A. (Ed.). (1984). *Development during middle childhood: The years from six to twelve.* Washington, DC: National Academy Press.

Colombo, J. (1993). *Infant cognition: Predicting later intellectual functioning.* Newbury Park, CA: Sage.

Colton, M., Buss, K., Mangelsdorf, S., Brooks, C., Sorenson, D., Stansbury, K., Harris, M., & Gunnar, M. (1992). *Relations between toddler coping strategies, temperament, attachment and adrenocortical stress responses.* Poster presented at the 8th International Conference on Infant Studies, Miami.

Compas, B. E., Ey, S., & Grant, K. E. (1993). Taxonomy, assessment, and diagnosis of depression during adolescence. *Psychological Bulletin, 114,* 323–344.

Comstock, G. (1991). *Television and the American child.* San Diego: Academic Press.

Conger, R. D., Conger, K. J., Elder, G. H., Jr., Lorenz, F. O., Simons, R. L., & Whitbeck, L. B. (1992). A family process model of economic hardship and adjustment of early adolescent boys. *Child Development, 63,* 526–541.

Conger, R. D., Ge, X., Elder, G. H., Jr., Lorenz, F. O., & Simons, R. L. (1994). Economic stress, coercive family process, and developmental problems of adolescence. *Child Development, 65,* 541–561.

Conger, R. D., Patterson, G. R., & Ge, X. (1995). It takes two to replicate: A mediational model for the impact of parents' stress on adolescent adjustment. *Child Development, 66,* 80–97.

Connolly, K., & Dalgleish, M. (1989). The emergence of a tool-using skill in infancy. *Developmental Psychology, 25,* 894–912.

Conrad, M., & Hammen, C. (1989). Role of maternal depression in perceptions of child maladjustment. *Journal of Consulting and Clinical Psychology, 57,* 663–667.

Cooper, R. P., & Aslin, R. N. (1994). Developmental differences in infant attention to the spectral properties of infant-directed speech. *Child Development, 65,* 1663–1677.

Costa, P. T., Jr., & McCrae, R. R. (1984). Personality as a life-long determinant of wellbeing. In C. Z. Malatesta & C. E. Izard (Eds.), *Emotion in adult development* (pp. 141–158). Beverly Hills, CA: Sage.

Costa, P. T., Jr., & McCrae, R. R. (1994). Set like plaster? Evidence for the stability of adult personality. In T. F. Hetherton & J. L. Weinberger (Eds.), *Can personality change?* (pp. 21–40). Washington, DC: American Psychological Association.

Costello, E. J., & Angold, A. (1995). Developmental epidemiology. In D. Cicchetti & D. J. Cohen (Eds.), *Developmental psychopathology: Vol. 1. Theory and methods* (pp. 23–56). New York: Wiley.

Cowan, B. R., & Underwood, M. K. (1995). *Sugar and spice and everything nice? A developmental investigation of social aggression among girls.* Paper presented at the biennial meetings of the Society for Research in Child Development, Indianapolis.

Crain-Thoreson, C., & Dale, P. S. (1995). *Parent vs. staff storybook reading as an intervention for language delay.* Paper presented at the biennial meetings of the Society for Research in Child Development, Indianapolis.

Crick, N. R., & Grotpeter, J. K. (1995). Relational aggression, gender, and social-psychological adjustment. *Child Development, 66,* 710–722.

Crisafi, M. A., & Brown, A. L. (1986). Analogical transfer in very young children: Combining two separately learned solutions to reach a goal. *Child Development, 57,* 953–968.

Crittenden, P. M., Partridge, M. F., & Claussen, A. H. (1991). Family patterns of relationship in normative and dysfunctional families. *Development and Psychopathology, 3,* 491–512.

Crnic, K. A., Greenberg, M. T., Ragozin, A. S., Robinson, N. M., & Basham, R. B. (1983). Effects of stress and social support on mothers and premature and full-term infants. *Child Development, 54,* 209–217.

Crockenberg, S. B. (1981). Infant irritability, mother responsiveness, and social support influences on the security of infant-mother attachment. *Child Development, 52,* 857–865.

Crockenberg, S. B. (1987). Predictors and correlates of anger toward and punitive control of toddlers by adolescent mothers. *Child Development, 58,* 964–975.

Crockenberg, S. B., & Litman, C. (1990). Autonomy as competence in 2-year-olds: Maternal correlates of child defiance, compliance, and self-assertion. *Developmental Psychology, 26,* 961–971.

Cromer, R. F. (1991). *Language and thought in normal and handicapped children.* Oxford, England: Basil Blackwell.

Crook, C. (1987). Taste and olfaction. In P. Salapatek & L. Cohen (Eds.), *Handbook of infant perception: Vol. 1. From sensation to perception* (pp. 237–264). Orlando, FL: Academic Press.

Crouter, A. C., & McHale, S. M. (1993). Familial economic circumstances: Implications for adjustment and development in early adolescence. In R. M. Lerner (Ed.), *Early adolescence:*

Perspectives on research, policy, and intervention (pp. 71–91). Hillsdale, NJ: Erlbaum.

Crystal, D. S., Chen, C., Fuligni, A. J., Stevenson, H. W., Hsu, C., Ko, H., Kitamura, S., & Kimura, S. (1994). Psychological maladjustment and academic achievement: A cross-cultural study of Japanese, Chinese, and American high school students. *Child Development, 65,* 738–753.

Crystal, D. S., & Stevenson, H. W. (1995). What is a bad kid? Answers of adolescents and their mothers in three cultures. *Journal of Research on Adolescence, 5,* 71–91.

Crystal, S., Shae, D., & Krishnaswami, S. (1992). Educational attainment, occupational history, and stratification: Determinants of later-life economic outcomes. *Journal of Gerontology: SOCIAL SCIENCES, 47,* S213–S221.

Cummings, E. M., & Davies, P. T. (1994). Maternal depression and child development. *Journal of Child Psychology and Psychiatry, 35,* 73–112.

Cunningham, A. S., Jelliffe, D. B., & Jelliffe, E. F. P. (1991). Breast-feeding and health in the 1980s: A global epidemiologic review. *Journal of Pediatrics, 118,* 659–666.

Cutrona, C. E., & Troutman, B. R. (1986). Social support, infant temperament, and parenting self-efficacy: A mediational model of postpartum depression. *Child Development, 57,* 1507–1518.

D'Alton, M. E., & DeCherney, A. H. (1993). Prenatal diagnosis. *New England Journal of Medicine, 328,* 114–118.

Damon, W. (1977). *The social world of the child.* San Francisco: Jossey-Bass.

Damon, W. (1983). The nature of social-cognitive change in the developing child. In W. F. Overton (Ed.), *The relationship between social and cognitive development* (pp. 103–142). Hillsdale, NJ: Erlbaum.

Danner, F. W., & Day, M. C. (1977). Eliciting formal operations. *Child Development, 48,* 1600–1606.

Dark, V. J., & Benbow, C. P. (1993). Cognitive differences among the gifted: A review and new data. In D. K. Detterman (Ed.), *Current topics in human intelligence: Vol. 3. Individual differences and cognition* (pp. 85–120). Norwood, NJ: Ablex.

Darling, N., & Steinberg, L. (1993). Parenting style as context: An integrative model. *Psychological Bulletin, 113,* 487–496.

Darlington, R. B. (1991). The long-term effects of model preschool programs. In L. Okagaki & R. J. Sternberg (Eds.), *Directors of development* (pp. 203–215). Hillsdale, NJ: Erlbaum.

Dasen, P. R. (1984). The cross-cultural study of intelligence: Piaget and the Baoule. *International Journal of Psychology, 19,* 407–434.

Davidson, E. S., Yasuna, A., & Tower, A. (1979). The effect of television cartoons on sex-role stereotyping in young girls. *Child Development, 50,* 597–600.

Davies, G. M. (1993). Children's memory for other people: An integrative review. In C. A. Nelson (Ed.), *The Minnesota Symposia on Child Psychology* (Vol. 26, pp. 123–157). Hillsdale, NJ: Erlbaum.

Davies, P. T., & Cummings, E. M. (1994). Marital conflict and child adjustment: An emotional security hypothesis. *Psychological Bulletin, 116,* 387–411.

Dawson, D. A. (1991). Family structure and children's health and well-being: Data from the 1988 National Health Interview Survey on child health. *Journal of Marriage and the Family, 53,* 573–584.

de Chateau, P. (1980). Effects of hospital practices on synchrony in the development of the infant-parent relationship. In P. M. Taylor (Ed.), *Parent-infant relationships* (pp. 137–168). New York: Grune & Stratton.

de Haan, M., Luciana, M., Maslone, S. M., Matheny, L. S., & Richards, M. L. M. (1994). Development, plasticity, and risk: Commentary on Huttenlocher, Pollit and Gorman, and Gottesman and Goldsmith. In C. A. Nelson (Ed.), *The Minnesota Symposia on Child Psychology* (Vol. 27, pp. 161–178). Hillsdale, NJ: Erlbaum.

de Jong-van den Berg, L. T. W., Waardenburg, C. M., Haaijer-Ruskamp, F. M., Dukes, M. N. G., & Wesseling, H. (1993). Drug use in pregnancy: A comparative appraisal of data collection methods. *European Journal of Clinical Pharmacology, 45,* 9–14.

de Villiers, P. A., & de Villiers, J. G. (1992). Language development. In M. H. Bornstein & M. E. Lamb (Eds.), *Developmental psychology: An advanced textbook* (3rd ed.) (pp. 337–418). Hillsdale, NJ: Erlbaum.

DeCasper, A. J., & Fifer, W. P. (1980). Of human bonding: Newborns prefer their mothers' voices. *Science, 208,* 1174–1176.

DeCasper, A. J., Lecaneut, J., Busnel, M., Granier-Deferre, C., & Maugeais, R. (1994). Fetal reactions to recurrent maternal speech. *Infant Behavior and Development, 17,* 159–164.

DeCasper, A. J., & Spence, M. J. (1986). Prenatal maternal speech influences newborns' perception of speech sounds. *Infant Behavior and Development, 9,* 133–150.

Delgado-Gaitan, C. (1994). Socializing young children in Mexican-American families: An intergenerational perspective. In P. M. Greenfield & R. R. Cocking (Eds.), *Cross-cultural roots of minority child development* (pp. 55–86). Hillsdale, NJ: Erlbaum.

DeLoache, J. S. (1989). The development of representation in young children. In H. W. Reese (Ed.), *Advances in child development and behavior* (Vol. 22, pp. 2–37). San Diego Academic Press.

DeLoache, J. S., & Brown, A. L. (1987). Differences in the memory-based searching of delayed and normally developing young children. *Intelligence, 11,* 277–289.

DeMeis, D. K., Hock, E., & McBride, S. L. (1986). The balance of employment and motherhood: Longitudinal study of mothers' feelings about separation from their first-born infants. *Developmental Psychology, 22,* 627–632.

Dempster, F. N. (1981). Memory span: Sources of individual and developmental differences. *Psychological Bulletin, 89,* 63–100.

Dennis, W. (1960). Causes of retardation among institutional children: Iran. *Journal of Genetic Psychology, 96,* 47–59.

DeRosier, M. E., Kupersmidt, J. B., & Patterson, C. J. (1994). Children's academic and behavioral adjustment as a function of the chronicity and proximity of peer rejection. *Child Development, 65,* 1799–1831.

Deter, H., & Herzog, W. (1994). Anorexia nervosa in a long-term perspective: Results of the Heidelberg-Mannheim study. *Psychosomatic Medicine, 56,* 20–27.

Deutsch, C. K., & Kinsbourne, M. (1990). Genetics and biochemistry in attention deficit disorder. In M. Lewis & S. M. Miller (Eds.), *Handbook of developmental psychopathology* (pp. 93–108). New York: Plenum Press.

The Diagram Group (1977). *Child's body.* New York: Paddington.

Diamond, A. (1991). Neuropsychological insights into the meaning of object concept development. In S. Carey & R. Gelman (Eds.), *The epigenesis of mind: Essays on biology and cognition* (pp. 67–110). Hillsdale, NJ: Erlbaum.

Dietz, W. H., & Gortmaker, S. L. (1985). Do we fatten our children at the television set? Obesity and television viewing in children and adolescents. *Pediatrics, 75,* 807–812.

Digman, J. M. (1990). Personality structure: Emergence of the five-factor model. *Annual Review of Psychology, 41,* 417–440.

Dishion, T. J. (1990). The family ecology of boys' peer relations in middle childhood. *Child Development, 61,* 874–892.

Dishion, T. J., Andrews, D. W., & Crosby, L. (1995). Antisocial boys and their friends in early adolescence: Relationship characteristics, quality, and interactional process. *Child Development, 66,* 139–151.

Dishion, T. J., Patterson, G. R., Stoolmiller, M., & Skinner, M. L. (1991). Family, school, and behavioral antecedents to early adolescent involvement with antisocial peers. *Developmental Psychology, 27,* 172–180.

Dodge, K. A. (1990). Developmental psychopathology in children of depressed mothers. *Developmental Psychology, 26,* 3–6.

Dodge, K. A., Coie, J. D., Pettit, G. S., & Price, J. M. (1990). Peer status and aggression in boys groups: Developmental and contextual analysis. *Child Development, 61,* 1289–1309.

Dodge, K. A., & Feldman, E. (1990). Issues in social cognition and sociometric status. In S. R. Asher & J. D. Coie (Eds.), *Peer rejection in childhood* (pp. 119–155). Cambridge, England: Cambridge University Press.

Dodge, K. A., Murphy, R. R., & Buchsbaum, K. (1984). The assessment of intention-cue detection skills in children: Implications for developmental psychopathology. *Child Development, 55,* 163–173.

Dodge, K. A., Pettit, G. S., & Bates, J. E. (1994). Socialization mediators of the relation between socioeconomic status and child conduct problems. *Child Development, 65,* 649–665.

Donnerstein, E., Slaby, R. G., & Eron, L. D. (1994). The mass media and youth aggression. In L. D. Eron, J. H. Gentry, & P. Schlegel (Eds.), *Reason to hope: A psychosocial perspective on violence and youth* (pp. 219–250). Washington, DC: American Psychological Association.

Donovan, J.E., & Jessor, R. (1985). Structure of problem behavior in adolescence and young adulthood. *Journal of Consulting and Clinical Psychology, 53,* 890–904.

Dornbusch, S. M., Gross, R. T., Duncan, P. D., & Ritter, P. L. (1987a). Stanford studies of adolescence using the National Health Examination Survey. In R. M. Lerner & T. T. Foch (Eds.), *Biological-psychosocial interactions in early adolescence* (pp. 189–206). Hillsdale, NJ: Erlbaum.

Dornbusch, S. M., Ritter, P. L., Liederman, P. H., Roberts, D. F., & Fraleigh, M. J. (1987b). The relation of parenting style to adolescent school performance. *Child Development, 58,* 1244–1257.

Downey, G., & Coyne, J. C. (1990). Children of depressed parents: An integrative review. *Psychological Bulletin, 108,* 50–76.

Doyle, A. B., & Aboud, F. E. (1995). A longitudinal study of white children's racial prejudice as a social-cognitive development. *Merrill-Palmer Quarterly, 41,* 209–228.

Dryfoos, J. (1990). *Adolescents at risk: Prevalence and prevention.* New York: Oxford University Press.

Duke, P. M., Carlsmith, J. M., Jennings, D., Martin, J. A., Dornbusch, S. M., Gross, R. T., & Siegel-Gorelick, B. (1982). Educational correlates of early and late sexual maturation in adolescence. *Journal of Pediatrics, 100,* 633–637.

Duncan, G. J. (1993). *Economic deprivation and childhood development.* Paper presented at the biennial meetings of the Society for Research in Child Development, New Orleans.

Duncan, G. J., Brooks-Gunn, J., & Klebanov, P. K. (1994). Economic deprivation and early childhood development. *Child Development, 65,* 296–318.

Dunham, P. J., Dunham, F., & Curwin, A. (1993). Joint-attentional states and lexical acquisition at 18 months. *Developmental Psychology, 29,* 827–831.

Dunn, J. (1992). Siblings and development. *Current Directions in Psychological Science, 1,* 6–9.

Dunn, J. (1993). *Young children's close relationships.* Newbury Park, CA: Sage.

Dunn, J. (1994). Experience and understanding of emotions, relationships, and membership in a particular culture. In P. Ekman & R. J. Davidson (Eds.), *The nature of emotion: Fundamental questions* (pp. 352–355). New York: Oxford University Press.

Dunn, J., & McGuire, S. (1994). Young children's nonshared experiences: A summary of studies in Cambridge and Colorado. In E. M. Hetherington, D. Reiss, & R. Plomin (Eds.), *Separate social worlds of siblings: The impact of nonshared environment on development* (pp. 111–128). Hillsdale, NJ: Erlbaum.

Dunphy, D. C. (1963). The social structure of urban adolescent peer groups. *Sociometry, 26,* 230–246.

Dyk, P. H. (1993). Anatomy, physiology, and gender issues in adolescence. In T. P. Gullotta, G. R. Adams, & R. Montemayor (Eds.), *Adolescent sexuality* (pp. 35–56). Newbury Park, CA: Sage.

Dykens, E. M., Hodapp, R. M., & Leckman, J. F. (1994). *Behavior and development in fragile X syndrome.* Thousand Oaks, CA: Sage.

Easterbrooks, M. A., Davidson, C. E., & Chazan, R. (1993). Psychosocial risk, attachment, and behavior problems among school-aged children. *Development and Psychopathology, 5,* 389–402.

Eaton, W. O., & Enns, L. R. (1986). Sex differences in human motor activity level. *Psychological Bulletin, 100,* 19–28.

Egeland, B., & Sroufe, L. A. (1981). Attachment and early maltreatment. *Child Development, 52,* 44–52.

Eisenberg, N. (1986). *Altruistic emotion, cognition, and behavior.* Hillsdale, NJ: Erlbaum.

Eisenberg, N. (1988). The development of prosocial and aggressive behavior. In M. H. Bornstein & M. E. Lamb (Eds.), *Developmental psychology: An advanced textbook* (2nd ed.) (pp. 461–496). Hillsdale, NJ: Erlbaum.

Eisenberg, N. (1990). Prosocial development in early and mid-adolescence. In R. Montemayor, G. R. Adams, & T. P. Gullotta (Eds.), *From childhood to adolescence: A transitional period?* (pp. 240–268). Newbury Park, CA: Sage.

Eisenberg, N. (1992). *The caring child.* Cambridge, MA: Harvard University Press.

Eisenberg, N., Fabes, R. A., Schaller, M., & Miller, P. A. (1989). Sympathy and personal distress: Development, gender differences, and interrelations of indexes. *New Directions for Child Development, 44,* 107–126.

Eisenberg, N., & Mussen, P. H. (1989). *The roots of prosocial behavior in children.* Cambridge, England: Cambridge University Press.

Eisenberg, N., Shell, R., Pasternack, J., Lennon, R., Beller, R., & Mathy, R. M. (1987). Prosocial development in middle childhood: A longitudinal study. *Developmental Psychology, 23,* 712–718.

Ekman, P. (1972). Universals and cultural differences in facial expressions of emotion. In J. Cole (Ed.), *Nebraska Symposium on Motivation, 1971* (pp. 207–282). Lincoln: University of Nebraska Press.

Ekman, P. (1973). Cross-cultural studies of facial expression. In P. Ekman (Ed.), *Darwin and facial expression* (pp. 169–222). New York: Academic Press.

Ekman, P. (1994). Strong evidence for universals in facial expressions: A reply to Russell's mistaken critique. *Psychological Bulletin, 115,* 268–287.

Elder, G. H., Jr. (1974). *Children of the Great Depression.* Chicago: University of Chicago Press.

Elder, G. H., Jr. (1981). Scarcity and prosperity in postwar childbearing: Explorations from a life course perspective. *Journal of Family History, 5,* 410–431.

Elder, G. H., Jr. (1984). Families, kin, and the life course: A sociological perspective. In R. D. Parke (Ed.), *Review of child development research: Vol. 7. The family* (pp. 80–136). Chicago: University of Chicago Press.

Elkind, D. (1967). Egocentrism in adolescence. *Child Development, 38,* 1025–1034.

Elkind, D., & Bowen, R. (1979). Imaginary audience behavior in children and adolescents. *Developmental Psychology, 15,* 38–44.

Elliott, R. (1988). Tests, abilities, race, and conflict. *Intelligence, 12,* 333–350.

Emde, R. N., Plomin, R., Robinson, J., Corley, R., DeFries, J., Fulker, D. W., Reznick, J. S., Campos, J., Kagan, J., & Zahn-Waxler, C. (1992). Temperament, emotion, and cognition at fourteen months: The MacArthur longitudinal twin study. *Child Development, 63,* 1437–1455.

Eme, R. F. (1979). Sex differences in childhood psychopathology: A review. *Psychological Bulletin, 86,* 374–395.

Emery, R. E. (1988). *Marriage, divorce, and children's adjustment.* Newbury Park, CA: Sage.

Entwisle, D. R. (1990). Schools and the adolescent. In S. S. Feldman & G. R. Elliott (Eds.), *At the threshold: The developing adolescent* (pp. 197–224). Cambridge, MA: Harvard University Press.

Entwisle, D. R., & Alexander, K. L. (1990). Beginning school math competence: Minority and majority comparisons. *Child Development, 61,* 454–471.

Entwisle, D. R., & Doering, S. G. (1981). *The first birth.* Baltimore: Johns Hopkins University Press.

Epstein, S. (1991). Cognitive-experiential self theory: Implications for developmental psychology. In M. R. Gunnar & L. A. Sroufe (Eds.), *The Minnesota Symposia on Child Development* (Vol. 23, pp. 79–123). Hillsdale, NJ: Erlbaum.

Erikson, E. H. (1963). *Childhood and society* (2nd ed.). New York: Norton.

Erikson, E. H. (1980). *Identity and the life cycle.* New York: Norton (originally published 1959).

Eron, L. D. (1987). The development of aggressive behavior from the perspective of a developing behaviorism. *American Psychologist, 42,* 435–442.

Eron, L. D. (1992). Testimony before the Senate Committee on Governmental Affairs. *Congressional Record, 88* (June 18), S8538–S8539.

Eron, L. D., Gentry, J. H., & Schlegel, P. (Eds.). (1994). *Reason to hope: A psychosocial perspective on violence and youth.* Washington, DC: American Psychological Association.

Eron, L. D., Huesmann, L. R., Dubow, E., Romanoff, R., & Yarmel, P. (1987). Aggression and its correlates over 22 years. In D. Crowell, I. Evans, & C. O'Donnell (Eds.), *Childhood aggression and violence: Sources of influence, prevention and control* (pp. 249–262). New York: Plenum Press.

Eron, L. D., Huesmann, L. R., & Zelli, A. (1991). The role of parental variables in the learning of aggression. In D. J. Pepler & K. H. Rubin (Eds.), *The development and treatment of childhood aggression* (pp. 169–188). Hillsdale, NJ: Erlbaum.

Escalona, K. S. (1981). The reciprocal role of social and emotional developmental advances and cognitive development during the second and third years of life. In E. K. Shapiro & E. Weber (Eds.), *Cognitive and affective growth: Developmental interaction* (pp. 87–108). Hillsdale, NJ: Erlbaum.

Eskes, T. K. A. B. (1992). Home deliveries in the Netherlands—perinatal mortality and morbidity. *International Journal of Gynecology and Obstetrics, 38,* 161–169.

Espinosa, M. P., Sigman, M. D., Neumann, C. G., Bwibo, N. O., & McDonald, M. A. (1992). Playground behaviors of school-age children in relation to nutrition, schooling, and family characteristics. *Developmental Psychology, 28,* 1188–1195.

Fabes, R. A., Knight, G. P., & Higgins, D. A. (1995). *Gender differences in aggression: A meta-analytic reexamination of time and age effects.* Paper presented at the biennial meetings of the Society for Research in Child Development, Indianapolis.

Fagan, J. F., III (1992). Intelligence: A theoretical viewpoint. *Current Directions in Psychological Science, 1,* 82–86.

Fagan, J. F., & Singer, L. T. (1983). Infant recognition memory as a measure of intelligence. In L. P. Lipsett (Ed.), *Advances in infancy research* (Vol. 2, pp. 31–78). Norwood, NJ: Ablex.

Fagard, J., & Jacquet, A. (1989). Onset of bimanual coordination and symmetry versus asymmetry of movement. *Infant Behavior and Development, 12,* 229–235.

Fagot, B. I., & Hagan, R. (1991). Observations of parent reactions to sex-stereotyped behaviors: Age and sex effects. *Child Development, 62,* 617–628.

Fagot, B. I., & Leinbach, M. D. (1989). The young child's gender schema: Environmental input, internal organization. *Child Development, 60,* 663–672.

Fagot, B. I., & Leinbach, M. D. (1993). Gender-role development in young children: From discrimination to labeling. *Developmental Review, 13,* 205–224.

Fagot, B. I., Leinbach, M. D., & O'Boyle, C. (1992). Gender labeling, gender stereotyping, and parenting behaviors. *Developmental Psychology, 28,* 225–230.

Falbo, T. (1992). Social norms and the one-child family: Clinical and policy implications. In F. Boer & J. Dunn (Eds.), *Children's sibling relationships: Developmental and clinical issues* (pp. 71–82). Hillsdale, NJ: Erlbaum.

Falbo, T., & Poston, D. L., Jr. (1993). The academic, personality, and physical outcomes of only children in China. *Child Development, 64,* 18–35.

Famularo, R., Stone, K., Barnum, R., & Whatron, R. (1986). Alcoholism and severe child maltreatment. *American Journal of Orthopsychiatry, 56,* 481–485.

Fantz, R. L. (1956). A method for studying early visual development. *Perceptual and Motor Skills, 6,* 13–15.

Farnham-Diggory, S. (1986). Time, now, for a little serious complexity. In S. J. Ceci (Ed.), *Handbook of cognitive, social, and neuropsychological aspects of learning disability* (Vol. 1). Hillsdale, NJ: Erlbaum.

Farnham-Diggory, S. (1992). *The learning-disabled child.* Cambridge, MA: Harvard University Press.

Farran, D. C., Haskins, R., & Gallagher, J. J. (1980). Poverty and mental retardation: A search for explanations. *New Directions for Exceptional Children, 1,* 47–66.

Farrar, M. J. (1992). Negative evidence and grammatical morpheme acquisition. *Developmental Psychology, 28,* 90–98.

Farrington, D. P. (1991). Childhood aggression and adult violence: Early precursors and later life outcomes. In D. J. Pepler & K. H. Rubin (Eds.), *The development and treatment of childhood aggression* (pp. 5–30). Hillsdale, NJ: Erlbaum.

Faust, M. S. (1983). Alternative constructions of adolescent growth. In J. Brooks-Gunn & A. C. Petersen (Eds.), *Girls at puberty: Biological and psychosocial perspectives* (pp. 105–126). New York: Plenum Press.

Featherstone, H. (1980). *A difference in the family.* New York: Basic Books.

Feldman, S. S. (1987). Predicting strain in mothers and fathers of 6-month-old infants: A short-term longitudinal study. In P. W. Berman & F. A. Pedersen (Eds.), *Men's transitions to parenthood* (pp. 13–36). Hillsdale, NJ: Erlbaum.

Feldman, S. S., & Elliott, G. R. (Eds.). (1990). *At the threshold: The developing adolescent.* Cambridge, MA: Harvard University Press.

Fennelly, K. (1993). Sexual activity and childbearing among Hispanic adolescents in the United States. In R. M. Lerner

(Ed.), *Early adolescence: Perspectives on research, policy, and intervention* (pp. 335–352). Hillsdale, NJ: Erlbaum.

Fenson, L., Dale, P. S., Reznick, J. S., Bates, E., Thal, D. J., & Pethick, S. J. (1994). Variability in early communicative development. *Monographs of the Society for Research in Child Development, 59* (5, Serial No. 242).

Fergusson, D. M., Horwood, L. J., & Lynskey, M. T. (1993). Maternal smoking before and after pregnancy: Effects on behavioral outcomes in middle childhood. *Pediatrics, 92,* 815–822.

Fernald, A. (1993). Approval and disapproval: Infant responsiveness to vocal affect in familiar and unfamiliar languages. *Child Development, 64,* 657–674.

Fernald, A., & Kuhl, P. (1987). Acoustic determinants of infant preference for motherese speech. *Infant Behavior and Development, 10,* 279–293.

Field, T. (1990). *Infancy.* Cambridge, MA: Harvard University Press.

Field, T., Healy, B., Goldstein, S., Perry, S., Bendell, D., Schanberg, S., Zimmerman, E. A., & Duhn, C. (1988). Infants of depressed mothers show "depressed" behavior even with nondepressed adults. *Child Development, 59,* 1569–1579.

Field, T. M. (1977). Effects of early separation, interactive deficits, and experimental manipulations on infant-mother face-to-face interaction. *Child Development, 48,* 763–771.

Field, T. M. (1978). Interaction behaviors of primary versus secondary caretaker fathers. *Developmental Psychology, 14,* 183–185.

Field, T. M. (1991). Quality infant day-care and grade school behavior and performance. *Child Development, 62,* 863–870.

Field, T. M., De Stefano, L., & Koewler, J. H. I. (1982). Fantasy play of toddlers and preschoolers. *Developmental Psychology, 18,* 503–508.

Field, T. M., Healy, B., Goldstein, S., & Guthertz, M. (1990). Behavior-state matching and synchrony in mother-infant interactions of nondepressed versus depressed dyads. *Developmental Psychology, 26,* 7–14.

Fields, S. A., & Wall, E. M. (1993). Obstetric analgesia and anesthesia. *Primary Care, 20,* 705–712.

Fish, M., Stifter, C. A., & Belsky, J. (1991). Conditions of continuity and discontinuity in infant negative emotionality: Newborn to five months. *Child Development, 62,* 1525–1537.

Flanagan, C. A., & Eccles, J. S. (1993). Changes in parents' work status and adolescents' adjustments at school. *Child Development, 64,* 246–257.

Flannery, D., Montemayor, R., Eberly, M., & Torquati, J. (1993). Unraveling the ties that bind: Affective expression and perceived conflict in parent-adolescent interactions. *Journal of Social and Personal Relations, 10,* 495–509.

Flannery, D. J., Montemayor, R., & Eberly, M. B. (1994). The influence of parent negative emotional expression on adolescents' perceptions of their relationships with their parents. *Personal Relationships, 1,* 259–274.

Flavell, J. H. (1985). *Cognitive development* (2nd ed.). Englewood Cliffs, NJ: Prentice Hall.

Flavell, J. H. (1986). The development of children's knowledge about the appearance-reality distinction. *American Psychologist, 41,* 418–425.

Flavell, J. H. (1992). Cognitive development: Past, present, and future. *Developmental Psychology, 28,* 998–1005.

Flavell, J. H. (1993). Young children's understanding of thinking and consciousness. *Current Directions in Psychological Science, 2,* 40–43.

Flavell, J. H., Green, F. L., & Flavell, E. R. (1989). Young children's ability to differentiate appearance-reality and level 2 perspectives in the tactile modality. *Child Development, 60,* 201–213.

Flavell, J. H., Green, F. L., & Flavell, E. R. (1990). Developmental changes in young children's knowledge about the mind. *Cognitive Development, 5,* 1–27.

Flavell, J. H., Green, F. L., & Flavell, E. R. (1995). Young children's knowledge about thinking. *Monographs of the Society for Research in Child Development, 60* (1, Serial No. 243).

Flavell, J. H., Green, F. L., Wahl, K. E., & Flavell, E. R. (1987). The effects of question clarification and memory aids on young children's performance on appearance-reality tasks. *Cognitive Development, 2,* 127–144.

Flavell, J. H., Zhang, X.-D., Zou, H., Dong, Q., & Qi, S. (1983). A comparison of the appearance-reality distinction in the People's Republic of China and the United States. *Cognitive Psychology, 15,* 459–466.

Fleming, A. S., Ruble, D. L., Flett, G. L., & Schaul, D. L. (1988). Postpartum adjustment in first-time mothers: Relations between mood, maternal attitudes, and mother-infant interactions. *Developmental Psychology, 24,* 71–81.

Fletcher, A. C., Darling, N. E., Steinberg, L., & Dornbusch, S. M. (1995). The company they keep: Relation of adolescents' adjustment and behavior to their friends' perceptions of authoritative parenting in the social network. *Developmental Psychology, 31,* 300–310.

Floyd, R. L., Rimer, B. K., Giovino, G. A., Mullen, P. D., & Sullivan, S. E. (1993). A review of smoking in pregnancy: Effects on pregnancy outcomes and cessation efforts. *Annual Review of Public Health, 14,* 379–411.

Folk, K. F., & Yi, Y. (1994). Piecing together child care with multiple arrangements: Crazy quilt or preferred pattern for employed parents of preschool children? *Journal of Marriage and the Family, 56,* 669–680.

Folven, R. J., & Bonvillian, J. D. (1991). The transition from nonreferential to referential language in children acquiring American Sign Language. *Developmental Psychology, 27,* 806–816.

Fox, N. A., Kimmerly, N. L., & Schafer, W. D. (1991). Attachment to mother/attachment to father: A meta-analysis. *Child Development, 62,* 210–225.

Fraiberg, S. (1974). Blind infants and their mothers: An examination of the sign system. In M. Lewis & L. A. Rosenblum (Eds.), *The effect of the infant on its caregiver* (pp. 215–232). New York: Wiley.

Fraiberg, S. (1975). The development of human attachments in infants blind from birth. *Merrill-Palmer Quarterly, 21,* 315–334.

Fraiberg, S. (1977). *Insights from the blind.* New York: New American Library (Meridian Books).

Francis, P. L., Self, P. A., & Horowitz, F. D. (1987). The behavioral assessment of the neonate: An overview. In J. D. Osofsky (Ed.), *Handbook of infant development* (2nd ed.) (pp. 723–779). New York: Wiley-Interscience.

Fraser, A. M., Brockert, J. E., & Ward, R. H. (1995). Association of young maternal age with adverse reproductive outcomes. *New England Journal of Medicine, 332,* 1113–1117.

Freedman, D. G. (1979). Ethnic differences in babies. *Human Nature, 2,* 36–43.

Freeman, E. W., & Rickels, K. (1993). *Early childbearing: Perspectives of black adolescents on pregnancy, abortion, and contraception.* Newbury Park, CA: Sage.

Freud, S. (1905). *The basic writings of Sigmund Freud* (A. A. Brill, Trans.). New York: Random House.

Freud, S. (1920). *A general introduction to psychoanalysis* (J. Riviere, Trans.). New York: Washington Square Press.

Frey, K. S., & Ruble, D. N. (1992). Gender constancy and the "cost" of sex-typed behavior: A test of the conflict hypothesis. *Developmental Psychology, 28,* 714–721.

Fu, Y., Pizzuti, A., Fenwick, R. G., Jr., King, J., Rajnarayan, S., Dune, P. W., Dubel, J., Nasser, G. A., Ashizawa, T., de Jong, P., Wieringa, B., Korneluk, R., Perryman, M. B., Epstein, H. F., & Caskey, C. T. (1992). An unstable triplet repeat in a gene related to myotonic muscular dystrophy. *Science, 225,* 1256–1258.

Furrow, D. (1984). Social and private speech at two years. *Child Development, 55,* 355–362.

Furstenberg, F. F., Jr. (1991). As the pendulum swings: Teenage childbearing and social concern. *Family Relations, 40,* 127–138.

Furstenberg, F. F., Jr., & Cherlin, A. J. (1991). *Divided families: What happens to children when parents part.* Cambridge, MA: Harvard University Press.

Ganchrow, J. R., Steiner, J. E., & Daher, M. (1983). Neonatal facial expressions in response to different qualities and intensities of gustatory stimuli. *Infant Behavior and Development, 6,* 189–200.

Garbarino, J., Dubrow, N., Kostelny, K., & Pardo, C. (1992). *Children in danger: Coping with the consequences of community violence.* San Francisco: Jossey-Bass.

Garbarino, J., Kostelny, K., & Dubrow, N. (1991). *No place to be a child. Growing up in a war zone.* Lexington, MA: Lexington Books.

Garbarino, J., & Sherman, D. (1980). High-risk neighborhoods and high-risk families: The human ecology of child maltreatment. *Child Development, 51,* 188–198.

Gardner, D., Harris, P. L., Ohmoto, M., & Hamasaki, T. (1988). Japanese children's understanding of the distinction between real and apparent emotion. *International Journal of Behavioral Development, 11,* 203–218.

Gardner, H. (1983). *Frames of mind: The theory of multiple intelligence.* New York: Basic Books.

Garland, A. F., & Zigler, E. (1993). Adolescent suicide prevention. Current research and social policy implications. *American Psychologist, 48,* 169–182.

Garmezy, N. (1993). Vulnerability and resilience. In D. C. Funder, R. D. Parke, C. Tomlinson-Keasey, & K. Widaman (Eds.), *Studying lives through time: Personality and development* (pp. 377–398). Washington, DC: American Psychological Association.

Garmezy, N., & Masten, A. S. (1991). The protective role of competence indicators in children at risk. In E. M. Cummings, A. L. Green, & K. H. Karraker (Eds.), *Life-span developmental psychology: Perspectives on stress and coping* (pp. 151–174). Hillsdale, NJ: Erlbaum.

Garmezy, N., & Rutter, M. (Eds.). (1983). *Stress, coping, and development in children.* New York: McGraw-Hill.

Garn, S. M. (1980). Continuities and change in maturational timing. In O. G. Brim, Jr., & J. Kagan (Eds.), *Constancy and change in human development* (pp. 113–162). Cambridge, MA: Harvard University Press.

Gazzaniga, J. M. (1993). Relationship between diet composition and body fatness, with adjustment for resting energy expenditure and physical activity, in preadolescent children. *American Journal of Clinical Nutrition, 58,* 21–28.

Geary, D. C., Bow-Thomas, C. C., Fan, L., & Siegler, R. S. (1993). Even before formal instruction, Chinese children outperform American children in mental addition. *Cognitive Development, 8,* 517–529.

Gecas, V., & Seff, M. A. (1990). Families and adolescents: A review of the 1980s. *Journal of Marriage and the Family, 52,* 941–958.

Gelman, R. (1972). Logical capacity of very young children: Number invariance rules. *Child Development, 43,* 75–90.

Genesee, F. (1993). Bilingual language development in preschool children. In D. Bishop & K. Mogford (Eds.), *Language development in exceptional circumstances* (pp. 62–79). Hove, England: Erlbaum.

Gentner, D. (1982). Why nouns are learned before verbs: Linguistic relativity versus natural partitioning. In S. A. Kuczaj II (Ed.), *Language development: Vol. 2. Language, thought, and culture* (pp. 301–334). Hillsdale, NJ: Erlbaum.

Georgieff, M. K. (1994). Nutritional deficiencies as developmental risk factors: Commentary on Pollitt and Gorman. In C. A. Nelson (Ed.), *The Minnesota Symposia on Child Development* (Vol. 27, pp. 145–159). Hillsdale, NJ: Erlbaum.

Gerson, R. P., & Damon, W. (1978). Moral understanding and children's conduct. *New Directions for Child Development, 2,* 41–60.

Gesell, A. (1925). *The mental growth of the preschool child.* New York: Macmillan.

Gibson, D. R. (1990). Relation of socioeconomic status to logical and sociomoral judgment of middle-aged men. *Psychology and Aging, 5,* 510–513.

Gibson, E. J. (1969). *Principles of perceptual learning and development.* New York: Appleton-Century-Crofts.

Gibson, E. J., & Spelke, E. S. (1983). The development of perception. In J. H. Flavell & E. M. Markman (Eds.), *Handbook of child psychology: Cognitive development* (Vol. 3, pp. 1–76). New York: Wiley.

Gibson, E. J., & Walk, R. D. (1960). The "visual cliff." *Scientific American, 202,* 80–92.

Gilbert, T. J., Percy, C. A., Sugarman, J. R., Benson, L., & Percy, C. (1992). Obesity among Navajo adolescents: Relationship to dietary intake and blood pressure. *American Journal of Diseases of Children, 146,* 289–295.

Gilligan, C. (1982). *In a different voice: Psychological theory and women's development.* Cambridge, MA: Harvard University Press.

Gilligan, C., & Wiggins, G. (1987). The origins of morality in early childhood relationships. In J. Kagan & S. Lamb (Eds.), *The emergence of morality in young children* (pp. 277–307). Chicago: University of Chicago Press.

Giordano, P. C., Cernkovich, S. A., & DeMaris, A. (1993). The family and peer relations of black adolescents. *Journal of Marriage and the Family, 55,* 277–287.

Gladue, B. A. (1994). The biopsychology of sexual orientation. *Current Directions in Psychological Science, 3,* 150–154.

Gleitman, L. R., & Gleitman, H. (1992). A picture is worth a thousand words, but that's the problem: The role of syntax in vocabulary acquisition. *Current Directions in Psychological Science, 1,* 31–35.

Gleitman, L. R., & Wanner, E. (1988). Current issues in language learning. In M. H. Bornstein & M. E. Lamb (Eds.), *Developmental psychology: An advanced textbook* (2nd ed.) (pp. 297–358). Hillsdale, NJ: Erlbaum.

Glenn, N. D. (1990). Quantitative research on marital quality in the 1980s: A critical review. *Journal of Marriage and the Family, 52,* 818–831.

Glueck, S., & Glueck, E. (1972). *Identification of pre-delinquents: Validation studies and some suggested uses of Glueck Table.* New York: Intercontinental Medical Book Corp.

Gnepp, J., & Chilamkurti, C. (1988). Children's use of personality attributions to predict other people's emotional and behavioral reactions. *Child Development, 50,* 743–754.

Goldberg, S. (1972). Infant care and growth in urban Zambia. *Human Development, 15,* 77–89.

Goldberg, W. A. (1990). Marital quality, parental personality, and spousal agreement about perceptions and expectations for children. *Merrill-Palmer Quarterly, 36,* 531–556.

Golden, M., & Birns, B. (1983). Social class and infant intelligence. In M. Lewis (Ed.), *Origins of intelligence: Infancy and early childhood* (2nd ed.) (pp. 347–398). New York: Plenum Press.

Goldfield, B. A., & Reznick, J. S. (1990). Early lexical acquisition: Rate, content, and the vocabulary spurt. *Journal of Child Language, 17,* 171–183.

Goldstein, J. H. (Ed.). (1994). *Toys, play, and child development.* Cambridge, England: Cambridge University Press.

Golinkoff, R. M., Mervis, C. B., & Hirsh-Pasek, K. (1994). Early object labels: The case for lexical principles. *Journal of Child Language, 21,* 125–155.

Golombok, S., & Fivush, R. (1994). *Gender development.* Cambridge, England: Cambridge University Press.

Good, T. L., & Weinstein, R. S. (1986). Schools make a difference. Evidence, criticisms, and new directions. *American Psychologist, 41,* 1090–1097.

Goodsitt, J. V., Morse, P. A., Ver Hoeve, J. N., & Cowan, N. (1984). Infant speech recognition in multisyllabic contexts. *Child Development, 55,* 903–910.

Gopnik, A., & Astington, J. W. (1988). Children's understanding of representational change and its relation to the understanding of false belief and the appearance-reality distinction. *Child Development, 59,* 26–37.

Gopnik, A., & Meltzoff, A. (1987). The development of categorization in the second year and its relation to other cognitive and linguistic developments. *Child Development, 58,* 1523–1531.

Gopnik, A., & Meltzoff, A. N. (1992). Categorization and naming: Basic-level sorting in eighteen-month-olds and its relation to language. *Child Development, 63,* 1091–1103.

Gopnik, A., & Wellman, H. M. (1994). The theory theory. In L. A. Hirschfeld & S. A. Gelman (Eds.), *Mapping the mind* (pp. 257–293). Cambridge, England: Cambridge University Press.

Gortmaker, S. L., Dietz, W. H., Sobol, A. M., & Welher, C. A. (1987). Increasing pediatric obesity in the United States.

American Journal of the Diseases of Children, 141, 535–540.

Gottesman, I. I., & Goldsmith, H. H. (1994). Developmental psychopathology of antisocial behavior: Inserting genes into its ontogenesis and epigenesis. In C. A. Nelson (Ed.), *The Minnesota Symposia on Child Psychology* (Vol. 27, pp. 69–104). Hillsdale, NJ: Erlbaum.

Gottfried, A. W., Gottfried, A. E., Bathurst, K., & Guerin, D. W. (1994). *Gifted IQ: Early developmental aspects.* New York: Plenum Press.

Gottlieb, G. (1976). Conceptions of prenatal development: Behavioral embryology. *Psychological Review, 83,* 215–234.

Gottman, J. M. (1986). The world of coordinated play: Same- and cross-sex friendship in young children. In J. M. Gottman & J. G. Parker (Eds.), *Conversations of friends: Speculations on affective development* (pp. 139–191). Cambridge, England: Cambridge University Press.

Graber, J. A., Brooks-Gunn, J., Paikoff, R. L., & Warren, M. P. (1994). Prediction of eating problems: An 8-year study of adolescent girls. *Developmental Psychology, 30,* 823–834.

Graham, S., & Hudley, C. (1994). Attributions of aggressive and nonaggressive African-American male early adolescents: A study of construct accessibility. *Developmental Psychology, 30,* 365–373.

Greenberg, J., & Kuczaj, S. A., II (1982). Towards a theory of substantive word-meaning acquisition. In S. A. Kuczaj II (Ed.), *Language development: Vol. I. Syntax and semantics* (pp. 275–312). Hillsdale, NJ: Erlbaum.

Greenberg, M. T., Siegel, J. M., & Leitch, C. J. (1983). The nature and importance of attachment relationships to parents and peers during adolescence. *Journal of Youth and Adolescence, 12,* 373–386.

Greenberg, M. T., Speltz, M. L., & DeKlyen, M. (1993). The role of attachment in the early development of disruptive behavior problems. *Development and Psychopathology, 5,* 191–213.

Greenberger, E., & Goldberg, W. A. (1989). Work, parenting, and the socialization of children. *Developmental Psychology, 25,* 22–35.

Greenberger, E., O'Neil, R., & Nagel, S. K. (1994). Linking workplace and homeplace: Relations between the nature of adults' work and their parenting behaviors. *Developmental Psychology, 30,* 990–1002.

Greenberger, E., & Steinberg, L. (1986). *When teenagers work: The psychological and social costs of adolescent employment.* New York: Basic Books.

Greenfield, P. (1995). Profile: On teaching. Culture, ethnicity, race, and development: Implications for teaching theory and research. *Society for Research in Child Development Newsletter* (Winter), 3–4, 12.

Greenfield, P. M. (1994). Independence and interdependence as developmental scripts: Implications for theory, research, and practice. In P. M. Greenfield & R. R. Cocking (Eds.), *Cross-cultural roots of minority child development* (pp. 1–37). Hillsdale, NJ: Erlbaum.

Greenfield, P. M., & Cocking, R. R. (Eds.). (1994). *Cross-cultural roots of minority child development.* Hillsdale, NJ: Erlbaum.

Greenough, W. T. (1991). Experience as a component of normal development: Evolutionary considerations. *Developmental Psychology, 27,* 11–27.

Greenough, W. T., Black, J. E., & Wallace, C. S. (1987). Experience and brain development. *Child Development, 58,* 539–559.

Gregg, V., Gibbs, J. C., & Basinger, K. S. (1994). Patterns of developmental delay in moral judgment by male and female delinquents. *Merrill-Palmer Quarterly, 40,* 538–553.

Grenier, G. (1985). Shifts to English as usual language by Americans of Spanish mother tongue. In R. O. de la Garza, F. D. Bean, C. M. Bonjean, R. Romo, & R. Alvarez (Eds.), *The Mexican American experience: An interdisciplinary anthology* (pp. 347–358). Austin: University of Texas Press.

Griffith, D. R., Azuma, S. D., & Chasnoff, I. J. (1994). Three-year outcome of children exposed prenatally to drugs. *Journal of the American Academy of Child and Adolescent Psychiatry, 33,* 20–27.

Grolnick, W. S., & Slowiaczek, M. L. (1994). Parents' involvement in children's schooling: A multidimensional conceptualization and motivational model. *Child Development, 65,* 237–252.

Grossmann, K., Grossmann, K. E., Spangler, G., Suess, G., & Unzner, L. (1985). Maternal sensitivity and newborns' orientation responses as related to quality of attachment in northern Germany. *Monographs of the Society of Research in Child Development, 50* (1–2, Serial No. 209), 233–256.

Grusec, J. E. (1992). Social learning theory and developmental psychology: The legacies of Robert Sears and Albert Bandura. *Developmental Psychology, 28,* 776–786.

Grusec, J. E., Saas-Kortsaak, P., & Simutis, Z. M. (1978). The role of example and moral exhortation in the training of altruism. *Child Development, 49,* 920–923.

Guerin, D. W., & Gottfried, A. W. (1994a). Temperamental consequences of infant difficultness. *Infant Behavior and Development, 17,* 413–421.

Guerin, D. W., & Gottfried, A. W. (1994b). Developmental stability and change in parent reports of temperament: A ten-year longitudinal investigation from infancy through preadolescence. *Merrill-Palmer Quarterly, 40,* 334–355.

Gullotta, T. P., Adams, G. R., & Montemayor, R. (Eds.). (1993). *Adolescent sexuality.* Newbury Park, CA: Sage.

Gunnar, M. R. (1994). Psychoendocrine studies of temperament and stress in early childhood: Expanding current models. In J. E. Bates & T. D. Wachs (Eds.), *Temperament:*

Individual differences at the interface of biology and behavior (pp. 175–198). Washington, DC: American Psychological Association.

Gunnar, M. R., Larson, M. C., Hertsgaard, L., Harris, M. L., & Brodersen, L. (1992). The stressfulness of separation among nine-month-old infants: Effects of social context variables and infant temperament. *Child Development, 63,* 290–303.

Guo, S. F. (1993). Postpartum depression. *Chung-Hua Fu Chan Ko Tsa Chi, 28,* 532–533, 569.

Guralnick, M. J., & Paul-Brown, D. (1984). Communicative adjustments during behavior-request episodes among children at different developmental levels. *Child Development, 55,* 911–919.

Guttentag, R. E., Ornstein, P. A., & Siemens, L. (1987). Children's spontaneous rehearsal: Transitions in strategy acquisition. *Cognitive Development, 2,* 307–326.

Gzesh, S. M., & Surber, C. F. (1985). Visual perspective-taking skills in children. *Child Development, 56,* 1204–1213.

Haan, N. (1981). Adolescents and young adults as producers of their own development. In R. M. Lerner & N. A. Busch-Rossnagel (Eds.), *Individuals as producers of their own development* (pp. 155–182). New York: Academic Press.

Haan, N. (1985). Processes of moral development: Cognitive or social disequilibrium? *Developmental Psychology, 21,* 996–1006.

Hack, M., Horbar, J. D., Mallow, M. H., Tyson, J. E., Wright, E., & Wright, L. (1991b). Very low birth weight outcomes of the National Institute of Child Health and Human Development Neonatal Network. *Prediatrics, 87,* 587–597.

Hack, M., Taylor, C. B. H., Klein, N., Eiben, R., Schatschneider, C., & Mercuri-Minich, N. (1994). School-age outcomes in children with birth weights under 750 g. *New England Journal of Medicine, 331,* 753–759.

Haddow, J. E., Palomaki, G. E., Knight, G. J., Cunningham, G. C., Lustig, L. S., & Boyd, P. A. (1994). Reducing the need for amniocentesis in women 35 years of age or older with serum markers for screening. *New England Journal of Medicine, 330,* 1114–1118.

Haith, M. M. (1980). *Rules that babies look by.* Hillsdale, NJ: Erlbaum.

Haith, M. M. (1990). Progress in the understanding of sensory and perceptual processes in early infancy. *Merrill-Palmer Quarterly, 36,* 1–26.

Hakuta, K. (1986). *Mirror on language: The debate on bilingualism.* New York: Basic Books.

Hakuta, K., & Garcia, E. E. (1989). Bilingualism and education. *American Psychologist, 44,* 374–379.

Halford, G. S., Maybery, M. T., O'Hare, A. W., & Grant, P. (1994). The development of memory and processing capacity. *Child Development, 65,* 1338–1356.

Halpern, C. T., Udry, J. R., Campbell, B., & Suchindran, C. (1993). Testosterone and pubertal development as predictors of sexual activity: A panel analysis of adolescent males. *Psychosomatic Medicine, 55,* 436–447.

Halpern, D. F. (1986). *Sex differences in cognitive abilities.* Hillsdale, NJ: Erlbaum.

Hamilton, C. E. (1995). *Continuity and discontinuity of attachment from infancy through adolescence.* Paper presented at the biennial meetings of the Society for Research in Child Development, Indianapolis.

Hammond, W. R., & Yung, B. (1993). Psychology's role in the public health response to assaultive violence among young African-American men. *American Psychologist, 48,* 142–154.

Hammond, W. R., & Yung, B. R. (1994). African Americans. In L. D. Eron, J. H. Gentry, & P. Schlegel (Eds.), *Reason to hope: A psychosocial perspective on violence and youth* (pp. 105–118). Washington, DC: American Psychological Association.

Hanna, E., & Meltzoff, A. N. (1993). Peer imitation by toddlers in laboratory, home, and day-care contexts: Implications for social learning and memory. *Developmental Psychology, 29,* 701–710.

Hansen, J., & Bowey, J. A. (1994). Phonological analysis skills, verbal working memory, and reading ability in second-grade children. *Child Development, 65,* 938–950.

Hanshaw, J. B., Scheiner, A. P., Moxley, A. W., Gaev, L., Abel, V., & Scheiner, B. (1976). School failure and deafness after "silent" congenital cytomegalovirus infection. *New England Journal of Medicine, 295,* 468–470.

Harkness, S., & Super, C. M. (1985). The cultural context of gender segregation in children's peer groups. *Child Development, 56,* 219–224.

Harris, B., Lovett, L., Newcombe, R. G., Read, G. F., Walker, R., & Riad-Fahmy, D. (1994). Maternity blues and major endocrine changes: Cardiff puerperal mood and hormone study II. *British Medical Journal, 308,* 949–953.

Harris, M. (1992). *Language experience and early language development: From input to uptake.* Hove, England: Erlbaum.

Harris, P. L. (1989). *Children and emotion: The development of psychological understanding.* Oxford: Basil Blackwell.

Harris, P. L., Olthof, T., & Terwogt, M. M. (1981). Children's knowledge of emotion. *Journal of Child Psychology and Psychiatry, 22,* 247–261.

Harrison, A. O., Wilson, M. N., Pine, C. J., Chan, S. Q., & Buriel, R. (1990). Family ecologies of ethnic minority children. *Child Development, 61,* 347–362.

Hart, B., & Risley, T. R. (1995). *Meaningful differences in the everyday experience of young American children.* Baltimore: Paul H. Brookes.

Harter, S. (1987). The determinations and mediational role of global self-worth in children. In N. Eisenberg (Ed.), *Contemporary topics in developmental psychology* (pp. 219–242). New York: Wiley-Interscience.

Harter, S. (1990). Processes underlying adolescent self-concept formation. In R. Montemayor, G. R. Adams, & T. P. Gullotta (Eds.), *From childhood to adolescence: A transitional period?* (pp. 205–239). Newbury Park, CA: Sage.

Harter, S., & Pike, R. (1984). The Pictorial Perceived Competence Scale for Young Children. *Child Development, 55,* 1969–1982.

Harter, S., & Whitesell, N. R. (1989). Developmental changes in children's understanding of single, multiple, and blended emotion concepts. In C. Saarni & P. L. Harris (Eds.), *Children's understanding of emotion* (pp. 81–116). Cambridge, England: Cambridge University Press.

Hartup, W. W. (1989). Social relationships and their developmental significance. *American Psychologist, 44,* 120–126.

Hartup, W. W., & Van Lieshout, C. F. M. (1995). Personality development in social context. *Annual Review of Psychology, 46,* 655–687.

Harvard Education Letter (1992, July/August). Youth sports: Kids are the losers, pp. 1–3.

Harwood, R. L. (1992). The influence of culturally derived values on Anglo and Puerto Rican mothers' perceptions of attachment behavior. *Child Development, 63,* 822–839.

Hashima, P. Y., & Amato, P. R. (1994). Poverty, social support, and parental behavior. *Child Development, 65,* 394–403.

Haskins, R. (1989). Beyond metaphor: The efficacy of early childhood education. *American Psychologist, 44,* 274–282.

Hatano, G., Siegler, R. S., Richards, D. D., Inagaki, K., Stavy, R., & Wax, N. (1993). The development of biological knowledge: A multi-national study. *Cognitive Development, 8,* 47–62.

Hatcher, P. J., Hulme, C., & Ellis, A. W. (1994). Ameliorating early reading failure by integrating the teaching of reading and phonological skills: The phonological linkage hypothesis. *Child Development, 65,* 41–57.

Hatchett, S. J., & Jackson, J. S. (1993). African American extended kin systems: An assessment. In H. P. McAdoo (Ed.), *Family ethnicity: Strength in diversity* (pp. 90–108). Newbury Park, CA: Sage.

Haviland, J. J., & Malatesta, C. Z. (1981). The development of sex differences in nonverbal signals: Fallacies, facts, and fantasies. In C. Mayo & N. M. Henley (Eds.), *Gender and nonverbal behavior* (pp. 183–208). New York: Springer-Verlag.

Haviland, J. M., & Lelwica, M. (1987). The induced affect response: 10-week-old infants' responses to three emotional expressions. *Developmental Psychology, 23,* 97–104.

Havill, V. L., Allen, K., Halverson, C. F., Jr., & Kohnstamm, G. A. (1994). Parents' use of Big Five categories in their natural language descriptions of children. In C. F. Halverson Jr., G. A. Kohnstamm, & R. P. Martin (Eds.), *The developing structure of temperament and personality from infancy to adulthood* (pp. 371–386). Hillsdale, NJ: Erlbaum.

Hawley, T. L., & Disney, E. R. (1992). Crack's children: The consequences of maternal cocaine abuse. *Social Policy Report, Society for Research in Child Development, 6*(4), 1–22.

Hawton, K., & Goldacre, M. (1982). Hospital admissions for adverse effects of medicinal agents (mainly self-poisoning) among adolescents in the Oxford region. *British Journal of Psychiatry, 141,* 166–170.

Hayes, C. D. (1987). *Risking the future: Vol. 1. Adolescent sexuality, pregnancy, and childbearing.* Washington, DC: National Academy Press.

Hazan, C., & Shaver, P. (1990). Love and work: An attachment-theoretical perspective. *Journal of Personality and Social Psychology, 59,* 270–280.

Heagarty, M. C. (1991). America's lost children: Whose responsibility? *Journal of Pediatrics, 118,* 8–10.

Henker, B., & Whalen, C. K. (1989). Hyperactivity and attention deficits. *American Psychologist, 44,* 216–223.

Henneborn, W. J., & Cogan, R. (1975). The effect of husband participation on reported pain and the probability of medication during labor and birth. *Journal of Psychosomatic Research, 19,* 215–222.

Hernandez, D. (1993). *America's Children.* New York: Russell Sage Foundation.

Hernandez, D. J. (1994). Children's changing access to resources: A historical perspective. *Social Policy Report, Society for Research in Child Development, 8*(1), 1–23.

Herrnstein, R. J., & Murray, C. (1994). *The bell curve: Intelligence and class structure in American life.* New York: Free Press.

Hess, E. H. (1972). "Imprinting" in a natural laboratory. *Scientific American, 227,* 24–31.

Hetherington, E. M. (1989). Coping with family transitions: Winners, losers, and survivors. *Child Development, 60,* 1–14.

Hetherington, E. M., & Camera, K. A. (1984). Families in transition: The process of dissolution and reconstitution. In R. D. Parke, R. N. Emde, H. P. McAdoo, & G. P. Sackett (Eds.), *Review of child development research: Vol. 7. The family* (pp. 398–440). Chicago: University of Chicago Press.

Hetherington, E. M., & Clingempeel, W. G. (1992). Coping with marital transitions: A family systems perspective. *Monographs of the Society for Research in Child Development, 57*(2–3, Serial No. 227).

Hickey, C. A., Cliver, S. P., Goldenberg, R. L., Kohatsu, J., & Hoffman, H. J. (1993). Prenatal weight gain, term birth weight, and fetal growth retardation among high-risk multi-parous black and white women. *Obstetrics and Gynecology, 81,* 529–535.

Higgins, A. (1991). The just community approach to moral education: Evolution of the idea and recent findings. In W. M. Kurtines & J. L. Gewirtz (Eds.), *Handbook of moral behavior and development: Vol. 3. Application* (pp. 111–141). Hillsdale, NJ: Erlbaum.

Higgins, A. T., & Turnure, J. E. (1984). Distractibility and concentration of attention in children's development. *Child Development, 55,* 1799–1810.

Hill, H. M., Soriano, F. I., Chen, S. A., & LaFromboise, T. D. (1994). Sociocultural factors in the etiology and prevention of violence among ethnic minority youth. In L. D. Eron, J. H. Gentry, & P. Schlegel (Eds.), *Reason to hope: A psychosocial perspective on violence and youth* (pp. 59–97). Washington, DC: American Psychological Association.

Hill, J. P., & Holmbeck, G. N. (1986). Attachment and autonomy. *Annals of Child Development, 3,* 145–189.

Hilts, P. J. (1995, April 19). Black teen-agers are turning away from smoking, but whites puff on. *The New York Times,* p. B7.

Hinde, R. A., Titmus, G., Easton, D., & Tamplin, A. (1985). Incidence of "friendship" and behavior toward strong associates versus nonassociates in preschoolers. *Child Development, 56,* 234–245.

Hines, M., & Kaufman, F. R. (1994). Androgen and the development of human sex-typical behavior: Rough-and-tumble play and sex of preferred playmates in children with congenital adrenal hyperplasia (CAH). *Child Development, 65,* 1042–1053.

Hinshaw, S. P., Lahey, B. B., & Hart, E. L. (1993). Issues of taxonomy and comorbidity in the development of conduct disorder. *Development and Psychopathology, 5,* 31–49.

Hirsch, H. V. B., & Tieman, S. B. (1987). Perceptual development and experience-dependent changes in cat visual cortex. In M. H. Bornstein (Ed.), *Sensitive periods in development: Interdisciplinary perspectives* (pp. 39–80). Hillsdale, NJ: Erlbaum.

Hirschfeld, L. A., & Gelman, S. A. (1994). Toward a topography of mind: An introduction to domain specificity. In L. A. Hirschfeld & S. A. Gelman (Eds.), *Mapping the mind* (pp. 3–35). Cambridge, England: Cambridge University Press.

Hirsh-Pasek, K., Trieman, R., & Schneiderman, M. (1984). Brown and Hanlon revisited: Mothers' sensitivity to ungrammatical forms. *Journal of Child Language, 11,* 81–88.

Hofferth, S. L. (1987a). Teenage pregnancy and its resolution. In S. L. Hofferth & C. D. Hayes (Eds.), *Risking the future: Adolescent sexuality, pregnancy, and childbearing. Working papers* (pp. 78–92). Washington, DC: National Academy Press.

Hofferth, S. L. (1987b). Social and economic consequences of teenage childbearing. In S. L. Hofferth & C. D. Hayes (Eds.), *Risking the future: Adolescent sexuality, pregnancy, and childbearing. Working papers* (pp. 123–144). Washington, DC: National Academy Press.

Hofferth, S. L., Boisjoly, J., & Duncan, G. (1995). *Does children's school attainment benefit from parental access to social capital?* Paper presented at the biennial meetings of the Society for Research in Child Development, Indianapolis.

Hoffman, H. J., & Hillman, L. S. (1992). Epidemiology of the sudden infant death syndrome: Maternal, neonatal, and postneonatal risk factors. *Clinics in Perinatology, 19*(4), 717–737.

Hoffman, L. W. (1989). Effects of maternal employment in the two-parent family. *American Psychologist, 44,* 283–292.

Hoffman, M. L. (1982). Development of prosocial motivation: Empathy and guilt. In N. Eisenberg (Ed.), *The development of prosocial behavior* (pp. 281–314). New York: Academic Press.

Hoffman, M. L. (1984). Empathy, its limitations, and its role in a comprehensive moral theory. In W. M. Kurtines & J. L. Gewirtz (Eds.), *Morality, moral behavior, and moral development* (pp. 283–302). New York: Wiley.

Hoffman, M. L. (1988). Moral development. In M. H. Bornstein & M. E. Lamb (Eds.), *Developmental psychology: An advanced textbook* (2nd ed.) (pp. 497–548). Hillsdale, NJ: Erlbaum.

Holahan, C. K. (1988). Relation of life goals at age 70 to activity participation and health and psychological well-being among Terman's gifted men and women. *Psychology and Aging, 3,* 286–291.

Holden, C. (1987). Genes and behavior: A twin legacy. *Psychology Today, 21*(9), 18–19.

Holloway, S. D., & Hess, R. D. (1985). Mothers' and teachers' attributions about children's mathematics performance. In I. E. Sigel (Ed.), *Parental belief systems: The psychological consequences for children* (pp. 177–200). Hillsdale, NJ: Erlbaum.

Holmbeck, G. N., & Hill, J. P. (1991). Conflictive engagement, positive affect, and menarche in families with seventh-grade girls. *Child Development, 62,* 1030–1048.

Honigfeld, L. S., & Kaplan, D. W. (1987). Native-American post-neonatal mortality. *Pediatrics, 80,* 575–578.

Honzik, M. P. (1986). The role of the family in the development of mental abilities: A 50-year study. In N. Datan, A. L. Greene, & H. W. Reese (Eds.), *Life-span developmental psychology: Intergenerational relations* (pp. 185–210). Hillsdale, NJ: Erlbaum.

Hopkins, J., Marcus, M., & Campbell, S. B. (1984). Postpartum depression: A critical review. *Psychological Bulletin, 95,* 498–515.

Horowitz, F. D. (1987). *Exploring developmental theories: Toward a structural/behavioral model of development.* Hillsdale, NJ: Erlbaum.

Horowitz, F. D. (1990). Developmental models of individual differences. In J. Colombo & J. Fagen (Eds.), *Individual differences in infancy: Reliability, stability, prediction* (pp. 3–18). Hillsdale, NJ: Erlbaum.

Hovell, M., Sipan, C., Blumberg, E., Atkins, C., Hofstetter, C. R., & Kreitner, S. (1994). Family influences on Latino and Anglo adolescents' sexual behavior. *Journal of Marriage and the Family, 56,* 973–986.

Howard, J. (1978). The influence of children's developmental dysfunctions on marital quality and family interaction. In R. M. Lerner & G. B. Spanier (Eds.), *Child influences on marital and family interaction: A life-span perspective* (pp. 275–298). New York: Academic Press.

Howes, C. (1983). Patterns of friendship. *Child Development, 54,* 1041–1053.

Howes, C. (1987). Social competence with peers in young children: Developmental sequences. *Developmental Review, 7,* 252–272.

Howes, C., & Matheson, C. C. (1992). Sequences in the development of competent play with peers: Social and pretend play. *Developmental Psychology, 28,* 961–974.

Howes, C., Phillips, D. A., & Whitebook, M. (1992). Thresholds of quality: Implications for the social development of children in center-based child care. *Child Development, 63,* 449–460.

Hubbard, F. O. A., & van IJzendoorn, M. H. (1987). Maternal unresponsiveness and infant crying. A critical replication of the Bell & Ainsworth study. In L. W. C. Tavecchio & M. H. v. IJzendoorn (Eds.), *Attachment in social networks* (pp. 339–378). Amsterdam: Elsevier/North-Holland.

Hubel, D. H., & Weisel, T. N. (1963). Receptive fields of cells in striate cortex of very young, visually inexperienced kittens. *Journal of Neurophysiology, 26,* 994–1002.

Hudley, C., & Graham, S. (1993). An attributional intervention to reduce peer-directed aggression among African-American boys. *Child Development, 64,* 124–138.

Huesmann, L. R., Lagerspetz, K., & Eron, L. D. (1984). Intervening variables in the television violence-aggression relation: Evidence from two countries. *Developmental Psychology, 20,* 746–775.

Huffman, L. C., Bryan, Y. E., Pedersen, F. A., Lester, B. M., Newman, J. D., & del Carmen, R. (1994). Infant cry acoustics and maternal ratings of temperament. *Infant Behavior and Development, 17,* 45–53.

Humphreys, L. G., Davey, T. C., & Park, R. K. (1985). Longitudinal correlation analysis of standing height and intelligence. *Child Development, 56,* 1465–1478.

Huntington, L., Hans, S. L., & Zeskind, P. S. (1990). The relations among cry characteristics, demographic variables, and developmental test scores in infants prenatally exposed to methadone. *Infant Behavior and Development, 13,* 533–538.

Hurwitz, E., Gunn, W. J., Pinsky, P. F., & Schonberger, L. B. (1991). Risk of respiratory illness associated with day-care attendance: A nationwide study. *Pediatrics, 87,* 62–69.

Huston, A. C. (Ed.). (1991). *Children in poverty: Child development and public policy.* Cambridge, England: Cambridge University Press.

Huston, A. C. (1994). Children in poverty: Designing research to affect policy. *Social Policy Report, Society for Research in Child Development, 8*(2), 1–12.

Huston, A. C., Greer, D., Wright, J. C., Welch, R., & Ross, R. (1984). Children's comprehension of televised formal features with masculine and feminine connotations. *Developmental Psychology, 20,* 707–716.

Huston, A. C., & Wright, J. C. (1994). Educating children with television: The forms of the medium. In D. Zillmann, J. Bryant, & A. C. Huston (Eds.), *Media, children, and the family: Social scientific, psychodynamic, and clinical perspectives* (pp. 73–84). Hillsdale, NJ: Erlbaum.

Huston, A. C., Wright, J. C., Rice, M. L., Kerkman, D., & St. Peters, M. (1990). Development of television viewing patterns in early childhood: A longitudinal investigation. *Developmental Psychology, 26,* 409–420.

Hutt, S. J., Lenard, H. G., & Prechtl, H. F. R. (1969). Psychophysiological studies in newborn infants. In L. P. Lipsitt & H. W. Reese (Eds.), *Advances in child development and behavior* (Vol. 4, pp. 128–173). New York: Academic Press.

Huttenlocher, P. R. (1994). Synaptogenesis, synapse elimination, and neural plasticity in human cerebral cortex. In C. A. Nelson (Ed.), *The Minnesota Symposia on Child Psychology* (Vol. 27, pp. 35–54). Hillsdale, NJ: Erlbaum.

Ingram, D. (1981). Early patterns of grammatical development. In R. E. Stark (Ed.), *Language behavior in infancy and early childhood* (pp. 327–358). New York: Elsevier/North-Holland.

Inhelder, B., & Piaget, J. (1958). *The growth of logical thinking from childhood to adolescence.* New York: Basic Books.

Inoff-Germain, G., Arnold, G. S., Nottelmann, E. D., Susman, E. J., Cutler, G. B., Jr., & Chrousos, G. P. (1988). Relations between hormone levels and observational measures of aggressive behavior of young adolescents in family interactions. *Developmental Psychology, 24,* 129–139.

Isabella, R. A. (1993). Origins of attachment: Maternal interactive behavior across the first year. *Child Development, 64,* 605–621.

Isabella, R. A., Belsky, J., & von Eye, A. (1989). Origins of infant-mother attachment: An examination of interactional synchrony during the infant's first year. *Developmental Psychology, 25,* 12–21.

Istvan, J. (1986). Stress, anxiety, and birth outcomes: A critical review of the evidence. *Psychological Bulletin, 100,* 331–348.

Izard, C. E., & Harris, P. (1995). Emotional development and developmental psychopathology. In D. Cicchetti & D. J. Cohen (Eds.), *Developmental psychopathology: Vol. 1: Theory and methods* (pp. 467–503). New York: Wiley.

Izard, C. E., & Malatesta, C. Z. (1987). Perspectives on emotional development I: Differential emotions theory of early emotional development. In J. D. Osofsky (Ed.), *Handbook of infant development* (2nd ed.) (pp. 494–554). New York: Wiley-Interscience.

Jacklin, C. N. (1989). Female and male: Issues of gender. *American Psychologist, 44,* 127–133.

Jadack, R. A., Hyde, J. S., Moore, C. F., & Keller, M. L. (1995). Moral reasoning about sexually transmitted diseases. *Child Development, 66,* 167–177.

Janos, P. M., & Robinson, N. M. (1985). Psychosocial development in intellectually gifted children. In F. D. Horowitz & M. O'Brien (Eds.), *The gifted and talented. Developmental perspectives* (pp. 149–196). Washington, DC: American Psychological Association.

Jensen, A. R. (1980). *Bias in mental testing.* New York: Free Press.

Jessor, R. (1992). Risk behavior in adolescence: A psychosocial framework for understanding and action. *Developmental Review, 12,* 374–390.

John, O. P., Caspi, A., Robins, R. W., Moffitt, T. E., & Stouthamer-Loeber, M. (1994). The "little five": Exploring the nomological network of the five-factor model of personality in adolescent boys. *Child Development, 65,* 160–178.

Johnston, J. R. (1985). Cognitive prerequisites: The evidence from children learning English. In D. I. Slobin (Ed.), *The crosslinguistic study of language acquisition: Vol. 2. Theoretical issues* (pp. 961–1004). Hillsdale, NJ: Erlbaum.

Jones, E. F., Forrest, J. D., Goldman, N., Henshaw, S. K., Lincoln, R., Rosoff, J. L., Westoff, C. F., & Wulf, D. (1986). *Teenage pregnancy in industrialized countries.* New Haven, CT: Yale University Press.

Jordan, N. C., Huttenlocher, J., & Levine, S. C. (1992). Differential calculation abilities in young children from middle- and low-income families. *Developmental Psychology, 28,* 644–653.

Jorgensen, S. R. (1993). Adolescent pregnancy and parenting. In T. P. Gullotta, G. R. Adams, & R. Montemayor (Eds.), *Adolescent sexuality* (pp. 103–140). Newbury Park, CA: Sage.

Joshi, M. S., & MacLean, M. (1994). Indian and English children's understanding of the distinction between real and apparent emotion. *Child Development, 65,* 1372–1384.

Jung, C. G. (1916). *Analytical psychology.* New York: Moffat, Yard.

Jung, C. G. (1939). *The integration of personality.* New York: Holt, Rinehart and Winston.

Jusczyk, P. W., Cutler, A., & Redanz, N. J. (1993). Infants' preference for the predominant stress patterns of English words. *Child Development, 64,* 675–687.

Kagan, J. (1971). *Change and continuity in infancy.* New York: Wiley.

Kagan, J. (1994). *Galen's prophecy.* New York: Basic Books.

Kagan, J., Arcus, D., Snidman, N., Feng, W. Y., Hendler, J., & Greene, S. (1994). Reactivity in infants: A cross-national comparison. *Developmental Psychology, 30,* 342–345.

Kagan, J., Kearsley, R., & Zelazo, P. (1978). *Infancy: Its place in human development.* Cambridge, MA: Harvard University Press.

Kagan, J., Reznick, J. S., & Snidman, N. (1990). The temperamental qualities of inhibition and lack of inhibition. In M. Lewis & S. M. Miller (Eds.), *Handbook of developmental psychopathology* (pp. 219–226). New York: Plenum Press.

Kagan, J., Snidman, N., & Arcus, D. (1993). On the temperamental categories of inhibited and uninhibited children. In K. H. Rubin & J. B. Asendorpf (Eds.), *Social withdrawal, inhibition, and shyness in childhood* (pp. 19–28). Hillsdale, NJ: Erlbaum.

Kail, R. (1991b). Processing time declines exponentially during childhood and adolescence. *Developmental Psychology, 27,* 259–266.

Kail, R., & Hall, L. K. (1994). Processing speed, naming speed, and reading. *Developmental Psychology, 30,* 949–954.

Kandel, D. B., & Wu, P. (1995). The contributions of mothers and fathers to the intergenerational transmission of cigarette smoking in adolescence. *Journal of Research on Adolescence, 5,* 225–252.

Karmiloff-Smith, A. (1993). NeoPiagetians: A theoretical misnomer? *Society for Research in Child Development Newsletter* (Spring), 3, 10–11.

Katz, P. A., & Ksansnak, K. R. (1994). Developmental aspects of gender role flexibility and traditionality in middle childhood and adolescence. *Developmental Psychology, 30,* 272–282.

Kaye, K. (1982). *The mental and social life of babies: How parents create persons.* Chicago: University of Chicago Press.

Kaye, K. L., & Bower, T. G. R. (1994). Learning and intermodal transfer of information in newborns. *Psychological Science, 5,* 286–288.

Keating, D. P. (1980). Thinking processes in adolescence. In J. Adelson (Ed.), *Handbook of adolescent psychology* (pp. 211–246). New York: Wiley.

Keating, D. P., List, J. A., & Merriman, W. E. (1985). Cognitive processing and cognitive ability: Multivariate validity investigation. *Intelligence, 9,* 149–170.

Keefe, S. E., & Padilla, A. M. (1987). *Chicano ethnicity.* Albuquerque: University of New Mexico Press.

Keeney, T. J., Cannizzo, S. R., & Flavell, J. H. (1967). Spontaneous and induced verbal rehearsal in a recall task. *Child Development, 38,* 935–966.

Kelley, M. L., Sanches-Hucles, J., & Walker, R. R. (1993). Correlates of disciplinary practices in working- to middle-class African-American mothers. *Merrill-Palmer Quarterly, 39,* 252–264.

Kempe, A., Wise, P. H., Barkan, S. E., Sappenfield, W. M., Sachs, B., Gortmaker, S. L., Sobol, A. M., First, L. R., Pursley, D., Reinhart, H., Kotelchuck, M., Cole, F. S., Gunter, N., & Stockbauer, J. W. (1992). Clinical determinants of the racial disparity in very low birth weight. *New England Journal of Medicine, 327,* 969–973.

Kendall-Tackett, K. A., Williams, L. M., & Finkelhor, D. (1993). Impact of sexual abuse on children: A review and synthesis of recent empirical studies. *Psychological Bulletin, 113,* 164–180.

Keniston, K. (1970). Youth: A "new" stage in life. *American Scholar, 8*(Autumn), 631–654.

Kestenbaum, R., Farber, E. A., & Sroufe, L. A. (1989). Individual differences in empathy among preschoolers: Relation to attachment history. *New Directions for Child Development, 44,* 51–64.

Killen, J. D., Hayward, C., Litt, I., Hammer, L. D., Wilson, D. M., Miner, B., Taylor, B., Varady, A., & Shisslak, C. (1992). Is puberty a risk factor for eating disorders? *American Journal of Diseases of Childhood, 146,* 323–325.

Kilpatrick, S. J., & Laros, R. K. (1989). Characteristics of normal labor. *Obstetrics and Gynecology, 74,* 85–87.

Kim, U., & Choi, S. (1994). Individualism, collectivism, and child development: A Korean perspective. In P. M. Greenfield & R. R. Cocking (Eds.), *Cross-cultural roots of minority child development* (pp. 227–257). Hillsdale, NJ: Erlbaum.

Kinney, D. A. (1993). From "nerds" to "normals": Adolescent identity recovery within a changing social system. *Sociology of Education, 66,* 21–40.

Klaus, H. M., & Kennell, J. H. (1976). *Maternal-infant bonding.* St. Louis: Mosby.

Klerman, L. V. (1991). The health of poor children: Problems and programs. In A. C. Huston (Ed.), *Children in poverty: Child development and public policy* (pp. 136–157). Cambridge, England: Cambridge University Press.

Klesges, R. C., Shelton, M. L., & Klesges, L. M. (1993). Effects of television on metabolic rate: Potential implications for childhood obesity. *Pediatrics, 91,* 281–286.

Kline, M., Tschann, J. M., Johnston, J. R., & Wallerstein, J. S. (1989). Children's adjustment in joint and sole physical custody families. *Developmental Psychology, 25,* 430–438.

Knight, G. P., Cota, M. K., & Bernal, M. E. (1993). The socialization of cooperative, competitive, and individualistic preferences among Mexican American children: The mediating role of ethnic identity. *Hispanic Journal of Behavioral Sciences, 15,* 291–309.

Kohlberg, L. (1964). Development of moral character and moral ideology. In M. L. Hoffman & L. W. Hoffman (Eds.), *Review of child development research* (Vol. 1, pp. 283–332). New York: Russell Sage Foundation.

Kohlberg, L. (1966). A cognitive-developmental analysis of children's sex-role concepts and attitudes. In E. E. Maccoby (Ed.), *The development of sex differences* (pp. 82–172). Stanford, CA: Stanford University Press.

Kohlberg, L. (1975). The cognitive-developmental approach to moral education. *Phi Delta Kappan,* pp. 670–677.

Kohlberg, L. (1976). Moral stages and moralization: The cognitive-developmental approach. In T. Lickona (Ed.), *Moral development and behavior: Theory, research, and social issues* (pp. 31–53). New York: Holt.

Kohlberg, L. (1978). Revisions in the theory and practice of moral development. *New Directions for Child Development, 2,* 83–88.

Kohlberg, L. (1981). *Essays on moral development: Vol. 1. The philosophy of moral development.* New York: Harper & Row.

Kohlberg, L. (1984). *Essays on moral development: Vol. II. The psychology of moral development.* San Francisco: Harper & Row.

Kohlberg, L., & Candee, D. (1984). The relationship of moral judgment to moral action. In W. M. Kurtines & J. L. Gewirtz (Eds.), *Morality, moral behavior, and moral development* (pp. 52–73). New York: Wiley.

Kohlberg, L., & Elfenbein, D. (1975). The development of moral judgments concerning capital punishment. *American Journal of Orthopsychiatry, 54,* 614–640.

Kohlberg, L., & Higgins, A. (1987). School democracy and social interaction. In W. M. Kurtines & J. L. Gewirtz (Eds.), *Moral development through social interaction* (pp. 102–130). New York: Wiley–Interscience.

Kohlberg, L., Levine, C., & Hewer, A. (1983). *Moral stages: A current formulation and a response to critics.* Basel: S. Karger.

Kohlberg, L., & Ullian, D. Z. (1974). Stages in the development of psychosexual concepts and attitudes. In R. C. Friedman, R. M. Richart, & R. L. Vande Wiele (Eds.), *Sex differences in behavior* (pp. 209–222). New York: Wiley.

Kohn, M. L. (1980). Job complexity and adult personality. In N. J. Smelser & E. H. Erikson (Eds.), *Themes of work and love in adulthood* (pp. 193–212). Cambridge, MA: Harvard University Press.

Kohn, M. L., & Schooler, C. (1983). *Work and personality: An inquiry into the impact of social stratification.* Norwood, NJ: Ablex Press.

Kohnstamm, G. A., Halverson, C. F., Jr., Havill, V. L., & Mervielde, I. (1994). Parents' free descriptions of child characteristics: A cross-cultural search for the roots of the big five. In S. Harkness & C. M. Super (Eds.), *Parents' cultural belief systems: Cultural origins and developmental consequences.* New York: Guilford Press.

Kolata, G. (1992, April 26). A parents' guide to kids' sports. *The New York Times Magazine,* pp. 12–15, 40, 44, 46.

Kopp, C. B. (1994). Trends and directions in studies of developmental risk. In C. A. Nelson (Ed.), *The Minnesota Symposia on Child Psychology* (Vol. 27, pp. 1–33). Hillsdale, NJ: Erlbaum.

Kopp, C. B., & Kaler, S. R. (1989). Risk in infancy: Origins and implications. *American Psychologist, 44,* 224–230.

Korner, A. F., Hutchinson, C. A., Koperski, J. A., Kraemer, H. C., & Schneider, P. A. (1981). Stability of individual differences of neonatal motor and crying patterns. *Child Development, 52,* 83–90.

Kortenhaus, C. M., & Demarest, J. (1993). Gender role stereotyping in children's literature: An update. *Sex Roles, 28,* 219–232.

Kuczaj, S. A., II (1977). The acquisition of regular and irregular past tense forms. *Journal of Verbal Learning and Verbal Behavior, 49,* 319–326.

Kuczaj, S. A., II (1978). Children's judgments of grammatical and ungrammatical irregular past tense verbs. *Child Development, 49,* 319–326.

Kuhl, P. K., & Meltzoff, A. N. (1984). The intermodal representation of speech in infants. *Infant Behavior and Development, 7,* 361–381.

Kuhn, D. (1992). Cognitive development. In M. H. Bornstein & M. E. Lamb (Eds.), *Developmental psychology: An advanced textbook* (3rd ed.) (pp. 211–272). Hillsdale, NJ: Erlbaum.

Kupersmidt, J. B., & Coie, J. D. (1990). Preadolescent peer status, aggression, and school adjustment as predictors of externalizing problems in adolescence. *Child Development, 61,* 1350–1362.

Kurdek, L. A., & Fine, M. A. (1994). Family acceptance and family control as predictors of adjustment in young adolescents: Linear, curvilinear, or interactive effects? *Child Development, 65,* 1137–1146.

Kurdek, L. A., & Krile, D. (1982). A developmental analysis of the relation between peer acceptance and both interpersonal understanding and perceived social self-competence. *Child Development, 53,* 1485–1491.

Kurtines, W. M., & Gewirtz, J. L. (Eds.). (1991). *Handbook of moral behavior and development: Vol. 1, Theory; Vol. 2, Research; Vol. 3, Application.* Hillsdale, NJ: Erlbaum.

La Freniere, P., Strayer, F. F., & Gauthier, R. (1984). The emergence of same-sex affiliative preferences among preschool peers: A developmental/ethological perspective. *Child Development, 55,* 1958–1965.

Lamb, M. E. (1981). The development of father-infant relationships. In M. E. Lamb (Ed.), *The role of the father in child development* (2nd ed.) (pp. 459–488). New York: Wiley.

Lamb, M. E., Frodi, A. M., Hwang, C., Frodi, M., & Steinberg, J. (1982). Mother- and father-infant interaction involving play and holding in traditional and nontraditional Swedish families. *Developmental Psychology, 18,* 215–221.

Lamb, M. E., Frodi, M., Hwang, C., & Frodi, A. M. (1983). Effects of paternal involvement on infant preferences for mothers and fathers. *Child Development, 54,* 450–458.

Lamb, M. E., Sternberg, K. J., & Prodromidis, M. (1992). Nonmaternal care and the security of infant-mother attachment: A reanalysis of the data. *Infant Behavior and Development, 15,* 71–83.

Lambert, C. (1993, March–April). The demand side of the health care crisis. *Harvard Magazine,* pp. 30–33.

Lamborn, S. D., Mounts, N. S., Steinberg, L., & Dornbusch, S. M. (1991). Patterns of competence and adjustment among adolescents from authoritative, authoritarian, indulgent, and neglectful families. *Child Development, 62,* 1049–1065.

Lamke, L. K. (1982a). Adjustment and sex-role orientation. *Journal of Youth and Adolescence, 11,* 247–259.

Lamke, L. K. (1982b). The impact of sex-role orientation on self-esteem in early adolescence. *Child Development, 53,* 1530–1535.

Langlois, J. H., Ritter, J. M., Roggman, L. A., & Vaughn, L. S. (1991). Facial diversity and infant preferences for attractive faces. *Developmental Psychology, 27,* 79–84.

Langlois, J. H., Roggman, L. A., Casey, R. J., Ritter, J. M., Rieser-Danner, L. A., & Jenkins, V. Y. (1987). Infant preferences for attractive faces: Rudiments of a stereotype? *Developmental Psychology, 23,* 263–369.

Langlois, J. H., Roggman, L. A., & Rieser-Danner, L. A. (1990). Infants' differential social responses to attractive and unattractive faces. *Developmental Psychology, 26,* 153–159.

Laub, J. H., & Sampson, R. J. (1995). The long-term effect of punitive discipline. In J. McCord (Ed.), *Coercion and punishment in long-term perspectives* (pp. 247–258). Cambridge, England: Cambridge University Press.

Laumann, E. O., Gagnon, J. H., Michael, R. T., & Michaels, S. (1994). *The social organization of sexuality: Sexual practices in the United States.* Chicago: University of Chicago Press.

Laursen, B. (1995). Conflict and social interaction in adolescent relationships. *Journal of Research on Adolescence, 5,* 55–70.

Leaper, C. (1991). Influence and involvement in children's discourse: Age, gender, and partner effects. *Child Development, 62,* 797–811.

Lebra, T. S. (1994). Mother and child in Japanese socialization: A Japan-U.S. comparison. In P. M. Greenfield & R. R. Cocking (Eds.), *Cross-cultural roots of minority child development* (pp. 259–274). Hillsdale, NJ: Erlbaum.

Lederberg, A. R., & Mobley, C. E. (1990). The effect of hearing impairment on the quality of attachment and mother-toddler interaction. *Child Development, 61,* 1596–1604.

Lee, C. C. (1985). Successful rural black adolescents: A psychological profile. *Adolescence, 20,* 129–142.

Lee, V. E., Burkham, D. T., Zimiles, H., & Ladewski, B. (1994). Family structure and its effect on behavioral and emotional problems in young adolescents. *Journal of Research on Adolescence, 4,* 405–437.

Lerner, J. V., & Galambos, N. L. (1986). Child development and family change: The influences of maternal employment in infants and toddlers. In L. P. Lipsitt & C. Rovee-Collier (Eds.), *Advances in infancy research* (Vol. 4, pp. 40–86). Norwood, NJ: Ablex.

Lerner, R. M. (1985). Adolescent maturational changes and psychosocial development: A dynamic interactional perspective. *Journal of Youth and Adolescence, 14,* 355–372.

Lerner, R. M. (1987). A life-span perspective for early adolescence. In R. M. Lerner & T. T. Foch (Eds.), *Biological-psychosocial interactions in early adolescence* (pp. 9–34). Hillsdale, NJ: Erlbaum.

Lester, B. M. (1987). Prediction of developmental outcome from acoustic cry analysis in term and preterm infants. *Pediatrics, 80,* 529–534.

Lester, B. M., Boukydis, C. F. Z., Garcia-Coll, C. T., Hole, W., & Peucker, M. (1992). Infantile colic: Acoustic cry characteristics, maternal perception of cry, and temperament. *Infant Behavior and Development, 15,* 15–26.

Lester, B. M., & Dreher, M. (1989). Effects of marijuana use during pregnancy on newborn cry. *Child Development, 60,* 765–771.

Levano, K. J., Cunningham, G., Nelson, S., Roark, M., Williams, M. L., Guzick, D., Dowling, S., Rosenfeld, C. R., & Buckley, A. (1986). A prospective comparison of selective and universal electronic fetal monitoring in 34,995 pregnancies. *New England Journal of Medicine, 315,* 615–619.

Levitt, M. J., Guacci-Franco, N., & Levitt, J. L. (1993). Convoys of social support in childhood and early adolescence: Structure and function. *Developmental Psychology, 29,* 811–818.

Levy, G. D., & Fivush, R. (1993). Scripts and gender: A new approach for examining gender-role development. *Developmental Review, 13,* 126–146.

Lewis, C. C. (1981). How adolescents approach decisions: Changes over grades seven to twelve and policy implications. *Child Development, 52,* 538–544.

Lewis, C. N., Freeman, N. H., & Maridaki-Kassotaki, K. (1995). *The social basis of theory of mind: Influences of siblings and, more importantly, interactions with adult kin.* Paper presented at the biennial meetings of the Society for Research in Child Development, Indianapolis.

Lewis, M. (1990). Social knowledge and social development. *Merrill-Palmer Quarterly, 36,* 93–116.

Lewis, M. (1991). Ways of knowing: Objective self-awareness of consciousness. *Developmental Review, 11,* 231–243.

Lewis, M., Allesandri, S. M., & Sullivan, M. W. (1992). Differences in shame and pride as a function of children's gender and task difficulty. *Child Development, 63,* 630–638.

Lewis, M., & Brooks, J. (1978). Self-knowledge and emotional development. In M. Lewis & L. A. Rosenblum (Eds.), *The development of affect* (pp. 205–226). New York: Plenum Press.

Lewis, M., & Brooks-Gunn, J. (1979). *Social cognition and the acquisition of self.* New York: Plenum Press.

Lewis, M., & Miller, S. M. (Eds.). (1990). *Handbook of developmental psychopathology.* New York: Plenum Press.

Lewis, M., & Sullivan, M. W. (1985). Infant intelligence and its assessment. In B. B. Wolman (Ed.), *Handbook of intelligence* (pp. 505–599). New York: Wiley-Interscience.

Lewis, M., Sullivan, M. W., Stanger, C., & Weiss, M. (1989). Self development and self-conscious emotions. *Child Development, 60,* 146–156.

Lewis, M. D. (1993). Early socioemotional predictors of cognitive competence at 4 years. *Developmental Psychology, 29,* 1036–1045.

Lewkowicz, D. J. (1994). Limitations on infants' response to rate-based auditory-visual relations. *Developmental Psychology, 30,* 880–892.

Lichter, D. T., & Eggebeen, D. J. (1994). The effect of parental employment on child poverty. *Journal of Marriage and the Family, 56,* 633–645.

Lickona, T. (1978). Moral development and moral education. In J. M. Gallagher & J. A. Easley Jr. (Eds.), *Knowledge and development* (Vol. 2, pp. 21–74). New York: Plenum Press.

Lickona, T. (1983). *Raising good children.* Toronto: Bantam Books.

Lieberman, M., Doyle, A., & Markiewicz, D. (1995). *Attachment to mother and father: Links to peer relations in children.* Paper presented at the biennial meetings of the Society for Research in Child Development, Indianapolis.

Lillard, A. S., & Flavell, J. H. (1992). Young children's understanding of different mental states. *Developmental Psychology, 28,* 626–634.

Lindsay, R., Feldkamp, M., Harris, D., Robertson, J., & Rallison, M. (1994). Utah Growth Study: Growth standards and the prevalence of growth hormone deficiency. *Journal of Pediatrics, 125,* 29–35.

Linney, J. A., & Seidman, E. (1989). The future of schooling. *American Psychologist, 44,* 336–340.

Livesley, W. J., & Bromley, D. B. (1973). *Person perception in childhood and adolescence.* London: Wiley.

Lockman, J. J., & Thelen, E. (1993). Developmental biodynamics: Brain, body, behavior connections. *Child Development, 64,* 953–959.

Loehlin, J. C. (1992). *Genes and environment in personality development.* Newbury Park, CA: Sage.

Loehlin, J. C., Horn, J. M., & Willerman, L. (1994). Differential inheritance of mental abilities in the Texas Adoption Project. *Intelligence, 19,* 325–336.

Long, J. V. F., & Vaillant, G. E. (1984). Natural history of male psychological health: Escape from the underclass. *American Journal of Psychiatry, 141,* 341–346.

Longo, D. C., & Bond, L. (1984). Families of the handicapped child: Research and practice. *Family Relations, 33,* 57–65.

Lore, R. K., & Schultz, L. A. (1993). Control of human aggression: A comparative perspective. *American Psychologist, 48,* 16–25.

Lubinski, D., & Benbow, C. P. (1992). Gender differences in abilities and preferences among the gifted: Implications for the math-science pipeline. *Current Directions in Psychological Science, 1,* 61–66.

Luke, B., & Murtaugh, M. (1993). The racial disparity in very low birth weight. *New England Journal of Medicine, 328,* 285–286.

Luke, B., Williams, C., Minogue, J., & Keith, L. (1993). The changing pattern of infant mortality in the US: The role of prenatal factors and their obstetrical implications. *International Journal of Gynecology and Obstetrics, 40,* 199–212.

Lundh, W., & Gyllang, C. (1993). Use of the Edinburgh Postnatal Depression Scale in some Swedish child health care centres. *Scandinavian Journal of Caring Sciences, 7,* 149–154.

Luster, T., Boger, R., & Hannan, K. (1993). Infant affect and home environment. *Journal of Marriage and the Family, 55,* 651–661.

Luster, T., & Small, S. A. (1994). Factors associated with sexual risk-taking behaviors among adolescents. *Journal of Marriage and the Family, 56,* 622–632.

Luthar, S. S., & Zigler, E. (1992). Intelligence and social competence among high-risk adolescents. *Development and Psychopathology, 4,* 287–299.

Lykken, D. T., McGue, M., Tellegen, A., & Bouchard, T. J., Jr. (1992). Emergenesis. Genetic traits that may not run in families. *American Psychologist, 47,* 1565–1577.

Lyon, T. D., & Flavell, J. H. (1994). Young children's understanding of "remember" and "forget." *Child Development, 65,* 1357–1371.

Lyons, N. P. (1983). Two perspectives: On self, relationships, and morality. *Harvard Educational Review, 53,* 125–145.

Lytton, H., & Romney, D. M. (1991). Parents' differential socialization of boys and girls: A meta-analysis. *Psychological Bulletin, 109,* 267–296.

Maccoby, E. E. (1980). *Social development: Psychological growth and the parent-child relationship.* New York: Harcourt Brace Jovanovich.

Maccoby, E. E. (1984). Middle childhood in the context of the family. In W. A. Collins (Ed.), *Development during middle childhood: The years from six to twelve* (pp. 184–239). Washington, DC: National Academy Press.

Maccoby, E. E. (1988). Gender as a social category. *Developmental Psychology, 24,* 755–765.

Maccoby, E. E. (1990). Gender and relationships: A developmental account. *American Psychologist, 45,* 513–520.

Maccoby, E. E., & Jacklin, C. N. (1974). *The psychology of sex differences.* Stanford, CA: Stanford University Press.

Maccoby, E. E., & Jacklin, C. N. (1987). Gender segregation in childhood. In H. W. Reese (Ed.), *Advances in child development and behavior* (Vol. 20, pp. 239–288). Orlando, FL: Academic Press.

Maccoby, E. E., & Martin, J. A. (1983). Socialization in the context of the family: Parent-child interaction. In E. M. Hetherington (Ed.), *Handbook of child psychology: Socialization, personality, and social development* (Vol. 4, pp. 1–102). New York: Wiley.

MacDonald, K. (1992). Warmth as a developmental construct: An evolutionary analysis. *Child Development, 63,* 753–773.

Macfarlane, A. (1977). *The psychology of childbirth.* Cambridge, MA: Harvard University Press.

MacGowan, R. J., MacGowan, C. A., Serdula, M. K., Lane, J. M., Joesoef, R. M., & Cook, F. H. (1991). Breast-feeding among women attending women, infants, and children clinics in Georgia, 1987. *Pediatrics, 87,* 361–366.

MacIver, D. J., Reuman, D. A., & Main, S. R. (1995). Social structuring of the school: Studying what is, illuminating what could be. *Annual Review of Psychology, 46,* 375–400.

Mack, V., Urberg, K., Lou, Q., & Tolson, J. (1995). *Ethnic, gender and age differences in parent and peer orientation during adolescence.* Paper presented at the biennial meetings of the Society for Research in Child Development, Indianapolis.

Maclean, M., Bryant, P., & Bradley, L. (1987). Rhymes, nursery rhymes, and reading in early childhood. *Merrill-Palmer Quarterly, 33,* 255–281.

Madsen, W. (1969). Mexican Americans and Anglo Americans: A comparative study of mental health in Texas. In S. C. Plog & R. B. Edgerton (Eds.), *Changing perspectives in mental illness* (pp. 217–247). New York: Holt, Rinehart and Winston.

Maffeis, C., Schutz, Y., Piccoli, R., Gonfiantini, E., & Pinelli, L. (1993). Prevalence of obesity in children in north-east Italy. *International Journal of Obesity, 14,* 287–294.

Magnusson, D., Stattin, H., & Allen, V. L. (1986). Differential maturation among girls and its relation to social adjustment: A longitudinal perspective. In P. B. Baltes, D. L. Featherman, & R. M. Lerner (Eds.), *Life-span development and behavior* (Vol. 7, pp. 136–173). Hillsdale, NJ: Erlbaum.

Main, M., & Hesse, E. (1990). Parents' unresolved traumatic experiences are related to infant disorganized attachment status: Is frightened and/or frightening parental behavior the linking mechanism? In M. T. Greenberg, D. Cicchetti, & E. M. Cummings (Eds.), *Attachment in the preschool years: Theory, research, and intervention* (pp. 161–182). Chicago: University of Chicago Press.

Main, M., Kaplan, N., & Cassidy, J. (1985). Security in infancy, childhood, and adulthood: A move to the level of representation. *Monographs of the Society for Research in Child Development, 50*(Serial No. 209), 66–104.

Main, M., & Solomon, J. (1990). Procedures for identifying infants as disorganized/disoriented during the Ainsworth Strange Situation. In M. T. Greenberg, D. Cicchetti, & E. M. Cummings (Eds.), *Attachment in the preschool years: Theory, research, and intervention* (pp. 121–160). Chicago: University of Chicago Press.

Malina, R. M. (1982). Motor development in the early years. In S. G. Moore & C. R. Cooper (Eds.), *The young child: Reviews of research* (Vol. 3, pp. 211–232). Washington, DC: National Association for the Education of Young Children.

Malina, R. M. (1990). Physical growth and performance during the transition years. In R. Montemayor, G. R. Adams, & T. P. Gullotta (Eds.), *From childhood to adolescence: A transitional period?* (pp. 41–62). Newbury Park, CA: Sage.

Malinosky-Rummell, R., & Hansen, D. J. (1993). Long-term consequences of childhood physical abuse. *Psychological Bulletin, 114,* 68–79.

Mangelsdorf, S. C. (1992). Developmental changes in infant-stranger interaction. *Infant Behavior and Development, 15,* 191–208.

Maratsos, M. (1983). Some current issues in the study of the acquisition of grammar. In J. H. Flavell & E. M. Markman (Eds.), *Handbook of child psychology: Cognitive development* (pp. 707–786). New York: Wiley.

Marcia, J. E. (1966). Development and validation of ego identity status. *Journal of Personality and Social Psychology, 3,* 551–558.

Marcia, J. E. (1980). Identity in adolescence. In J. Adelson (Ed.), *Handbook of adolescent psychology* (pp. 159–187). New York: Wiley.

Marcus, G. F., Pinker, S., Ullman, M., Hollander, M., Rosen, T. J., & Fei, X. (1992). Overregularization in language acquisition. *Monographs of the Society for Research in Child Development, 57*(4, Serial No. 228).

Marcus, R. F. (1986). Naturalistic observation of cooperation, helping, and sharing and their association with empathy and affect. In C. Zahn-Waxler, E. M. Cummings, & R. Iannotti (Eds.), *Altruism and aggression: Biological and social origins* (pp. 256–279). Cambridge, England: Cambridge University Press.

Marean, G. C., Werner, L. A., & Kuhl, P. K. (1992). Vowel categorization by very young infants. *Developmental Psychology, 28,* 396–405.

Markman, E. M. (1992). Constraints on word learning: Speculations about their nature, origins, and domain specificity. In M. R. Gunnar & M. Maratsos (Eds.), *The Minnesota Symposia on Child Psychology* (Vol. 25, pp. 59–101). Hillsdale, NJ: Erlbaum.

Marschark, M. (1993). *Psychological development of deaf children.* New York: Oxford University Press.

Martin, C. L. (1991). The role of cognition in understanding gender effects. In H. W. Reese (Ed.), *Advances in child development and behavior* (Vol. 23, pp. 113–150). San Diego: Academic Press.

Martin, C. L. (1993). New directions for investigating children's gender knowledge. *Developmental Review, 13,* 184–204.

Martin, C. L., & Halverson C. F., Jr. (1981). A schematic processing model of sex typing and stereotyping in children. *Child Development, 52,* 1119–1134.

Martin, C. L., & Little, J. K. (1990). The relation of gender understanding to children's sex-typed preferences and gender stereotypes. *Child Development, 61,* 1427–1439.

Martin, C. L., Wood, C. H., & Little, J. K. (1990). The development of gender stereotype components. *Child Development, 61,* 1891–1904.

Martin, E. P., & Martin, J. M. (1978). *The black extended family.* Chicago: University of Chicago Press.

Martin, R. P., Wisenbaker, J., & Huttunen, M. (1994). Review of factor analytic studies of temperament measures based on the Thomas-Chess structural model: Implications for the Big Five. In C. F. Halverson Jr., G. A. Kohnstamm, & R. P. Martin (Eds.), *The developing structure of temperament and personality from infancy to adulthood* (pp. 157–172). Hillsdale, NJ: Erlbaum.

Martorano, S. C. (1977). A developmental analysis of performance on Piaget's formal operations tasks. *Developmental Psychology, 13,* 666–672.

Masataka, N. (1992). Motherese in a signed language. *Infant Behavior and Development, 15,* 453–460.

Mason, C. A., Cauce, A. M., Gonzales, N., Hiraga, Y., & Grove, K. (1994). An ecological model of externalizing behaviors in

African-American adolescents: No family is an island. *Journal of Research on Adolescence, 4,* 639–655.

Massad, C. M. (1981). Sex role identity and adjustment during adolescence. *Child Development, 52,* 1290–1298.

Masten, A. S. (1989). Resilience in development: Implications of the study of successful adaptation for developmental psychopathology. In D. Cicchetti (Ed.), *The emergence of a discipline: Rochester Symposium on Developmental Psychopathology* (Vol. 1, pp. 261–294). Hillsdale, NJ: Erlbaum.

Masten, A. S., Best, K. M., & Garmezy, N. (1990). Resilience and development: Contributions from the study of children who overcome adversity. *Development and Psychopathology, 2,* 425–444.

Matarazzo, J. D. (1992). Biological and physiological correlates of intelligence. *Intelligence, 16,* 257–258.

Mather, P. L., & Black, K. N. (1984). Heredity and environmental influences on preschool twins' language skills. *Developmental Psychology, 20,* 303–308.

Mathew, A., & Cook, M. (1990). The control of reaching movements by young infants. *Child Development, 61,* 1238–1257.

Maughan, B., Pickles, A., & Quinton, D. (1995). Parental hostility, childhood behavior, and adult social functioning. In J. McCord (Ed.), *Coercion and punishment in long-term perspectives* (pp. 34–58). Cambridge, England: Cambridge University Press.

Maurer, D., & Maurer, C. (1988). *The world of the newborn.* New York: Basic Books.

McAdoo, H. P. (Ed.). (1993). *Family ethnicity: Strength in diversity.* Newbury Park, CA: Sage.

McBride, G. (1991). Nontraditional inheritance: II. The clinical implications. *Mosaic, 22* (Fall), 12–25.

McCall, R. B. (1993). Developmental functions for general mental performance. In D. K. Detterman (Ed.), *Current topics in human intelligence: Vol. 3. Individual differences and cognition* (pp. 3–30). Norwood, NJ: Ablex.

McCall, R. B., Evahn, C., & Kratzer, L. (1992). *High school underachievers.* Newbury Park, CA: Sage.

McCarthy, J., & Hardy, J. (1993). Age at first birth and birth outcomes. *Journal of Research on Adolescence, 3,* 374–392.

McCord, J. (1982). A longitudinal view of the relationship between parental absence and crime. In J. Gunn & D. P. Farrington (Eds.), *Abnormal offenders, delinquency, and the criminal justice system* (pp. 113–128). London: Wiley.

McCord, J. (1991). Questioning the value of punishment. *Social Problems, 38,* 167–178.

McCord, W., McCord, J., & Zola, I. K. (1959). *Origins of crime.* New York: Columbia University Press.

McCrae, R. R., & John, O. P. (1992). An introduction to the Five-Factor Model and its applications. *Journal of Personality, 60,* 175–215.

McCune, L. (1995). A normative study of representational play at the transition to language. *Developmental Psychology, 31,* 198–206.

McFalls, J. A., Jr. (1990). The risks of reproductive impairment in the later years of childbearing. *Annual Review of Sociology, 16,* 491–519.

McGue, M. (1994). Why developmental psychology should find room for behavior genetics. In C. A. Nelson (Ed.), *The Minnesota Symposia on Child Development* (Vol. 27, pp. 105–119). Hillsdale, NJ: Erlbaum.

McGue, M., & Lykken, D. T. (1992). Genetic influence on risk of divorce. *Psychological Science, 3,* 368–373.

McHale, S. M., & Lerner, R. M. (1990). Stages of human development. In R. M. Thomas (Ed.), *The encyclopedia of human development and education* (pp. 163–166). Oxford: Pergamon Press.

McLanahan, S., & Sandefur, G. (1994). *Growing up with a single parent: What hurts, what helps.* Cambridge, MA: Harvard University Press.

McLaughlin, B. (1984). *Second-language acquisition in childhood: Vol. 1. Preschool children* (2nd ed.). Hillsdale, NJ: Erlbaum.

McLoyd, V. C., Jayaratne, T. E., Ceballo, R., & Borquez, J. (1994). Unemployment and work interruption among African American single mothers: Effects on parenting and adolescent socioemotional functioning. *Child Development, 65,* 562–589.

McLoyd, V., & Wilson, L. (1991). The strain of living poor: Parenting, social support, and child mental health. In A. C. Huston (Ed.), *Children in poverty: Child development and public policy* (pp. 105–135). Cambridge, England: Cambridge University Press.

McCrae, R. R., & Costa, P. T., Jr. (1990). *Personality in adulthood.* New York: Guilford Press.

Mehana, M., & Reynolds, A. J. (1995). *The effects of school mobility on scholastic achievement.* Paper presented at the biennial meetings of the Society for Research on Child Development, Indianapolis.

Melson, G. F., Ladd, G. W., & Hsu, H. (1993). Maternal support networks, maternal cognitions, and young children's social and cognitive development. *Child Development 64,* 1401–1417.

Meltzoff, A. N. (1988). Infant imitation and memory: Nine-month-olds in immediate and deferred tasks. *Child Development, 59,* 217–225.

Meltzoff, A. N., & Borton, R. W. (1979). Intermodal matching by human neonates. *Nature, 282,* 403–404.

Menaghan, E. G., & Parcel, T. L. (1995). Social sources of change in children's home environments: The effects of parental occupational experiences and family conditions. *Journal of Marriage and the Family, 57,* 69–84.

Merikangas, K. R., & Angst, J. (1995). The challenge of depressive disorders in adolescence. In M. Rutter (Ed.), *Psychosocial disturbances in young people: Challenges for prevention* (pp. 131–165). Cambridge, England: Cambridge University Press.

Mervis, C. B., & Bertrand, J. (1994). Acquisition of the novel name–nameless category (N3C) principle. *Child Development, 65,* 1646–1662.

Mervis, C. B., Bertrand, J., Robinson, B. F., Armstrong, S. C., Klein, B. P., Turner, N. D., Baker, D. E., & Reinberg, J. (1995). *Early language development of children with Williams syndrome.* Paper presented at the biennial meetings of the Society for Research in Child Development, Indianapolis.

Mervis, C. B., & Mervis, C. A. (1982). Leopards are kitty-cats: Object labeling by mothers for their thirteen-month-olds. *Child Development, 53,* 267–273.

Meyer-Bahlburg, H. F. L., Ehrhardt, A. A., & Feldman, J. F. (1986). Long-term implications of the prenatal endocrine milieu for sex-dimorphic behavior. In L. Erlenmeyer-Kimling & N. E. Miller (Eds.), *Life-span research on the prediction of psychopathology* (pp. 17–30). Hillsdale, NJ: Erlbaum.

Meyer-Bahlburg, H. F. L., Ehrhardt, A. A., Rosen, L. R., Gruen, R. S., Veridiano, N. P., Vann, F. H., & Neuwalder, H. F. (1995). Prenatal estrogens and the development of homosexual orientation. *Developmental Psychology, 31,* 12–21.

Miller, B. C., Christopherson, C. R., & King, P. K. (1993). Sexual behavior in adolescence. In T. P. Gullotta, G. R. Adams, & R. Montemayor (Eds.), *Adolescent sexuality* (pp. 57–76). Newbury Park, CA: Sage.

Miller, B. C., & Moore, K. A. (1990). Adolescent sexual behavior, pregnancy, and parenting: Research through the 1980s. *Journal of Marriage and the Family, 52,* 1025–1044.

Miller, K. E., & Pedersen-Randall, P. (1995). *Work, farm work, academic achievement and friendship: A comparison of rural and urban 10th, 11th and 12th graders.* Paper presented at the biennial meetings of the Society for Research in Child Development, Indianapolis.

Mischel, W. (1966). A social learning view of sex differences in behavior. In E. E. Maccoby (Ed.), *The development of sex differences* (pp. 56–81). Stanford, CA: Stanford University Press.

Mischel, W. (1970). Sex typing and socialization. In P. H. Mussen (Ed.), *Carmichael's manual of child psychology* (Vol. 2, pp. 3–72). New York: Wiley.

Mitchell, E. A., Ford, R. P. K., Steward, A. W., Taylor, B. J., Becroft, D. M. O., Thompson, J. M. D., Scragg, R., Hassall, I. B., Barry, D. M. J., Allen, E. M., & Roberts, A. P. (1993). Smoking and sudden infant death syndrome. *Pediatrics, 91,* 893–896.

Mitchell, P. R., & Kent, R. D. (1990). Phonetic variation in multisyllable babbling. *Journal of Child Language, 17,* 247–265.

Mitchell, R. (1992). *Testing for learning: How new approaches to evaluation can improve American schools.* New York: Free Press.

Moffitt, T. E. (1990). Juvenile delinquency and attention deficit disorder: Boys' developmental trajectories from age 3 to age 15. *Child Development, 61,* 893–910.

Money, J. (1987). Sin, sickness, or status? Homosexual gender identity and psychoneuroendocrinology. *American Psychologist, 42,* 384–399.

Montemayor, R., Adams, G. R., & Gullotta, T. P. (Eds.). (1994). *Personal relationships during adolescence.* Thousand Oaks, CA: Sage.

Montemayor, R., & Eisen, M. (1977). The development of self-conceptions from childhood to adolescence. *Developmental Psychology, 13,* 314–319.

Montpetit, R. R., Montoye, H. J., & Laeding, L. (1967). Grip strength of school children, Saginaw, Michigan—1964. *Research Quarterly, 38,* 231–240.

Moon, C., & Fifer, W. P. (1990). Syllables as signals for 2-day-old infants. *Infant Behavior and Development, 13,* 377–390.

Moore, E. G. J. (1986). Family socialization and the IQ test performance of traditionally and transracially adopted black children. *Developmental Psychology, 22,* 317–326.

Moore, K. A., Myers, D. E., Morrison, D. R., Nord, C. W., Brown, B., & Edmonston, B. (1993). Age at first childbirth and later poverty. *Journal of Research on Adolescence, 3,* 393–422.

Moore, K. L., & Persaud, T. V. N. (1993). *The developing human: Clinically oriented embryology* (5th ed.). Philadelphia: W. B. Saunders.

Morgan, J. L. (1994). Converging measures of speech segmentation in preverbal infants. *Infant Behavior and Development, 17,* 389–403.

Morgan, J. L., Bonamo, K. M., & Travis, L. L. (1995). Negative evidence on negative evidence. *Developmental Psychology, 31,* 180–197.

Morgan, M. (1982). Television and adolescents' sex role stereotypes: A longitudinal study. *Journal of Personality and Social Psychology, 43,* 947–955.

Morgan, M. (1987). Television, sex-role attitudes, and sex-role behavior. *Journal of Early Adolescence, 7,* 269–282.

Morrison, D. M. (1985). Adolescent contraceptive behavior: A review. *Psychological Bulletin, 98,* 538–568.

Morrongiello, B. A. (1988). Infants' localization of sounds along the horizontal axis: Estimates of minimum audible angle. *Developmental Psychology, 24,* 8–13.

Morrongiello, B. A., Fenwick, K. D., & Chance, G. (1990). Sound localization acuity in very young infants: An observer-based testing procedure. *Developmental Psychology, 26,* 75–84.

Morse, P. A., & Cowan, N. (1982). Infant auditory and speech perception. In T. M. Field, A. Houston, H. C. Quay, L. Troll, & G. E. Finley (Eds.), *Review of human development* (pp. 32–61). New York: Wiley.

Mortimer, J. T., Finch, M. D., Dennehy, K., Lee, C., & Beebe, T. (1995). *Work experience in adolescence.* Paper presented at the biennial meetings of the Society for Research in Child Development, Indianapolis.

Muller, C. (1995). Maternal employment, parent involvement, and mathematics achievement among adolescents. *Journal of Marriage and the Family, 57,* 85–100.

Munro, G., & Adams, G. R. (1977). Ego-identity formation in college students and working youth. *Developmental Psychology, 13,* 523–524.

Munroe, R. H., Shimmin, H. S., & Munroe, R. L. (1984). Gender understanding and sex role preference in four cultures. *Developmental Psychology, 20,* 673–682.

Murray, J. L., & Bernfield, M. (1988). The differential effect of prenatal care on the incidence of low birth weight among blacks and whites in a prepaid health care plan. *New England Journal of Medicine, 319,* 1385–1391.

Murray, J. P. (1980). *Television & youth. 25 years of research and controversy.* Stanford, CA: The Boys Town Center for the Study of Youth Development.

Musick, J. S. (1994). Capturing the childrearing context. *Society for Research in Child Development Newsletter* (Fall), 1, 6–7.

Myers, B. J. (1987). Mother-infant bonding as a critical period. In M. H. Bornstein (Ed.), *Sensitive periods in development: Interdisciplinary perspectives* (pp. 223–246). Hillsdale, NJ: Erlbaum.

Nachmias, M. (1993). *Maternal personality relations with toddler's attachment classification, use of coping strategies, and adrenocortical stress response.* Paper presented at the biennial meetings of the Society for Research in Child Development, New Orleans.

Neimark, E. D. (1982). Adolescent thought: Transition to formal operations. In B. B. Wolman (Ed.), *Handbook of developmental psychology* (pp. 486–502). Englewood Cliffs, NJ: Prentice Hall.

Nelson, C. A. (1987). The recognition of facial expression in the first two years of life: Mechanisms of development. *Child Development, 58,* 889–909.

Nelson, C. A. (1994). Neural bases of infant temperament. In J. E. Bates & T. D. Wachs (Eds.), *Temperament. Individual differences at the interface of biology and behavior* (pp. 47–82). Washington, DC: American Psychological Association.

Nelson, K. (1973). Structure and strategy in learning to talk. *Monographs of the Society for Research in Child Development, 38*(Serial No. 149).

Nelson, K. (1977). Facilitating children's syntax acquisition. *Developmental Psychology, 13,* 101–107.

Nelson, K. (1985). *Making sense: The acquisition of shared meaning.* New York: Academic Press.

Nelson, K. (1988). Constraints on word learning. *Cognitive Development, 3,* 221–246.

Newcomb, A. F., & Bagwell, C. L. (1995). Children's friendship relations: A meta-analytic review. *Psychological Bulletin, 117,* 306–347.

Newcomb, A. F., Bukowski, W. M., & Pattee, L. (1993). Children's peer relations: A meta-analytic review of popular, rejected, neglected, controversial, and average sociometric status. *Psychological Bulletin, 113,* 99–128.

Newcombe, N. S., & Baenninger, M. (1989). Biological change and cognitive ability in adolescence. In G. R. Adams, R. Montemayor, & T. P. Gullotta (Eds.), *Biology of adolescent behavior and development* (pp. 168–194). Newbury Park, CA: Sage.

New York Times, The (1994, September 14). Students cite pregnancies as a reason to drop out, p. B7.

Nightingale, E. O., & Goodman, M. (1990). *Before birth: Prenatal testing for genetic disease.* Cambridge, MA: Harvard University Press.

Nilsson, L. (1990). *A child is born.* New York: Delacorte Press.

Nisan, M., & Kohlberg, L. (1982). Universality and variation in moral judgment: A longitudinal and cross-sectional study in Turkey. *Child Development, 53,* 865–876.

Nolen-Hoeksema, S. (1994). An interactive model for the emergence of gender differences in depression in adolescence. *Journal of Research on Adolescence, 4,* 519–534.

Nolen-Hoeksema, S., & Girgus, J. S. (1994). The emergence of gender differences in depression during adolescence. *Psychological Bulletin, 115,* 424–443.

Nottelmann, E. D., Susman, E. J., Blue, J. H., Inoff-Germain, G., Dorn, L. D., Loriaux, D. L., Cutler, G. B., Jr., & Chrousos, G. P. (1987). Gonadal and adrenal hormone correlates of adjustment in early adolescence. In R. M. Lerner & T. T. Foch (Eds.), *Biological-psychosocial interactions in early adolescence* (pp. 303–324). Hillsdale, NJ: Erlbaum.

Notzon, F. C., Cnattingius, S., Pergsjø, P., Cole, S., Taffel, S., Irgens, L., & Dalveit, A. K. (1994). Cesarean section delivery in the 1980s: International comparison by indication. *American Journal of Obstetrics and Gynecology, 170,* 495–504.

Novacek, J., Raskin, R., & Hogan, R. (1991). Why do adolescents use drugs? Age, sex, and user differences. *Journal of Youth and Adolescence, 20,* 475–492.

Nowakowski, R. S. (1987). Basic concepts of CNS development. *Child Development, 58,* 568–595.

Nsamenang, A. B., & Lamb, M. E. (1994). Socialization of Nso children in the Bamenda grassfields of northwest Cameroon. In P. M. Greenfield & R. R. Cocking (Eds.), *Cross-cultural roots of minority child development* (pp. 133–146). Hillsdale, NJ: Erlbaum.

O'Beirne, H., & Moore, C. (1995). *Attachment and sexual behavior in adolescence.* Paper presented at the biennial meetings of the Society for Research in Child Development, Indianapolis.

O'Brien, M. (1992). Gender identity and sex roles. In V. B. Van Hasselt & M. Hersen (Eds.), *Handbook of social development. A lifespan perspective* (pp. 325–345). New York: Plenum Press.

O'Brien, S. F., & Bierman, K. L. (1988). Conceptions and perceived influence of peer groups: Interviews with preadolescents and adolescents. *Child Development, 59,* 1360–1365.

O'Connor, S., Vietze, P. M., Sandler, H. M., Sherrod, K. B., & Altemeier, W. A. (1980). Quality of parenting and the mother-infant relationships following rooming-in. In P. M. Taylor (Ed.), *Parent-infant relationships* (pp. 349–368). New York: Grune & Stratton.

Offord, D. R., Boyle, M. H., & Racine, Y. A. (1991). The epidemiology of antisocial behavior in childhood and adolescence. In D. J. Pepler & K. H. Rubin (Eds.), *The development and treatment of childhood aggression* (pp. 31–54). Hillsdale, NJ: Erlbaum.

Ogbu, J. U. (1994). From cultural differences to differences in cultural frame of reference. In P. M. Greenfield & R. R. Cocking (Eds.), *Cross-cultural roots of minority child development* (pp. 365–391). Hillsdale, NJ: Erlbaum.

O'Hara, M. W., Schlechte, J. A., Lewis, D. A., & Varner, M. W. (1992). Controlled prospective study of postpartum mood disorders: Psychological, environmental, and hormonal variables. *Journal of Abnormal Psychology, 100,* 63–73.

Okamoto, E., Davidson, L. L., & Conner, D. R. (1993). High prevalence of overweight in inner-city schoolchildren. *American Journal of Diseases of Children, 147,* 155–159.

Oller, D. K. (1981). Infant vocalizations: Exploration and reflectivity. In R. E. Stark (Ed.), *Language behavior in infancy and early childhood* (pp. 85–104). New York: Elsevier/North-Holland.

Olshan, A. F., Baird, P. A., & Teschke, K. (1989). Paternal occupational exposures and the risk of Down syndrome. *American Journal of Human Genetics, 44,* 646–651.

Olson, H. C., Sampson, P. D., Barr, H., Streissguth, A. P., & Bookstein, F. L. (1992). Prenatal exposure to alcohol and school problems in late childhood: A longitudinal prospective study. *Development and Psychopathology, 4,* 341–359.

Olson, S. L., Bates, J. E., & Kaskie, B. (1992). Caregiver-infant interaction antecedents of children's school-age cognitive ability. *Merrill-Palmer Quarterly, 38,* 309–330.

O'Neill, D. K., Astington, J. W., & Flavell, J. H. (1992). Young children's understanding of the role that sensory experiences play in knowledge acquisition. *Child Development, 63,* 474–490.

Osofsky, J. D. (Ed.). (1987). *Handbook of infant development.* New York: Wiley-Interscience.

Osofsky, J. D., Hann, D. M., & Peebles, C. (1993). Adolescent parenthood: Risks and opportunities for mothers and infants. In C. H. Zeanah, Jr. (Ed.), *Handbook of infant mental health* (pp. 106–119). New York: Guilford Press.

Overton, W. F., & Reese, H. W. (1973). Models of development: Methodological implications. In J. R. Nesselroade & H. W. Reese (Eds.), *Life-span developmental psychology: Methodological issues* (pp. 65–86). New York: Academic Press.

Overton, W. F., Ward, S. L., Noveck, I. A., Black, J., & O'Brien, D. P. (1987). Form and content in the development of deductive reasoning. *Developmental Psychology, 23,* 22–30.

Padilla, A. M., Lindholm, K. J., Chen, A., Duran, R., Hakuta, K., Lambert, W., & Tucker, G. R. (1991). The English-only movement: Myths, reality, and implications for psychology. *American Psychologist, 46,* 120–130.

Page, D. C., Mosher, R., Simpson, E. M., Fisher, E. M. C., Mardon, G., Pollack, J., McGillivray, B., de la Chapelle, A., & Brown, L. G. (1987). The sex-determining region of the human Y chromosome encodes a finger protein. *Cell, 51,* 1091–1104.

Paik, H., & Comstock, G. (1994). The effects of television violence on antisocial behavior: A meta-analysis. *Communication Research, 21,* 516–546.

Paikoff, R. L., & Brooks-Gunn, J. (1990). Physiological processes: What role do they play during the transition to adolescence? In R. Montemayor, G. R. Adams, & T. P. Gullotta (Eds.), *From childhood to adolescence: A transitional period?* (pp. 63–81). Newbury Park, CA: Sage.

Palkovitz, R. (1985). Fathers' birth attendance, early contact, and extended contact with their newborns: A critical review. *Child Development, 56,* 392–406.

Palla, B., & Litt, I. R. (1988). Medical complications of eating disorders in adolescents. *Pediatrics, 81,* 613–623.

Panel on High Risk Youth (1993). *Losing generations: Adolescents in high risk settings.* Commission on Behavioral and Social Sciences and Education, National Research Council. Washington, DC: National Academy Press.

Papousek, H., & Papousek, M. (1991). Innate and cultural guidance of infants' integrative competencies: China, the United States, and Germany. In M. H. Bornstein (Ed.), *Cultural approaches to parenting* (pp. 23–44). Hillsdale, NJ: Erlbaum.

Parcel, T. L., & Menaghan, E. G. (1994). *Parents' jobs and children's lives.* New York: Aldine de Gruyter.

Parke, R. D., & Tinsley, B. R. (1981). The father's role in infancy: Determinants of involvement in caregiving and play. In M. E. Lamb (Ed.), *The role of the father in child development* (2nd ed.) (pp. 429–458). New York: Wiley.

Parke, R. D., & Tinsley, B. R. (1984). Fatherhood: Historical and contemporary perspectives. In K. A. McCluskey & H. W. Reese (Eds.), *Life-span developmental psychology: Historical and generational effects* (pp. 203–248). Orlando, FL: Academic Press.

Parmelee, A. H., Jr. (1986). Children's illnesses: Their beneficial effects on behavioral development. *Child Development, 57,* 1–10.

Parmelee, A. H., Jr., Wenner, W. H., & Schulz, H. R. (1964). Infant sleep patterns from birth to 16 weeks of age. *Journal of Pediatrics, 65,* 576–582.

Parsons, J. E., Adler, T. F., & Daczala, C. M. (1982). Socialization of achievement attitudes and beliefs: Parental influences. *Child Development, 53,* 310–321.

Passman, R. H., & Longeway, K. P. (1982). The role of vision in maternal attachment: Giving 2-year-olds a photograph of their mother during separation. *Developmental Psychology, 18,* 530–533.

Patterson, G. R. (1975). *Families: Applications of social learning to family life.* Champaign, IL: Research Press.

Patterson, G. R., Capaldi, D., & Bank, L. (1991). An early starter model for predicting delinquency. In D. J. Pepler & K. H. Rubin (Eds.), *The development and treatment of childhood aggression* (pp. 139–168). Hillsdale, NJ: Erlbaum.

Patterson, G. R., DeBarsyshe, B. D., & Ramsey, E. (1989). A developmental perspective on antisocial behavior. *American Psychologist, 44,* 329–335.

Paxton, S. J., Wertheim, E. H., Gibbons, K., Szmukler, G. I., Hillier, L., & Petrovich, J. L. (1991). Body image satisfaction, dieting beliefs, and weight loss behaviors in adolescent girls and boys. *Journal of Youth and Adolescence, 20,* 361–379.

Peckham, C. S. (1994). Human immunodeficiency virus infection and pregnancy. *Sexually Transmitted Diseases, 21*(No. 2 Suppl.), S28–S31.

Pedersen, N. L., Plomin, R., McClearn, G. E., & Friberg, L. (1988). Neuroticism, extraversion and related traits in adult twins reared apart and reared together. *Journal of Personality and Social Psychology, 55,* 950–957.

Pederson, D. R., Moran, G., Sitko, C., Campbell, K., Ghesquire, K., & Acton, H. (1990). Maternal sensitivity and the security of infant-mother attachment: A Q-sort study. *Child Development, 61,* 1974–1983.

Pedlow, R., Sanson, A., Prior, M., & Oberklaid, F. (1993). Stability of maternally reported temperament from infancy to 8 years. *Developmental Psychology, 29,* 998–1007.

Pegg, J. E., Werker, J. F., & McLeod, P. J. (1992). Preference for infant-directed over adult-directed speech: Evidence from 7-week-old infants. *Infant Behavior and Development, 15,* 325–345.

Penrod, S. (1993). The child witness, the courts, and psychological research. In C. A. Nelson (Ed.), *The Minnesota Symposia on Child Psychology* (Vol. 26, pp. 159–170). Hillsdale, NJ: Erlbaum.

Perlman, M., Claris, O., Hao, Y., Pandid, P., Whyte, H., Chipman, M., & Liu, P. (1995). Secular changes in the outcomes to eighteen to twenty-four months of age of extremely low birth weight infants, with adjustment for changes in risk factors and severity of illness. *Journal of Pediatrics, 126,* 75–87.

Perner, J., & Wimmer, H. (1985). "John thinks that Mary thinks that . . .": Attribution of second-order beliefs by 5- to 10-year-old children. *Journal of Experimental Child Psychology, 39,* 437–471.

Petersen, A. C. (1987). The nature of biological-psychosocial interactions: The sample case of early adolescence. In R. M. Lerner & T. T. Foch (Eds.), *Biological-psychosocial interactions in early adolescence* (pp. 35–62). Hillsdale, NJ: Erlbaum.

Petersen, A. C., Compas, B. C., Brooks-Gunn, J., Stemmler, M., Ey, S., & Grant, K. E. (1993). Depression in adolescence. *American Psychologist, 48,* 155–168.

Petersen, A. C., Sarigiani, P. A., & Kennedy, R. E. (1991). Adolescent depression: Why more girls? *Journal of Youth and Adolescence, 20,* 247–272.

Petersen, A. C., & Taylor, B. (1980). The biological approach to adolescence. In J. Adelson (Ed.), *Handbook of adolescent psychology* (pp. 117–158). New York: Wiley.

Peterson, G. H., Mehl, L. E., & Leiderman, P. H. (1979). The role of some birth-related variables in father attachment. *American Journal of Orthopsychiatry, 49,* 330–338.

Petitto, L. A. (1988). "Language" in the prelinguistic child. In F. S. Kessell (Ed.), *The development of language and language researchers: Essays in honor of Roger Brown* (pp. 187–222). Hillsdale, NJ: Erlbaum.

Phinney, J. S. (1990). Ethnic identity in adolescents and adults: Review of research. *Psychological Bulletin, 108,* 499–514.

Phinney, J. S., & Rosenthal, D. A. (1992). Ethnic identity in adolescence: Process, context, and outcome. In G. R. Adams, T. P. Gullotta, & R. Montemayor (Eds.), *Adolescent identity formation* (pp. 145–172). Newbury Park, CA: Sage.

Piaget, J. (1932). *The moral judgment of the child.* New York: Macmillan.

Piaget, J. (1952). *The origins of intelligence in children.* New York: International Universities Press.

Piaget, J. (1954). *The construction of reality in the child.* New York: Basic Books. (Originally published 1937.)

Piaget, J. (1970). Piaget's theory. In P. H. Mussen (Ed.), *Carmichael's manual of child psychology* (Vol. 1, 3rd ed.) (pp. 703–732). New York: Wiley.

Piaget, J. (1977). *The development of thought: Equilibration of cognitive structures.* New York: Viking Press.

Piaget, J., & Inhelder, B. (1959). *La gènese des structures logiques élémentaires: Classifications et seriations [The origin of elementary logical structures: Classification and seriation].* Neuchâtel: Delachaux et Niestlé.

Piaget, J., & Inhelder, B. (1969). *The psychology of the child.* New York: Basic Books.

Pianta, R. C., & Egeland, B. (1994). Predictors of instability in children's mental test performance at 24, 48, and 96 months. *Intelligence, 18,* 145–163.

Pianta, R., Egeland, B., & Erickson, M. F. (1989). The antecedents of maltreatment: Results of the Mother-Child Interaction Research Project. In D. Cicchetti & V. Carlson (Eds.), *Child maltreatment* (pp. 203–253). Cambridge, England: Cambridge University Press.

Pick, H. L., Jr. (1986). Reflections on the data and theory of cross-modal infancy research. In L. P. Lipsitt & C. Rovee-Collier (Eds.), *Advances in infancy research* (Vol. 4, pp. 230–239). Norwood, NJ: Ablex.

Pickens, J. (1994). Perception of auditory-visual distance relations by 5-month-old infants. *Developmental Psychology, 30,* 537–544.

Pickens, J., & Field, T. (1993). Facial expressivity in infants of depressed mothers. *Developmental Psychology, 29,* 986–988.

Pinker, S. (1987). The bootstrapping problem in language acquisition. In B. MacWhinney (Ed.), *Mechanisms of language acquisition* (pp. 399–442). Hillsdale, NJ: Erlbaum.

Pinker, S. (1994). *The language instinct: How the mind creates language.* New York: Morrow.

Plomin, R. (1989). Environment and genes: Determinants of behavior. *American Psychologist, 44,* 105–111.

Plomin, R. (1995). Genetics and children's experiences in the family. *Journal of Child Psychology and Psychiatry, 36,* 33–68.

Plomin, R., & DeFries, J. C. (1985). *Origins of individual differences in infancy: The Colorado Adoption Project.* Orlando, FL: Academic Press.

Plomin, R., Emde, R. N., Braungart, J. M., Campos, J., Corley, R., Fulker, D. W., Kagan, J., Reznick, J. S., Robinson, J., Zahn-Waxler, C., & DeFries, J. C. (1993). Genetic change and continuity from fourteen to twenty months: The MacArthur longitudinal twin study. *Child Development, 64,* 1354–1376.

Plomin, R., Loehlin, J. C., & DeFries, J. C. (1985). Genetic and environmental components of "environmental" influences. *Developmental Psychology, 21,* 391–402.

Plomin, R., & McClearn, G. E. (Eds.). (1993). *Nature, nurture & psychology.* Washington, DC: American Psychological Association.

Plomin, R., Reiss, D., Hetherington, E. M., & Howe, G. W. (1994). Nature and nurture: Genetic contributions to measures of the family environment. *Developmental Psychology, 30,* 32–43.

Plomin, R., & Rende, R. (1991). Human behavioral genetics. *Annual Review of Psychology, 42,* 161–190.

Plumert, J. M. (1994). Flexibility in children's use of spatial and categorical organizational strategies in recall. *Developmental Psychology, 30,* 738–747.

Polka, L., & Werker, J. F. (1994). Developmental changes in perception of nonnative vowel contrasts. *Journal of Experimental Psychology: Human Perception and Performance, 20,* 421–435.

Pollitt, E., & Gorman, K. S. (1994). Nutritional deficiencies as developmental risk factors. In C. A. Nelson (Ed.), *The Minnesota Symposia on Child Development* (Vol. 27, pp. 121–144). Hillsdale, NJ: Erlbaum.

Ponsonby, A., Dwyer, T., Gibbons, L. E., Cochrane, J. A., & Wang, Y. (1993). Factors potentiating the risk of sudden infant death syndrome associated with the prone position. *New England Journal of Medicine, 329,* 377–382.

Poole, D. A., & Warren, A. R. (1995). *Recent challenges to three commonly held assumptions about children's eyewitness testimony.* Paper presented at the biennial meetings of the Society for Research in Child Development, Indianapolis.

Poole, D. A., & White, L. T. (1993). Two years later: Effects of question repetition and retention interval on the eyewitness testimony of children and adults. *Developmental Psychology, 29,* 844–853.

Porter, J. R., & Washington, R. E. (1993). Minority identity and self-esteem. *Annual Review of Sociology, 19,* 139–161.

Poulin-Dubois, D., Serbin, L. A., Kenyon, B., & Derbyshire, A. (1994). Infants' intermodal knowledge about gender. *Developmental Psychology, 30,* 436–442.

Poulson, C. L., Nunes, L. R. D., & Warren, S. F. (1989). Imitation in infancy: A critical review. In H. W. Reese (Ed.), *Advances in child development and behavior* (Vol. 22, pp. 272–298). San Diego: Academic Press.

Powell, B., & Steelman, L. C. (1982). Testing an undertested comparison: Maternal effects on sons' and daughters' attitudes toward women in the labor force. *Journal of Marriage and the Family, 44,* 349–355.

Powlishta, K. K., Serbin, L. A., Doyle, A., & White, D. R. (1994). Gender, ethnic, and body type biases: The generality of prejudice in childhood. *Developmental Psychology, 30,* 526–536.

Prechtl, H. F. R., & Beintema, D. J. (1964). *The neurological examination of the full-term newborn infant: Clinics in Developmental Medicine, 12.* London: Hinemann.

Pulkkinen, L. (1982). Self-control and continuity from childhood to late adolescence. In P. Baltes & O. G. Brim, Jr. (Eds.), *Life span development and behavior* (Vol. 4, pp. 64–107). New York: Academic Press.

Pye, C. (1986). Quiche Mayan speech to children. *Journal of Child Language, 13,* 85–100.

Quiggle, N. L., Garber, J., Panak, W. F., & Dodge, K. A. (1992). Social information processing in aggressive and depressed children. *Child Development, 63,* 1305–1320.

Raja, S. N., McGee, R., & Stanton, W. R. (1992). Perceived attachments to parents and peers and psychological well-being in adolescence. *Journal of Youth and Adolescence, 21,* 471–485.

Ramey, C. T. (1993). A rejoinder to Spitz's critique of the Abecedarian experiment. *Intelligence, 17,* 25–30.

Ramey, C. T., & Campbell, F. A. (1987). The Carolina Abecedarian Project: An educational experiment concerning human malleability. In J. J. Gallagher & C. T. Ramey (Eds.), *The malleability of children* (pp. 127–140). Baltimore: Paul H. Brookes.

Rappoport, L. (1972). *Personality development: The chronology of experience.* Glenview, IL: Scott, Foresman.

Ree, M. J., & Earles, J. A. (1992). Intelligence is the best predictor of job performance. *Current Directions in Psychological Science, 1,* 86–89.

Reinherz, H. Z., Giaconia, R. M., Pakiz, B., Silverman, A. B., Frost, A. K., & Lefkowitz, E. S. (1993). Psychosocial risks for major depression in late adolescence: A longitudinal community study. *Journal of the American Academy of Child and Adolescent Psychiatry, 32,* 1155–1163.

Reisman, J. E. (1987). Touch, motion, and proprioception. In P. Salapatek & L. Cohen (Eds.), *Handbook of infant perception: Vol. 1. From sensation to perception* (pp. 265–304). Orlando, FL: Academic Press.

Reisman, J. M., & Shorr, S. I. (1978). Friendship claims and expectations among children and adults. *Child Development, 49,* 913–916.

Remafedi, G. (1987a). Adolescent homosexuality: Psychosocial and medical implications. *Pediatrics, 79,* 331–337.

Remafedi, G. (1987b). Male homosexuality: The adolescent's perspective. *Pediatrics, 79,* 326–330.

Remafedi, G., Farrow, J. A., & Deisher, R. W. (1991). Risk factors for attempted suicide in gay and bisexual youth. *Pediatrics, 87,* 869–875.

Remafedi, G., Resnick, M., Blum, R., & Harris, L. (1992). Demography of sexual orientation in adolescents. *Pediatrics, 89,* 714–721.

Renouf, A. G., & Harter, S. (1990). Low self-worth and anger as components of the depressive experience in young adolescents. *Development and Psychopathology, 2,* 293–310.

Report of National Institute (1993). Report of National Institute of Child Health and Human Development workshop on Chorionic Villus Sampling and limb and other defects, October 20, 1992. *Teratology, 48,* 7–13.

Rest, J. R. (1983). Morality. In J. H. Flavell & E. M. Markman (Eds.), *Handbook of child psychology: Cognitive development* (Vol. 3, pp. 556–629). New York: Wiley.

Rest, J. R., & Thoma, S. J. (1985). Relation of moral judgment development to formal education. *Developmental Psychology, 21,* 709–714.

Reynolds, A. J. (1994). Effects of a preschool plus follow-on intervention for children at risk. *Developmental Psychology, 30,* 787–804.

Reynolds, A. J., & Bezruczko, N. (1993). School adjustment of children at risk through fourth grade. *Merrill-Palmer Quarterly, 39,* 457–480.

Rholes, W. S., & Ruble, D. N. (1984). Children's understanding of dispositional characteristics of others. *Child Development, 55,* 550–560.

Ricciuti, H. N. (1993). Nutrition and mental development. *Current Directions in Psychological Science, 2,* 43–46.

Rice, M. L., Huston, A. C., Truglio, R., & Wright, J. (1990). Words from "Sesame Street": Learning vocabulary while viewing. *Developmental Psychology, 26,* 421–428.

Richards, H. C., Bear, G. G., Stewart, A. L., & Norman, A. D. (1992). Moral reasoning and classroom conduct: Evidence of a curvilinear relationship. *Merrill-Palmer Quarterly, 38,* 176–190.

Richardson, G. A., & Day, N. L. (1994). Detrimental effects of prenatal cocaine exposure: Illusion or reality? *Journal of the American Academy of Child and Adolescent Psychiatry, 33,* 28–34.

Richman, A. L., Miller, P. M., & LeVine, R. A. (1992). Cultural and educational variations in maternal responsiveness. *Developmental Psychology, 28,* 614–621.

Richters, J., & Pellegrini, D. (1989). Depressed mothers' judgments about their children: An examination of the depression-distortion hypothesis. *Child Development, 60,* 1068–1075.

Riegel, K. F. (1975). Adult life crises: A dialectic interpretation of development. In N. Datan & L. H. Ginsberg (Eds.), *Lifespan developmental psychology: Normative life crises* (pp. 99–128). New York: Academic Press.

Rierdan, J., & Koff, E. (1993). Developmental variables in relation to depressive symptoms in adolescent girls. *Development and Psychopathology, 5,* 485–496.

Rierdan, J., Koff, E., & Stubbs, M. L. (1989). Timing of menarche, preparation, and initial menstrual experience: Replication and further analysis in a prospective study. *Journal of Youth and Adolescence, 18,* 413–426.

Roberts, C. W., Green, R., Williams, K., & Goodman, M. (1987). Boyhood gender identity development: A statistical contrast of two family groups. *Developmental Psychology, 23*, 544–557.

Roberts, R. E., & Sobhan, M. (1992). Symptoms of depression in adolescence: A comparison of Anglo, African, and Hispanic Americans. *Journal of Youth and Adolescence, 21*, 639–651.

Robins, L. N., & McEvoy, L. (1990). Conduct problems as predictors of substance abuse. In L. N. Robins & M. Rutter (Eds.), *Straight and devious pathways from childhood to adulthood* (pp. 182–204). Cambridge, England: Cambridge University Press.

Robinson, H. B. (1981). The uncommonly bright child. In M. Lewis & L. A. Rosenblum (Eds.), *The uncommon child* (pp. 57–82). New York: Plenum Press.

Robinson, N. M., & Janos, P. M. (1986). Psychological adjustment in a college-level program of marked academic acceleration. *Journal of Youth and Adolescence, 15*, 51–60.

Roche, A. F. (1979). Secular trends in human growth, maturation, and development. *Monographs of the Society for Research in Child Development, 44*(3–4, Serial No. 179).

Rogers, J. (1991). Nontraditional inheritance: I. Mechanisms Mendel never knew. *Mosaic, 22*(Fall), 3–11.

Rogers, J. L. (1984). Confluence effects: Not here, not now! *Developmental Psychology, 20*, 321–331.

Rogers, J. L., Rowe, D. C., & May, K. (1994). DF analysis of NLSY IQ/Achievement data: Nonshared environmental influences. *Intelligence, 19*, 157–177.

Roggman, L. A., Langlois, J. H., Hubbs-Tait, L., & Rieser-Danner, L. A. (1994). Infant day-care, attachment, and the "file drawer problem." *Child Development, 65*, 1429–1443.

Rohner, R. P., Kean, K. J., & Cournoyer, D. E. (1991). Effects of corporal punishment, perceived caretaker warmth, and cultural beliefs on the psychological adjustment of children in St. Kitts, West Indies. *Journal of Marriage and the Family, 53*, 681–693.

Rolls, B. J., Fedoroff, I. C., & Guthrie, J. F. (1991). Gender differences in eating behavior and body weight regulation. *Health Psychology, 20*, 133–142.

Rooks, J. P., Weatherby, N. L., Ernst, E. K. M., Stapleton, S., Rosen, D., & Rosenfield, A. (1989). Outcomes of care in birth centers: The National Birth Center Study. *New England Journal of Medicine, 321*, 1804–1811.

Rose, R. J. (1995). Genes and human behavior. *Annual Review of Psychology, 56*, 625–54.

Rose, S. A., & Ruff, H. A. (1987). Cross-modal abilities in human infants. In J. D. Osofsky (Ed.), *Handbook of infant development* (2nd ed.) (pp. 318–362). New York: Wiley-Interscience.

Rosenbaum, J. E. (1984). *Career mobility in a corporate hierarchy.* New York: Academic Press.

Rosenberg, M. (1986). Self-concept from middle childhood through adolescence. In J. Suls & A. G. Greenwald (Eds.), *Psychological perspectives on the self* (Vol. 3, pp. 107–136). Hillsdale, NJ: Erlbaum.

Rosenblith, J. F. (1992). *In the beginning* (2nd ed.). Thousand Oaks, CA: Sage.

Rosenthal, R. (1994). Interpersonal expectancy effects: A 30-year perspective. *Current Directions in Psychological Science, 3*, 176–179.

Ross, G., Kagan, J., Zelazo, P., & Kotelchuck, M. (1975). Separation protest in infants in home and laboratory. *Developmental Psychology, 11*, 256–257.

Rothbart, M. K., Ahadi, S. A., & Hershey, K. L. (1994). Temperament and social behavior in childhood. *Merrill-Palmer Quarterly, 40*, 21–39.

Rothbart, M. K., Derryberry, D., & Posner, M. I. (1994). A psychobiological approach to the development of temperament: In J. E. Bates & T. D. Wachs (Eds.), *Temperament: Individual differences at the interface of biology and behavior* (pp. 83–116). Washington, DC: American Psychological Association.

Rothbart, M. K., Posner, M. I., & Hershey, K. L. (1995). Temperament, attention, and developmental psychopathology. In D. Cicchetti & D. J. Cohen (Eds.), *Developmental psychopathology: Vol. 1. Theory and methods* (pp. 315–340). New York: Wiley.

Rothbaum, F., Pott, M., & Morelli, G. (1995). *Ties that bind: Cultural differences in the development of family closeness.* Paper presented at the biennial meetings of the Society for Research in Child Development, Indianapolis.

Rotheram-Borus, M. J., Rosario, M., & Koopman, C. (1991). Minority youths at high risk: Gay males and runaways. In M. E. Colten & S. Gore (Eds.), *Adolescent stress: Causes and consequences* (pp. 181–200). New York: Aldine de Gruyter.

Rovee-Collier, C. (1986). The rise and fall of infant classical conditioning research: Its promise for the study of early development. In L. P. Lipsitt & C. Rovee-Collier (Eds.), *Advances in infancy research* (Vol. 4, pp. 139–162). Norwood, NJ: Ablex.

Rovee-Collier, C. (1993). The capacity for long-term memory in infancy. *Current Directions in Psychological Science, 2*, 130–135.

Rovet, J., & Netley, C. (1983). The triple X chromosome syndrome in childhood: Recent empirical findings. *Child Development, 54*, 831–845.

Rowe, D. C. (1994). *The limits of family influence: Genes, experience, and behavior.* New York: Guilford Press.

Rowe, I., & Marcia, J. E. (1980). Ego identity status, formal operations, and moral development. *Journal of Youth and Adolescence, 9*, 87–99.

Rubin, K. H., Fein, G. G., & Vandenberg, B. (1983). Play. In E. M. Hetherington (Ed.), *Handbook of child psychology: Socialization, personality, and social development* (Vol. 4, pp. 693–774). New York: Wiley.

Rubin, K. H., Hymel, S., Mills, R. S. L., & Rose-Krasnor, L. (1991). Conceptualizing different developmental pathways to and from social isolation in childhood. In D. Cicchetti & S. L. Toth (Eds.), *Internalizing and externalizing expressions of dysfunction: Rochester symposium on developmental psychopathology* (Vol. 2, pp. 91–122). Hillsdale, NJ: Erlbaum.

Ruble, D. N. (1987). The acquisition of self-knowledge: A self-socialization perspective. In N. Eisenberg (Ed.), *Contemporary topics in developmental psychology* (pp. 243–270). New York: Wiley-Interscience.

Russell, G. (1982). Shared-caregiving families: An Australian study. In M. E. Lamb (Ed.), *Nontraditional families* (pp. 139–172). Hillsdale, NJ: Erlbaum.

Russell, J. A. (1989). Culture, scripts, and children's understanding of emotion. In C. Saarni & P. L. Harris (Eds.), *Children's understanding of emotion* (pp. 293–318). Cambridge, England: Cambridge University Press.

Rutter, D. R., & Durkin, K. (1987). Turn-taking in mother-infant interaction: An examination of vocalizations and gaze. *Developmental Psychology, 23,* 54–61.

Rutter, M. (1978). Early sources of security and competence. In J. S. Bruner & A. Garton (Eds.), *Human growth and development* (pp. 33–61). London: Oxford University Press.

Rutter, M. (1983). School effects on pupil progress: Research findings and policy implications. *Child Development, 54,* 1–29.

Rutter, M. (1987). Continuities and discontinuities from infancy. In J. D. Osofsky (Ed.), *Handbook of infant development* (2nd ed.) (pp. 1256–1296). New York: Wiley-Interscience.

Rutter, M. (1989). Isle of Wight revisited: Twenty-five years of child psychiatric epidemiology. *Journal of the American Academy of Child and Adolescent Psychiatry, 28,* 633–653.

Rutter, M. (1990). Commentary: Some focus and process considerations regarding effects of parental depression on children. *Developmental Psychology, 26,* 60–67.

Rutter, M., & Garmezy, N. (1983). Developmental psychopathology. In E. M. Hetherington (Ed.), *Handbook of child psychology: Vol 4. Socialization, personality, and social development* (pp. 775–912). New York: Wiley.

Rutter, M., Tizard, J., & Whitmore, K. (1981). *Education, health and behaviour.* Huntington, NY: Krieger. (Originally published 1970.)

Ryan, A. S., Rush, D., Krieger, F. W., & Lewandowski, G. E. (1991). Recent declines in breast-feeding in the United States, 1984 through 1989. *Pediatrics, 88,* 719–727.

Saccuzzo, D. P., Johnson, N. E., & Guertin, T. L. (1994). Information processing in gifted versus nongifted African American, Latino, Filipino, and White children: Speeded versus nonspeeded paradigms. *Intelligence, 19,* 219–243.

Sack, W. H., Mason, R., & Higgins, J. E. (1985). The single parent family and abusive child punishment. *American Journal of Orthopsychiatry, 55,* 252–259.

Sadowski, M. (1995). The numbers game yields simplistic answers on the link between spending and outcomes. *Harvard Education Letter, 11*(2), 1–4.

Sagi, A. (1990). Attachment theory and research from a cross-cultural perspective. *Human Development, 33,* 10–22.

Sagi, A., van IJzendoorn, M. H., & Koren-Karie, N. (1991). Primary appraisal of the strange situation: A cross-cultural analysis of preseparation episodes. *Developmental Psychology, 27,* 587–596.

Saigal, S., Szatmari, P., Rosenbaum, P., Campbell, D., & King, S. (1991). Cognitive abilities and school performance of extremely low birth weight children and matched term control children at age 8 years: A regional study. *Journal of Pediatrics, 118,* 751–760.

Sameroff, A. J. (1995). General systems theories and developmental psychopathology. In D. Cicchetti & D. J. Cohen (Eds.), *Developmental psychopathology: Vol. 1. Theory and methods* (pp. 659–695). New York: Wiley.

Sameroff, A., Seifer, R., Barocas, R., Zax, M., & Greenspan, S. (1987). Intelligence quotient scores of 4-year-old children: Social-environmental risk factors. *Pediatrics, 79,* 343–350.

Sampson, R. J., & Laub, J. H. (1994). Urban poverty and the family context of delinquency: A new look at structure and process in a classic study. *Child Development, 65,* 523–540.

Sapir, E. (1929). The status of linguistics as a science. *Language, 5,* 207–214.

Sattler, J. M. (1988). *Assessment of children* . San Diego: Jerome M. Sattler.

Saunders, W. L., & Shepardson, D. (1987). A comparison of concrete and formal science instruction upon science achievement and reasoning ability of sixth grade students. *Journal of Research in Science Teaching, 24,* 39–51.

Savage-Rumbaugh, E. S., Murphy, J., Sevcik, R. A., Brakke, K. E., Williams, S. L., & Rumbaugh, D. M. (1993). Language comprehension in ape and child. *Monographs of the Society for Research in Child Development, 58*(3–4, Serial No. 223).

Scafidi, F. A., Field, T. M., Schanberg, S. M., Bauer, C. R., Tucci, K., Roberts, J., Morrow, C., & Kuhn, C. M. (1990). Massage stimulates growth in preterm infants: A replication. *Infant Behavior and Development, 13,* 167–188.

Scarr, S., & Eisenberg, M. (1993). Child care research: Issues, perspectives, and results. *Annual Review of Psychology, 44,* 613–644.

Scarr, S., & Kidd, K. K. (1983). Developmental behavior genetics. In M. M. Haith & J. J. Campos (Eds.), *Handbook of child psychology: Vol. 2. Infancy and developmental psychobiology* (pp. 345–434). New York: Wiley.

Scarr, S., & McCartney, K. (1983). How people make their own environments: A theory of genotype → environment effects. *Child Development, 54,* 424–435.

Scarr, S., Weinberg, R. A., & Waldman, I. D. (1993). IQ correlations in transracial adoptive families. *Intelligence, 17,* 541–555.

Scarr-Salapatek, S. (1976). An evolutionary perspective on infant intelligence: Species patterns and individual variations. In M. Lewis (Ed.), *Origins of intelligence* (pp. 165–198). New York: Plenum Press.

Schaefli, A., Rest, J. R., & Thoma, S. J. (1985). Does moral education improve moral judgment? A meta-analysis of intervention studies using the Defining Issues Test. *Review of Educational Research, 55,* 319–352.

Schaie, K. W. (1983). What can we learn from the longitudinal study of adult psychological development? In K. W. Schaie (Ed.), *Longitudinal studies of adult psychological development* (pp. 1–19). New York: Guilford Press.

Schank, R. C., & Abelson, R. (1977). *Scripts, plans, goals, and understanding.* Hillsdale, NJ: Erlbaum.

Schlesinger, H. S., & Meadow, K. P. (1972). *Sound and sign.* Berkeley: University of California Press.

Schneider, B., Hieshima, J. A., Lee, S., & Plank, S. (1994). East-Asian academic success in the United States: Family, school, and community explanations. In P. M. Greenfield & R. R. Cocking (Eds.), *Cross-cultural roots of minority child development* (pp. 323–350). Hillsdale, NJ: Erlbaum.

Schneider, M. L. (1992). The effect of mild stress during pregnancy on birthweight and neuromotor maturation in rhesus monkey infants (*Macaca mulatta*). *Infant Behavior and Development, 15,* 389–403.

Schneider, W., & Bjorklund, D. F. (1992). Expertise, aptitude, and strategic remembering. *Child Development, 63,* 461–473.

Schneider, W., & Pressley, M. (1989). *Memory development between 2 and 20.* New York: Springer-Verlag.

Schoendorf, K. C., Hogue, C. J. R., Kleinman, J. C., & Rowley, D. (1992). Mortality among infants of black as compared with white college-educated parents. *New England Journal of Medicine, 326,* 1522–1526.

Schoendorf, K. C., & Kiely, J. L. (1992). Relationship of Sudden Infant Death Syndrome to maternal smoking during and after pregnancy. *Pediatrics, 90,* 905–908.

Schonfeld, I. S., Shaffer, D., O'Connor, P., & Portny, S. (1988). Conduct disorder and cognitive functioning: Testing three causal hypotheses. *Child Development, 59,* 993–1007.

Schramm, W. F., Barnes, D. E., & Bakewell, J. M. (1987). Neonatal mortality in Missouri home births, 1978–84. *American Journal of Public Health, 77,* 930–935.

Scollon, R. (1976). *Conversations with a one-year-old.* Honolulu: University of Hawaii Press.

Sears, R. R., Maccoby, E. E., & Levin, H. (1977). *Patterns of child rearing.* Stanford, CA: Stanford University Press. (Originally published 1957 by Row, Peterson.)

Seidman, E., Allen, L., Aber, J. L., Mitchell, C., & Feinman, J. (1994). The impact of school transitions in early adolescence on the self-system and perceived social context of poor urban youth. *Child Development, 65,* 507–522.

Seitz, V. (1988). Methodology. In M. H. Bornstein & M. E. Lamb (Eds.), *Developmental psychology: An advanced textbook* (pp. 51–84). Hillsdale, NJ: Erlbaum.

Selman, R. L. (1980). *The growth of interpersonal understanding.* New York: Academic Press.

Senchak, M., & Leonard, K. E. (1992). Attachment styles and marital adjustment among newlywed couples. *Journal of Social and Personal Relationships, 9,* 51–64.

Serbin, L., Moskowitz, D. S., Schwartzman, A. E., & Ledingham, J. E. (1991). Aggressive, withdrawn, and aggressive/withdrawn children in adolescence: Into the next generation. In D. J. Pepler & K. H. Rubin (Eds.), *The development and treatment of childhood aggression* (pp. 55–70). Hillsdale, NJ: Erlbaum.

Serbin, L. A., Powlishta, K. K., & Gulko, J. (1993). The development of sex typing in middle childhood. *Monographs of the Society for Research in Child Development, 58*(2, Serial No. 232).

Serdula, M. K., Ivery, D., Coates, R. J., Freedman, D. S., Williamson, D. F., & Byers, T. (1993). Do obese children become obese adults? A review of the literature. *Preventive Medicine, 22,* 167–177.

Shaffer, D., Garland, A., Gould, M., Fisher, P., & Trautman, P. (1988). Preventing teenage suicide: A critical review. *Journal of the American Academy of Child and Adolescent Psychiatry, 27,* 675–687.

Shaffer, D., Garland, A., Vieland, V., Underwood, M., & Busner, C. (1991). The impact of curriculum-based suicide prevention programs for teenagers. *Journal of the American Academy of Child and Adolescent Psychiatry, 30,* 588–596.

Shantz, C. U. (1983). Social cognition. In J. H. Flavell & E. M. Markman (Eds.), *Handbook of child psychology: Vol. 3. Cognitive development* (pp. 495–555). New York: Wiley.

Shaw, D. S., Kennan, K., & Vondra, J. I. (1994). Developmental precursors of externalizing behavior: Ages 1 to 3. *Developmental Psychology, 30,* 355–364.

Sheldon, W. H. (1940). *The varieties of human physique.* New York: Harper.

Sherry, B., Springer, D. A., Connell, F. A., & Garrett, S. M. (1992). Short, thin, or obese? Comparing growth indexes of children from high- and low-poverty areas. *Journal of the American Dietetic Association, 92,* 1092–1095.

Shonkoff, J. P. (1984). The biological substrate and physical health in middle childhood. In W. A. Collins (Ed.), *Development during middle childhood. The years from six to twelve* (pp. 24–69). Washington, DC: National Academy Press.

Shore, C. (1986). Combinatorial play, conceptual development, and early multiword speech. *Developmental Psychology, 22,* 184–190.

Shore, C. M. (1995). *Individual differences in language development.* Thousand Oaks, CA: Sage.

Shweder, R. A., Mahapatra, M., & Miller, J. G. (1987). Culture and moral development. In J. Kagan & S. Lamb (Eds.), *The emergence of morality in young children* (pp. 1–82). Chicago: University of Chicago Press.

Siegal, M. (1987). Are sons and daughters treated more differently by fathers than by mothers? *Developmental Review, 7,* 183–209.

Siegler, R. S. (1976). Three aspects of cognitive development. *Cognitive Psychology, 8,* 431–520.

Siegler, R. S. (1978). The origins of scientific reasoning. In R. S. Siegler (Ed.), *Children's thinking: What develops?* (pp. 109–150). Hillsdale, NJ: Erlbaum.

Siegler, R. S. (1981). Developmental sequences within and between concepts. *Monographs of the Society for Research in Child Development, 46* (2, Serial No. 189).

Siegler, R. S. (1994). Cognitive variability: A key to understanding cognitive development. *Current Directions in Psychological Science, 3,* 1–5.

Sigman, M., Neumann, C., Carter, E., Cattle, D. J., D'Souza, S., & Bwibo, N. (1988). Home interactions and the development of Embu toddlers in Kenya. *Child Development, 59,* 1251–1261.

Silbereisen, R. K., & Kracke, B. (1993). Variations in maturational timing and adjustment in adolescence. In S. Jackson & H. Rodrigues-Tom (Eds.), *Adolescence and its social worlds* (pp. 67–94). Hove, England: Erlbaum.

Simmons, R. G., Blyth, D. A., & McKinney, K. L. (1983). The social and psychological effects of puberty on white females. In J. Brooks-Gunn & A. C. Petersen (Eds.), *Girls at puberty: Biological and psychosocial perspectives* (pp. 229–272). New York: Plenum Press.

Simmons, R. G., Burgeson, R., & Reef, M. J. (1988). Cumulative change at entry to adolescence. In M. R. Gunnar & W. A. Collins (Eds.), *The Minnesota Symposia on Child Psychology* (Vol. 21, pp. 123–150). Hillsdale, NJ: Erlbaum.

Simons, R. L., Robertson, J. F., & Downs, W. R. (1989). The nature of the association between parental rejection and delinquent behavior. *Journal of Youth and Adolescence, 18,* 297–309.

Simpson, J. A. (1990). Influence of attachment styles on romantic relationships. *Journal of Personality and Social Psychology, 59,* 971–980.

Skinner, B. F. (1957). *Verbal behavior.* New York: Prentice Hall.

Slaby, R. G., & Frey, K. S. (1975). Development of gender constancy and selective attention to same-sex models. *Child Development, 46,* 849–856.

Slater, A. (1995). Individual differences in infancy and later IQ. *Journal of Child Psychology and Psychiatry, 36,* 69–112.

Slobin, D. I. (1985a). Introduction: Why study acquisition crosslinguistically? In D. I. Slobin (Ed.), *The crosslinguistic study of language acquisition: Vol. 1. The data* (pp. 3–24). Hillsdale, NJ: Erlbaum.

Slobin, D. I. (1985b). Crosslinguistic evidence for the language-making capacity. In D. I. Slobin (Ed.), *The crosslinguistic study of language acquisition: Vol. 2. Theoretical issues* (pp. 1157–1256). Hillsdale, NJ: Erlbaum.

Small, S. A., & Luster, T. (1994). Adolescent sexual activity: An ecological, risk-factor approach. *Journal of Marriage and the Family, 56,* 181–192.

Smetana, J. G. (1990). Morality and conduct disorders. In M. Lewis & S. M. Miller (Eds.), *Handbook of developmental psychopathology* (pp. 157–180). New York: Plenum Press.

Smetana, J. G., Killen, M., & Turiel, E. (1991). Children's reasoning about interpersonal and moral conflicts. *Child Development, 62,* 629–644.

Smith, D. W. (1978). Prenatal life. In D. W. Smith, E. L. Bierman, & N. M. Robinson (Eds.), *The biologic ages of man* (2nd ed.) (pp. 42–62). Philadelphia: Saunders.

Smock, P. J. (1993). The economic costs of marital disruption for young women over the past two decades. *Demography, 30,* 353–371.

Smoll, F. L., & Schutz, R. W. (1990). Quantifying gender differences in physical performance: A developmental perspective. *Developmental Psychology, 26,* 360–369.

Snarey, J. R. (1985). Cross-cultural universality of social-moral development: A critical review of Kohlbergian research. *Psychological Bulletin, 97,* 202–232.

Snarey, J. R., Reimer, J., & Kohlberg, L. (1985). Development of social-moral reasoning among kibbutz adolescents: A longitudinal cross-sectional study. *Developmental Psychology, 21,* 3–17.

Snyder, J., Edwards, P., McGraw, K., Kilgore, K., & Holton, A. (1994). Escalation and reinforcement in mother-child conflict: Social processes associated with the development of physical aggression. *Development and Psychopathology, 6,* 305–321.

Soken, N. H., & Pick, A. D. (1992). Intermodal perception of happy and angry expressive behaviors by seven-month-old infants. *Child Development, 63,* 787–795.

Sonnenschein, S. (1986). Development of referential communication skills: How familiarity with a listener affects a speaker's production of redundant messages. *Developmental Psychology, 22,* 549–552.

Sosa, R., Kennell, J. H., Klaus, M. H., Robertson, S., & Urrutia, J. (1980). The effect of a supportive companion on perinatal problems, length of labor and mother-infant interaction. *New England Journal of Medicine, 303,* 597–600.

Spelke, E. S. (1979). Exploring audible and visible events in infancy. In A. D. Pick (Ed.), *Perception and its development: A tribute to Eleanor J. Gibson* (pp. 221–236). Hillsdale, NJ: Erlbaum.

Spelke, E. S. (1982). Perceptual knowledge of objects in infancy. In J. Mehler, E. C. T. Walker, & M. Garrett (Eds.), *Perspectives on mental representation* (pp. 409–430). Hillsdale, NJ: Erlbaum.

Spelke, E. S. (1985). Perception of unity, persistence, and identity: Thoughts on infants' conceptions of objects. In J. Mehler & R. Fox (Eds.), *Neonate cognition* (pp. 89–113). Hillsdale, NJ: Erlbaum.

Spelke, E. S. (1991). Physical knowledge in infancy: Reflections on Piaget's theory. In S. Carey & R. Gelman (Eds.), *The epigenesis of mind: Essays on biology and cognition* (pp. 133–169). Hillsdale, NJ: Erlbaum.

Spelke, E. S., & Owsley, C. J. (1979). Intermodal exploration and knowledge in infancy. *Infant Behavior and Development, 2,* 13–27.

Spelke, E. S., von Hofsten, C., & Kestenbaum, R. (1989). Object perception in infancy: Interaction of spatial and kinetic information for object boundaries. *Developmental Psychology, 25,* 185–196.

Spence, J. T., & Helmreich, R. L. (1978). *Masculinity and femininity.* Austin: University of Texas Press.

Spencer, M. B., & Dornbusch, S. M. (1990). Challenges in studying minority youth. In S. S. Feldman & G. R. Elliott (Eds.), *At the threshold: The developing adolescent* (pp. 123–146). Cambridge, MA: Harvard University Press.

Spieker, S. J., & Booth, C. L. (1988). Maternal antecedents of attachment quality. In J. Belsky & T. Nezworski (Eds.), *Clinical implications of attachment* (pp. 95–135). Hillsdale, NJ: Erlbaum.

Spiers, P. S., & Guntheroth, W. G. (1994). Recommendations to avoid the prone sleeping position and recent statistics for Sudden Infant Death Syndrome in the United States. *Archives of Pediatric and Adolescent Medicine, 148,* 141–146.

Spiker, D. (1990). Early intervention from a developmental perspective. In D. Cicchetti & M. Beeghly (Eds.), *Children with Down syndrome: A developmental perspective* (pp. 424–448). Cambridge, England: Cambridge University Press.

Spiker, D., Ferguson, J., & Brooks-Gunn, J. (1993). Enhancing maternal interactive behavior and child social competence in low birth weight, premature infants. *Child Development, 64,* 754–768.

Spitze, G. (1988). Women's employment and family relations: A review. *Journal of Marriage and the Family, 50,* 595–618.

Sroufe, L. A. (1979). The coherence of individual development: Early care, attachment, and subsequent developmental issues. *American Psychologist, 34,* 834–841.

Sroufe, L. A. (1983). Infant-caregiver attachment and patterns of adaptation in preschool: The roots of maladaption and competence. In M. Perlmutter (Ed.), *The Minnesota Symposium on Child Psychology* (Vol. 16, pp. 41–84). Hillsdale, NJ: Erlbaum.

Sroufe, L. A. (1988). The role of infant-caregiver attachment in development. In J. Belsky & T. Nezworski (Eds.), *Clinical implications of attachment* (pp. 18–40). Hillsdale, NJ: Erlbaum.

Sroufe, L. A. (1989). Pathways to adaptation and maladaptation: Psychopathology as developmental deviation. In D. Cicchetti (Ed.), *The emergence of a discipline: Rochester symposium on developmental psychopathology* (pp. 13–40). Hillsdale, NJ: Erlbaum.

Sroufe, L. A. (1990). A developmental perspective on day care. In N. Fox & G. G. Fein (Eds.), *Infant day care: The current debate* (pp. 51–60). Norwood, NJ: Ablex.

Sroufe, L. A., Carlson, E., & Schulman, S. (1993). Individuals in relationships: Development from infancy through adolescence. In D. C. Funder, R. D. Parke, C. Tomlinson-Keasey, & K. Widaman (Eds.), *Studying lives through time: Personality and development* (pp. 315–342). Washington, DC: American Psychological Association.

Sroufe, L. A., Egeland, B., & Kreutzer, T. (1990). The fate of early experience following developmental change: Longitudinal approaches to individual adaptation in childhood. *Child Development, 61,* 1363–1373.

Sroufe, L. A., & Rutter, M. (1984). The domain of developmental psychopathology. *Child Development, 55,* 17–29.

Starfield, B. (1991). Childhood morbidity: Comparisons, clusters, and trends. *Pediatrics, 88,* 519–526.

Stattin, H., & Klackenberg-Larsson, I. (1993). Early language and intelligence development and their relationship to future criminal behavior. *Journal of Abnormal Psychology, 102,* 369–378.

Steele, H., Holder, J., & Fonagy, P. (1995). *Quality of attachment to mother at one year predicts belief-desire reasoning at five years.* Paper presented at the biennial meetings of the Society for Research in Child Development, Indianapolis.

Stein, Z., Susser, M., Saenger, G., & Morolla, F. (1975). *Famine and human development: The Dutch hunger winter of 1944–1945.* New York: Oxford University Press.

Steinberg, L. (1988). Reciprocal relation between parent-child distance and pubertal maturation. *Developmental Psychology, 24,* 122–128.

Steinberg, L. (1990). Autonomy, conflict and harmony in the parent-adolescent relationship. In S. S. Feldman & G. R. Elliott (Eds.), *At the threshold: The developing adolescent* (pp. 255–276). Cambridge, MA: Harvard University Press.

Steinberg, L., & Dornbusch, S. M. (1991). Negative correlates of part-time employment during adolescence: Replication and elaboration. *Developmental Psychology, 27,* 304–313.

Steinberg, L., Dornbusch, S. M., & Brown, B. B. (1992). Ethnic differences in adolescent achievement: An ecological perspective. *American Psychologist, 47,* 723–729.

Steinberg, L., Elmen, J. D., & Mounts, N. S. (1989). Authoritative parenting, psychosocial maturity, and academic success among adolescents. *Child Development, 60,* 1424–1436.

Steinberg, L., Fegley, S., & Dornbusch, S. M. (1993). Negative impact of part-time work on adolescent adjustment: Evidence from a longitudinal study. *Developmental Psychology, 29,* 171–180.

Steinberg, L., Lamborn, S. D., Dornbusch, S. M., & Darling, N. (1992). Impact of parenting practices on adolescent achievement: Authoritative parenting, school involvement, and encouragement to succeed. *Child Development, 63,* 1266–1281.

Steinberg, L., Lambron, S. D., Darling, N., Mounts, N. S., & Dornbusch, S. M. (1994). Over-time changes in adjustment and competence among adolescents from authoritative, authoritarian, indulgent, and neglectful families. *Child Development, 65,* 754–770.

Steinberg, L., Mounts, N. S., Lamborn, S. D., & Dornbusch, S. D. (1991). Authoritative parenting and adolescent adjustment across varied ecological niches. *Journal of Research on Adolescence, 1,* 19–36.

Steiner, J. E. (1979). Human facial expressions in response to taste and smell stimulation. In H. W. Reese & L. P. Lipsitt (Eds.), *Advances in child development and behavior* (Vol. 13, pp. 257–296). New York: Academic Press.

Sternberg, R. J. (1986). *Intelligence applied.* New York: Harcourt Brace Jovanovich.

Sternberg, R. J., & Davidson, J. E. (1985). Cognitive development in the gifted and talented. In F. D. Horowitz & M. O'Brien (Eds.), *The gifted and talented: Developmental perspectives* (pp. 37–74). Washington, DC: American Psychological Association.

Sternberg, R. J., & Davidson, J. E. (Eds.). (1986). *Conceptions of giftedness.* Cambridge, England: Cambridge University Press.

Sternberg, R. J., & Suben, J. G. (1986). The socialization of intelligence. In M. Perlmutter (Ed.), *The Minnesota Symposia on Child Psychology* (Vol. 19, pp. 201–236). Hillsdale, NJ: Erlbaum.

Sternberg, R. J., & Wagner, R. K. (1993). The g-ocentric view of intelligence and job performance is wrong. *Current Directions in Psychological Science, 2,* 1–5.

Stevenson, H. (1994). Moving away from stereotypes and preconceptions: Students and their education in East Asia and the United States. In P. M. Greenfield & R. R. Cocking (Eds.), *Cross-cultural roots of minority child development* (pp. 315–322). Hillsdale, NJ: Erlbaum.

Stevenson, H. W. (1988). Culture and schooling: Influences on cognitive development. In E. M. Hetherington, R. M. Lerner, & M. Perlmutter (Eds.), *Child development in life span perspective* (pp. 241–258). Hillsdale, NJ: Erlbaum.

Stevenson, H. W., & Chen, C. (1989). Schooling and achievement: A study of Peruvian children. *International Journal of Educational Research, 13,* 883–894.

Stevenson, H. W., Chen, C., Lee, S., & Fuligni, A. J. (1991). Schooling, culture, and cognitive development. In L. Okagaki & R. J. Sternberg (Eds.), *Directors of development* (pp. 243–268). Hillsdale, NJ: Erlbaum.

Stevenson, H. W., & Lee, S. (1990). Contexts of achievement: A study of American, Chinese, and Japanese children. *Monographs of the Society for Research in Child Development, 55*(1–2, Serial No. 221).

Stevenson, H. W., Lee, S., Chen, C., Lummis, M., Stigler, J., Fan, L., & Ge, F. (1990). Mathematics achievement of children in China and the United States. *Child Development, 61,* 1053–1066.

Steward, M. S. (1993). Understanding children's memories of medical procedures: "He didn't touch me and it didn't hurt!" In C. A. Nelson (Ed.), *The Minnesota Symposia on Child Psychology* (Vol. 26, pp. 171–225). Hillsdale, NJ: Erlbaum.

Stewart, J. F., Popkin, B. M., Guilkey, D. K., Akin, J. S., Adair, L., & Flieger, W. (1991). Influences on the extent of breastfeeding: A prospective study in the Philippines. *Demography, 28,* 181–199.

Stewart, R. B., Cluff, L. E., & Philp, R. (1977). *Drug monitoring: A requirement for responsible drug use.* Baltimore: Williams & Wilkins.

Stigler, J. W., Lee, S., & Stevenson, H. W. (1987). Mathematics classrooms in Japan, Taiwan, and the United States. *Child Development, 58,* 1272–1285.

Stigler, J. W., & Stevenson, H. W. (1991). How Asian teachers polish each lesson to perfection. *American Educator* (Spring), 12–20, 43–47.

Stipek, D. (1992). The child at school. In M. H. Bornstein & M. E. Lamb (Eds.), *Developmental psychology: An advanced textbook* (3rd ed.) (pp. 579–625). Hillsdale, NJ: Erlbaum.

Stipek, D., & Gralinski, H. (1991). Gender differences in children's achievement-related beliefs and emotional responses to success and failure in math. *Journal of Educational Psychology, 83,* 361–371.

Storfer, M. D. (1990). *Intelligence and giftedness.* San Francisco: Jossey-Bass.

Story, M., Rosenwinkel, K., Himes, J. H., Resnick, M., Harris, L. J., & Blum, R. W. (1991). Demographic and risk factors associated with chronic dieting in adolescents. *American Journal of Diseases of Childhood, 145,* 994–998.

Stoutjesdyk, D., & Jevne, R. (1993). Eating disorders among high performance athletes. *Journal of Youth and Adolescence, 22,* 271–282.

St. Peters, M., Fitch, M., Huston, A. C., Wright, J. C., & Eakins, D. J. (1991). Television and families: What do young children watch with their parents? *Child Development, 62,* 1409–1423.

Strassberg, Z., Dodge, K. A., Bates, J. E., & Pettit, G. S. (1992). The longitudinal relation between parental conflict strategies and children's sociometric standing in kindergarten. *Merrill-Palmer Quarterly, 38,* 4777–493.

Strassberg, Z., Dodge, K. A., Pettit, G. S., & Bates, J. E. (1994). Spanking in the home and children's subsequent aggression toward kindergarten peers. *Development and Psychopathology, 6,* 445–461.

Straus, M. A. (1991a). Discipline and deviance: Physical punishment of children and violence and other crime in adulthood. *Social Problems, 38,* 133–152.

Straus, M. A. (1991b). New theory and old canards about family violence research. *Social Problems, 38,* 180–194.

Straus, M. A. (1995). Corporal punishment of children and adult depression and suicidal ideation. In J. McCord (Ed.), *Coercion and punishment in long-term perspectives* (pp. 59–77). Cambridge, England: Cambridge University Press.

Straus, M. A., & Donnelly, D. A. (1993). Corporal punishment of adolescents by American parents. *Youth and Society, 24,* 419–442.

Streissguth, A. P., Aase, J. M., Clarren, S. K., Randels, S. P., LaDue, R. A., & Smith, D. F. (1991). Fetal alcohol syndrome in adolescents and adults. *Journal of the American Medical Association, 265,* 1961–1967.

Streissguth, A. P., Barr, H. M., & Sampson, P. D. (1990). Moderate prenatal alcohol exposure: Effects on child IQ and learning problems at age 7½ years. *Alcoholism. Clinical and Experimental Research, 14,* 662–669.

Streissguth, A. P., Barr, H. M., Sampson, P. D., Darby, B. L., & Martin, D. C. (1989). IQ at age 4 in relation to maternal alcohol use and smoking during pregnancy. *Developmental Psychology, 25,* 3–11.

Streissguth, A. P., Landesman-Dwyer, S., Martin, J. C., & Smith, D. W. (1980). Teratogenic effects of alcohol in humans and laboratory animals. *Science, 209,* 353–361.

Streissguth, A. P., Martin, D. C., Barr, H. M., Sandman, B. M., Kirchner, G. L., & Darby, B. L. (1984). Intrauterine alcohol and nicotine exposure: Attention and reaction time in 4-year-old children. *Developmental Psychology, 20,* 533–541.

Streissguth, A. P., Martin, D. C., Martin, J. C., & Barr, H. M. (1981). The Seattle longitudinal prospective study on alcohol and pregnancy. *Neurobehavioral Toxicology and Teratology, 3,* 223–233.

Striegel-Moore, R. H., Silberstein, L. R., & Rodin, J. (1986). Toward an understanding of risk factors for bulimia. *American Psychologist, 41,* 246–263.

Stringfield, S., & Teddlie, C. (1991). Observers as predictors of schools' multiyear outlier status on achievement tests. *The Elementary School Journal, 91,* 357–376.

Stunkard, A. J., Harris, J. R., Pedersen, N. L., & McClearn, G. E. (1990). The body-mass index of twins who have been reared apart. *New England Journal of Medicine, 322,* 1483–1487.

Stunkard, A. J., Sorensen, T. I. A., Hanis, C., Teasdale, T. W., Chakraborty, R., Schull, W. J., & Schulsinger, F. (1986). An adoption study of human obesity. *New England Journal of Medicine, 314,* 193–198.

Sue, S., & Okazaki, S. (1990). Asian-American educational achievements: A phenomenon in search of an explanation. *American Psychologist, 45,* 913–920.

Sullivan, K., Zaitchik, D., & Tager-Flusberg, H. (1994). Preschoolers can attribute second-order beliefs. *Developmental Psychology, 30,* 395–402.

Super, C. M., & Harkness, S. (1982). The infant's niche in rural Kenya and metropolitan America. In L. Adler (Ed.), *Issues in cross-cultural research* (pp. 47–56). New York: Academic Press.

Swedo, S. E., Rettew, D. C., Kuppenheimer, M., Lum, D., Dolan, S., & Goldberger, E. (1991). Can adolescent suicide attempters be distinguished from at-risk adolescents? *Pediatrics, 88,* 620–629.

Taffel, S. M., Keppel, K. G., & Jones, G. K. (1993). Medical advice on maternal weight gain and actual weight gain. Results from the 1988 National Maternal and Infant Health Survey. *Annals of the New York Academy of Sciences, 678,* 293–305.

Takei, Y., & Dubas, J. S. (1993). Academic achievement among early adolescents: Social and cultural diversity. In R. M. Lerner (Ed.), *Early adolescence: Perspectives on research, policy, and intervention* (pp. 175–190). Hillsdale, NJ: Erlbaum.

Tamis-LeMonda, C., & Bornstein, M. H. (1987). Is there a "sensitive period" in human mental development? In M. H. Bornstein (Ed.), *Sensitive periods in development: Interdisciplinary perspectives* (pp. 163–182). Hillsdale, NJ: Erlbaum.

Tannen, D. (1990). *You just don't understand.* New York: Morrow.

Tanner, J. M. (1978). *Fetus into man: Physical growth from conception to maturity.* Cambridge, MA: Harvard University Press.

Tanner, J. M., Hughes, P. C. R., & Whitehouse, R. H. (1981). Radiographically determined widths of bone, muscle and fat in the upper arm and calf from 3 to 18 years. *Annals of Human Biology, 8,* 495–517.

Taylor, M., Cartwright, B. S., & Carlson, S. M. (1993). A developmental investigation of children's imaginary companions. *Developmental Psychology, 29,* 276–285.

Taylor, R. D., Casten, R., & Flickinger, S. M. (1993). Influence of kinship social support on the parenting experiences and psychosocial adjustment of African-American adolescents. *Developmental Psychology, 29,* 382–388.

Taylor, R. D., Casten, R., Flickinger, S. M., Roberts, D., & Fulmore, C. D. (1994). Explaining the school performance of African-American adolescents. *Journal of Research on Adolescence, 4,* 21–44.

Tellegen, A., Lykken, D. T., Bouchard, T. J., Jr., Wilcox, K. J., Segal, N. L., & Rich, S. (1988). Personality similarity in twins reared apart and together. *Journal of Personality and Social Psychology, 54,* 1031–1039.

Terman, L. (1916). *The measurement of intelligence.* Boston: Houghton Mifflin.

Terman, L. (1925). *Mental and physical traits of a thousand gifted children: Vol. 1. Genetic studies of genius.* Stanford, CA: Stanford University Press.

Terman, L., & Merrill, M. A. (1937). *Measuring intelligence: A guide to the administration of the new revised Stanford-Binet tests.* Boston: Houghton Mifflin.

Terman, L., & Oden, M. (1959). *Genetic studies of genius: Vol. 5. The gifted group at mid-life.* Stanford, CA: Stanford University Press.

Tesman, J. R., & Hills, A. (1994). Developmental effects of lead exposure in children. *Social Policy Report, Society for Research in Child Development, 8*(3), 1–16.

Teti, D. M., Gelfand, D. M., Messinger, D. S., & Isabella, R. (1995). Maternal depression and the quality of early attachment: An examination of infants, preschoolers, and their mothers. *Developmental Psychology, 31,* in press.

Tew, M. (1985). Place of birth and perinatal mortality. *Journal of the Royal College of General Practitioner, 35,* 390–394.

Thal, D., & Bates, E. (1990). Continuity and variation in early language development. In J. Colombo & J. Fagen (Eds.), *Individual differences in infancy: Reliability, stability, prediction* (pp. 359–385). Hillsdale, NJ: Erlbaum.

Thelen, E. (1981). Rhythmical behavior in infancy: An ethological perspective. *Developmental Psychology, 17,* 237–257.

Thelen, E. (1995). Motor development: A new synthesis. *American Psychologist, 50,* 79–95.

Thelen, E., & Adolph, K. E. (1992). Arnold L. Gesell: The paradox of nature and nurture. *Developmental Psychology, 28,* 368–380.

Thomas, A., & Chess, S. (1977). *Temperament and development.* New York: Brunner/Mazel.

Thomas, R. M. (Ed.). (1990). *The encyclopedia of human development and education: Theory, research, and studies.* Oxford: Pergamon Press.

Thomas, R. M. (1990a). Motor development. In R. M. Thomas (Ed.), *The encyclopedia of human development and education: Theory, research, and studies* (pp. 326–330). Oxford: Pergamon Press.

Thomas, R. M. (1990b). Basic concepts and applications of Piagetian cognitive development theory. In R. M. Thomas (Ed.), *The encyclopedia of human development and education: Theory, research, and studies* (pp. 53–55). Oxford: Pergamon Press.

Thompson, S. K. (1975). Gender labels and early sex role development. *Child Development, 46,* 339–347.

Thorne, B. (1986). Girls and boys together . . . but mostly apart: Gender arrangements in elementary schools. In W. W. Hartup & Z. Rubin (Eds.), *Relationships and development* (pp. 167–184). Hillsdale, NJ: Erlbaum.

Thornton, A. (1990). The courtship process and adolescent sexuality. *Journal of Family Issues, 11,* 239–273.

Timmer, S. G., Eccles, J., & O'Brien, K. (1985). How children use time. In F. T. Juster & F. P. Stafford (Eds.), *Time, goods, and well-being* (pp. 353–369). Ann Arbor: Institute for Social Research, The University of Michigan.

Tobin-Richards, M. H., Boxer, A. M., & Petersen, A. C. (1983). The psychological significance of pubertal change: Sex differences in perceptions of self during early adolescence. In J. Brooks-Gunn & A. C. Petersen (Eds.), *Girls at puberty: Biological and psychosocial perspectives* (pp. 127–154). New York: Plenum Press.

Todd, R. D., Swarzenski, B., Rossi, P. G., & Visconti, P. (1995). Structural and functional development of the human brain. In D. Cicchetti & D. J. Cohen (Eds.), *Developmental psychopathology: Vol. 1. Theory and methods* (pp. 161–194). New York: Wiley.

Tomasello, M., & Mannle, S. (1985). Pragmatics of sibling speech to one-year-olds. *Child Development, 56,* 911–917.

Tomlinson-Keasey, C., Eisert, D. C., Kahle, L. R., Hardy-Brown, K., & Keasey, B. (1979). The structure of concrete operational thought. *Child Development, 50,* 1153–1163.

Trehub, S. E., Bull, D., & Thorpe, L. A. (1984). Infants' perception of melodies: The role of melodic contour. *Child Development, 55,* 821–830.

Trehub, S. E., & Rabinovitch, M. S. (1972). Auditory-linguistic sensitivity in early infancy. *Developmental Psychology, 6,* 74–77.

Trehub, S. E., Thorpe, L. A., & Morrongiello, B. A. (1985). Infants' perception of melodies: Changes in a single tone. *Infant Behavior and Development, 8,* 213–223.

Tremblay, R. E. (1991). Commentary. Aggression, prosocial behavior, and gender: Three magic words, but no magic wand. In D. J. Pepler & K. H. Rubin (Eds.), *The development and treatment of aggression* (pp. 71–78). Hillsdale, NJ: Erlbaum.

Tremblay, R. E., Kurtz, L., Mâsse, L. C., Vitaro, F., & Pihl, R. O. (1995). A bimodal preventive intervention for disruptive kindergarten boys: Its impact through mid-adolescence. *Journal of Consulting and Clinical Psychology,* in press.

Tronick, E. Z., Morelli, G. A., & Ivey, P. K. (1992). The Efe forager infant and toddler's pattern of social relationships: Multiple and simultaneous. *Developmental Psychology, 28,* 568–577.

Tuna, J. M. (1989). Mental health services for children: The state of the art. *American Psychologist, 44,* 188–199.

Tunmer, W. E., Herriman, M. L., & Nesdale, A. R. (1988). Metalinguistic abilities and beginning reading. *Reading Research Quarterly, 23,* 134–158.

Turiel, E. (1966). An experimental test of the sequentiality of developmental stages in the child's moral judgment. *Journal of Personality and Social Psychology, 3,* 611–618.

Turkheimer, E., & Gottesman, I. I. (1991). Individual differences and the canalization of human behavior. *Developmental Psychology, 27,* 18–22.

Udry, J. R., & Campbell, B. C. (1994). Getting started on sexual behavior. In A. S. Rossi (Ed.), *Sexuality across the life course* (pp. 187–208). Chicago: University of Chicago Press.

Umberson, D., & Gove, W. R. (1989). Parenthood and psychological well-being. Theory, measurement, and stage in the family life course. *Journal of Family Issues, 10,* 440–462.

Underwood, M. K., Coie, J. D., & Herbsman, C. R. (1992). Display rules for anger and aggression in school-age children. *Child Development, 63,* 366–380.

Ungerer, J. A., & Sigman, M. (1984). The relation of play and sensorimotor behavior to language in the second year. *Child Development, 55,* 1448–1455.

U.S. Bureau of the Census (1994). *Statistical abstract of the United States: 1994* (114th ed.). Washington, DC: U.S. Government Printing Office.

U.S. Department of Health and Human Services (1994). Health risk behaviors among adolescents who do and do not attend school—United States, 1992. *Morbidity and Mortality Weekly Report, 43,* 129–132.

Upchurch, D. M. (1993). Early schooling and childbearing experiences: Implications for post-secondary school attendance. *Journal of Research on Adolescence, 3,* 423–443.

Urban, J., Carlson, E., Egeland, B., & Sroufe, L. A. (1991). Patterns of individual adaptation across childhood. *Development and Psychopathology, 3,* 445–460.

Uribe, F. M. T., LeVine, R. A., & LeVine, S. E. (1994). Maternal behavior in a Mexican community: The changing environments of children. In P. M. Greenfield & R. R. Cocking (Eds.), *Cross-cultural roots of minority child development* (pp. 41–54). Hillsdale, NJ: Erlbaum.

Valdez-Menchaca, M. C., & Whitehurst, G. J. (1992). Accelerating language development through picture book reading: A systematic extension to Mexican day care. *Developmental Psychology, 28,* 1106–1114.

Van de Perre, P., Simonen, A., Msellati, P., Hitimana, D., Vaira, D., Bazebagira, A., Van Goethem, C., Stevens, A., Karita, E., Sondag-Thull, D., Dabis, F., & Lepage, P. (1991). Postnatal transmission of human immunodeficiency virus type 1 from mother to infant. *New England Journal of Medicine, 325,* 593–598.

van den Boom, D. C. (1994). The influence of temperament and mothering on attachment and exploration: An experimental manipulation of sensitive responsiveness among lower-class mothers with irritable infants. *Child Development, 65,* 1457–1477.

van IJzendoorn, M. H., Goldberg, S., Kroonenberg, P. M., & Frenkel, O. J. (1992). The relative effects of maternal and child problems on the quality of attachment: A meta-analysis of attachment in clinical samples. *Child Development, 63,* 840–858.

van IJzendoorn, M. H., & Kroonenberg, P. M. (1988). Cross-cultural patterns of attachment: A meta-analysis of the Strange Situation. *Child Development, 59,* 147–156.

van Lieshout, C. F. M., & Haselager, G. J. T. (1994). The big five personality factors in Q-sort descriptions of children and adolescents. In C. F. Halverson, Jr., G. A. Kohnstamm, & R. P. Martin (Eds.), *The developing structure of temperament and personality from infancy to adulthood* (pp. 293–318). Hillsdale, NJ: Erlbaum.

van Wel, F. (1994). "I count my parents among my best friends": Youths' bonds with parents and friends in the Netherlands. *Journal of Marriage and the Family, 56,* 835–843.

Vandenberg, B. (1984). Developmental features of exploration. *Developmental Psychology, 20,* 3–8.

Vernon, P. A. (Ed.). (1987). *Speed of information-processing and intelligence.* Norwood, NJ: Ablex.

Vernon, P. A. (1993). Intelligence and neural efficiency. In D. K. Detterman (Ed.), *Current topics in human intelligence: Vol. 3. Individual differences and cognition* (pp. 171–187). Norwood, NJ: Ablex.

Vernon, P. A., & Mori, M. (1992). Intelligence, reaction times, and peripheral nerve conduction velocity. *Intelligence, 16,* 273–288.

Victorian Infant Collaborative Study Group (1991). Eight-year outcome in infants with birth weight of 500–999 grams: Continuing regional study of 1979 and 1980 births. *Journal of Pediatrics, 118,* 761–767.

Vihko, R., & Apter, D. (1980). The role of androgens in adolescent cycles. *Journal of Steroid Biochemistry, 12,* 369–373.

Vorhees, C. F., & Mollnow, E. (1987). Behavioral teratogenesis: Long-term influences on behavior from early exposure to environmental agents. In J. D. Osofsky (Ed.), *Handbook of infant development* (2nd ed.) (pp. 913–971). New York: Wiley-Interscience.

Voyer, D., Voyer, S., & Bryden, M. P. (1995). Magnitude of sex differences in spatial abilities: A meta-analysis and consideration of critical variables. *Psychological Bulletin, 117,* 250–270.

Vuchinich, S., Bank, L., & Patterson, G. R. (1992). Parenting, peers, and the stability of antisocial behavior in preadolescent boys. *Developmental Psychology, 28,* 510–521.

Vygotsky, L. S. (1962). *Thought and language.* New York: Wiley.

Wachs, T. D., Bishry, Z., Sobhy, A., McCabe, G., Galal, O., & Shaheen, F. (1993). Relation of rearing environment to adaptive behavior of Egyptian toddlers. *Child Development, 64,* 586–604.

Waddington, C. H. (1957). *The strategy of the genes.* London: Allen & Son.

Waddington, C. H. (1974). A catastrophe theory of evolution. *Annals of the New York Academy of Sciences, 231,* 32–41.

Wahlström, J. (1990). Gene map of mental retardation. *Journal of Mental Deficiency Research, 34,* 11–27.

Walden, T. A. (1991). Infant social referencing. In J. Garber & K. A. Dodge (Eds.), *The development of emotion regulation and dysregulation* (pp. 69–88). Cambridge, England: Cambridge University Press.

Waldrop, M. F., & Halverson, C. F., Jr. (1975). Intensive and extensive peer behavior: Longitudinal and cross-sectional analysis. *Child Development, 46,* 19–26.

Walker, H., Messinger, D., Fogel, A., & Karns, J. (1992). Social and communicative development in infancy. In V. B. V. Hasselt & M. Hersen (Eds.), *Handbook of social development: A lifespan perspective* (pp. 157–181). New York: Plenum Press.

Walker, L. J. (1980). Cognitive and perspective-taking prerequisites for moral development. *Child Development, 51,* 131–139.

Walker, L. J. (1989). A longitudinal study of moral reasoning. *Child Development, 60,* 157–160.

Walker, L. J., de Vries, B., & Trevethan, S. D. (1987). Moral stages and moral orientations in real-life and hypothetical dilemmas. *Child Development, 58,* 842–858.

Walker-Andrews, A. S., & Lennon, E. (1991). Infants' discrimination of vocal expressions: Contributions of auditory and visual information. *Infant Behavior and Development, 14,* 131–142.

Wallerstein, J. (1989). Children after divorce: Wounds that don't heal. *The New York Times Magazine* (January 22), 19–21, 41–44.

Wallerstein, J. S. (1984). Children of divorce: Preliminary report of a ten-year follow-up of young children. *American Journal of Orthopsychiatry, 54,* 444–458.

Walters, R. H., & Brown, M. (1963). Studies of reinforcement of aggression. III. Transfer of responses to an interpersonal situation. *Child Development, 34,* 563–571.

Walton, G. E., Bower, N. J. A., & Bower, T. G. R. (1992). Recognition of familiar faces by newborns. *Infant Behavior and Development, 15,* 265–269.

Walton, G. E., & Bower, T. G. R. (1993). Amodal representation of speech in infants. *Infant Behavior and Development, 16,* 233–253.

Wang, P. P., & Bellugi, U. (1993). Williams Syndrome, Down Syndrome, and cognitive neuroscience. *American Journal of Diseases of Children, 147,* 1246–1251.

Ward, M. J., & Carlson, E. A. (1995). Associations among adult attachment representations, maternal sensitivity, and infant-mother attachment in a sample of adolescent mothers. *Child Development, 66,* 69–79.

Wartner, U. B., Grossman, K., Fremmer-Bombik, E., & Suess, G. (1994). Attachment patterns at age six in south Germany: Predictability from infancy and implications for preschool behavior. *Child Development, 65,* 1014–1027.

Waterman, A. S. (1985). Identity in the context of adolescent psychology. *New Directions for Child Development, 30,* 5–24.

Watson, J. D., & Crick, F. H. C. (1953). Molecular structure of nucleic acid: A structure for deoxyribose nucleic acid. *Nature, 171,* 737–738.

Watson, M. W., & Getz, K. (1990a). Developmental shifts in Oedipal behaviors related to family role understanding. *New Directions for Child Development, 48,* 5–28.

Watson, M. W., & Getz, K. (1990b). The relationship between Oedipal behaviors and children's family role concepts. *Merrill-Palmer Quarterly, 36,* 487–506.

Waxman, S., & Gelman, R. (1986). Preschoolers' use of superordinate relations in classification and language. *Cognitive Development, 1,* 139–156.

Waxman, S. R., & Hall, D. G. (1993). The development of a linkage between count nouns and object categories: Evidence from fifteen- to twenty-one-month-old infants. *Child Development, 64,* 1224–1241.

Waxman, S. R., & Kosowski, T. D. (1990). Nouns mark category relations: Toddlers' and preschoolers' word-learning biases. *Child Development, 61,* 1461–1473.

Webster, M. L., Thompson, J. M., Mitchell, E. A., & Werry, J. S. (1994). Postnatal depression in a community cohort. *Australian & New Zealand Journal of Psychiatry, 28,* 42–49.

Webster-Stratton, C. (1988). Mothers' and fathers' perceptions of child deviance: Roles of parent and child adjustment and child deviance. *Journal of Consulting and Clinical Psychology, 56,* 909–915.

Webster-Stratton, C., & Hammond, M. (1988). Maternal depression and its relationship to life stress, perceptions of child behavior problems, parenting behaviors and child conduct problems. *Journal of Abnormal Child Psychology, 16,* 299–315.

Wechsler, D. (1974). *Manual for the Wechsler Intelligence Scale for Children—Revised.* New York: Psychological Corporation.

Wegman, M. E. (1992). Annual summary of vital statistics—1991. *Pediatrics, 90,* 835–845.

Wegman, M. E. (1993). Annual summary of vital statistics—1992. *Pediatrics, 82,* 743–754.

Wegman, M. E. (1994). Annual summary of vital statistics—1993. *Pediatrics, 94,* 792–803.

Weinberg, R. A. (1989). Intelligence and IQ: Landmark issues and great debates. *American Psychologist, 44,* 98–104.

Weisner, T. S. (1984). Ecocultural niches of middle childhood: A cross-cultural perspective. In W. A. Collins (Ed.), *Development during middle childhood: The years from six to twelve* (pp. 335–369). Washington, DC: National Academy Press.

Weiss, B., Dodge, K. A., Bates, J. E., & Pettit, G. S. (1992). Some consequences of early harsh discipline: Child aggression and a maladaptive social information processing style. *Child Development, 63,* 1321–1335.

Weisz, J. R., Sigman, M., Weiss, B., & Mosk, J. (1993). Parent reports of behavioral and emotional problems among children in Kenya, Thailand, and the United States. *Child Development, 64,* 98–109.

Wellman, H. M. (1982). The foundations of knowledge: Concept development in the young child. In S. G. Moore & C. C. Cooper (Eds.), *The young child: Reviews of research* (Vol. 3, pp. 115–134). Washington, DC: National Association for the Education of Young Children.

Wellman, H. M., & Hickling, A. K. (1994). The mind's "I": Children's conception of the mind as an active agent. *Child Development, 65,* 1564–1580.

Wen, S. W., Goldenberg, R. L., Cutter, G. R., Hoffman, H. J., Cliver, S. P., Davis, R. O., & DuBard, M. D. (1990). Smoking, maternal age, fetal growth, and gestational age at delivery. *American Journal of Obstetrics and Gynecology, 162,* 53–58.

Werker, J. F., Pegg, J. E., & McLeod, P. J. (1994). A cross-language investigation of infant preference for infant-directed communication. *Infant Behavior and Development, 17,* 323–333.

Werker, J. F., & Tees, R. C. (1984). Cross-language speech perception: Evidence for perceptual reorganization during the first year of life. *Infant Behavior and Development, 7,* 49–63.

Werner, E. E. (1986). A longitudinal study of perinatal risk. In D. C. Farran & J. D. McKinney (Eds.), *Risk in intellectual and psychosocial development* (pp. 3–28). Orlando, FL: Academic Press.

Werner, E. E., & Smith, R. S. (1992). *Overcoming the odds: High risk children from birth to adulthood.* Ithaca, NY: Cornell University Press.

Werner, H. (1948). *Comparative psychology of mental development.* Chicago: Follett.

Werner, L. A., & Gillenwater, J. M. (1990). Pure-tone sensitivity of 2- to 5-week old infants. *Infant Behavior and Development, 13,* 355–375.

Whitam, F. L., Diamond, M., & Martin, J. (1993). Homosexual orientation in twins: A report on 61 pairs and three triplet sets. *Archives of Sexual Behavior, 22,* 187–206.

Whitehurst, G. J. (1995). *Levels of reading readiness and predictors of reading success among children from low-income families.* Paper presented at the biennial meetings of the Society for Research in Child Development, Indianapolis.

Whitehurst, G. J., Arnold, D. S., Epstein, J. N., Angell, A. L., Smith, M., & Fischel, J. E. (1994). A picture book reading intervention in day care and home for children from low-income families. *Developmental Psychology, 30,* 679–689.

Whitehurst, G. J., Falco, F. L., Lonigan, C. J., Fischel, J. E., DeBaryshe, B. D., Valdez-Menchaca, M. C., & Caulfield, M. (1988). Accelerating language development through picture book reading. *Developmental Psychology, 24,* 552–559.

Whitehurst, G. J., Fischel, J. E., Crone, D. A., & Nania, O. (1995). *First year outcomes of a clinical trial of an emergent literacy intervention in Head Start homes and classrooms.* Paper presented at the biennial meetings of the Society for Research in Child Development, Indianapolis.

Whiting, B. B., & Edwards, C. P. (1988). *Children of different worlds: The formation of social behavior.* Cambridge, MA: Harvard University Press.

Whitney, M. P., & Thoman, E. B. (1994). Sleep in premature and fullterm infants from 24-hour home recordings. *Infant Behavior and Development, 17,* 223–234.

Wierson, M., & Forehand, R. (1994). Parent behavioral training for child noncompliance: rational, concepts, and effectiveness. *Current Directions in Psychological Science, 3,* 146–150.

Wiesenfeld, A. R., Malatesta, C. Z., & DeLoach, L. L. (1981). Differential parental response to familiar and unfamiliar infant distress signals. *Infant Behavior and Development, 4,* 281–296.

Wilcox, A. J., Weinberg, C. R., O'Connor, J. F., Baird, D. D., Schlatterer, J. P., Canfield, R. E., Armstrong, E. G., & Nisula, B. C. (1988). Incidence of early loss of pregnancy. *New England Journal of Medicine, 319,* 189–194.

Williams, E., Radin, N., & Allegro, T. (1992). Sex role attitudes of adolescents reared primarily by their fathers: An 11-year follow-up. *Merrill-Palmer Quarterly, 38,* 457–476.

Williams, J. E., & Best, D. L. (1990). *Measuring sex stereotypes: A multination study* (rev. ed.). Newbury Park, CA: Sage.

Willig, A. (1985). Meta-analysis of studies on bilingual education. *Review of Educational Research, 55,* 269–317.

Wilson, M. N. (1986). The black extended family: An analytical consideration. *Developmental Psychology, 22,* 246–258.

Wilson, M. N. (1989). Child development in the context of the black extended family. *American Psychologist, 44,* 380–385.

Winick, M. (1980). *Nutrition in health and disease.* New York: Wiley.

World Health Organization (1981). *Contemporary patterns of breast-feeding. Report on the WHO collaborative study on breast-feeding.* Geneva: World Health Organization.

Yonas, A. (1981). Infants' responses to optical information for collision. In R. N. Aslin, J. R. Alberts, & M. R. Peterson (Eds.), *Development of perception: Psychobiological perspectives: Vol. 2. The visual system* (pp. 313–334). New York: Academic Press.

Yonas, A., & Owsley, C. (1987). Development of visual space perception. In P. Salapatek & L. Cohen (Eds.), *Handbook of infant perception: Vol. 2. From perception to cognition* (pp. 80–122). Orlando, FL: Academic Press.

Youniss, J., McLellan, J. A., & Strouse, D. (1994). "We're popular, but we're not snobs": Adolescents describe their crowds. In R. Montemayor, G. R. Adams, & T. P. Gullotta (Eds.), *Personal relationships during adolescence* (pp. 101–122). Thousand Oaks, CA: Sage.

Zahn-Waxler, C., & Radke-Yarrow, M. (1982). The development of altruism: Alternative research strategies. In N. Eisenberg (Ed.), *The development of prosocial behavior* (pp. 109–138). New York: Academic Press.

Zajonc, R. B. (1983). Validating the confluence model. *Psychological Bulletin, 93,* 457–480.

Zajonc, R. B., & Marcus, G. B. (1975). Birth order and intellectual development. *Psychological Review, 82,* 74–88.

Zametkin, A. J., Nordahl, T. E., Gross, M., King, A. C., Semple, W. E., Rumsey, J., Hamburger, S., & Cohen, R. M. (1990). Cerebral glucose metabolism in adults with hyperactivity of childhood onset. *New England Journal of Medicine, 323,* 1361–1366.

Zani, B. (1993). Dating and interpersonal relationships in adolescence. In S. Jackson & H. Rodrigues-Tomé (Eds.), *Adolescence and its social worlds* (pp. 95–119). Hove, England: Erlbaum.

Zaslow, M. J., & Hayes, C. D. (1986). Sex differences in children's responses to psychosocial stress: Toward a cross-context analysis. In M. E. Lamb, A. L. Brown, & B. Rogoff (Eds.), *Advances in developmental psychology* (Vol. 4, pp. 285–238). Hillsdale, NJ: Erlbaum.

Zelazo, N. A., Zelazo, P. R., Cohen, K. M., & Zelazo, P. D. (1993). Specificity of practice effects on elementary neuromotor patterns. *Developmental Psychology, 29,* 686–691.

Zeskind, P. S., & Ramey, C. T. (1981). Preventing intellectual and interactional sequelae of fetal malnutrition: A longitudinal, transactional, and synergistic approach to development. *Child Development, 52,* 213–218.

Zigler, E., & Hall, N. W. (1989). Physical child abuse in America: Past, present, and future. In D. Cicchetti & V. Carlson (Eds.), *Child maltreatment* (pp. 38–75). Cambridge, England: Cambridge University Press.

Zigler, E., & Hodapp, R. M. (1991). Behavioral functioning in individuals with mental retardation. *Annual Review of Psychology, 42,* 29–50.

Zigler, E., & Styfco, S. J. (1993). Using research and theory to justify and inform Head Start expansion. *Social Policy Report, Society for Research in Child Development, 7*(2), 1–21.

Zill, N., & Nord, C. W. (1994). *Running in place: How American families are faring in a changing economy and an individualistic society.* Washington, DC: Child Trends.

Zoccolillo, M. (1993). Gender and the development of conduct disorder. *Development and Psychopathology, 5,* 65–78.

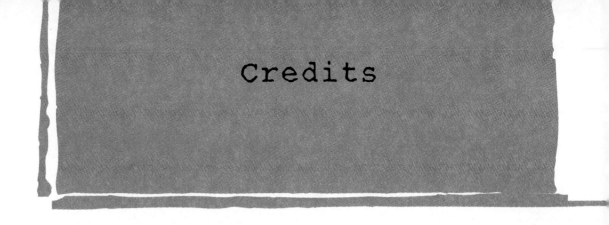

Credits

Note: Unless otherwise acknowledged, all photographs are the property of Scott, Foresman and Company.
Page abbreviations are (t) top, (c) center, (b) bottom, (r) right, and (l) left.

1: Mary Kate Denny/PhotoEdit; **2:** Paul Conklin; **9:** David Young-Wolff/PhotoEdit; **13(t):** Bob Daemmrich/Image Works; **13(b):** Laura Dwight; **16:** Paul Conklin; **18:** Laura Dwight; **19:** Don Smetzer/Tony Stone Images; **30:** Laura Dwight; **36:** Ricardo e Aratanha/Image Bank; **37:** Photo Researchers; **38:** Gabe Palmer/Stock Market; **47:** Laura Dwight; **54(both):** George Steinmetz; **58:** Laura Dwight; **66:** Jerry Koontz/Picture Cube, Inc.; **70:** S.I.U./Peter Arnold, Inc.; **71:** David Young-Wolff/PhotoEdit; **74:** Hyman/Stock Boston; **80(t,both):** From *Neurological Examination of the Full-Term Newborn Infant,* Second Edition, by Heinz F. R. Prechtl; *A Manual for Clinical Use* from the Department of Developmental Neurology, University of Groningen: Clinics in Developmental Medicine, Nos. 63, 977. Spastics International Medical Publications, now Mackeith Press; London: William Heinemann Medical Books Ltd.; Philadelphia: J. B. Lippincott Co. Printed in England by The Lavenham Press Ltd., Lavenham, Suffolk.; **80(b):** Laura Dwight; **81:** Laura Dwight; **82:** Laura Dwight; **83:** Ursula Markus/Photo Researchers; **87:** L. Johnson, *Hi Mom! Hi Dad! 101 Cartoons for New Parents* (Meadowbrook Press); **90:** Laura Dwight; **94:** Merritt Vincent/PhotoEdit; **95(t):** Myrleen Ferguson/PhotoEdit; **95(b):** Bob Daemmrich/Image Works; **108(all):** Laura Dwight; **111:** Bob Daemmrich/Stock Boston; **116:** Brent Jones; **117:** Okoniewski/Image Works; **119(l):** Michael Newman/PhotoEdit; **119(r):** Robert Brenner/PhotoEdit; **121:** William Thompson/Picture Cube, Inc.; **125:** Tom McCarthy/PhotoEdit; **128:** Laura Dwight; **131:** Michael Newman/PhotoEdit; **133(all):** J. E. Steiner, Human facial expressions in response to taste and smell stimulation. In H. W. Reese & L. P. Lipsett (Eds.), *Advances in child development and behavior,* Vol. 13. New York: Academic Press, 1979, Figure 1, p. 269; **134:** Laura Dwight; **135:** Enrico Ferorelli; **138:** Bob Daemmrich; **142:** Laura Dwight; **151:** Myrleen F. Cate/PhotoEdit; **152:** David Young-Wolff/PhotoEdit; **155:** Paul Conklin/PhotoEdit; **157:** Laura Dwight; **158(t):** Bob Daemmrich; **158(b):** Laura Dwight; **159:** Bob Daemmrich/Stock Boston; **163:** Paul Conklin/PhotoEdit; **164:** R. Crandall/Stock Boston; **168:** David Young-Wolff/PhotoEdit; **171:** Bob Daemmrich/Stock Boston; **181:** David Young-Wolff/PhotoEdit; **182:** Tony Freeman/PhotoEdit; **183:** Laura Dwight; **185(both):** Laura Dwight; **186:** Sam Falk/NYT Pictures; **188:** Arthur Tilley/Tony Stone Images; **192:** From Carolyn Rovee-Collier, *Current Directions in Psychological Science,* 2(4): 130–135, 1993; **194:** Laura Dwight; **198:** Laura Dwight; **204:** R. Sidney/Image Works; **205:** John Eastcott/YVA Momatiuk/Image Works; **207(t):** Laura Dwight; **207(c):** Elizabeth Crews/Image Works; **207(b):** John Eastcott/YVA Momatiuk/Image Works; **211:** Laura Dwight; **217:** David Young-Wolff/PhotoEdit; **219:** H. S. Terrace/Anthro-Photo File; **221:** Elizabeth Crews/Image Works; **231:** Laura Dwight; **232(t):** Roy Kirby/Stock Boston; **232(b):** Miro Vintoniv/Stock Boston; **234:** Laura Dwight; **242:** Laura Dwight; **243:** Laura Dwight; **244:** Laura Dwight; **247:** Tom Pettyman/PhotoEdit; **248:** Bob Daemmrich; **252:** Jerry Howard/Positive Images; **256:** David Young-Wolff/PhotoEdit; **262:** Laura Dwight; **263:** David Young-Wolff/PhotoEdit; **265:** Laura Dwight; **267:** Myrleen Ferguson/PhotoEdit; **269:** M. Heron/Monkmeyer Press Photo Service, Inc.; **278:** Rhoda Sidney/PhotoEdit; **280:** Laura Dwight; **282:** Jeffry W. Myers/Stock Boston; **286:** Daniel Laine/Actuality, Inc.; **288:** Bob Daemmrich/Stock Boston; **290:** Michael Newman/PhotoEdit; **292:** Lawrence Migdale/Photo Researchers; **293:** Willie Hill/Image Works; **296:** Robert W. Ginn/Picture Cube, Inc.; **299:** Kim Robbie/Stock Market; **304:** Elizabeth Crews; **306:** Frank Siteman/Picture Cube, Inc.; **308(tl):** Laura Dwight; **308(tr):** R. Pasley/Stock Boston; **308(b):** Jeffry Myers/Stock Boston; **313:** Winter/Image Bank; **315:** Laura Dwight; **321:** Laura Dwight; **322:** Myrleen Ferguson/PhotoEdit; **324:** Jerry Howard/Positive Images; **326:** Laura Dwight; **329:** Bob Daemmrich/Image Works; **332:** Laura Dwight; **337:** Nancy Sheehan/PhotoEdit; **340:** David Young-Wolff/PhotoEdit; **341:** Photos from *Unmasking the Face* by Paul Ekman and Wallace V. Friesen, Prentice Hall, 1975; **343:** Esther Shapiro/Photo Researchers; **349:** Peter Menzel/Stock Boston; **350:** J. C. Francolon/Gamma-Liaison; **355:** Willie Hill/Image Works; **357:** Tony Freeman/PhotoEdit; **359:** MacDonald/PhotoEdit; **364:** Myrleen Ferguson/PhotoEdit; **367:** Liane Enkelis/Stock Boston; **368:** Myrleen Ferguson/PhotoEdit; **372:** Brent Jones; **378:** Susan Kuklin/Photo Researchers; **382:** Timothy Eagan/Woodfin Camp & Associates; **384:** Bill Aron/PhotoEdit; **385(t):** Gilles Peress/PhotoEdit; **385(b):** April Saul; **389:** David Young-Wolff/PhotoEdit; **390:** Joyce Marshall/*Fort Worth Star-Telegram*/Sipa Press; **395:** John Eastcott/YVA Momatiuk/Image Works; **398:** Jim Harrison/Stock Boston; **400:** Bob Daemmrich/Stock Boston; **403:** Bob Daemmrich/Image Works; **405:** Bob Daemmrich; **408(both):** Bob Daemmrich; **410:** Hache/Photo Researchers; **419:** Burt Glinn/Magnum Photos; **420:** Robert Brenner/PhotoEdit; **424:** Bob Daemmrich; **426:** Laura Dwight; **431:** Bob Collins/Image Works; **436:** Laura Dwight; **437:** J. P. Laffont/Sygma; **442:** Cleo/PhotoEdit; **443:** Tom and Deeann McCarthy/Stock Market; **447:** Laura Dwight; **449:** Stephen Shames/Matrix International, Inc.; **452(t):** Dal Bayles/*The New York Times;* **452(b):** Gaye Hilsenrath/Picture Cube, Inc.; **453:** Tony Freeman/PhotoEdit; **460:** Michael Newman/PhotoEdit; **463:** Laura Dwight; **467:** Tom Prettyman/PhotoEdit; **471:** Michael Newman/PhotoEdit; **472:** David R. Frazier/Photo Researchers; **474:** Myrleen Ferguson/PhotoEdit; **476:** Laura Dwight; **477:** Tony Freeman/PhotoEdit; **483:** Bruce Roberts/Photo Researchers.

Name Index

Subject Index